ACSM's Resources for the Exercise Physiologist

SENIOR EDITOR

Gary Liguori, PhD, FACSM, ACSM-CES
Department Head, Health and Human Performance
University of Tennessee Chattanooga
Chattanooga, Tennessee

ASSOCIATE EDITORS

Gregory B. Dwyer, PhD, FACSM, ACSM-PD, ACSM-CES, ACSM-ETT, ACSM-RCEP
Professor of Exercise Science
East Stroudsburg University
East Stroudsburg, Pennsylvania

Teresa C. Fitts, DPE, FACSM, ACSM-HFS
Professor of Movement Science
Co-Program Director, Exercise Science Program
Westfield State University
Westfield, Massachusetts

Beth Lewis, PhD
Associate Professor of Kinesiology
University of Minnesota
Minneapolis, Minnesota

ADDITIONAL RESOURCES

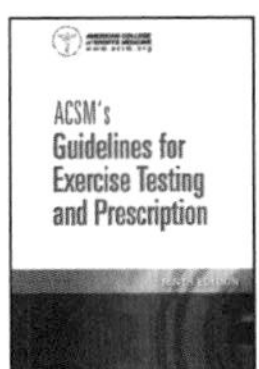

ACSM's Guidelines for Exercise Testing and Prescription

NINTH EDITION

This text has long been considered the Gold Standard in sports medicine, exercise science, and health and fitness. It enables you to test and evaluate individuals to prescribe effective exercise programs tailored to their particular needs and based on the latest evidence.

Highlights include:

- A new chapter on behavior strategies to help keep clients motivated and committed to lifelong exercise
- Expanded coverage of special populations
- As always, the latest guidelines and recommendations from ACSM and other professional organizations

978-1-60913-605-5 (spiral) / 480 pp / 2013
978-1-60913-955-1 (perfectbound) / 480 pp / 2013

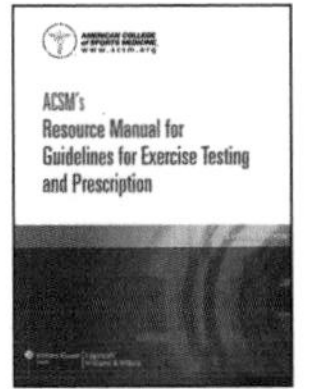

ACSM's Resource Manual for Guidelines for Exercise Testing and Prescription

SEVENTH EDITION

The perfect companion to *ACSM's Guidelines for Exercise Testing and Prescription*, this resource enables you to explore in depth the links between exercise and health.

Highlights include:

- An expanded behavior change section with the tools needed to motivate people to begin exercise and then adhere to a program
- Content reflects the most recent research findings in the field as well as ACSM position stands

978-1-60913-956-8 / 896 pp / 2013

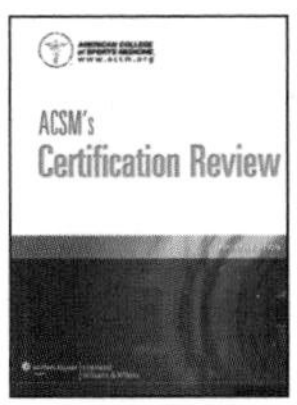

ACSM's Certification Review

FOURTH EDITION

ACSM's Certification Review is the ultimate resource to help you pass the exam to become a Certified Personal Trainer (CPT), Certified Health Fitness Specialist (HFS), or Certified Clinical Exercise Specialist (CES).

Highlights include:

- Case studies that reinforce concepts, organized by KSA domains
- Practice Exams that contain questions for each certification level
- Job Task Analysis tables that provide breakdowns of all the KSAs by certification level and domain

978-1-60913-954-4 / 320 pp / 2013

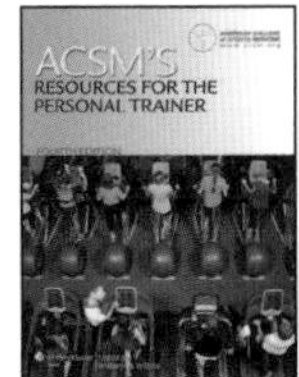

ACSM's Resources for the Personal Trainer

FOURTH EDITION

This essential resource is the official ACSM preparatory tool for the ACSM Certified Personal Trainer exam. It provides crucial information for both beginning and experienced personal trainers, presenting an introduction to the profession along with coverage of exercise physiology, biomechanics, anatomy, motor learning, and nutrition.

978-1-4511-0859-0 / 656 pp / 2013

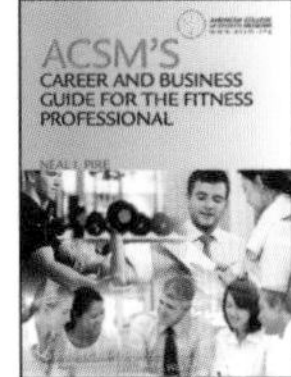

ACSM's Career and Business Guide for the Fitness Professional

This book covers the practical aspects of running a successful fitness business and having a successful fitness career. Fitness professionals will have the information they need to start planning their own business and make wise career choices. The book is designed to be very practical and provides forms and succinct how-to instructions for successful business planning.

978-1-60831-195-8 / 240 pp / 2012

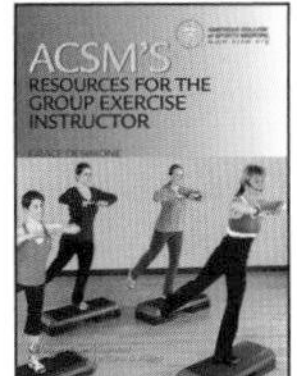

ACSM's Resources for the Group Exercise Instructor

This book includes the knowledge and the skills needed to effectively lead group exercise, and can be used in preparation to become an ACSM Certified Group Exercise Instructor. Topics covered include leadership, class design, legal issues and responsibilities, and how to take advantage of group dynamics to improve health and well-being. It provides details on how to adapt the skills to different environments, including gyms, studios, recreational facilities, and clubs.

978-1-60831-196-5 / 336 pp / 2011

It's easy to order!
Call 1-800-486-5643 or visit http://lww.com

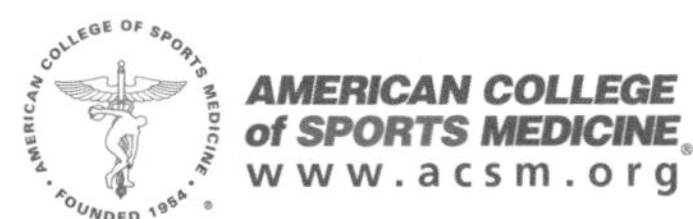

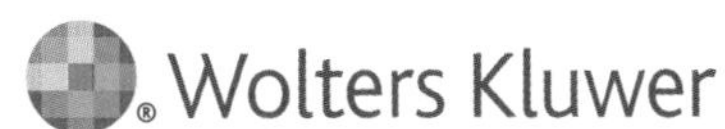

ACSM's Resources for the Exercise Physiologist

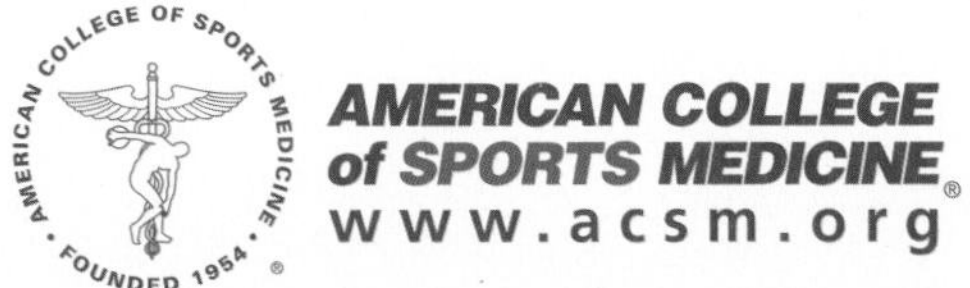

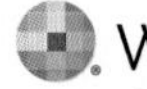

Wolters Kluwer | Lippincott Williams & Wilkins
Health
Philadelphia • Baltimore • New York • London
Buenos Aires • Hong Kong • Sydney • Tokyo

Acquisitions Editor: Emily Lupash
Product Manager: Andrea M. Klingler
Marketing Manager: Sarah Schuessler
Vendor Manager: Marian Bellus
Creative Director: Doug Smock
Compositor: S4Carlisle Publishing Services
ACSM Committee on Certification and Registry Boards Chair: Deborah Riebe, PhD, FACSM, ACSM-HFS
ACSM Publications Committee Chair: Walter R. Thompson, PhD, FACSM, ACSM-PD, ACSM-RCEP
ACSM Group Publisher: Kerry O'Rourke
Umbrella Editor: Jonathan K. Ehrman, PhD, FACSM, ACSM-PD, ACSM-CES

First Edition

Printed in China

9 8 7 6 5 4 3 2 1

978-1-4963-2926-4
Library of Congress Cataloging-in-Publication Data
available upon request

DISCLAIMER

Care has been taken to confirm the accuracy of the information present and to describe generally accepted practices. However, the authors, editors, and publisher are not responsible for errors or omissions or for any consequences from application of the information in this book and make no warranty, expressed or implied, with respect to the currency, completeness, or accuracy of the contents of the publication. Application of this information in a particular situation remains the professional responsibility of the practitioner; the clinical treatments described and recommended may not be considered absolute and universal recommendations.

The authors, editors, and publisher have exerted every effort to ensure that drug selection and dosage set forth in this text are in accordance with the current recommendations and practice at the time of publication. However, in view of ongoing research, changes in government regulations, and the constant flow of information relating to drug therapy and drug reactions, the reader is urged to check the package insert for each drug for any change in indications and dosage and for added warnings and precautions. This is particularly important when the recommended agent is a new or infrequently employed drug.

Some drugs and medical devices presented in this publication have Food and Drug Administration (FDA) clearance for limited use in restricted research settings. It is the responsibility of the health care provider to ascertain the FDA status of each drug or device planned for use in their clinical practice.

To purchase additional copies of this book, call our customer service department at (800) 638-3030 or fax orders to (301) 223-2320. International customers should call (301) 223-2300.

Visit Lippincott Williams & Wilkins on the Internet: http://www.lww.com. Lippincott Williams & Wilkins customer service representatives are available from 8:30 am to 6:00 pm, EST.

Dedication

This book is dedicated to all of the outstanding individuals, past and present, associated with the American College of Sports Medicine.

Acknowledgments

I give a special thank you to Larry Durstine for all he has done for me over the years. I thank my many friends, colleagues, and former graduate students who have assisted with this and many other projects, particularly Walt Thompson, Amanda Lewis, Ronda Klubben, and Arupendra Mozumdar, along with the great staff at Lippincott, Williams & Wilkins for their belief in this project and all the wonderful assistance they provided along the way. Greg, Teresa, and Beth are not simply my associate editors, but my friends and colleagues without whom this book would never had happened. To say this was a group effort would be an understatement. Most importantly, I thank my dear wife, Heidi, for her patience with this and every other project I originally promised to say "no" to. Your support and encouragement guide my every step. Finally, to my three wonderful children: dream big, and don't be surprised at what you can achieve.

Gary Liguori, Senior Editor

Foreword

In early 2009, ACSM's Committee on Certification and Registry Board (CCRB) began the periodic task of updating the knowledge, skills, and assessments (KSAs) for each level of its health fitness and clinical certifications. At that time, the committee initiated a new process of evaluating and validating job-related proficiencies, called a job task analysis (JTA).

JTA is a performance-based process that provides a basis for the development of standardized national examinations for evaluating job proficiencies. The JTA process for all ACSM certifications took many months and resulted from the tireless efforts of many committee volunteers, ACSM staff members, and working certified professionals. All aspects of the tasks performed daily by Personal Trainers, Health Fitness Specialists, Clinical Exercise Professionals, and Registered Clinical Exercise Physiologists were evaluated and ranked on the basis of their frequency and importance. The job tasks were grouped into broader performance domains, which for the Health Fitness Specialist (HFS) included health and fitness assessment, exercise prescription and implementation, exercise counseling and behavioral strategies, legal/professional considerations, and management.

The concept for this book was a natural extension of the JTA process. *ACSM's Resources for the Exercise Physiologist* (formerly titled *ACSM's Resources for the Health Fitness Specialist*) is an excellent evidence-based resource for the practicing ACSM-certified HFS and a valuable study tool for those aspiring to attain the certification. A unique feature of this text is case studies, which have been contributed by practicing professionals from across the United States. Finally, a description of the Exercise is Medicine global health initiative and the interaction with the HFS professional is discussed throughout the book. The HFS professional is uniquely qualified to work with medical professionals to ensure that all people are participating in some type of physical activity program.

I would like to personally thank past and present members of the CCRB HFS subcommittee, Dr. Deb Riebe, Dr. Meir Magel, Dr. Matt Parrot, Ms. Nancy Belli, Dr. Teresa Fitts, and finally Dr. Gary Liguori, for all their hard work and dedication in making the HFS credential a highly valued commodity in the health fitness marketplace.

To the editors — Dr. Liguori, Dr. Greg Dwyer, Dr. Fitts, and Dr. Beth Lewis — thank you for your initiative and innovation in bringing this concept to print. Your vision and enthusiasm for the health and fitness profession serves as an inspiration to all of us. I hope current and future fitness professionals will appreciate and enjoy this valuable resource.

Madeline Paternostro-Bayles, PhD, FACSM, ACSM-CES, PD
Chair of ACSM CCRB, 2008–2011
Professor, Health and Physical Education
Undergraduate/Graduate Exercise Science Coordinator
Indiana University of Pennsylvania
Indiana, Pennsylvania

Preface

The purpose of this text is to serve as the key resource for Health Fitness Specialists (HFSs), with particular regard to the ACSM HFS. To accomplish this, *ACSM's Resources for the Exercise Physiologist* (formerly titled *ACSM's Resources for the Health Fitness Specialist*) provides information about the theory and practice that forms the basis of the HFS scope of practice. This book is able to stand alone as a classroom text or serve as a supplement to many existing texts. The array and strength of the chapter contributors, many of whom are renowned experts in their fields, is a key aspect that adds to the value of this text.

The primary audience for *ACSM's Resources for the Exercise Physiologist* is the student or professional studying for the ACSM-EP-C certification exam. Secondary markets include HFSs and personal trainers who wish to broaden their knowledge base. Other health care providers (nurses, physical therapists, etc.) looking to expand their understanding of exercise, exercise prescription, and best practices related to exercise also will find valuable information here.

Organization

This book is organized around the scope of practice domains identified for the ACSM-EP-C. We begin with an introductory section focused on understanding exercise and physical activity along with preexercise screening. Part I includes assessment and programming for healthy populations. Part II covers a similar underlying theme, but focuses on special populations, including those with metabolic disorders, pregnant women, children, and the elderly. Part III includes counseling and behavioral strategies for encouraging and sustaining exercise, a critical need for all exercise professionals. The final section, Part IV, covers legal, management, and professional issues relevant to all exercise professionals, especially those interested in owning a business or ascending the leadership ladder. The information within this text is based on *ACSM's Guidelines for Exercise Testing and Prescription, Ninth Edition.*

Features

Each of the chapters begins with **objectives** and ends with **open-ended questions** directly related to the objectives. Chapters contain **How To boxes,** which provide step-by-step instructions for different types of assessments an HFS regularly encounters, and an **Exercise is Medicine Connection,** which describes research about the role of exercise in improving health. **Case Studies** (submitted by ACSM-certified individuals from around the country) are also a key feature as they detail real-life situations HFSs face, with suggestions on how to best address them. **Icons** highlight relevant video clips that are available on the book's Web site.

Additional Resources

ACSM's Resources for the Exercise Physiologist includes additional resources for students and instructors that are available on the book's companion Web site at http://thepoint.lww.com/activate.

Students

- Full text online
- Video clips

Instructors

Approved adopting instructors will be given access to the following additional resources:

- Brownstone test generator
- PowerPoint presentations
- Image bank
- Case study answers
- WebCT/Angel/Blackboard ready cartridge

In addition, purchasers of the text can access the searchable full text online by going to the *ACSM's Resources for the Exercise Physiologist* Web site at http://thepoint.lww.com/activate. See the inside front cover of this text for more details, including the passcode you will need to gain access to the Web site.

Contributors

Anthony A. Abbott, EdD, FACSM
Fitness Institute International, Inc.
Lighthouse Point, Florida
Chapter 13

Keith Burns, MS
Kent State University
Kent, Ohio
Chapter 7

Dino Costanzo, MA, ACSM-RCEP, FACSM, ACSM-PD, ACSM-ETT
The Hospital of Central Connecticut
New Britain, Connecticut
Appendix A

Katrina DuBose, PhD, FACSM
East Carolina University
Greenville, North Carolina
Chapter 6

J. Larry Durstine, PhD, FACSM
University of South Carolina
Columbia, South Carolina
Chapter 7

Gregory B. Dwyer, PhD, FACSM ACSM-PD, ACSM-CES, ACSM-ETT, ACSM-RCEP
East Stroudsburg University
East Stroudsburg, Pennsylvania
Chapter 2

Chris Eschbach, PhD, ACSM-HFS
Valencell, Inc
Raleigh, North Carolina
Chapter 5

Avery Faigenbaum, EdD, FACSM
The College of New Jersey
Ewing, New Jersey
Chapter 4

Diana Ferris, MS, ACSM-HFS
ACSM/NPAS-PAPHS
Public Health Specialist
Stratford, Connecticut
Chapter 15

Teresa C. Fitts, DPE, FACSM, ACSM-HFS
Westfield State University
Westfield, Massachusetts
Chapter 17

Charles Fountaine, PhD
University of Minnesota Duluth
Duluth, Minnesota
Chapter 3

Benjamin Gordon, MS, ACSM-CES
The University of South Carolina
Columbia, South Carolina
Chapter 7

Sarah T. Henes, PhD, RD, LDN
East Carolina University
Greenville, North Carolina
Chapter 6

Ernestine Jennings, PhD
Warren Alpert Medical School,
Brown University
Providence, Rhode Island
Chapter 11

Betsy Keller, PhD, FACSM
Ithaca College
Ithaca, New York
Chapter 8

Riggs Klika, PhD, FACSM
Cancer Survivor Center
Aspen, Colorado
Chapter 9

Matthew Kutz, PhD, ATC, ACSM-CES
Bowling Green State University
Bowling Green, Ohio
Chapter 14

Beth Lewis, PhD
University of Minnesota
Minneapolis, Minnesota
Chapter 10

Gary Liguori, PhD, FACSM, ACSM-CES
University of Tennessee Chattanooga
Chattanooga, Tennessee
Chapters 1 and 7

Sarah Linke, PhD, MPH
University of California, San Diego
La Jolla, California
Chapter 11

Randi Lite, MA, ACSM-RCEP
Simmons College
Boston, Massachusetts
Chapter 17

Meir Magal, PhD, ACSM-CES
North Carolina Wesleyan College
Rocky Mount, North Carolina
Chapter 5

Bess Marcus, PhD, FACSM
University of California, San Diego
La Jolla, California
Chapter 11

Jessica Meendering, PhD, ACSM-HFS, ATC
South Dakota State University
Brookings, South Dakota
Chapter 3

Laurie Milliken, PhD, FACSM
University of Massachusetts Boston
Boston, Massachusetts
Chapter 9

Rob Motl, PhD
University of Illinois
Urbana, Illinois
Chapter 12

Mark Nutting, ACSM HFD, ACSM HFS
Saco Sport & Fitness
Saco, Maine
Chapter 16

Matthew W. Parrott, PhD, ACSM-HFS
H-P Fitness, LLC
Leawood, Kansas
Chapter 16

Neal I. Pire, MA, FACSM
Inspire Training Systems
Ridgewood, New Jersey
Chapter 15

Deborah Riebe, PhD, FACSM, ACSM-HFS
University of Rhode Island
Kingston, Rhode Island
Chapter 6

John M. Schuna, Jr, PhD
Pennington Biomedical Research Center
Baton Rouge, Louisiana
Chapter 1

Katie Schuver, MS
University of Minnesota
Minneapolis, Minnesota
Chapter 10

John Sigg, PhD
Ithaca College
Ithaca, New York
Chapter 8

Madeline Weikert, MS
Human Kinetics
Champaign, Illinois
Chapter 12

Molly Winke, PhD
Hanover College
Hanover, Indiana
Chapter 2

Case Study Contributors

Sarah Burnham, BS, ACSM-HFS
Somers, Connecticut
Chapter 3

Travis Michael Combest, MS, ACSM-RCEP
Walter Reed National Military Medical Center
Bethesda, Maryland
Chapter 8

Carol Jean Dale, MS, ACSM-HFS
NMMC — Pontotoc Wellness Center
Pontotoc, Michigan
Chapter 14

Kim DeLaFuente, MA, ACSM-PD
Spectrum Health
Grand Rapids, Michigan
Chapter 9

Joyce Dendy, MS, RD, ACSM-HFS
Affirmative Fitness
Waltham, Massachusetts
Chapter 11

J. Larry Durstine, PhD, FACSM
University of South Carolina
Columbia, South Carolina
Chapter 7

Teresa C. Fitts, DPE, FACSM, ACSM-HFS
Westfield State University
Westfield, Massachusetts
Chapter 15

Benjamin Gleason, MSEd, ACSM-HFS
Military Fitness Program Liaison
Eglin AFB, Florida
Chapter 4

Benjamin Gordon, MS, ACSM-CES
University of South Carolina
Columbia, South Carolina
Chapter 7

Len Haggerty, MS
Strides Human Performance Institute
Northampton, Massachusetts
Chapter 17

Leah Hantman, BS, ACSM-HFS
Franklin, Massachusetts
Chapter 3

Nancy R. Hudson, BS, ACSM-HFS
Baystate Health
Springfield, Massachusetts
Chapter 15

James R. Mazzapica, Jr., BS, ACSM-HFS
Tewksbury, Massachusetts
Chapter 2

Steve McClaran, PhD, ACSM-HFS
Colorado State University
Pueblo, Colorado
Chapter 10

Stephanie Marie Otto, PhD, ACSM-HFS
Gustavus Adolphus College
St. Peter, Minnesota
Chapter 5

Melissa W. Roti, PhD, ACSM-HFS
Westfield State University
Westfield, Massachusetts
Chapter 17

Geoff Sullivan, BS, ACSM-HFS
Continuum Performance Center
East Longmeadow, Massachusetts
Chapter 16

Kaitlin Teser, MS, ACSM-HFS
South Dartmouth, Massachusetts
Chapter 1

William Raymond VanWye, PT, DPT, ACSM-RCEP
Active Physical Therapy
Hilliard, Ohio
Chapter 12

Linda Vaughn, MS, MBA, ACSM-HFS
YMCA of Metropolitan Atlanta
Atlanta, Georgia
Chapter 6

Chris Worrell, BS, ACSM-HFS
Continuum Performance Center
East Longmeadow, Massachusetts
Chapter 16

ACSM CCRB Reviewers

Sherry A. Barkley, PhD, ACSM-RCEP, ACSM-CES
Augustana College
Sioux Falls, South Dakota

Clinton A. Brawner, MS, FACSM, ACSM-RCEP
Henry Ford Hospital
Detroit, Michigan

Mindy E. Caplan, AS, ACSM-HFS
Personal Training, Yoga, and Wellness Coaching
Austin, Texas

Brian J. Coyne, MEd, ACSM-RCEP, ACSM/NCPAD-CIFT
Duke University Health System
Morrisville, North Carolina

Lana K. Dench, BS, BA, BPE, ACSM-HFS
Y of Central Maryland
Catonsville, Maryland

Grace DeSimone, BA, ACSM-CPT, ACSM-GEI
Plus One Health Management
New York, New York

Sabrina Fairchild, MA, ACSM-HFS
California State University, Chico
Durham, California

Yuri Feito, PhD, MPH, ACSM-RCEP, ACSM-CES
Barry University
Miami, Florida

Sharon L. McGoff, BS, JD, ACSM-HFS
Fit 4 Life Coaching, LLC
Indianapolis, Indiana

Deborah Riebe, PhD, FACSM, ACSM-HFS
University of Rhode Island
Kingston, Rhode Island

Benjamin Thompson, PhD, ACSM-HFS
Metropolitan State College of Denver
Denver, Colorado

Paul Sorace, MS, ACSM-CES
Hackensack University Medical Center
Bayonne, New Jersey

Mark S. Zaleskiewicz, MS, FAACVPR, ACSM-CES
Shore Medical Center
Mays Landing, New Jersey

Reviewers

Laura Abbott, MS
Georgia State University
Atlanta, Georgia

Ken Alan, BS
California State University at Fullerton
Fullerton, California

Mike Bates, MBA
University of Windsor
Refine Fitness Studio
Windsor, ON, Canada
Chapter 15

Kelly Brooks, PhD
Texas A&M at Corpus Christi
Corpus Christi, Texas

Jeffrey Burnett, EdD
Fort Hays State University
Hays, Kansas

Christian Cianfrani, BS, MS
Bryan University
Los Angeles, California

Angela Dougall, PhD
University of Texas, Arlington
Arlington, Texas
Chapter 12

JoAnn Eickhoff-Shemek, PhD, FACSM
University of South Florida
Tampa, Florida
Chapter 13

Scott Eide, BS, MS
Minnesota School of Business
Waite Park, Minnesota

Chris Eschbach, PhD, FACSM, ACSM-HFS
Valencell, Inc.
Raleigh, North Carolina
Chapter 3

Anthony Gencarelli, DC
Institute for Therapeutic Massage
Haskell, New Jersey

Bonnie Goodwin, MS
Capital University
Columbus, Ohio

Douglas Hill, MS
Broadview University
Layton, Utah

Ernestine Jennings, PhD
Brown University
Providence, Rhode Island
Chapter 1

Marcus Kilpatrick, PhD, ACSM-HFS
University of South Florida
Tampa, Florida
Chapter 10

Matt Kutz, PhD
Bowling Green State University
Bowling Green, Ohio
Chapter 17

Michelle Martin, PhD
University of Alabama, Birmingham
Birmingham, Alabama
Chapter 11

Colleen McGlone, PhD
Costal Carolina University
Conway, South Carolina
Chapter 16

Gavin Moir, PhD
East Stroudsburg University
East Stroudsburg, Pennsylvania
Chapter 8

Laura O'Neil, PhD
Westfield State University
Westfield, Massachusetts
Chapter 14

Gail Sas
Health Quest Unlimited
Buellton, California

Emily Sauers, PhD
East Stroudsburg University
East Stroudsburg, Pennsylvania
Chapter 7

Christopher Scott, PhD
University of Southern Maine
Goreham, Maine
Chapter 4

Julie Snyder, MS
Keiser University
Port St Lucie, Florida

Jared Tucker, PhD
Helen DeVos Children's Hospital
Grand Rapids, Michigan
Chapter 6

Eric Wickel, PhD
University of Tulsa
Tulsa, Oklahoma
Chapter 9

Danielle Wigmore, PhD
Fitchburg State University
Fitchburg, Massachusetts
Chapter 2

Chad Witmer, PhD
East Stroudsburg University
East Stroudsburg, Pennsylvania
Chapter 5

Brief Contents

Detailed Contents

PART I

Overview

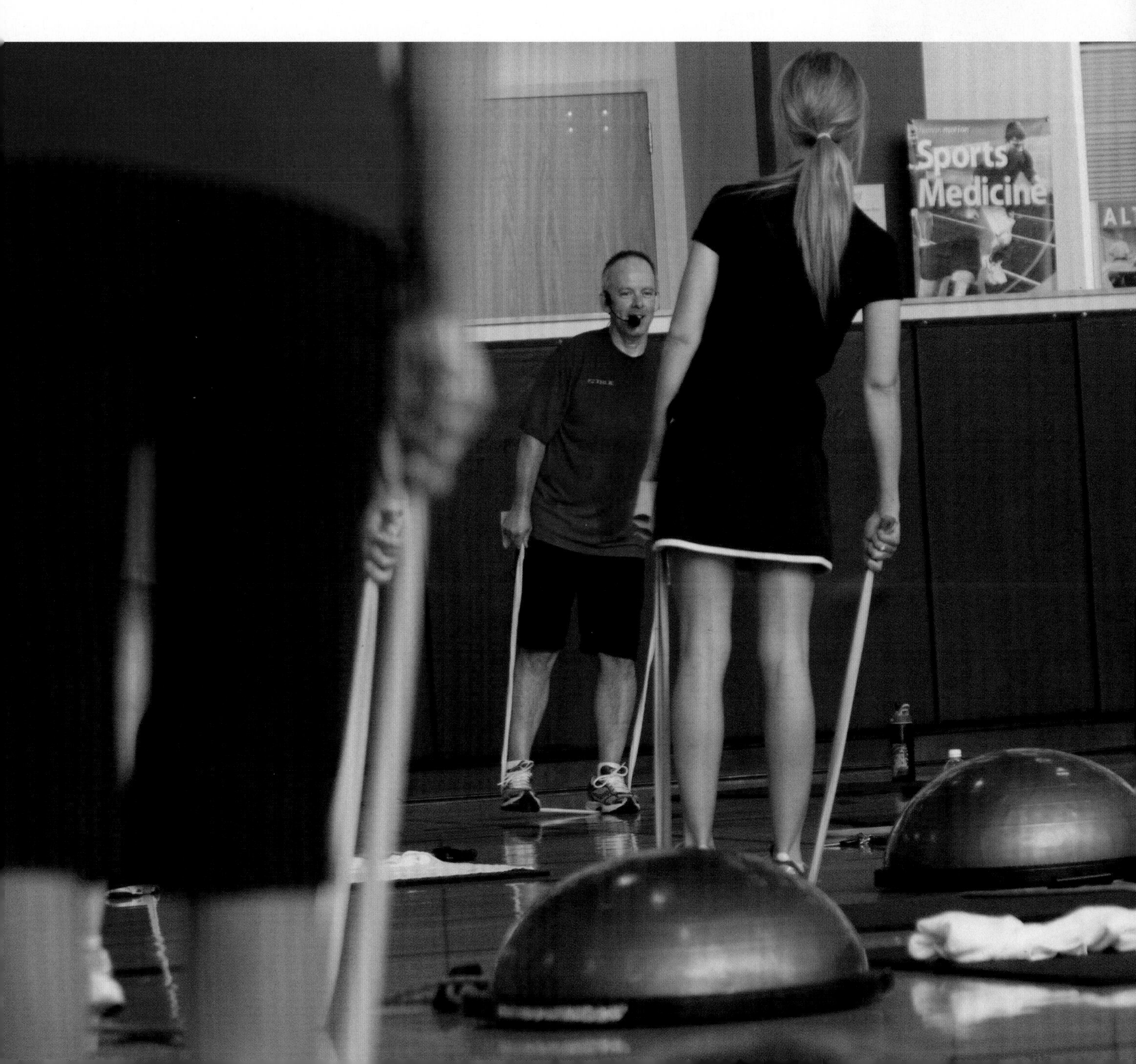

CHAPTER

1 Understanding Physical Activity and Exercise

Gary Liguori • John Schuna

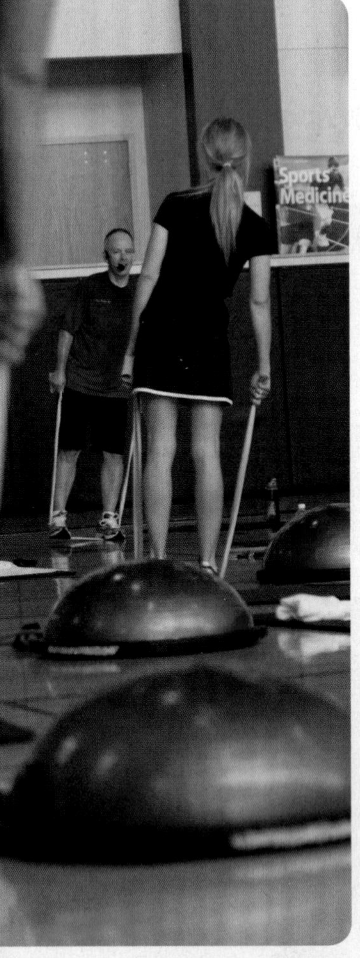

CHAPTER OBJECTIVES

- Define physical activity, exercise, health-related fitness, and skill-related fitness
- Identify several key historical individuals and landmark research that were instrumental in building the current knowledge base regarding the health benefits of physical activity and physical fitness
- Know how physical activity can positively impact health across the lifespan
- Understand the general health risks associated with physical activity and exercise

A practicing health fitness specialist (HFS) should be able to distinguish between physical activity (PA), exercise, health-related fitness, and skill-related fitness. Although all of these are closely intertwined, they all have distinguishing features to make them unique. This chapter discusses some of the unique features that help define each. In addition, this chapter will review important historical landmarks in the evolution of fitness, including well-cited research studies and key individuals, all leading to today's understanding of the health benefits and risks of exercise. Finally, there is an overview of current guidelines and recommendations for using exercise and PA to promote better health.

DEFINING PHYSICAL ACTIVITY, EXERCISE, HEALTH-RELATED FITNESS, AND SKILL-RELATED FITNESS

Physical activity (PA) is by far the broadest of all the terms mentioned in the introduction. By definition, PA is any bodily movement produced by contracting skeletal muscles, with a concomitant increase in energy expenditure (9). Although energy expenditure is increased during PA, it does not always reflect exercise, health-related fitness, or skill-related fitness.

Muscle contraction, which is necessary during PA, can be static or dynamic. Static, or isometric, contractions produce no change in the affected joint angle, such as seen when pressing against a wall. With static contractions, muscle strength is gained in only one joint position, not across a range of motion, which limits the application of the strength. In addition, static strength gains are lost very quickly if not practiced daily. Conversely, a dynamic or isotonic contraction produces a change in the affected joint angle, such as a squat causing a change in knee angle or a pull-up resulting in a change in elbow angle. Dynamic movement also allows muscle strength gains to occur across the full range of motion and can better mimic daily activities or sport movements, each of which is an example of functional strength.

PA can be a blend of aerobic (oxygen dependent) and anaerobic (oxygen independent) activities, depending on the intensity. Within any one given activity, both aerobic and anaerobic processes may be present, as can both static and dynamic muscle contractions.

PA can also be categorized by its environmental context: leisure time, occupational, household, and transportation. The purpose of any given bout of PA can vary by environment, and can also change from day to day. For instance, transportation for some might mean using public transport and walking to and from the bus station and workplace. This type of PA is likely to provide some health-related benefits. Others might cycle vigorously to and from work as part of an exercise training program, or to prepare for an upcoming triathlon event. Both activities are transportation-related PA, but are for a different purpose and with different outcomes.

One of the largest components of PA-related energy expenditure is occupational PA. A substantial portion of many Americans' waking day is spent working, with recent estimates indicating that employed individuals work an average of 7.5 hours$\cdot$day^{-1} (85). However, during the past 50 years, there has been a dramatic reduction in the percentage of Americans working in occupations that require moderate-intensity PA, as the nature of work has become more sedentary (11). Moreover, it has been estimated that occupational energy expenditure has declined by more than 100 calories$\cdot$day^{-1} over the past 5 decades. The increase in obesity prevalence among American adults may be partly related to this overall decrease in occupational PA.

Similarly to occupational PA, though more anecdotally, household PA has also decreased. Gardening, home repairs, cleaning (house and vehicle), and childcare are just some means of accumulating household PA throughout the day, and many have been made "easier" by technology.

Although there are numerous ways of accumulating PA, and reaping the inherent health benefits, it remains difficult for many adults to find the necessary time (see Table 1.1). Chapters 10 through 12 address different behavioral strategies to help initiate and sustain meaningful PA.

Exercise training may be considered a component of PA. Although exercise and PA are often used interchangeably, it is important to be able to clearly distinguish the two. Compared with PA, exercise is more specific and quantifiable in its definition: any planned, structured, repetitive, and purposeful activity that seeks to improve or maintain any component of fitness (9). While exercise is certainly a form of PA, PA does not always include exercise. Household chores and using public transport are PAs, although typically not considered exercise. Conversely, daily 5-km training runs clearly meet the definition of exercise and are also PA.

Physical fitness is a factor that directly relates to the quantity and type of PA an individual can perform. Physical fitness, however, includes different domains from health-related fitness. Physical fitness is defined as "a set of attributes that people have or achieve that relates to the ability to

TABLE 1.1 POPULAR PAS AND COMMON BARRIERS TO PA

Popular PAs	Common Barriers to PA
Walking	Lack of time/inconvenience
Gardening	Lack of motivation
Calisthenics	Not enjoyable/boring
Strength training	Fear of injury
Swimming	Lack of support/access
Jogging	Lack of encouragement

perform physical activity" (9). Physical fitness includes cardiorespiratory endurance; muscle strength, endurance, and power; flexibility; agility; balance; reaction time; and body composition. Physical fitness also implies specificity of training toward a particular goal. The majority of these attributes lend themselves to athletic performance, or the subcomponent of physical fitness known as performance-related fitness.

Health-related fitness is another subcomponent of physical fitness. Although health- and performance-related fitness share certain attributes, they tend to appeal to individuals with very different interests and needs. In addition, health-related fitness is confined to cardiorespiratory fitness, muscular endurance, muscular strength, flexibility, and body composition.

Skill-related fitness is the third aspect of PA and can also be thought of as performance-related fitness. Skill-related fitness comprises agility, balance, coordination, power, reaction time, and speed and can result in an increased desire to participate in physical activities. Overall, skill-related fitness contributes to one's ability to function in a more skilled and efficient manner (43).

The underlying premise is that PA will maintain or improve health, with an emphasis on improving each kind of PA. This is in contrast to those individuals choosing to remain relatively sedentary and putting themselves at greater risk for premature morbidity and mortality. Therefore, when the HFS develops an exercise prescription, or motivates an individual to initiate an exercise program, knowledge of these guiding principles is essential.

HISTORIC TRENDS IN PA

Ancient Times and the Rise of Exercise Physiology

The importance of PA as a means to promote health and well-being is not a new concept. In ancient China, records of exercise for health promotion date back to approximately 2500 BC (45). Following this, teachings of the Greek physician Hippocrates, of the fifth and fourth centuries BC, detailed the importance of exercise for health and well-being (28). Despite this ancient knowledge that PA confers health benefits, an understanding of the pathways and mechanisms through which PA influences health and well-being remained poorly understood until recent times. Much of our current understanding in these areas evolved out of advancements in human physiology, in particular, exercise physiology.

Moving forward from ancient times to the early 20th century, pioneers such as A.V. Hill and D.B. Dill, among many others, contributed vastly to the field of exercise physiology. Hill is perhaps best known for his work studying muscle mechanics and physiology, while Dill and numerous colleagues at the Harvard Fatigue Laboratory extensively studied exercise responses in varying environmental conditions. Collectively, developments in exercise physiology during this period laid the groundwork for our understanding of how PA and conditioning influences physical fitness.

T.K. Cureton and the Physical Fitness Movement

Building upon earlier advancements in the field of exercise physiology, T.K. Cureton's work during the 1940s focused on assessing physical fitness and the importance of physical conditioning. Cureton acted as a driving force behind the physical fitness movement in the United States while developing strong research and service programs at the University of Illinois. As a result, Cureton drew significant academic attention to the topics of physical fitness and physical conditioning (5). The cumulative contributions from Cureton and his graduate students provided much of the scientific basis for modern exercise prescription.

In addition to his scientific accomplishments, Cureton made a number of service contributions pertinent to the physical fitness movement. Several of his notable contributions included, but were not limited to, fitness training and testing of soldiers during World War II, assistance in the design of physical fitness training programs for Federal Bureau of Investigation trainees, and instrumental support in the development of the President's Council on Physical Fitness (5). Moreover, Cureton was one of the original 54 charter members of the American College of Sports Medicine® (ACSM) at the time of its founding in 1954.

One of Cureton's many distinguished students who made substantial contributions to exercise physiology and the physical fitness movement was the late Michael Pollock. Pollock is perhaps most remembered as a prominent researcher who made notable contributions in the areas of exercise prescription and cardiac rehabilitation. Pollock was the lead author of the ACSM's first position statement regarding the mode and quantity of exercise necessary to elicit fitness improvements (2). In addition, Pollock was instrumental in legitimizing the role of cardiac rehabilitation as an integral part of medical treatment for patients with heart disease. Many of Pollock's significant contributions were made during his tenure at the well-known Cooper Institute for Aerobics Research in the mid-1970s.

Historical Evolution of PA Epidemiology

Although research developments in exercise physiology during the early to mid-20th century led to an improved understanding of how physical fitness could be impacted by PA, the relationships between PA and certain chronic conditions (*e.g.*, cardiovascular disease [CVD] and obesity) remained largely unknown. This was especially problematic considering the dramatic increase in CVD-related mortality that occurred during the first half of the 20th century. In an attempt to identify and understand the underlying causes of heart disease and other chronic conditions, a number of large-scale epidemiological studies (*e.g.*, Framingham Heart Study and Harvard Alumni Health Study) were initiated during the middle decades of the century.

The first epidemiological evidence indicating that greater amounts of PA were associated with reduced risks of CVD was presented by Morris and colleagues after studying double-decker bus workers in London, England (55). The major finding from this line of research was that physically active bus conductors suffered roughly half the coronary events than did more sedentary bus drivers. Further illustrating the potential health benefits of being physically active, later work by Paffenbarger and coworkers demonstrated that work-related caloric expenditure and the risk of death from coronary heart disease were inversely related among longshoremen in San Francisco, California (61).

A number of subsequent large-scale epidemiological investigations demonstrated an inverse relationship between PA and CVD incidence and mortality (40–42, 56, 73, 76). In general, these investigations showed a dose-response relationship as greater levels of PA were associated with reduced risks of developing CVD (see Fig. 1.1).

Besides PA, research has shown that physical fitness is also inversely related to CVD incidence and mortality (7, 15, 39, 71) (Fig. 1.1). An important project related to this research area is the ongoing Aerobics Center Longitudinal Study (ACLS) conducted at the Cooper Clinic in Dallas, Texas. Men and women who visited the preventive medicine clinic completed a maximal treadmill test and were rated as having low, moderate, or high physical fitness based on their gender, age, and treadmill exercise time. Blair and colleagues published one of the landmark papers in this research area using

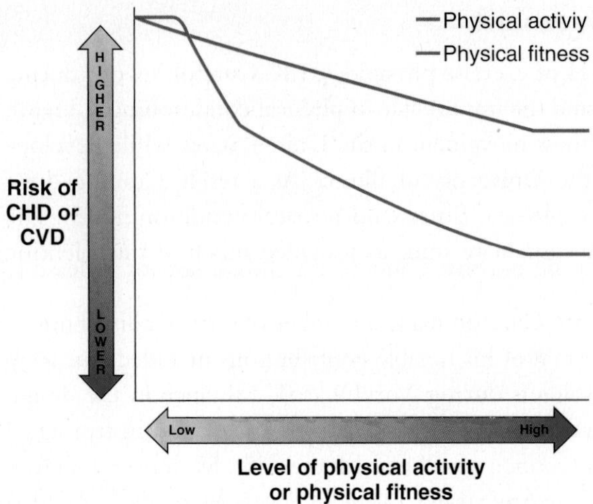

FIGURE 1.1. General relationships between PA or physical fitness level and relative risk of coronary heart disease (CHD) and cardiovascular disease (CVD). (Adapted with permission from Williams PT. Physical fitness and activity as separate heart disease risk factors: A meta-analysis. *Med Sci Sports Exerc.* 2001;33(5):754–61.)

data from the ACLS, which demonstrated that higher levels of objectively measured physical fitness from the maximal treadmill test were associated with reduced risks of CVD mortality (7).

Development of PA Guidelines and Recommendations

The eventual accumulation of evidence pointing to the beneficial and protective role of PA on health-related outcomes resulted in the publication of a joint position statement by the ACSM and Centers for Disease Control and Prevention (CDC) in 1995 regarding PA and public health (62). Based on the current literature at the time, the joint position statement from the ACSM/CDC recommended that every adult accumulate 30 minutes or more of moderate-intensity PA on most, preferably all, days of the week. Soon to follow the ACSM/CDC joint position statement, the U.S. Department of Health and Human Services published the Surgeon General's Report on Physical Activity and Health in 1996 (87). This report presented a thorough review of the available evidence regarding PA and its relation to numerous health problems while restating the PA guidelines put forth by the joint ACSM/CDC position statement. Figure 1.2 shows the trend of US adults

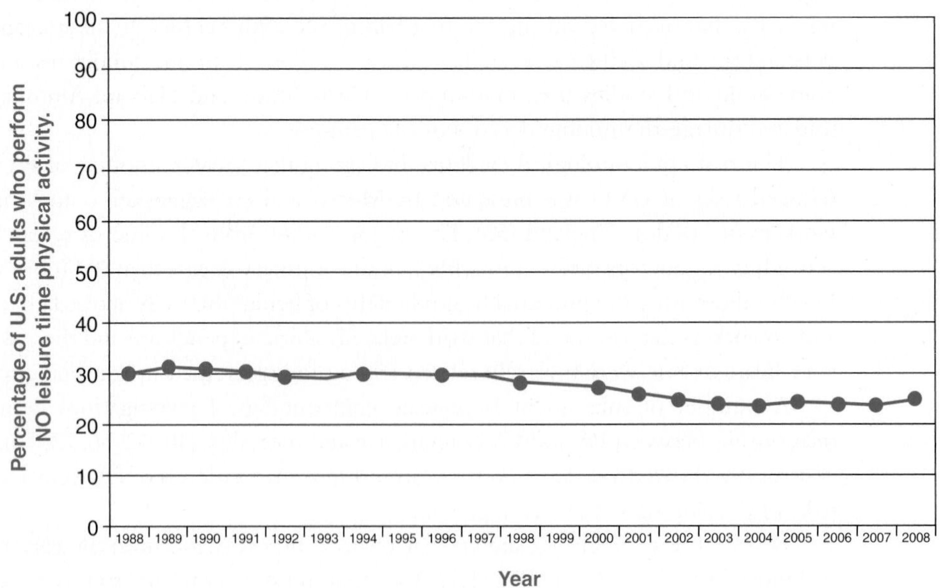

FIGURE 1.2. Trend line showing percentage of Americans completing no leisure-time PA. (Adapted from Centers for Disease Control and Prevention, National Center for Chronic Disease Prevention and Health Promotion, Division of Nutrition. *Physical Activity and Obesity*. Available from: http://www.cdc.gov/nccdphp/dnpa/physical/stats/leisure_time.htm. Retrieved 23 June, 2011.)

reporting no leisure time PA, which has remained steady to slightly declining, since the release of the Surgeon General's Report in 1996.

Twelve years after the joint position statement by the ACSM/CDC, an update regarding PA and public health was issued in 2007 (24). The updated position statement further clarified the recommendations made in 1995. One of the main changes was the more specific frequency recommendation for moderate-intensity PA as the "most, preferably all, days of the week" qualification was changed to "five days each week." In addition, the update incorporated guidelines for meeting the recommendation with vigorous PA and indicated that bouts of PA should last for at least 10 minutes in duration to be counted toward the 30-minute daily goal. Specifics relating to muscle strengthening were also incorporated into the updated recommendation.

One year after the updated ACSM/CDC PA recommendations, the U.S. Department of Health Human Services published the 2008 Physical Activity Guidelines for Americans (88). This document represented the first comprehensive PA guidelines put forth by the US government. These guidelines presented recommendations for three different age groups (children and adolescents, adults, and older adults) and incorporated specifics regarding aerobic, muscle-strengthening, and flexibility activities. Unlike the ACSM/CDC guidelines, the 2008 Physical Activity Guidelines for Americans did not specify a weekly frequency for aerobic activity (*e.g.*, $\geq$5 d·wk^{-1}). Instead, the guidelines simply called for an accumulation of 150 minutes of moderate-intensity PA on a weekly basis, and suggested that the cumulative duration be spread throughout the week.

RELATIONSHIP BETWEEN PA/EXERCISE AND HEALTH ACROSS THE LIFESPAN

Until recently, attempts to quantify daily durations of PA in free-living conditions often relied on subjective self-report methods (*e.g.*, PA questionnaires and PA logs). However, the best estimates for county by county leisure-time PA were based on CDC self-report data and give a clear picture of which regions of the United States are least and most physically active (Fig. 1.3). In 2008, however, Troiano and colleagues (84) published a landmark paper detailing the first objective assessment of PA among a nationally representative sample of Americans. This objective assessment was conducted using specialized PA accelerometers, which can measure the duration and intensity of accumulated PA. Alarming among the findings from this assessment were the extremely low daily durations of moderate to vigorous PA ($\geq$3 METs) among Americans across all ranges. This research revealed that less than 4% of American adults 20 years of age and older were meeting public health recommendations for PA. It is difficult to explain the discrepancy between the self-report and the objective measures of PA, yet this provokes concern that most Americans are not as active as they might think.

The low levels of PA demonstrated among the majority of Americans are particularly problematic, especially when considering the numerous health benefits associated with regular PA. Across

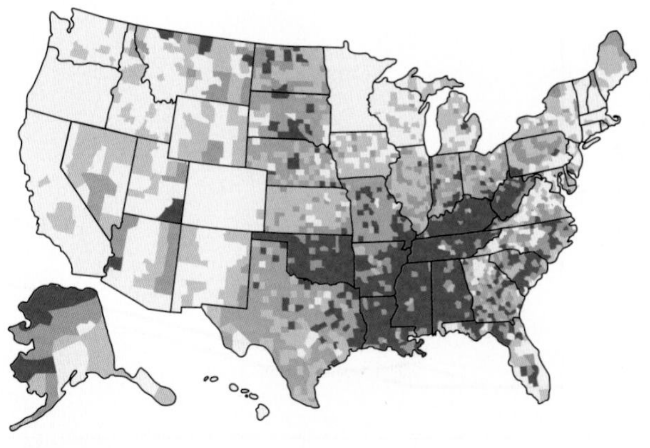

FIGURE 1.3. 2008 estimates of leisure-time physical inactivity among adults 20 years of age or older. (Adapted from Centers for Disease Control and Prevention. National Diabetes Surveillance System. Available from: http://apps.nccd.cdc.gov/DDTSTRS/default.aspx. Retrieved 23 June, 2011.)

the age continuum, PA can have positive impacts in biological, psychological, and social domains. Moreover, the therapeutic and prophylactic benefits of PA can often be obtained at little to no cost and in nearly any environment.

PA and Health in Children and Adolescents

In addition to healthy eating habits, incorporating regular PA into the lives of children and adolescents (17 yr of age and younger) provides an early starting point to aid in the prevention of numerous chronic diseases. Chapters 10 through 12 discuss the importance of establishing positive health behaviors early in life as a means of lifelong healthy living. An increasingly prevalent chronic disease among America's youth is obesity. Data from the early 1970s indicated that 5.0% of 2- to 5-year-olds, 4.0% of 6- to 11-year-olds, and 6.1% of 12- to 19-year-olds were obese (60). However, two- to fourfold increases in obesity prevalence have been observed over the past four decades as current estimates indicate that 10.4% of 2- to 5-year-olds, 19.6% of 6- to 11-year-olds, and 18.1% of 12- to 19-year-olds are obese (Fig. 1.4). This has become a major health concern, as childhood obesity increases the risk for a host of other chronic diseases such as diabetes, hyperlipidemia, and hypertension (57). In addition, childhood obesity may result in detrimental behavioral, social, and economic effects (21, 72, 79).

PA has been one of many modalities suggested as a means to address the rising obesity epidemic among children and adolescents. Among youth, lower levels of PA are associated with a greater risk of being overweight or obese (35, 74). Moreover, evidence suggests that being physically active during childhood and adolescence positively influences metabolic risk factors related to Type 2 diabetes (38, 67), which has become an emerging health problem among America's youth (1).

Adequate PA is also important for normal musculoskeletal development during childhood. An adequate stimulus via structured exercise and/or PA can help increase bone accretion during youth and adolescence (4). In turn, greater peak bone mineral density in early adulthood may be attained, which reduces the risk or delays the onset of osteoporosis in later adulthood (26).

PA and Health in Adults

Adults who engage in regular PA can enjoy many health benefits from being regularly physically active. Among adults, research has shown that increases in PA energy expenditure are associated with significant weight reduction (66, 69, 70, 77). This has become especially pertinent, as approximately 68% of the US general population is either overweight or obese (18). However, regular PA carries health benefits regardless of any changes in body composition that occur as a result of increased PA energy expenditure (34). Additional health benefits of regular PA include, but are not limited to, reduced risks of Type 2 diabetes (32, 49), hypertension (25, 64), CVD (30, 48), colon cancer (53), and all-cause mortality (31).

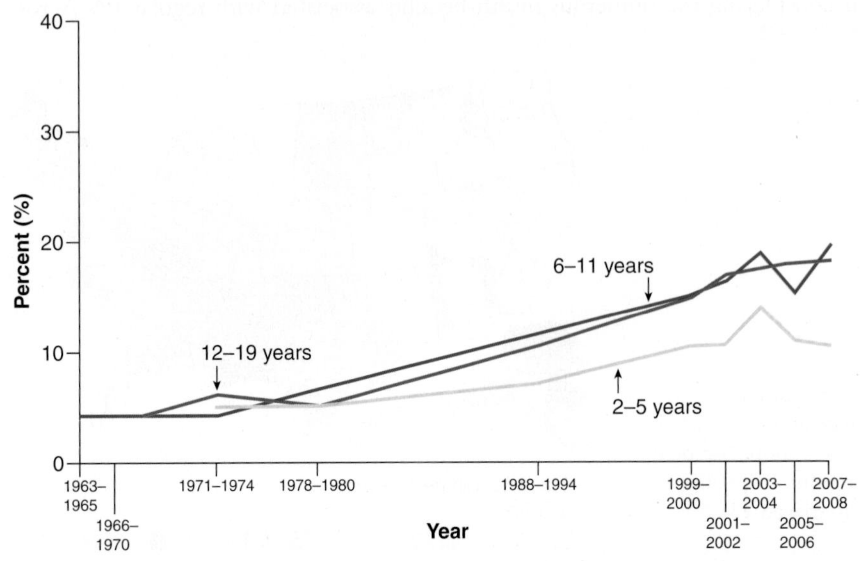

FIGURE 1.4. Childhood obesity trends since the early 1960s. (Adapted from Ogden C, Carroll M. *Prevalence of Obesity among Children and Adolescents: United States, Trends 1963–1965 through 2007–2008*. Hyattsville (MD): Centers for Disease Control and Prevention, National Center for Health Statistics; 2010.)

Of particular interest regarding PA among adults is the role it can play in the prevention of future CVD. The economic cost associated with CVD has grown substantially in recent times, with current estimates of the direct and indirect costs associated with CVD and stroke in the United States exceeding $500 billion in 2010 (44). Current estimates among adults 20 to 59 years of age indicate that only 3.5% are meeting public health recommendations for PA (84). Substantially increasing the proportion of adults meeting current PA guidelines would undoubtedly have positive effects on CVD prevalence and its associated costs.

PA and Health in Older Adults

Recent evidence has shown that PA levels in America tend to decline as age increases and are lower among persons with chronic diseases (84). This age-related decline in PA may be partly attributable to limitations resulting from common chronic diseases. However, like younger adults and children, older individuals can also reap health benefits by being physically active (87, 88). Interestingly, some research has demonstrated that leisure-time PA is a more important protective measure against heart disease in older adults (older than 65 yr) than in younger adults (81).

In comparison with younger individuals, older adults are more likely to have a chronic condition (*e.g.*, CVD). However, PA still confers health benefits on those individuals suffering from one or more chronic diseases. As an example, PA after first nonfatal myocardial infarction (MI) has been shown to reduce the risk for a second MI (78). In addition, regular PA has also been shown to be an effective treatment for osteoarthritis among older adults (8, 63).

Particularly important to older adults, a physically active lifestyle can help them maintain physical function during later years (10). Much of this benefit is due to greater levels of functional capacity that can be achieved through PA (16). These higher levels of functional capacity can allow older individuals to live independently and make it easier to carry out activities of daily living. In addition, PA during later adulthood is associated with decreased risks of falls and osteoporotic fractures (17, 27).

GENERAL RISKS ASSOCIATED WITH PA/EXERCISE

It is the inherent responsibility of a HFS to take reasonable precautions when working with individuals who wish to become physically active or to increase their current activity level. In healthy individuals free of CVD diagnosis, exercise does not present a risk for CVD-related events, particularly with moderate-intensity exercise (90). In addition, the 2008 Physical Activity Guidelines emphasize the importance of regular PA across all age groups, almost regardless of current health status, as the benefits are far reaching (88).

Most sedentary individuals can safely begin a low- to moderate-intensity PA program without the need for baseline exercise testing or prior medical clearance. However, individuals with known or suspected cardiovascular, pulmonary, or metabolic disease should obtain medical clearance before beginning a vigorous-intensity exercise program. Chapter 2 will discuss this in greater detail. The HFS responsible for supervising vigorous-intensity exercise programs, regardless of the population, should have current training in basic and/or advanced cardiac life support and emergency procedures, while also being keenly aware of the signs and symptoms of CVD.

Risks of Sudden Cardiac Death

Despite the known benefits of PA and exercise, inherent risk does exist. Sudden cardiac death associated with exercise is widely publicized, especially in children or adolescents. In truth, sudden cardiac death related to moderate exercise is extremely rare (75, 83). For young individuals (younger than 30 yr), the most common causes of sudden cardiac death are congenital and hereditary abnormalities; however, there is no clear consensus on the actual rate of sudden death in young individuals (14, 50, 89). High school and college athletes are typically required to have a preparticipation screening, which is one means of detecting potential cardiac issues.

Sudden cardiac death risk increases with age and prevalence of known or unknown CVD (20, 23, 54, 75, 82, 90, 92). Further, the rates of sudden cardiac death, and acute MI, are disproportionately higher in the most sedentary individuals performing infrequent exercise (3), such as a generally sedentary person shoveling heavy snow.

Although the exact mechanism of sudden cardiac death or MI remains elusive, there appears to be an acute arterial insult that dislodges already present plaque, resulting in platelet aggregation or thrombosis (6, 12, 22). The HFS should have a basic understanding of this sequela and the inherent risks of sudden cardiac death or MI any one individual may carry. Appropriate screening is critical for minimizing this risk (see Chapter 2).

The Risk of Cardiac Events during Exercise Testing

A practicing HFS is likely to suggest and perform baseline and follow-up exercise tests across a wide variety of individuals. While submaximal exercise testing is generally considered safe for most, maximal- or vigorous-intensity exercise testing does pose some risk (19, 36, 52, 68, 80). Similar to exercise, exercise testing is also rather safe when performed properly. Overall, the risk of cardiac events during symptom-limited exercise testing in a clinical environment is low (~6 cardiac events per 10,000 tests), and given proper screening and attention, most tests can be performed with a high degree of safety (58, 59).

Musculoskeletal Injury Associated with Exercise

In addition to the acute risk of sudden cardiac death or MI, there is also an increased risk of musculoskeletal injury associated with exercise. Typically, the highest risk is associated with activities that are weight-bearing or involve repetitive motion: jogging, walking, cycling, weightlifting, and the like. The most common musculoskeletal injuries, regardless of gender, occur in the lower body, particularly at the knee or foot (29). The rate of musculoskeletal injury is highest in team and contact sports, and includes injuries of all types, not just lower-body injuries (22).

The annual rate of musculoskeletal injury associated with running and jogging is significant, ranging from 35% to 65% (37, 46). However, only about 7% of US adults use jogging or running as their regular form of exercise. Walking for exercise, which is performed by approximately 30% of adults, is the most popular exercise in the United States (86). The musculoskeletal risk associated with walking is considerably lower than that with jogging, with about 1.5% of people reporting an injury in the previous month (65). Compared with joggers, walkers of both genders are at 25% to 30% lower risk for incurring an acute or chronic musculoskeletal injury (13).

Aerobic dance and resistance training are two other popular types of exercise with a documented musculoskeletal injury rate. Resistance training includes weightlifting, body weight exercises, and the like, and was shown to have a 1-month injury rate of 2.4% (65).

Although certainly not life-threatening, musculoskeletal injuries present a real and present issue. Preventing and minimizing injury will lead to greater opportunities to remain physically active, although, unfortunately, those previously injured from exercise are at higher risk for reinjury (33, 37, 47, 51, 91). Therefore, to minimize musculoskeletal injury from the outset, the HFS should consider the following:

- Be diligent in choosing exercise modes and prescribing exercise that are based on an individual's current fitness level and desires, along with any past exercise experiences.
- Start at a low level of intensity, frequency, and duration, and progress slowly.
- Be aware and make clients aware of early signs of potential injury (*i.e.*, increasing muscle soreness, bone and joint pain, excessive fatigue, and performance decrements). When noted, take appropriate precautions, which may include temporarily ceasing the activity, more frequent rest days, or simply decreasing the frequency, intensity, or duration of exercise.
- Set realistic exercise goals to avoid overexercising (see Chapter 11 for goal setting).

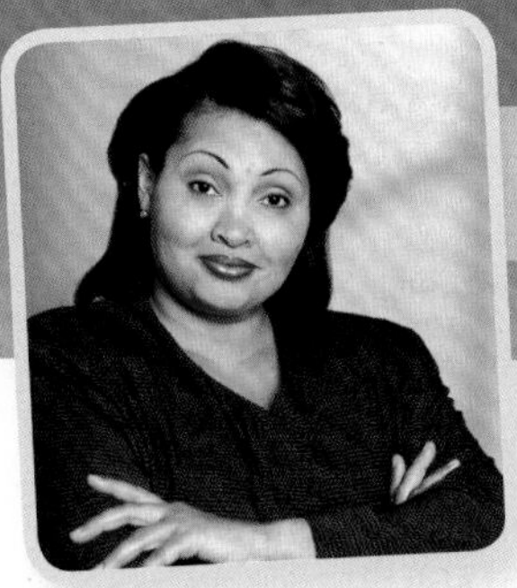

The Case of Rachel

Submitted by **Kaitlin Teser, MS, ACSM-HFS, Brookline Hebrew Senior Life Center, Brookline, MA**

Rachel is a 43-year-old, low-risk, moderately active mom. Rachel's initial goal of losing 10 lb shifted to wanting to incorporate a more active lifestyle habits into her daily routine.

Narrative

Rachel is a 43-year old, low-risk woman who works 40 hours a week in a sedentary office job. Rachel's original goal was to lose 10 lb in 12 weeks. She was moderately active. Her two children, Zach, age 10, and Emily, age 8, are involved in karate. In addition to a walk around the local track with coworkers twice a week, Rachel also took a cardio kickboxing class on Saturday mornings.

Fitness Testing Results

The results of Rachel's fitness assessment were as follows:

Resting blood pressure	110/85 mm Hg	Good
Resting heart rate	81 bpm	Good
Body fat (%)	28.7	Fair
Body mass index	25.5	Average
Sit and reach (box)	29 cm	Fair
Muscular endurance (YMCA bench press)	16 reps	Low-average
Aerobic fitness (YMCA submaximal bike test)	23.3 $mL \cdot kg^{-1} \cdot min^{-1}$	Very poor

Although Rachel's first wellness vision seemed like it related to active living, she was really focused on weight loss. I was careful to "meet her where she was" and encourage her use of the term *active living* in her wellness vision.

Rachel's First Wellness Vision

"My wellness vision is to be healthy, energetic, and vital. I am motivated by my desire to stay active with my children and continue to be active as I age. I am challenged by my demanding schedule and multiple commitments, but have been a regular exerciser in the past and know the importance of active living as a way of life. I am confident that with increased social support, a regular routine and a realistic weight management plan, I will achieve success."

Rachel's program followed the FITT principle and incorporated both health-related and skill-related fitness components. She added another cardio kickboxing class to her week and convinced her coworkers to walk on the track an additional day. My work with Rachel focused on increasing strength and range of motion. I introduced Rachel to a variety of modalities that could be used both at home and at the office to provide brief workouts throughout the day. The more I put myself in Rachel's shoes and developed programs that were fun, efficient, and effective, the more she seemed to be engaged in the session. I learned that Rachel often went home and tried out a modified version of our activities with her children. After 4 weeks, Rachel's attitude started to shift. When talking about food, I heard less about her examples of "willpower," and more about healthy choices. Externally,

continues

***The Case of Rachel* cont.**

one of the first changes I noticed was how she was dressed. Rachel had begun to wear work clothes that enabled her to perform a set of "tricep dips" at her desk. Her fitness indicators were all improving, and she genuinely seemed to have more pep in her step!

On completion of the 12-week program, Rachel had lost 6 lb and increased her strength, flexibility, and aerobic fitness. What was more exciting, however, was that Rachel had gained a real appreciation of the value of daily practices of active living. She was able to restructure her work schedule to allow her to walk to school once a week with her children. She incorporated stretch breaks into the start of every meeting at work. She used the stairs instead of the elevator, and always opened a door with her own strength (without assistance from an automatic door). It was only in retrospect that Rachel realized that the choices she and her family were making for recreation had shifted from inside activities, such as shopping and the movies, to hiking, cycling, and swimming. Rachel also realized that her new choices had resulted in meeting new friends who shared similar interests in being active and enjoying family activities that involved movement.

Rachel's New Wellness Vision

"My wellness vision is to move and keep moving—to move freely through a full range of motion and to move in a way that enables me to do all the things that I need to do in my life and have energy left over. I want to move with and for my children and grandchildren. I may be challenged by old habits of acting on misguided priorities, but I know that with the help of my friends and family and by incorporating brief workout breaks into my day and committing to at least one act of active living every day, I will be able to sustain and maintain my newfound joy."

Rachel was able to achieve her new goal of moving more by small choices and daily practices that reflected a new attitude about exercise. She set an achievable goal of incorporating one act of active living into every day. Rachel also became willing to meet new people who were like-minded and would support her efforts to be active. To an outside observer, Rachel's changes may seem like minor adjustments in her schedule, but to anyone who really knows her, a seismic shift took place that will enable Rachel to realize her wellness vision and goals for the future.

Questions

1. What did the HFS do to support Rachel's goals? The HFS had a key role in actively listening to Rachel. The HFS was skilled in not only being able to identify Rachel's interest in losing weight, but also wanting to incorporate active living. As a facilitator of motivation, the HFS was able to encourage Rachel to identify ways in which active living techniques could be incorporated into daily life. The HFS also provided a sound exercise program that encouraged competence, confidence, and relatedness.
2. What role did social support play in Rachel's success? Rachel was able to establish herself as a leader and learner. She was encouraged to be creative in the completion of her goals. By including coworkers, Rachel was able to share the benefits of exercise and have support when she was challenged to work through lunch. Rachel was also able to enlist the help of her children by creating time for a walk to school morning.
3. How can one act of active living a day make a difference in someone's life? A shift in attitude and expectations enabled Rachel to evaluate her original goals in a way that sustained her adherence to the program. By committing to one act of active living, Rachel was able to cultivate other habits of behavior around both exercise and nutrition that further aided her in reaching her weight loss and fitness goals.

References

Brownson RC, Eyler AA, King AC, Brown DR, Shyu, Y, Sallis, JF. Patterns and correlates of physical activity among US women 40 years and older. *Am J Public Health*. 2000;90:264–70.

Kerr J, Norman GJ, Sallis JF, Patrick K. Exercise aids, neighborhood safety, and physical activity in adolescents and parents. *Med Sci Sports Exerc*. 2008;40(7):1244–8.

Moore M, Tschannen-Moran B. *Coaching Psychology Manual*. Baltimore (MD): Lippincott Williams & Wilkins; 2009. 208 p.

Moustaka FC, Vlachopoulos SP, Kabitsis C, Theodorakis Y. Effects of an autonomy-supportive exercise instructing style on exercise motivation, psychological well-being, and exercise attendance in middle-age women. *J Phys Act Health*. 2012;9(1):138–50.

SUMMARY

As discussed earlier in this chapter, the notion that PA can improve and/or maintain health is by no means novel. However, it was not until substantial scientific advancements during the 20th century, in fields such as exercise physiology and epidemiology, that our understanding of how PA could treat and/or prevent common chronic diseases (*e.g.*, CVD, hypertension, and Type 2 diabetes mellitus) became known. Despite these advancements, there remain many unanswered questions regarding the exact pathways and mechanisms through which PA influences health.

Although there is still much to learn, the current evidence strongly indicates that regular PA and exercise can have tremendous benefits for an individual's physical, metabolic, and mental health. However, overexercising, doing too much too soon, or exercising at an unsafe intensity can bring negative consequences, even as severe as sudden death. Although the risks associated with exercise are proportional to the amount and intensity of exercise, both acute and chronic, the benefits of habitual exercise far outweigh the risks.

This Resource Manual is intended to prepare the HFS with the necessary tools to assess fitness and prescribe exercise for populations able to exercise without medical supervision. While no manual is completely comprehensive, the information within should serve as an outstanding resource for both the new and the experienced exercise professional.

STUDY QUESTIONS

1. Compare and contrast PA, exercise, health-related fitness, and skill-related fitness.
2. Describe at least two individuals and two landmark research studies that made significant contributions to the current body of knowledge regarding PA/physical fitness and associated health benefits.
3. Describe the health benefits and health risks associated with acute and chronic PA.

REFERENCES

1. Amed S, Daneman D, Mahmud FH, Hamilton J. Type 2 diabetes in children and adolescents. *Expert Rev Cardiovasc Ther.* 2010;8(3):393–406.
2. American College of Sports Medicine. The recommended quality and quantity of exercise for developing and maintaining fitness in healthy adults. *Med Sci Sports Exerc.* 1978;10(3):vii–x.
3. American College of Sports Medicine, American Heart Association. Exercise and acute cardiovascular events: Placing the risks into perspective. *Med Sci Sports Exerc.* 2007;39(5):886–97.
4. Bailey DA, McKay HA, Mirwald RL, Crocker PRE, Faulkner RA. A six-year longitudinal study of the relationship of physical activity to bone mineral accrual in growing children: The University of Saskatchewan bone mineral accrual study. *J Bone Miner Res.* 1999;14(10):1672–9.
5. Berryman JW. Thomas K. Cureton, Jr.: Pioneer researcher, proselytizer, and proponent for physical fitness. *Res Q Exerc Sport.* 1996;67(1):1–12.
6. Black A, Black MM, Gensini G. Exertion and acute coronary artery injury. *Angiology.* 1975;26(11):759–83.
7. Blair SN, Kohl HW III, Paffenbarger RS Jr, Clark DG, Cooper KH, Gibbons LW. Physical fitness and all-cause mortality: A prospective study of healthy men and women. *JAMA.* 1989;262(17):2395–401.
8. Brosseau L, Pelland L, Wells G, Macleay L, Lamothe C, Michaud G. Efficacy of aerobic exercises for osteoarthritis. Part II. A meta-analysis. *Phys Ther Rev.* 2004;9:125–45.
9. Caspersen CJ, Powell KE, Christenson GM. Physical activity, exercise, and physical fitness: Definitions and distinctions for health-related research. *Public Health Rep.* 1985;100(2):126–31.
10. Chodzko-ZajkoW, Schwingel A, Park CH. Successful aging: The role of physical activity. *Am J Lifestyle Med.* 2009;3(1):20–8.
11. Church TS, Thomas DM, Tudor-Locke C, et al. Trends over 5 decades in U.S. occupation-related physical activity and their associations with obesity. *PLoS One.* 2011;6(5):e19657.

12. Ciampricotti R, Deckers JW, Taverne R, el Gamal M, Relik-van Wely L, Pool J. Characteristics of conditioned and sedentary men with acute coronary syndromes. *Am J Cardiol.* 1994;73(4):219–22.
13. Colbert LH, Hootman JM, Macera CA. Physical activity-related injuries in walkers and runners in the aerobics center longitudinal study. *Clin J Sport Med.* 2000;10(4):259–63.
14. Drezner JA, Chun JS, Harmon KG, Derminer L. Survival trends in the United States following exercise-related sudden cardiac arrest in the youth: 2000–2006. *Heart Rhythm.* 2008;5(6):794–9.
15. Ekelund LG, Haskell WL, Johnson JL, Whaley FS, Criqui MH, Sheps DS. Physical fitness as a predictor of cardiovascular mortality in asymptomatic North American men. The lipid research clinics mortality follow-up study. *N Engl J Med.*1988;319(21):1379–84.
16. Evans WJ. Effects of exercise on body composition and functional capacity of the elderly. *J Gerontol A Biol Sci Med Sci.* 1995;50(special issue):147–50.
17. Feskanich D, Willett W, Colditz G. Walking and leisure-time activity and risk of hip fracture in postmenopausal women. *JAMA.* 2002;288(18):2300–6.
18. Flegal KM, Carroll MD, Ogden CL, Curtin LR. Prevalence and trends in obesity among U.S. adults, 1999–2008. *JAMA.* 2010;303(3):235–41.
19. Gibbons L, Blair SN, Kohl HW, Cooper K. The safety of maximal exercise testing. *Circulation.* 1989;80(4):846–52.
20. Giri S, Thompson PD, Kiernan FJ, et al. Clinical and angiographic characteristics of exertion-related acute myocardial infarction. *JAMA.* 1999;282(18):1731–6.
21. Gortmaker SL, Must A, Perrin JM, Sobol AM, Dietz WH. Social and economic consequences of overweight in adolescence and young adulthood. *N Engl J Med.* 1993;329(14):1008–12.
22. Centers for Disease Control and Prevention (CDC). Nonfatal sports-and recreation-related injuries treated in emergency departments—United States, July 2000–June 2001. *MMWR Morb Mortal Wkly Rep.*2002;51(33):736–40.
23. Hammoudeh AJ, Haft JI. Coronary-plaque rupture in acute coronary syndromes triggered by snow shoveling. *N Engl J Med.* 1996;335(26):2001–2.
24. Haskell WL, Lee IM, Pate RR, et al. Physical activity and public health: Updated recommendation for adults from the American College of Sports Medicine and the American Heart Association. *Med Sci Sports Exerc.* 2007;39(8):1423–34.
25. Hayashi T, Tsumura K, Suematsu C, Okada K, Fujii S, Endo G. Walking to work and the risk for hypertension in men: The Osaka Health Survey. *Ann Intern Med.* 1999;131(1):21–6.
26. Hernandez CJ, Beaupre GS, Carter DR. A theoretical analysis of the relative influences of peak BMD, age-related bone loss and menopause on the development of osteoporosis. *Osteoporos Int.* 2003;14(10):843–7.
27. Heesch KC, Byles JE, Brown WJ. Prospective association between physical activity and falls in community-dwelling older women. *J Epidemiol Community Health.* 2008;62(5):421–6.
28. Hippocrates. *Jones WHS, Translation. Regimen I.* Cambridge (MA): Harvard University Press; 1952. 229 p.
29. Hootman JM, Macera CA, Ainsworth BE, Addy CL, Martin M, Blair SN. Epidemiology of musculoskeletal injuries among sedentary and physically active adults. *Med Sci Sports Exerc.* 2002;34(5):838–44.
30. Hu G, Tuomilehto J, Silventoinen K, Barengo NC, Jousilahti P. Joint effects of physical activity, body mass index, waist circumference and waist-to-hip ratio with the risk of cardiovascular disease among middle-aged Finnish men and women. *Eur Heart J.* 2004;25(24):2212–9.
31. Hu G, Tuomilehto J, Silventoinen K, Barengo NC, Peltonen M, Jousilahti P. The effects of physical activity and body mass index on cardiovascular, cancer and all-cause mortality among 47,212 middle-aged Finnish men and women. *Int J Obes.* 2005;29(8):894–902.
32. Hu FB, Sigal RJ, Rich-Edwards JW, et al. Walking compared with vigorous physical activity and risk of type 2 diabetes in women: A prospective study. *JAMA.*1999;282(15):1433–9.
33. Jacobs SJ, Berson BL. Injuries to runners: A study of entrants to a 10,000 meter race. *Am J Sports Med.* 1986;14(2):151–5.
34. Janiszewski PM, Ross R. Physical activity in the treatment of obesity: Beyond body weight reduction. *Appl Physiol Nutr Metab.* 2007;32(3):512–22.
35. Janssen I, Katmarzyk PT, Boyce WF, et al. Comparison of overweight and obesity prevalence in school-aged youth from 34 countries and their relationships with physical activity and dietary patterns. *Obes Rev.* 2005;6(2):123–32.
36. Knight JA, Laubach CA Jr, Butcher RJ, Menapace FJ. Supervision of clinical exercise testing by exercise physiologists. *Am J Cardiol.* 1995;75(5):390–1.
37. Koplan JP, Powell KE, Sikes RK, Shirley RW, Campbell CC. An epidemiologic study of the benefits and risks of running. *JAMA.* 1982;248(23):3118–21.
38. Ku CY, Gower BA, Hunter GR, Goran MI. Racial differences in insulin secretion and sensitivity in prepubertal children: Role of physical fitness and physical activity. *Obes Res.* 2000;8(7):506–15.
39. Lakka TA, Venäläinen JM, Rauramaa R, Salonen R, Tuomilehto J, Salonen JT. Relation of leisure-time physical activity and cardiorespiratory fitness to the risk of acute myocardial infarction. *N Engl J Med.* 1994;330(22):1549–54.
40. Lee IM, Paffenbarger RS Jr. Associations of light, moderate, and vigorous intensity physical activity with longevity: The Harvard alumni health study. *Am J Epidemiol.* 2000;151(3):293–9.
41. Lee IM, Rexrode KM, Cook NR, Manson JE, Buring JE. Physical activity and coronary heart disease in women: Is "no pain, no gain" passé? *JAMA.* 2001;285(11):1447–54.
42. Leon AS, Connett J, Jacobs DR Jr, Rauramaa R. Leisure-time physical activity levels and risk of coronary heart disease and death: The multiple risk factor intervention trial. *JAMA.*1987;258(17):2388–95.
43. Liguori G, Carroll-Cobb S. *FitWell: Questions and Answers.* New York (NY): McGraw-Hill; 2011. 66 p.
44. Lloyd-Jones D, Adams RJ, Brown TM, et al. Executive summary: Heart disease and stroke statistics—2010 update. *Circulation.*2010;121(7):948–54.
45. Lyons AS, Petrucelli RJ. *Medicine: An Illustrated History.* New York (NY): Abradale Press, Harry N. Abrams Inc.; 1978. 130 p.
46. Lysholm J, Wiklander J. Injuries in runners. *Am J Sports Med.* 1987;15(2):168–71.
47. Macera CA, Pate RR, Powell KE, Jackson KL, Kendrick JS, Craven TE. Predicting lower-extremity injuries among habitual runners. *Arch Intern Med.* 1989;149(11):2565–8.
48. Manson JE, Hu FB, Rich-Edwards JW, et al. A prospective study of walking as compared with vigorous exercise in the prevention of coronary heart disease in women. *N Engl J Med.* 1999;341(9):650–8.
49. Manson JE, Nathan DM, Krolewski AS, Stampfer MJ, Willett WC, Hennekens CH. A prospective study of exercise and incidence of diabetes among US male physicians. *JAMA.* 1992;268(1):63–7.
50. Maron BJ, Doerer JJ, Haas TS, Tierney DM, Mueller FO. Sudden deaths in young competitive athletes: Analysis of

1866 deaths in the United States, 1980–2006. *Circulation.* 2009;119(8):1085–92.

51. Marti B. Benefits and risks of running among women: An epidemiologic study. *Int J Sports Med.* 1988;9(2):92–8.
52. McHenry PL. Risks of graded exercise testing. *Am J Cardiol.* 1977;39(6):935–7.
53. McTiernan A, Ulrich C, Slate S, Potter J. Physical activity and cancer etiology: Associations and mechanisms. *Cancer Causes Control.* 1998;9:487–509.
54. Mittleman MA, Maclure M, Tofler GH, Sherwood JB, Goldberg RJ, Muller JE. Triggering of acute myocardial infarction by heavy physical exertion. Protection against triggering by regular exertion. Determinants of Myocardial Infarction Onset Study Investigators. *N Engl J Med.* 1993;329(23):1677–83.
55. Morris JN, Heady JA, Raffle PA, Roberts CG, Parks JW. Coronary heart-disease and physical activity of work. *Lancet.* 1953;265(6795):1053–7.
56. Morris JN, Pollard R, Everitt MG, Chave SPW, Semmence AM. Vigorous exercise in leisure-time: Protection against coronary heart disease. *Lancet.* 1980;316(8206):1207–10.
57. Must A, Anderson SE. Effects of obesity on morbidity in children and adolescents. *Nutr Clin Care.* 2003;6(1):4–12.
58. Myers J, Prakash M, Froelicher V, Do D, Partington S, Atwood JE. Exercise capacity and mortality among men referred for exercise testing. *N Engl J Med.* 2002;346(11):793–801.
59. Myers J, Voodi L, Umann T, Froelicher VF. A survey of exercise testing: methods, utilization, interpretation, and safety in the VAHCS. *J Cardiopulm Rehabil.* 2000;20(4):251–8.
60. Ogden C, Carroll M. *Prevalence of Obesity among Children and Adolescents: United States, Trends 1963–1965 through 2007–2008.* Hyattsville (MD): Centers for Disease Control and Prevention, National Center for Health Statistics; 2010.
61. Paffenbarger RS Jr, Laughlin ME, Gima AS, Black RA. Work activity of longshoremen as related to death from coronary heart disease and stroke. *N Engl J Med.* 1970;282(20):1109–14.
62. Pate RR, Pratt M, Blair SN, et al. Physical activity and public health. A recommendation from the Centers for Disease Control and Prevention and the American College of Sports Medicine. *JAMA.* 1995;273(5):402–7.
63. Pelland L, Brosseau L, Wells G, et al. Efficacy of strengthening exercises for osteoarthritis. Part I. A meta-analysis. *Phys Ther Rev.* 2004;9(2):77–108.
64. Pereira MA, Folsom AR, McGovern PG, et al. Physical activity and incident hypertension in black and white adults: The atherosclerosis risk in communities study. *Prev Med.* 1999;28(3):304–12.
65. Powell KE, Heath GW, Kresnow MJ, Sacks JJ, Branche CM. Injury rates from walking, gardening, weightlifting, outdoor bicycling, and aerobics. *Med Sci Sports Exerc.* 1998;30(8):1246–9.
66. Racette SB, Weiss EP, Villareal DT, et al. One year caloric restriction in humans: Feasibility and effects on body composition and abdominal adipose tissue. *J Gerontol A Biol Sci Med Sci.* 2006;61(9):943–50.
67. Raitakari OT, Porkka KV, Taimela S, Telama R, Rasanen L, Viikari JS. Effects of persistent physical activity and inactivity on coronary risk factors in children and young adults. The cardiovascular risk in young Finns study. *Am J Epidemiol.* 1994;140(3):195–205.
68. Rochmis P, Blackburn H. Exercise tests. A survey of procedures, safety, and litigation experience in approximately 170,000 tests. *JAMA.* 1971;217(8):1061–6.
69. Ross R, Dagnone D, Jones PJ, et al. Reduction in obesity and related comorbid conditions after diet-induced weight loss or exercise-induced weight loss in men: A randomized, controlled trial. *Ann Intern Med.* 2000;133(2):92–103.
70. Ross R, Janssen I, Dawson J, et al. Exercise-induced reduction in obesity and insulin resistance in women: A randomized controlled trial. *Obes Res.* 2004;12(5):789–98.
71. Sandvik L, Erikssen J, Thaulow E, Erikssen G, Mundal R, Rodahl K. Physical fitness as a predictor of mortality among healthy, middle-aged Norwegian men. *N Engl J Med.* 1993;328(8):533–7.
72. Schwimmer JB, Burwinkle TM, Varni JW. Health-related quality of life of severely obese children and adolescents. *JAMA.* 2003;289(14):1813–9.
73. Sesso HD, Paffenbarger RS Jr, Lee IM. Physical activity and coronary heart disease in men. *Circulation.* 2000;102(9):975–80.
74. Singh GK, Kogan MD, Van Dyck PC, Siahpush M. Racial/ethnic, socioeconomic, and behavioral determinants of childhood and adolescent obesity in the United States: Analyzing independent and joint associations. *Ann Epidemiol.* 2008;18(9):682–95.
75. Siscovick DS, Weiss NS, Fletcher RH, Lasky T. The incidence of primary cardiac arrest during vigorous exercise. *N Engl J Med.* 1984;311(14):874–7.
76. Slattery ML, Jacobs DR Jr, Nichaman MZ. Leisure time physical activity and coronary heart disease death: The US railroad study. *Circulation.* 1989;79(2):304–11.
77. Slentz CA, Duscha BD, Johnson JL, et al. Effects of the amount of exercise on body weight, body composition, and measures of central obesity: STRRIDE — a randomized controlled study. *Arch Intern Med.* 2004;164(1):31–9.
78. Steffen-Batey L, Nichaman MZ, Goff DC Jr, et al. Change in level of physical activity and risk of all-cause mortality or reinfarction: The Corpus Christi Heart Project. *Circulation.* 2000;102(18):2204–9.
79. Pediatrics Web site [Internet]. Elk Grove Village (IL): American Academy of Pediatrics; [cited 2011 May 15]. Available from: http://pediatrics.aappublications.org/
80. Stuart RJ Jr, Ellestad MH. National survey of exercise stress testing facilities. *Chest.* 1980;77(1):94–7.
81. Talbot LA, Morrell CH, Metter EJ, Fleg JL. Comparison of cardiorespiratory fitness versus leisure time physical activity as predictors of coronary events in men aged 65 years. *Am J Cardiol.* 2002;89(10):1187–92.
82. Thompson PD, Funk EJ, Carleton RA, Sturner WQ. Incidence of death during jogging in Rhode Island from 1975 through 1980. *JAMA.* 1982;247(18):2535–8.
83. Thompson PD, Stern MP, Williams P, Duncan K, Haskell WL, Wood PD. Death during jogging or running. A study of 18 cases. *JAMA.* 1979;242(12):1265–7.
84. Troiano RP, Berrigan D, Dodd KW, Mâsse LC, Tilert T, McDowell M. Physical activity in the United States measured by accelerometer. *Med Sci Sports Exerc.* 2008;40(1):181–8.
85. U.S. Bureau of Labor Statistics. Economic news release: American Time Use Survey — 2010 results. Washington (DC): U.S. Bureau of Labor Statistics. Available from: http://www.bls.gov/news.release/atus.nr0.htm. Last accessed March 2012.
86. U.S. Bureau of Labor Statistics. Spotlight on statistics: Sports and exercise. Washington (DC): U.S. Bureau of Labor Statistics; 2008. Available from: http://www.bls.gov/spotlight/2008/sports/pdf/sports_bls_spotlight.pdf. Last accessed May 2011.
87. U.S. Department of Health and Human Services. *Physical Activity and Health: A Report of the Surgeon General.* DHHS Publication No. 017-023-00196-5. 1996.

88. U.S. Department of Health and Human Services. Office of Disease Prevention & Health Promotion. *2008 Physical Activity Guidelines for Americans*. ODPHP Publication No. U0036. 2008.
89. Van Camp SP, Bloor CM, Mueller FO, Cantu RC, Olson HG. Nontraumatic sports death in high school and college athletes. *Med Sci Sports Exerc.* 1995;27(5):641–7.
90. Vuori I. The cardiovascular risks of physical activity. *Acta Med Scand.* 1986;220(S711):205–14.
91. Walter SD, Hart LE, McIntosh JM, Sutton JR. The Ontario cohort study of running-related injuries. *Arch Intern Med.* 1989;149(11):2561–4.
92. Willich SN, Lewis M, Lowel H, Arntz HR, Schubert F, Schroder R. Physical exertion as a trigger of acute myocardial infarction. Triggers and mechanisms of myocardial infarction study group. *N Engl J Med.* 1993;329(23):1684–90.

CHAPTER

2 Physical Activity Preparticipation Screening Guidelines

Gregory B. Dwyer • Molly Winke

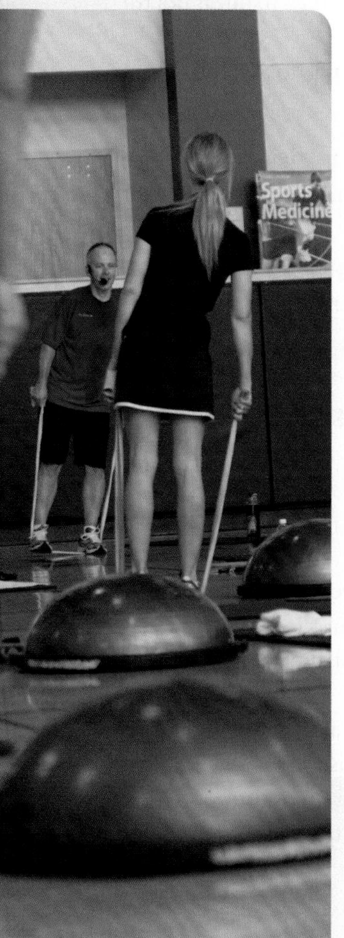

CHAPTER OBJECTIVES

- To explore the importance of and issues with pre-physical activity participation screening, including the Physical Activity Readiness Questionnaire (PAR-Q), AHA/ACSM Health/Fitness Facility Pre-participation Screening Questionnaire, and a Health History Questionnaire.
- To understand the process and outcomes of the ACSM Risk Classification and the American Heart Association Risk Stratification process.
- To learn the process of determining exercise testing recommendations based on client risk classification and fitness goals.
- To discuss the concept of absolute and relative contraindications to exercise testing and exercise programming.

As the formal promotion of physical activity (PA) has increased, there has also been an increasing emphasis on pre-PA participation screening ("screening") to minimize the risks associated with PA (9). The process of pre-PA participation screening has been increasingly professionalized over the years. The American College of Sports Medicine® (ACSM) introduced the concept of "risk stratification," now called "risk classification" (1), which considers coronary risk factors and PA contraindications. This chapter will explore the screening concept, so the health fitness specialist (HFS) can make informed decisions as to the physical readiness of an individual undertaking a new PA program.

IMPORTANCE OF PRE-PA PARTICIPATION SCREENING

To reduce the likelihood of untoward or unwanted event(s) during a fitness assessment or PA program, it is prudent to conduct some form of screening on each client as a first step (38). Each screening involves gathering and analyzing demographic and health-related information as well as completing medical/health assessments such as resting blood pressure and heart rate. This information is then used to make informed decisions regarding a client's activity assessment and PA prescription (1). The screening is a dynamic process that may vary in its scope and components depending on the client's needs (including the presence of various disease states), the type of fitness assessments to be conducted (*e.g.*, submaximal vs. maximal cardiorespiratory endurance tests), the PA program goals (*e.g.*, moderate vs. vigorous PA and/or exercise), and the equipment and policies of a given facility (*i.e.*, medical doctor or HFS to conduct the test).

The following is a selected list of reasons for conducting an initial screening for clients interested in fitness assessments and/or PA programs (1, 3):

- To identify those with medical contraindications (exclusion criteria) to PA participation.
- To identify those who should receive a medical/physical evaluation/examination prior to PA or assessments.
- To identify those who should participate in a medically supervised PA program.
- To identify those with significant but nonlimiting health/medical concerns (*e.g.*, orthopedic injuries).
- To provide benchmark data as an effective motivational tool for client goal setting.
- To provide normative data for screening assessments and to determine meaningful fitness assessment choices.

HISTORY OF PRE-PA PARTICIPATION SCREENING

There are several national and international organizations with suggested screening guidelines, including the ACSM (2, 4, 5, 14). While these guidelines are only suggested and not legally mandated, the HFS should always offer screenings and have a screening scheme that best meets the needs of his or her clients and environment.

The US Surgeon General in the 1996 report on Physical Activity and Health stated that (38): Previously inactive men over age 40, women over age 50, and people at high risk for CVD (cardiovascular disease) should first consult a physician before embarking on a program of vigorous physical activity to which they are unaccustomed. People with disease should be evaluated by a physician first. . . . In addition, a "caution" listed on most commercially available exercise equipment, exercise books, and exercise videos include statements such as:

- "First consult your physician before starting an exercise program."
- "This is especially important for:
  - Men ≥45 years old; women ≥55 years old
  - Those who are going to perform vigorous physical activity
  - And for those who are new to exercise or are unaccustomed to exercise"

The two most widely recognized sets of formal screening guidelines for apparently healthy individuals are published by the ACSM and the American Heart Association (AHA). The ACSM screening was first published in the *Guidelines for Exercise Testing and Prescription* (GETP), 4th edition, in 1991, and is updated every 5 years. The AHA publishes screening guidelines, with the most recent revisions in 2001 (1, 14).

Although the AHA and ACSM screening guidelines share many components, the AHA guidelines make some additional suggestions related to PA restrictions, monitoring, and supervision during exercise on the basis of the individual's risk category (14).

LEVELS OF SCREENING

According to the ACSM, there are two basic approaches to pre-PA participation screening: self-guided and professional (1). These two levels of screening are not mutually exclusive; for instance, an individual may first practice some self-guided methods before consulting an HFS for professional guidance.

Self-Guided Screenings

Self-guided approaches to screening have been suggested by many organizations, including ACSM and AHA, as a minimum starting point for anyone wishing to increase their PA (1). Two questionnaires, the Physical Activity Readiness Questionnaire and the AHA/ACSM Health/Fitness Facility Preparticipation Screening Questionnaire, have been suggested for use in self-guided screening and are discussed below.

Physical Activity Readiness Questionnaire

The Physical Activity Readiness Questionnaire (PAR-Q), presented in Figure 2.1, was developed as a brief, concise tool for initial screening (31). The PAR-Q contains seven YES/NO questions that are both readable and understandable for most individuals. The PAR-Q is designed to identify clients for whom strenuous PA is not recommended or who would benefit from physician clearance prior to exercise. The PAR-Q, which is widely used, has been recommended as a minimal standard for entry into moderate-intensity exercise programs. Thus, the PAR-Q may be considered a useful tool for individuals to gauge their own "medical" readiness to participate in PA assessments and programs (1). One limitation of the PAR-Q is its limited effectiveness as a screening tool for low- to moderate-risk clients (2).

AHA/ACSM Health/Fitness Facility Preparticipation Screening Questionnaire

In addition to the PAR-Q, the AHA and the ACSM have developed the AHA/ACSM Health/Fitness Facility Preparticipation Screening Questionnaire (AHA/ACSM Questionnaire), which is presented in Figure 2.2. This questionnaire is also useful for clients to gauge their own readiness and therefore suggested as a self-guided screening tool. Unlike the simplicity of the PAR-Q, the AHA/ACSM Questionnaire is more comprehensive and surveys recognized signs and symptoms suggestive of CVD and other ACSM-established risk factor thresholds (7). Since the signs and symptoms and thresholds are modified on a regular basis (*i.e.*, with the publication of a new edition of the GETP), it is important for the HFS to use the most current set of published guidelines.

The HFS should suggest, at minimum, that their clients complete a PAR-Q prior to participation in any self-guided activity or assessment program (1, 37). Furthermore, the client may want to consider using the AHA/ACSM Questionnaire for a more detailed self-guided screening.

Effectiveness of PAR-Q and AHA/ACSM Health/Fitness Facility Preparticipation Screening Questionnaire

Currently, there are no available data on the sensitivity or specificity of the AHA/ACSM Questionnaire for identifying high-risk individuals. The PAR-Q, however, has been found to be a useful screening tool (31). de Oliveira Luz and colleagues found the PAR-Q to have high sensitivity (89%), or true positives, for identifying potential medical conditions in older adults that might be exacerbated during exercise. Conversely, the specificity, or true negative rate (42%), was not as high (12). Thus, the PAR-Q may be effective in identifying clients at high risk, but not necessarily reliable in identifying those at little or no risk. Because of this discrepancy in sensitivity and specificity, the HFS should consider the ACSM Risk Classification when interpreting these initial self-guided screenings (19).

Physical Activity Readiness Questionnaire - PAR-Q (revised 2002)

PAR-Q & YOU

(A Questionnaire for People Aged 15 to 69)

Regular physical activity is fun and healthy, and increasingly more people are starting to become more active every day. Being more active is very safe for most people. However, some people should check with their doctor before they start becoming much more physically active.

If you are planning to become much more physically active than you are now, start by answering the seven questions in the box below. If you are between the ages of 15 and 69, the PAR-Q will tell you if you should check with your doctor before you start. If you are over 69 years of age, and you are not used to being very active, check with your doctor.

Common sense is your best guide when you answer these questions. Please read the questions carefully and answer each one honestly: check YES or NO.

YES	NO	
☐	☐	**1. Has your doctor ever said that you have a heart condition and that you should only do physical activity recommended by a doctor?**
☐	☐	**2. Do you feel pain in your chest when you do physical activity?**
☐	☐	**3. In the past month, have you had chest pain when you were not doing physical activity?**
☐	☐	**4. Do you lose your balance because of dizziness or do you ever lose consciousness?**
☐	☐	**5. Do you have a bone or joint problem (for example, back, knee or hip) that could be made worse by a change in your physical activity?**
☐	☐	**6. Is your doctor currently prescribing drugs (for example, water pills) for your blood pressure or heart condition?**
☐	☐	**7. Do you know of any other reason why you should not do physical activity?**

If you answered

YES to one or more questions

Talk with your doctor by phone or in person BEFORE you start becoming much more physically active or BEFORE you have a fitness appraisal. Tell your doctor about the PAR-Q and which questions you answered YES.

- You may be able to do any activity you want — as long as you start slowly and build up gradually. Or, you may need to restrict your activities to those which are safe for you. Talk with your doctor about the kinds of activities you wish to participate in and follow his/her advice.
- Find out which community programs are safe and helpful for you.

NO to all questions

If you answered NO honestly to all PAR-Q questions, you can be reasonably sure that you can:

- start becoming much more physically active – begin slowly and build up gradually. This is the safest and easiest way to go.
- take part in a fitness appraisal – this is an excellent way to determine your basic fitness so that you can plan the best way for you to live actively. It is also highly recommended that you have your blood pressure evaluated. If your reading is over 144/94, talk with your doctor before you start becoming much more physically active.

→ **DELAY BECOMING MUCH MORE ACTIVE:**

- if you are not feeling well because of a temporary illness such as a cold or a fever – wait until you feel better; or
- if you are or may be pregnant – talk to your doctor before you start becoming more active.

PLEASE NOTE: If your health changes so that you then answer YES to any of the above questions, tell your fitness or health professional. Ask whether you should change your physical activity plan.

Informed Use of the PAR-Q: The Canadian Society for Exercise Physiology, Health Canada, and their agents assume no liability for persons who undertake physical activity, and if in doubt after completing this questionnaire, consult your doctor prior to physical activity.

No changes permitted. You are encouraged to photocopy the PAR-Q but only if you use the entire form.

NOTE: If the PAR-Q is being given to a person before he or she participates in a physical activity program or a fitness appraisal, this section may be used for legal or administrative purposes.

"I have read, understood and completed this questionnaire. Any questions I had were answered to my full satisfaction."

NAME ____

SIGNATURE ____ DATE ____________________

SIGNATURE OF PARENT
or GUARDIAN (for participants under the age of majority) ____ WITNESS ____________________

Note: This physical activity clearance is valid for a maximum of 12 months from the date it is completed and becomes invalid if your condition changes so that you would answer YES to any of the seven questions.

CSEP SCPE Supported by: Health Canada Santé Canada

continued on other side...

FIGURE 2.1. The PAR-Q (used with permission from the Canadian Society for Exercise Physiology. Physical Activity Readiness Questionnaire [PAR-Q]. 2002. www.csep.ca).

...continued from other side

PAR-Q & YOU

Physical Activity Readiness Questionnaire - PAR-Q (revised 2002)

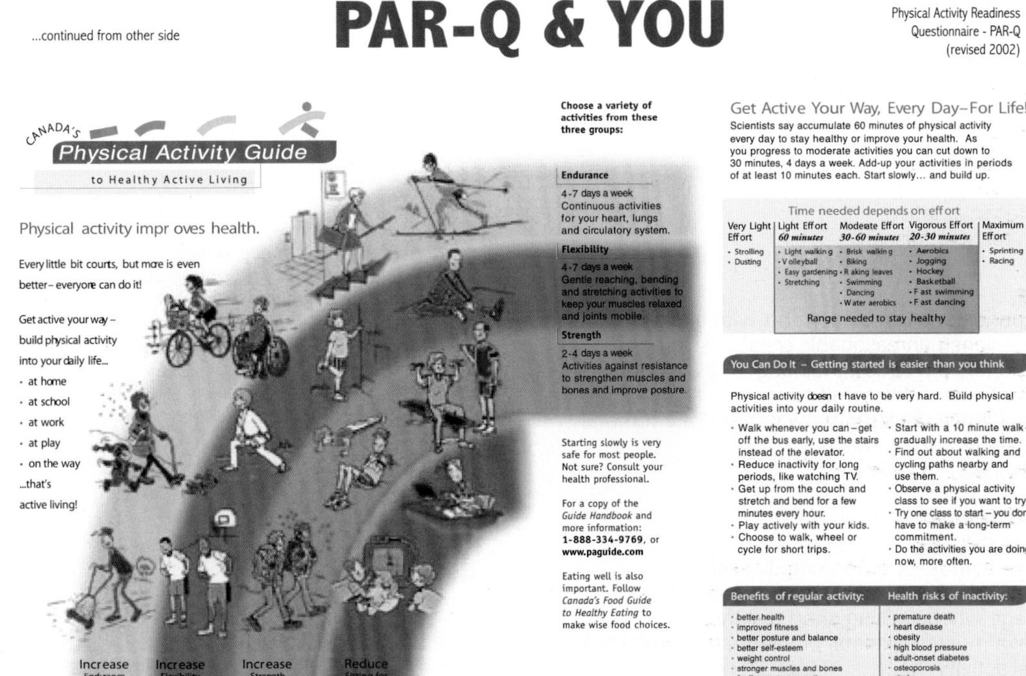

Canada's Physical Activity Guide to Healthy Active Living

Physical activity improves health.

Every little bit counts, but more is even better– everyone can do it!

Get active your way – build physical activity into your daily life...

- at home
- at school
- at work
- at play
- on the way

...that's active living!

Increase Endurance Activities | Increase Flexibility Activities | Increase Strength Activities | Reduce Sitting for long periods

Choose a variety of activities from these three groups:

Endurance
4-7 days a week
Continuous activities for your heart, lungs and circulatory system.

Flexibility
4-7 days a week
Gentle reaching, bending and stretching activities to keep your muscles relaxed and joints mobile.

Strength
2-4 days a week
Activities against resistance to strengthen muscles and bones and improve posture.

Starting slowly is very safe for most people. Not sure? Consult your health professional.

For a copy of the *Guide Handbook* and more information: **1-888-334-9769**, or **www.paguide.com**

Eating well is also important. Follow *Canada's Food Guide to Healthy Eating* to make wise food choices.

Get Active Your Way, Every Day–For Life!

Scientists say accumulate 60 minutes of physical activity every day to stay healthy or improve your health. As you progress to moderate activities you can cut down to 30 minutes, 4 days a week. Add-up your activities in periods of at least 10 minutes each. Start slowly... and build up.

Time needed depends on effort

Very Light Effort	Light Effort *60 minutes*	Moderate Effort *30-60 minutes*	Vigorous Effort *20-30 minutes*	Maximum Effort
• Strolling • Dusting	• Light walking • Volleyball • Easy gardening • Stretching	• Brisk walking • Biking • Raking leaves • Swimming • Dancing • Water aerobics	• Aerobics • Jogging • Hockey • Basketball • Fast swimming • Fast dancing	• Sprinting • Racing
	Range needed to stay healthy			

You Can Do It – Getting started is easier than you think

Physical activity doesn t have to be very hard. Build physical activities into your daily routine.

- Walk whenever you can – get off the bus early, use the stairs instead of the elevator.
- Reduce inactivity for long periods, like watching TV.
- Get up from the couch and stretch and bend for a few minutes every hour.
- Play actively with your kids.
- Choose to walk, wheel or cycle for short trips.
- Start with a 10 minute walk – gradually increase the time.
- Find out about walking and cycling paths nearby and use them.
- Observe a physical activity class to see if you want to try it.
- Try one class to start – you don t have to make a long-term commitment.
- Do the activities you are doing now, more often.

Benefits of regular activity:	Health risks of inactivity:
• better health • improved fitness • better posture and balance • better self-esteem • weight control • stronger muscles and bones • feeling more energetic • relaxation and reduced stress • continued independent living in later life	• premature death • heart disease • obesity • high blood pressure • adult-onset diabetes • osteoporosis • stroke • depression • colon cancer

Health Canada Santé Canada | Canadian Society for Exercise Physiology | Active Living

Source: Canada's Physical Activity Guide to Healthy Active Living, Health Canada, 1998 http://www.hc-sc.gc.ca/hppb/paguide/pdf/guideEng.pdf

FITNESS AND HEALTH PROFESSIONALS MAY BE INTERESTED IN THE INFORMATION BELOW:

The following companion forms are available for doctors' use by contacting the Canadian Society for Exercise Physiology (address below):

The **Physical Activity Readiness Medical Examination (PARmed-X)** – to be used by doctors with people who answer YES to one or more questions on the PAR-Q.

The **Physical Activity Readiness Medical Examination for Pregnancy (PARmed-X for Pregnancy)** – to be used by doctors with pregnant patients who wish to become more active.

References:

Arraix, G.A., Wigle, D.T., Mao, Y. (1992). Risk Assessment of Physical Activity and Physical Fitness in the Canada Health Survey Follow-Up Study. **J. Clin. Epidemiol.** 45:4 419-428.

Mottola, M., Wolfe, L.A. (1994). Active Living and Pregnancy, In: A. Quinney, L. Gauvin, T. Wall (eds.), **Toward Active Living: Proceedings of the International Conference on Physical Activity, Fitness and Health**. Champaign, IL: Human Kinetics.

PAR-Q Validation Report, British Columbia Ministry of Health, 1978.

Thomas, S., Reading, J., Shephard, R.J. (1992). Revision of the Physical Activity Readiness Questionnaire (PAR-Q). **Can. J. Spt. Sci.** 17:4 338-345.

For more information, please contact the:

Canadian Society for Exercise Physiology
202-185 Somerset Street West
Ottawa, ON K2P 0J2
Tel. 1-877-651-3755 • FAX (613) 234-3565
Online: www.csep.ca

The original PAR-Q was developed by the British Columbia Ministry of Health. It has been revised by an Expert Advisory Committee of the Canadian Society for Exercise Physiology chaired by Dr. N. Gledhill (2002).

Disponible en français sous le titre «Questionnaire sur l'aptitude à l'activité physique - Q-AAP (revisé 2002)».

Supported by: Health Canada Santé Canada

FIGURE 2.1. Continued

Assess your health status by marking all *true* statements

History

You have had:

___ a heart attack
___ heart surgery
___ cardiac catheterization
___ coronary angioplasty (PTCA)
___ pacemaker/implantable cardiac defibrillator/rhythm disturbance
___ heart valve disease
___ heart failure
___ heart transplantation
___ congenital heart disease

Symptoms

___ You experience chest discomfort with exertion
___ You experience unreasonable breathlessness
___ You experience dizziness, fainting, or blackouts
___ You experience ankle swelling
___ You experience unpleasant awareness of a forceful or rapid heart rate
___ You take heart medications

Other health issues

___ You have diabetes
___ You have asthma or other lung disease
___ Y ou have burning or cramping sensation in your lower legs when walking short distance
___ Y ou have musculoskeletal problems that limit your physical activity
___ You have concerns about the safety of exercise
___ You take prescription medications
___ You are pregnant

If you marked any of these statements in this section, consult your physician or other appropriate health care provider before engaging in exercise. You may need to use a facility with a ***medically qualified staff****.*

Cardiovascular risk factors

___ You are a man ≥45 yr
___ You are a woman ≥55 yr
___ You smoke or quit smoking within the previous 6 mo
___ Your blood pressure is ≥140/90 mm Hg
___ You do not know your blood pressure
___ You take blood pressure medication
___ Your blood cholesterol level is ≥200 mg · dL^{-1}
___ You do not know your cholesterol level
___ You have a close blood relative who had a heart attack or heart surgery before age 55 (father or brother) or age 65 (mother or sister)
___ You are physically inactive (*i.e.*, you get <30 min of physical activity on at least 3 d per week)
___ You have a body mass index ≥30 kg · m^{-2}
___ You have prediabetes
___ You do not know if you have prediabetes

If you marked two or more of the statements in this section you should consult your physician or other appropriate health care as part of good medical care and progress gradually with your exercise program. You might benefit from using a facility with a ***professionally qualified exercise staff***[a] *to guide your exercise program.*

___ None of the above

You should be able to exercise safely without consulting your physician or other appropriate health care provider in a self-guide program or almost any facility that meets your exercise program needs.

[a]Professionally qualified exercise staff refers to appropriately trained individuals who possess academic training, practical and clinical knowledge, skills, and abilities commensurate with the credentials defined in *Appendix D*.

FIGURE 2.2. AHA/ACSM Health/Fitness Facility Preparticipation Screening Questionnaire. Modified from American College of Sports Medicine Position Stand and American Heart Association. (1998). Recommendations for cardiovascular screening, staffing, and emergency policies at health/fitness facilities. *Med Sci Sports Exerc.* 1018; American College of Sports Medicine. (2014). *ACSM's Guidelines for Exercise Testing and Prescription* (9th ed.). Baltimore (MD): Lippincott Williams & Wilkins, with permission.

Professional Screenings

Self-analysis of PA participation risk is important given the large number of individuals who are currently physically inactive and being encouraged to engage in activity. It would be professionally naive, however, to assume that every individual should complete a professional screening before starting an exercise program. In fact, it would likely present a serious public health deterrent to PA if this were indeed a national policy. Therefore, while self-guided screening (*e.g.*, PAR-Q) can and should be used by all, there are many individuals, especially those at medical risk, who should also consult an experienced exercise professional (*e.g.*, HFS) for a more thorough screening. Professional screening, under the guidance of an HFS, may involve collecting a health history and a medical evaluation, ideally in accordance with the ACSM Risk Classification process (1) (Fig. 2.3).

Health History Questionnaire

Some form of a Health History Questionnaire (HHQ) is necessary to use with a client to establish his or her medical/health risks for both activity assessment and activity participation (2, 16). An example of an HHQ is presented in Figure 2.4. The risk classification process also includes the HHQ along with other medical/health data, and will be discussed later in this chapter. The HHQ, however, should be tailored to fit the needs of both the program and the client. In general, the HHQ should minimally assess a client's (1):

- Family history
- History of various diseases and illnesses, including CVD
- Surgical history
- Past and present health behaviors/habits (such as history of cigarette smoking and PA)
- Current use of various drugs/medications
- Specific history of various signs and symptoms suggested of cardiovascular and other chronic or metabolic disease.

The latest edition of the GETP contains a more detailed list of the specifics of the health and medical evaluation, including desirable laboratory tests (1).

Medical Examination

A medical examination led by a physician (or other qualified medical professional) may be desired by individuals at higher risk for untoward events and should be guided by local laws and policies along with decisions by the attending health care provider. In addition, it may be desirable to perform some routine laboratory assessments (*e.g.*, blood cholesterol and blood glucose) on each client before performing more extensive health-related fitness assessments (2).

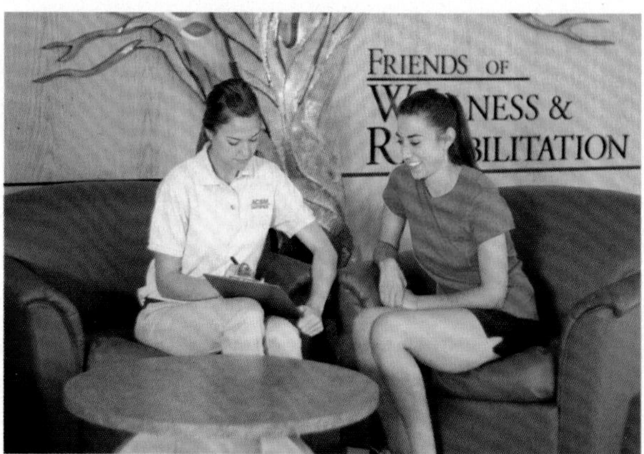

FIGURE 2.3. A prescreening consultation session.

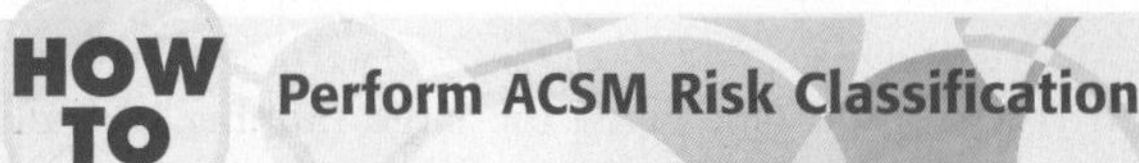

HOW TO Perform ACSM Risk Classification

Your client Sam decides that he wants to exercise in your program. You take him through your routine preactivity screening. He presents to you with the following information: his father died of a heart attack at the age of 52. His mother was put on medication for hypertension 2 years ago at the age of 69. He presents no signs or symptoms of cardiovascular, pulmonary, and/or metabolic (CPM) disease and is a nonsmoker. His personal data show that he is 38 years old. He weighs 170 lb and is 5 ft 8 in. His body fat percentage was found to be 22 via skinfolds. His cholesterol is 270 $mg{\cdot}dL^{-1}$, high-density lipoprotein (HDL) is 46 $mg{\cdot}dL^{-1}$, and resting blood glucose is 84 $mg{\cdot}dL^{-1}$. His resting heart rate is 74 bpm, and his resting blood pressure measured 132/82 and 130/84 mm Hg on two separate occasions. He has a sedentary job in a factory and stands on his feet all day. He complains that as a supervisor on the job, he never gets a rest throughout his shift and is often required to work overtime. He routinely plays basketball once a week with his work buddies and then goes out for a few beers.

	ACSM Risk Factor Thresholds	Comment
+	Family history	Father had heart attack (myocardial infarction) at the age of 52; mother with hypertension does not count
−	Cigarette smoking	Okay, nonsmoker (not sure about passive smoking)
−	Hypertension	Okay, blood pressures measured are "fine" (132/84 mm Hg)
+	Dyslipidemia	TC = 270 $mg{\cdot}dL^{-1}$ (LDL-C unknown)
−	Prediabetes	Okay, (FBG = 82 $mg{\cdot}dL^{-1}$)
−	Obesity	Okay, (BMI = 25.8 $kg{\cdot}m^{-2}$)
+	Sedentary lifestyle	Sedentary
	High HDL-C	Not positive (HDL = 46 $mg{\cdot}dL^{-1}$); cannot subtract
3	(+) Risk factors	

Major symptoms or signs suggestive of CPM disease: none noted

ACSM Risk Classification: moderate risk (has two or more risk factors)

Need for medical examination and exercise testing: Could have a medical examination before starting a vigorous exercise program (it's recommended). Of note, a diagnostic exercise test is not recommended. All of this may not be as necessary if he is to start and continue in a low-to-moderate intensity exercise program.

Exercise test: A maximal exercise test, if performed, should be physician supervised (physician in proximity, and available, if needed) for this client. Remember, a competent nonphysician health care professional could supervise the exercise test.

Contraindications

Sam has the recommended medical evaluation with his personal physician before joining your vigorous exercise program. His physician performs a medical evaluation (physical examination) and reports the following: Sam has no signs and symptoms of CPM disease and has the known risk factors you already uncovered (dyslipidemia and sedentary lifestyle as well as a family history). His physical examination results are unremarkable except for asymptomatic rheumatoid arthritis and periodic lower back pain.

HOW TO Perform ACSM Risk Classification *(continued)*

Absolute Contraindications: NONE

Relative Contraindications: Sam suffers some from rheumatoid arthritis that is not usually made worse by exercise. In addition, Sam suffered a musculoskeletal injury to his low back last year that forced him to miss a week of work. However, his low back area has been problem free over the past 6 months.

Analysis

Sam may not suffer from any contraindications that would prevent him from performing an exercise test for exercise prescription purposes as well as participating in an exercise program. Remember, relative contraindications are considered in terms of cost and benefit to your client. Certainly, as a prudent HFS, you will want to conduct the exercise test for prescriptive purposes, being careful not to exacerbate Sam's previous back injury. In addition, having rheumatoid arthritis should signal you to take ease with your client. A submaximal exercise test may be preferable to a maximal test to allow for an effective exercise prescription to be written.

ACSM Coronary Artery Disease Risk Factor Thresholds

Using the client's health history and AHA/ACSM Preparticipation Screening Questionnaires, the HFS would total the number of positive risk factors to determine which threshold they meet. Below is a summary of the current ACSM risk factor thresholds (1, 13, 6, 10, 11, 14, 22, 26, 27, 36, 38):

- Client's age of ≥45 for men and ≥55 for women.
- Family history of specific cardiovascular events, including myocardial infarction (heart attack), coronary revascularization (bypass surgery or angioplasty), or sudden cardiac death. This applies to first-degree relatives only (biological parents, siblings, and children). The risk factor threshold is met when at least one male relative (≤55 years) or one female relative (≤65 years) has had one of these specific events.
- Current cigarette smoker or having quit smoking in the past 6 months or regular exposure to secondhand smoke.
- A sedentary lifestyle.
- Obesity, as defined by body mass index (BMI ≥ 30 $kg \cdot m^{-2}$) or waist circumference (<102 cm, or 40 in, for men and >88 cm, or 35 in, for women). If available, body fat percentage values could also be used with appropriate judgment.
- Hypertension, which is defined as resting blood pressure equal to or above 140 mm Hg systolic or equal to or above 90 mm Hg diastolic, or currently taking antihypertensive medication.
- Dyslipidemia, defined as elevated low-density lipoprotein cholesterol (LDL-C ≥ 130 $mg \cdot dL^{-1}$), depressed high-density lipoprotein cholesterol (HDL-C ≤ 40 $mg \cdot dL^{-1}$), or currently taking a lipid-lowering medication. If total cholesterol is the only value available, the risk threshold is ≥200 $mg \cdot dL^{-1}$.
- Prediabetes, which is defined as having a fasting blood glucose (FBG) between 100 and 125 $mg \cdot dL^{-1}$ or a 2-hour value in oral glucose tolerance test ≥140 $mg \cdot dL^{-1}$ but <200 $mg \cdot dL^{-1}$. A FBG of 126 $mg \cdot dL^{-1}$ or greater would indicate that the individual has diabetes, which would automatically place him or her in the high risk classification.

There is also one negative risk factor used in the ACSM Risk Classification. If the client meets this one criterion, then subtract one from the total sum of the positive risk factors.

- High-serum HDL-C, which is defined as ≥60 $mg \cdot dL^{-1}$. HDL-C participates in reverse cholesterol transport and may thus lower the risk of CVD.

HEALTH HISTORY QUESTIONNAIRE

NAME______________________________AGE_______DATE________DATE OF BIRTH____________
First M.I. Last day/month/yr day/month/yr

ADDRESS____
Street City/State/Zip

TELEPHONE (home)__________________(business)__________________(cell)__________________

OCCUPATION__________________________PLACE OF EMPLOYMENT______________________

MARITAL STATUS: (circle one) SINGLE MARRIED DIVORCED WIDOWED

SPOUSE:______________________________

EDUCATION: (check highest level) ELEMENTARY______ HIGH SCHOOL______ COLLEGE______

GRADUATE_________

ETHNICITY:______________________________ PERSONAL PHYSICIAN____________________________

LOCATION______________________________

Reason for last doctor visit?__________________________ Date of last physician exam__________________

Have you previously been tested for an exercise program? YES _____ NO _____ YEAR(s) _____

LOCATION OF TEST__________________________

Person to contact in case of an emergency__________________________ Phone #__________________

(relationship)______________________________

PLEASE CHECK YES or NO

Title Title part 2			Title Title part 2			Title Title part 2		
Xahdhfiauwehasdjfhdk	☐	☐	Xahdhfiauwehasdjfhdk	☐	☐	Xahdhfiauwehasdjfhdk	☐	☐
Xahdhfiauwehasdjfhdk	☐	☐	Xahdhfiauwehasdjfhdk	☐	☐	Xahdhfiauwehasdjfhdk	☐	☐
Xahdhfiauwehasdjfhdk	☐	☐	Xahdhfiauwehasdjfhdk	☐	☐	Xahdhfiauwehasdjfhdk	☐	☐
Xahdhfiauwehasdjfhdk	☐	☐	Xahdhfiauwehasdjfhdk	☐	☐	Xahdhfiauwehasdjfhdk	☐	☐
Xahdhfiauwehasdjfhdk	☐	☐	Xahdhfiauwehasdjfhdk	☐	☐	Xahdhfiauwehasdjfhdk	☐	☐
Xahdhfiauwehasdjfhdk	☐	☐	Xahdhfiauwehasdjfhdk	☐	☐	Xahdhfiauwehasdjfhdk	☐	☐
Xahdhfiauwehasdjfhdk	☐	☐	Xahdhfiauwehasdjfhdk	☐	☐	Xahdhfiauwehasdjfhdk	☐	☐
Xahdhfiauwehasdjfhdk	☐	☐	Xahdhfiauwehasdjfhdk	☐	☐	Xahdhfiauwehasdjfhdk	☐	☐
Xahdhfiauwehasdjfhdk	☐	☐	Xahdhfiauwehasdjfhdk	☐	☐	Xahdhfiauwehasdjfhdk	☐	☐
Xahdhfiauwehasdjfhdk	☐	☐	Xahdhfiauwehasdjfhdk	☐	☐	Xahdhfiauwehasdjfhdk	☐	☐
Xahdhfiauwehasdjfhdk	☐	☐	Xahdhfiauwehasdjfhdk	☐	☐	Xahdhfiauwehasdjfhdk	☐	☐

(FOR STAFF COMMENTS)

FIGURE 2.4. Sample HHQ. (Courtesy of Gregory BD. East Stroudsburg University of Pennsylvania.)

HEALTH HISTORY QUESTIONNAIRE

Are you currently following a weight reduction diet plan? Yes_____ No_____ Name:________________________

If so, how long have you been dieting? _____months Is the plan prescribed by your doctor? Yes_____ No_____

Have you used weight reduction diets in the past? Yes_____ No_____; If yes, how often and which type(s)?

Please indicate the reasons why you want to join the exercise program.

To lose weight __________ Doctor's recommendation__________ For good health __________ Enjoyment_________

Release of tension__________ Improve physical appearance __________ Other ______________________________

FOR STAFF USE:

HOSPITALIZATIONS: Please list recent hospitalizations (Women: do not list normal pregnancies)
Year Location Reason

Any other medical problems/concerns not already identified? Yes_____ No_____ (Please list below)

Have you ever had your cholesterol measures? Yes_____ No_____; If yes, (valve)_____ (Date)_____

Are you taking any Prescription or Non-Prescription medication? Yes_____ No_____ (include birth control pills)
Medication Reason for Taking For How Long?

Do you currently smoke? Yes_____ No_____ If so, what? Cigarettes_____ Cigars_____ Pipe_____

How much per day: < .5 pack_____ 0.5 to 1pack_____ 1.5 to 2 packs_____ > 2 packs_____

Have you ever quit smoking? Yes_____ No_____ When?_____ How many years and how much did you smoke?

Do you drink any alcoholic beverages? Yes_____ No_____ If Yes, how much in 1 week?

Beer_________(cans) Wine_________(glasses) Hard liquor_________(drinks)

Do you drink any caffeinated beverages? Yes_____ No_____ If Yes, how much in 1 week?

Coffee_________(cups) Tea_________(glasses) Soft drinks_________(cans)

ACTIVITY LEVEL EVALUATION

What is your occupational activity level? sedentary______; light______; moderate______; heavy______

Do you currently engage in vigorous physical activity on a regular basis? Yes_____ No_____

If so, what type?____ How many days per week?_________

How much time per day? (check one) < 15 min_____ 15-30 min_____ 30-45 min_____ > 60 min_____

Do you ever have an uncomfortable shortness of breath during exercise? Yes_____ No_____

Do you ever have check discomfort during exercise? Yes_____ No_____ If so, does it go away with rest?

Do you engage in any recreational or leisure-time physical activities on a regular basis? Yes_____ No_____

If so, what activities?____

On average: How often?______________times/week; For how long?______________time/session

FIGURE 2.4. Continued

ACSM Major Signs or Symptoms Suggestive of CVD

There are several outward signs or symptoms that may indicate a client has current CPM disease, as indicated below. If a client has any of these signs or symptoms, then according to the ACSM, he or she is considered high risk regardless of the number of CPM disease risk factors present, and the client should be immediately referred to a physician before proceeding any further with exercise testing or programming.

Major Signs or Symptoms of CPM Diseases

- Pain or discomfort in the chest, neck, jaw, arms, or other areas that may be due to ischemia or lack of oxygenated blood flow (32).
- Dyspnea, or shortness of breath (32). Dyspnea is expected in most individuals during moderate-to-severe exertion, such as stair climbing. However, shortness of breath at rest or at mild exertion may be an indication of underlying cardiac and/or pulmonary disease.
- Syncope, or fainting, and dizziness during exercise may indicate poor blood flow to the brain because of inadequate cardiac output from a number of cardiac disorders (32). However, syncope and dizziness on sudden cessation of exercise is not entirely uncommon, even among healthy individuals, and is usually not a sign of latent disease. However, exercise programming should be so designed as to avoid postexercise syncope at all times, as this does present a dangerous situation to the exercising client.
- Orthopnea, which refers to trouble breathing while lying down, and paroxysmal nocturnal dyspnea, which is difficulty breathing while asleep (32). Both are indicative of poor left ventricular function and pose a hindrance to and danger during exercise.
- Ankle edema or swelling, if not resulting from injury, may be suggestive of heart failure, a blood clot, insufficiency of the veins, or a lymph system blockage (32). Generalized edema may indicate a more severe metabolic disorder.
- Palpitations and tachycardia, which both refer to rapid beating or fluttering of the heart (32). Feelings of anxiety and/or distress may accompany this heart rhythm.
- Intermittent claudication or severe calf pain when walking (32). This pain is reproducible with increasing exercise intensity and indicates a lack of oxygenated blood flow to the working muscles, similar in origin to angina pain.
- Heart murmurs, which are unusual sounds caused by blood flowing through the heart (32). The causes of some heart murmurs are harmless, whereas other murmurs are caused by CVD such as a valve disorder. Unless previously diagnosed and determined to be safe, all murmurs should be evaluated by a physician.
- Unusual fatigue or shortness of breath that occurs during light exertion or normal activity (32). "Unusual" indicates that an average person would not be fatigued or short of breath while performing such activity.

Known Disease

Clients with CPM disease are automatically determined to be at high risk and must be evaluated by a physician prior to exercise testing or training. However, two exceptions may be considered. First, a client with well-controlled exercise-induced asthma is often able to participate in activity without physician clearance, assuming they are otherwise healthy and do not meet the criteria for moderate or high risk. Second, newly diagnosed clients with diabetes may also be able to participate in PA programs, including testing given they do not meet criteria for moderate or high risk (1). For both of these exceptions, vigorous exercise training should be approached cautiously (1).

Missing Information

When information regarding a specific risk factor is not available, the HFS is encouraged to consider the missing risk factor as positive. The exception is prediabetes in which the risk factor is positive only if (1):

1. The client is ≥45 years old OR
2. The client's BMI is 25 kg·m^{-2} or more, and they have an additional risk factor for prediabetes such as a family history of diabetes, hypertension, a high waist circumference, or a sedentary lifestyle.

RISK CLASSIFICATION

The process of classifying individuals who may need further medical evaluation before performing fitness assessments or starting PA programs has been renamed Risk Classification (1). As the broad field of exercise science continues to evolve through research and practice, the HFS needs to be attentive to the dynamic nature of the risk classification criteria and process.

ACSM Risk Classification

The overall purpose of risk classification is to prevent the occurrence of exercise-related problems during exercise testing or training. Once the risk level or strata has been established, the appropriate course of action can then be determined (1). It is important to remember that these are suggested guidelines and that the HFS must use professional judgment as to whether a client should be formally cleared by a physician prior to activity. ACSM Risk Classification Decisions are presented in Figure 2.5. ACSM Risk Classification strata (low, moderate, and high) can be determined using the ACSM risk stratification process.

As can be seen in Figure 2.5, the process of risk classification can help determine three issues concerning exercise testing and training: (a) when a client should have a medical examination prior to exercise testing or training, (b) when an exercise test is recommended prior to exercise training, and (c) when a physician or competent nonphysician health care professional needs to supervise the exercise test. A competent nonphysician health care professional is one who has advanced training in clinical exercise testing and credentials such as the AHA Advanced Cardiac Life Support certification (25, 29). Each of these factors is influenced by risk strata (low, moderate, or high) of each individual. This can be seen in Figure 2.6 (1).

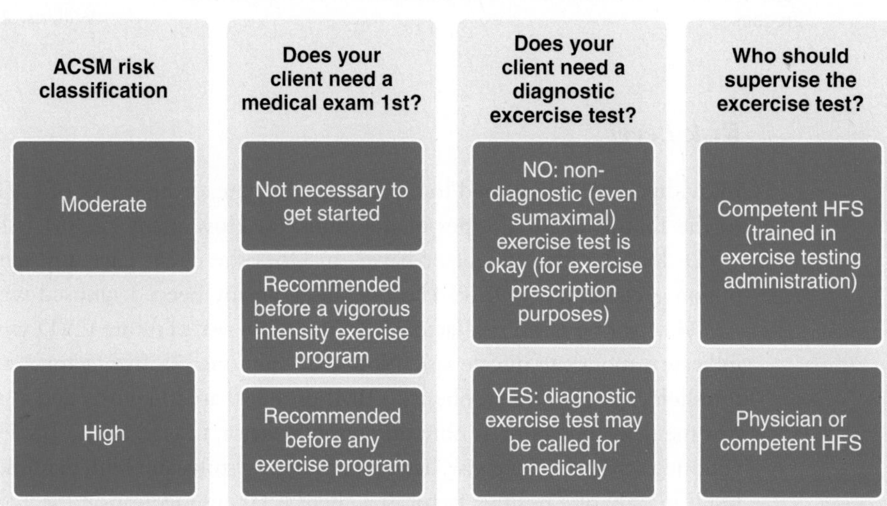

FIGURE 2.5. ACSM Risk Classification decisions. (Reprinted from Pescatello L, editor. *ACSM's Guidelines for Exercise Testing and Prescription*. 9th ed. Baltimore (MD): Lippincott Williams & Wilkins; 2014.)

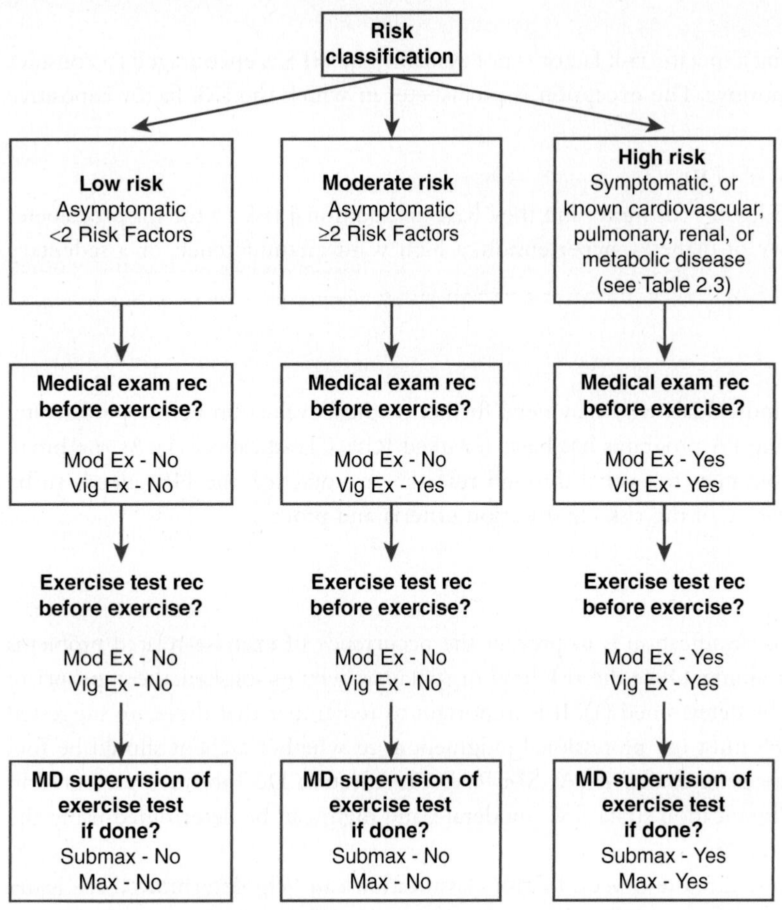

FIGURE 2.6. Exercise testing and test supervision recommendations based on risk stratification. (Reprinted from Pescatello L, editor. *ACSM's Guidelines for Exercise Testing and Prescription*. 9th ed. Baltimore (MD): Lippincott Williams & Wilkins; 2014.)

Risk Level

Individuals are determined to be at low, moderate, or high risk of CVD on the basis of the answers to the following three types of questions: (a) How many ACSM risk factor thresholds for future CVD does the client meet or have? (b) Does the client have any signs or symptoms indicative of ongoing, current, CVD? (c) Has the client already been diagnosed with CPM disease?

Having one or no risk factors indicates a low risk of future CVD, whereas two or more risk factors indicate a moderate disease risk. Note that only one positive factor is assigned per ACSM risk factor threshold. For instance, in obesity, a BMI greater than 30 $kg \cdot m^{-2}$ and a waist circumference of 105 cm (for men) would count as only one positive factor, instead of the BMI and waist circumference each counting separately. Likewise, having both high systolic and high diastolic resting blood pressure would result in only one positive factor. If a client is taking medication for hypertension or high cholesterol, they are considered positive for the associated risk factor, regardless of their actual resting blood pressure or blood cholesterol. The HFS will need to take a different course of action depending on how these questions are answered and if the client is determined to be low, moderate, or high risk.

What to Do Once Risk Level Has Been Established

The risk factor decision tree presented in Figure 2.5 can aid in determining the best course of action for clients engaged in the ACSM Risk Classification process. The HFS should always keep in mind that the ACSM Risk Classification process is a guideline and may need to be modified on the basis of many other issues such as local laws or policies, facility design and staffing, and the like. Client safety must come first.

A medical examination by a physician is suggested to be just one part of the screening, especially if a client is at moderate or high risk. However, for moderate-risk individuals, it is acceptable to start them in a low- to moderate-intensity exercise program prior to a medical examination. Vigorous exercise is typically defined as greater than or equal to 60% of functional capacity (60% of $V0_{2max}$ reserve; ≤6 METS), whereas low-to-moderate exercise programs would be less than 60% of capacity and safe for the untested, low-risk client (8, 15, 18, 28).

Nondiagnostic exercise testing is commonly performed in nonmedical or nonclinical settings. Also within these settings, submaximal exercise tests are common and can be a useful tool in generating an initial exercise prescription and for measuring programmatic progress. Diagnostic exercise testing is typically performed to assess the presence or impact of CVD (39); however, research and expert opinion has more recently questioned the value of the diagnostic exercise test as a precursor to starting an exercise program (15, 21).

The supervision criterion of exercise testing has also been recently revised by the ACSM and other professional organizations (1). Although the HFS may supervise some forms of exercise testing, these tests might be primarily conducted in individuals at low to moderate risk (according to ACSM). The ACSM Clinical Exercise Specialist® and Registered Clinical Exercise Physiologist® should be consulted when testing at-risk clients. Exercise test supervision requires the ability to deliver a level of emergency care (such as Advanced Cardiac Life Support) as well as experience in exercise testing interpretation and emergency plan practice (15, 20, 21). Acute exercise may present a risk of untoward events, including sudden death, and thus a diagnostic exercise test may be desirable as a preventive measure (23, 24, 30, 40).

ACSM recommends a diagnostic exercise test for clients with: (1)

- Previously diagnosed CVD
- New or changing symptoms suggestive of CVD
- Diabetes mellitus and at least one of the following:
  - Age older than 35 years
  - Type 2 diabetes mellitus greater than 10 years' duration
  - Type 1 diabetes mellitus greater than 15 years' duration
  - Any additional atherosclerotic CVD risk factor
  - Microvascular disease evidenced by vision impairment and poor renal function
  - Autonomic dysfunction (inappropriate heart rate and blood pressure response)
- End-stage renal disease
- Patients with pulmonary disease

AHA Risk Stratification

The AHA has also contributed to the field of risk stratification with guidelines most recently revised in 2007 (14, 18). The guidelines are similar to ACSM guidelines, with the notable exceptions below:

1. AHA lists four strata or classes (Class A, B, C, and D) as opposed to the ACSM's three (low, moderate, and high).
2. AHA lists PA guidelines for each of the four classes, whereas ACSM lists exercise-testing guidelines.

3. AHA lists supervision needs during exercise for each of the four classes, whereas ACSM does not.
4. AHA lists the special ECG and BP monitoring needs during exercise for each of the four classes, whereas ACSM does not.

The AHA Risk Stratification Guidelines are listed in Table 2.1 (18). The AHA Risk Stratification scheme may serve as an additional tool for the HFS to utilize when evaluating clients.

Pitfalls of Risk Classification

Perhaps the greatest danger in the routine use of risk classification is overlooking a sign or symptom of ongoing CVD, resulting in the client experiencing a cardiac event. Although the incidence of such events is rare (see the Exercise is Medicine box), the HFS should exercise caution to minimize such risk (17, 33–35). To reduce the risk of such an event, the HFS should obtain as much medical history information as possible through questionnaires and client interviews. When in doubt, particularly in a moderate- or high-risk client, the ACSM recommends consulting with a medical professional for advice on how to proceed. Remember it is better to be conservative and prudent than to endanger your client's health (15).

The need for activity preparticipation screening must be balanced by the public health need to increase PA without undue obstacles or barriers. Simplifying and tailoring the preactivity screening process can be used as an effective motivational tool to increase PA, especially in low-risk individuals. A moderate-risk client might be encouraged, particularly with a negative self-guided screening, to begin a low- to moderate-intensity exercise program with the guidance of an HFS (1). It is perhaps important for all individuals beginning an exercise program to start with low- to moderate-intensity exercise and increase intensity only if desired and in the absence of signs or symptoms suggestive of disease.

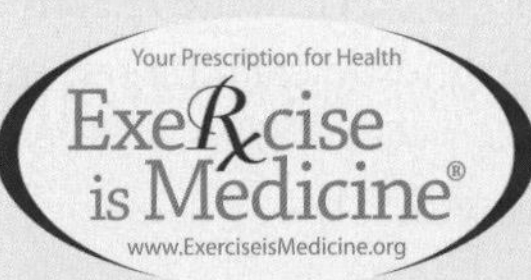

EXERCISE IS MEDICINE CONNECTION

Thompson, PD. Cardiovascular complications of vigorous physical activity. *Arch Int Med.* 1996;156(20):2297-302.

Thompson PD, Franklin BA, Balady GJ, et al. Exercise and acute cardiovascular events placing the risks into perspective: A scientific statement from the American Heart Association Council on Nutrition, Physical Activity, and Metabolism and the Council on Clinical Cardiology.*Circulation*. 2007;115(17):2358-68.

"Don't exercise too much, you may have a heart attack." How often have you heard that before? Dr. Paul Thompson and his colleagues from around the world have conducted many studies over the years to help refute that claim. In one particular study, published in the *Archives of Internal Medicine* in 1996, Dr. Thompson studied the complications that may occur from participation in exercise (33). That study found that only 6 per 100,000 men die of exertion each year. In this article, Dr. Thompson suggested that the routine use of cardiovascular exercise tests has little diagnostic value for CVD because of the rarity of sudden cardiac death in the population. In a scientific statement from the AHA published in Circulation in 2007, the writing team (Dr. Thompson and his colleagues) further suggested that the risk of sudden death from exercise is greatest in those least accustomed to PA (35). This lends further support to the concepts of performing diagnostic exercise tests only on those at high risk for CVD as well as using the principle of progressive overload in exercise training by starting those who are unaccustomed to exercise at a lower exercise load (intensity and duration) and gradually increasing the exercise load as he or she becomes more accustomed to exercise. Thus, the incidence of sudden cardiac death is lessened in your client.

TABLE 2.1 AHA RISK STRATIFICATION

Class	Description	Population	Clinical Characteristics	Activity Guidelines	ECG and Blood Pressure Monitoring	Supervision Requirements
A	Apparently healthy individuals	(1) Children, adolescents, men older than age 45, and women older than age 55 who have no symptoms of or known presence of heart disease or major coronary risk factors (2) Men ≥45 years and women ≥55 years who have no symptoms or known presence of heart disease and with <2 major cardiovascular risk factors (3) Men ≥45 years and women ≥55 years who have no symptoms or known presence of heart disease and with ≥2 major cardiovascular risk factors	—	No restrictions other than basic guidelines	Not required	None, although it is suggested that persons classified as Class A(2) and particularly Class A(3) undergo a medical examination and possibly a medically supervised exercise test before engaging in vigorous exercise
B	Presence of known, stable CVD with low risk for complications with vigorous exercise, but slightly greater than for apparently healthy individuals	(1) Coronary artery disease (CAD) (MI, CABGS, PTCA, angina pectoris, abnormal exercise test, and abnormal coronary angiograms) whose condition is stable and who have the clinical characteristics outlined below (2) Valvular heart disease, excluding severe valvular stenosis or regurgitation, with the clinical characteristics outlined below (3) Congenital heart disease; risk stratification should be guided by the 27th Bethesda Conference recommendations (24)	(1) New York Heart Association (NYHA) class 1 or 2 (2) Exercise capacity ≤6 METs (3) No evidence of congestive heart failure (4) No evidence of myocardial ischemia or angina at rest or on the exercise test at or below 6 METs (5) Appropriate rise in systolic blood pressure during exercise	Activity should be individualized, with exercise prescription by qualified individuals and approved by primary health care provider	Useful during the early prescription phase of training, usually 6 to 12 sessions	Medical supervision during initial prescription session is beneficial. Supervision by appropriate trained nonmedical personnel for other exercise sessions should occur until the individual understands how to monitor his or her activity. Medical personnel should be trained and certified in Advanced Cardiac Life Support. Nonmedical personnel should be trained and certified in Basic Life Support (which includes CPR)

(continued)

TABLE 2.1 AHA RISK STRATIFICATION (CONTINUED)

Class	Description	Population	Clinical Characteristics	Activity Guidelines	ECG and Blood Pressure Monitoring	Supervision Requirements
		(4) Cardiomyopathy; ejection fraction ≤30%; includes stable patients with heart failure with any of the clinical characteristics as outlined below but not hypertrophic cardiomyopathy or recent myocarditis (5) Exercise test abnormalities that do not meet the criteria outlined in Class C	(6) Absence of sustained or nonsustained ventricular tachycardia at rest or with exercise (7) Ability to satisfactorily self-monitor intensity of activity			
C	Those at moderate-to-high risk for cardiac complications during exercise and/or unable to self-regulate activity or to understand recommended activity level	(1) CAD with the clinical characteristics outlined below (2) Valvular heart disease, excluding severe valvular stenosis or regurgitation with the clinical characteristics outlined below. (3) Congenital heart disease; risk stratification should be guided by the 27th Bethesda Conference recommendations [24] (4) Cardiomyopathy; ejection fraction ≤30%; includes stable patients with heart failure with any of the clinical characteristics as outlined below but not hypertrophic cardiomyopathy or recent myocarditis (5) Complex ventricular arrhythmias not well controlled	(1) NYHA class 3 or 4 (2) Exercise test results: exercise capacity <6 METs angina or ischemia ST depression at workload <6 METs fall in systolic blood pressure below resting levels with exercise nonsustained ventricular tachycardia with exercise (3) Previous episode of primary cardiac arrest (*i.e.*, cardiac arrest that did not occur in the presence of an acute myocardial infarction or during a cardiac procedure) (4) A medical problem that the physician believes may be life-threatening	Activity should be individualized, with exercise prescription provided by qualified individuals and approved by primary health care provider	Continuous during exercise sessions until safety is established, usually ≥12 sessions	Medical supervision during all exercise sessions until safety is established

D	Unstable disease with activity restriction[a]	(1) Unstable ischemia (2) Severe and symptomatic valvular stenosis or regurgitation (3) Congenital heart disease; criteria for risk that would prohibit exercise conditioning should be guided by the 27th Bethesda Conference recommendations [24] (4) Heart failure that is not compensated (5) Uncontrolled arrhythmias (6) Other medical conditions that could be aggravated by exercise	—	No activity is recommended for conditioning purposes. Attention should be directed to treating the patient and restoring the patient to class C or better. Daily activities must be prescribed on the basis of individual assessment by the patient's personal physician	—

[a]Exercise for conditioning purposes is not recommended.

Recommendations versus Requirements

It is important to remember that the goal of participant screening is to proceed with fitness assessments and PA programming in the safest possible manner. In all cases, the HFS should exercise caution and use his or hers best judgment when working with an individual client. When in doubt, referring a client for a physician evaluation is always in good judgment.

It is interesting to note that to date there are no published reports on the effectiveness of the ACSM or the AHA Risk Classification schemes. Thus, although it is prudent to recommend that the HFS follow or adopt such a risk classification scheme, it is difficult to suggest this as a requirement, given the lack of an evidence base (19).

CONTRAINDICATIONS TO PA

The process of evaluating risk (through a medical examination, health history, or risk classification) may identify individual clinical characteristics that make PA risky. In certain cases, the risks may outweigh the benefits, and thereby the activity is considered contraindicated, or not recommended. There are a host of clinical characteristics that have been identified and published by ACSM, AHA, and others, and these are termed contraindications (Table 2.2). Most of the contraindications, relative and absolute, are CVD related and are typically identified in the presence of a physician. However, the HFS should make every effort to be aware of any possible conditions that make exercise risky.

What Does Contraindication Really Mean?

Just like risk classification, contraindications provide a guide that may be followed to ensure a safer exercise environment. A contraindication is an individual's clinical characteristic that may make PA

TABLE 2.2 CONTRAINDICATIONS TO EXERCISE TESTING

Absolute Contraindications	Relative Contraindications
A recent significant change in the resting ECG suggesting significant ischemia, recent myocardial infarction (within 2 d), or other acute cardiac event	Left main coronary stenosis
Unstable angina	Moderate stenotic valvular heart disease
Uncontrolled cardiac dysrhythmias causing symptoms or hemodynamic compromise	Electrolyte abnormalities (*e.g.*, hypokalemia or hypomagnesemia)
Symptomatic severe aortic stenosis	Severe arterial hypertension (*i.e.*, systolic blood pressure of >200 mm Hg, a diastolic BP of >110 mm Hg, or both) at rest
Uncontrolled symptomatic heart failure	Tachydysrhythmia or bradydysrhythmia.
Acute pulmonary embolus or pulmonary infarction	Hypertrophic cardiomyopathy and other forms of outflow tract obstruction
Acute myocarditis or pericarditis	Neuromotor, musculoskeletal, or rheumatoid disorders that are exacerbated by exercise
Suspected or known dissecting aneurysm	Uncontrolled metabolic disease (*e.g.*, diabetes, thyrotoxicosis, or myxedema)
Acute systemic infection, accompanied by fever, body aches, or swollen lymph glands	Chronic infectious disease (*e.g.*, HIV)
	Mental or physical impairment leading to inability to exercise adequately
	High-degree atrioventricular block Ventricular aneurysm

more risky. For instance, if an individual has unstable angina, or chest pain that is not well controlled or predictable, exercise may induce ischemia or even a heart attack. Although it is important to note that the incidence of cardiovascular complications is rare during exercise, the HFS is strongly advised to follow the contraindications listed to minimize this incidence (1, 35).

Absolute versus Relative

The list of contraindications is often divided between "absolute" and "relative." Essentially, absolute refers to those criteria that are "nonnegotiable"; individuals with those biomarkers should not be allowed to participate in any form of PA program and/or assessment, and should instead consult with his or her physician directly for medical care. Persons with relative contraindications, however, may be accepted or allowed into a fitness assessment and/or PA program if it is deemed that the individual benefits outweigh the potential risks (1). For instance, if the individual had a resting blood pressure of 210/105 mm Hg, his or her physician may decide that an exercise test is beneficial to determine cardiovascular responses to the exercise. An important consideration of applying contraindications is to account for the unique situation of each individual case and to always consult with the client's physician, especially if there is any doubt on the part of the HFS.

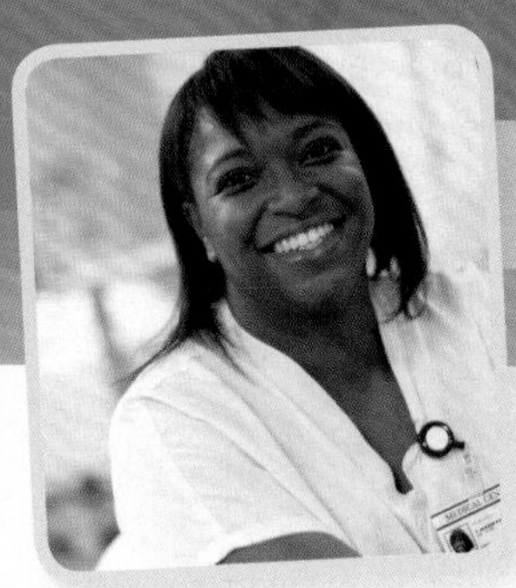

The Case of Donna

Submitted by: **James Mazzapica, BS, ACSM-HFS, Boston Sports Club, Boston, MA.**

Donna is a 34-year-old, moderate-risk woman with a history of bariatric surgery.

Donna's initial goal was to lose another 100 lb after surgery by incorporating exercise and good eating habits into her daily routine. Her day consists of 8 to 9 hours of work in a sedentary desk job. Donna found time to keep her activity level moderate to intense by including cardiovascular exercise, strength training, and flexibility training into her weekly routine. The health appraisal was the first step in creating an effective program for Donna.

Health Appraisal Forms

PAR-Q Responses

1. Has your doctor ever said that you have a heart condition and that you should only do PA recommended by a doctor? ***no***
2. Do you feel pain in your chest when you do PA? ***no***
3. In the past month, have you had chest pain when you were not doing PA? ***no***
4. Do you lose your balance because of dizziness or do you ever lose consciousness? ***no***
5. Do you have a bone or joint problem, for example back, knee, or hip, that could be made worse by a change in your PA? ***no***
6. Is your doctor currently prescribing drugs for your blood pressure or heart condition? ***no***
7. Do you know of any other reason why you should not do PA? ***no***

The Case of Donna cont.

AHA/ACSM Preparticipation Health Screening and Risk Classification Responses

History

You have had:

___ A heart attack
___ Heart surgery
___ Cardiac catheterization
___ Coronary angioplasty (PTCA)
___ Pacemaker/implantable cardiac defibrillator/ rhythm disturbance
___ Heart valve disease

Other health issues:

___ Heart failure
___ You have diabetes
___ Heart transplantation
___ You have asthma or other lung disease
___ Congenital heart disease
___ You have burning or cramping in your lower legs when walking short distances

Symptoms

___ You have musculoskeletal problems that limit your PA
___ You experience chest discomfort with exertion
___ You experience unreasonable breathlessness
___ You have concerns about the safety of exercise
___ You experience dizziness, fainting, blackouts
___ You take prescription medication(s)
___ You take heart medications
___ You are pregnant

Cardiovascular risk factors

___ You are a man older than 45 years
___ You are a woman older than 55 years, you have had a hysterectomy, or you are postmenopausal
___ You smoke, or quite within the previous 6 months
_X_ Your BP is greater than 140/90
___ You don't know your BP
___ You take BP medication
___ Your blood cholesterol level is greater than 200 $mg \cdot dL^{-1}$
___ You don't know your cholesterol level
___ You have a close blood relative who had a heart attack before age 55 (father or brother) or age 65 (mother or sister)
___ You are physically inactive (*i.e.*, you get <30 min of PA on at least 3 $d \cdot wk^{-1}$)
_X_ You are more than 20 lb overweight

If you marked any of the statements in this section, consult your physician or other appropriate health care provider before engaging in exercise. You may need to use a facility with a medically qualified staff.

If you marked two or more of the statements in this section, you should consult your physician or other appropriate health care provider before engaging in exercise. You might benefit by using a facility with a professionally qualified exercise staff to guide your exercise program.

Physical Assessment Data

Resting blood pressure: 144/95 mm Hg
Resting heart rate: 85 bpm
Weight: 267 lb
Height: 68.5 in
BMI: 42 $kg \cdot m^{-2}$

Risk Factor Analysis

Positive risk factors: high blood pressure and obesity
Negative risk factors: none
Medications: none
Risk classification: moderate

***The Case of Donna** cont.*

Wellness Vision Summary (2)

Donna's wellness vision is about looking forward to continuing on the journey she's been on for several years. Since her surgery, she has been able to change her lifestyle to include daily exercise. She finds joy in exercise. Donna likes to keep her routines fun and exciting, with high-intensity levels. She wants to incorporate more weight training, muscle building, and various plateau-busting workouts such as boxing and swimming. She has a very strong support system including her brother, who competes in natural bodybuilding competitions. Her motivation will stay strong even if she is pressured by work, home, or life in general. Her efforts will not be overshadowed by other obligations. Donna will write down her goals and post them in prominent places. She is determined to change, and although her dedication to reaching a certain bodyweight is important, it is not her ultimate desire. Her joy day in and day out comes from working hard to live a happy and healthy life.

Goal Setting

Long-term goal: Lose 15 to 20 lb by December 15
Short-term goal: Consistently lose 1 to 2 lb·week^{-1}
Strategy: Keep food diary on smartphone
Strategy: Use new Brita water bottle, 3 refills per day
Strategy: Take multivitamin daily
Short-term goal: Exercise minimum 5 to 6 days·week^{-1}, moderate intensity, 60 minutes
Strategy: Schedule exercise for lunch
Strategy: Bring workout partner to gym—call Kate
Strategy: Schedule weekly session with James

Donna's program followed the FITT principle and incorporated both health-related and skill-related fitness components. She enjoyed lifting weights, especially when she was feeling stressed out. Cardiovascular activity was her main focus to aid in her weight loss, but activities such as boxing, shadow boxing, jumping rope, playing basketball, and playing outside were incorporated to add some variety to her workouts. She enjoyed the fitness center because she felt she went there to work hard. Receiving feedback from the machines such as calories burned, duration, and the like helped her track numbers and data. My work with Donna in the weight room was also tracked and increased her motivation by seeing her strength increase month by month.

Donna's dedication and intense nature, moderate-risk classification, and history of bariatric surgery provided a great combination for success with a scientifically sound, supervised exercise program, which all began with the initial health screening and evaluation.

Questions

- What is the importance of risk classification?
- What do I do now that risk level has been established?
- What are some contraindications to PA?
- Do these guidelines prohibit people from exercising?

References

1. American College of Sports Medicine. *ACSM's Guidelines for Exercise Testing and Prescription*. 9th ed. Baltimore (MD): Lippincott Williams & Wilkins; 2013.
2. Moore M, Tschannen-Moran R. *Coaching Psychology Manual*. Baltimore (MD): Lippincott Williams & Wilkins; 2009.

SUMMARY

Pre-PA participation screening is a process that may include evaluating self-guided questionnaires as well as obtaining a health/medical history to determine the risk classification of an individual client. Although there are several examples or models that can be utilized in the screening process, the need to evaluate a client's medical readiness to undertake the health-related physical fitness assessments as well as a PA program is most critical. Thus, the pre-PA participation screening gives the relative assurance that the client is ready and able to participate in the rigors of the exercise assessment and training. Therefore, while the process may vary from site to site and even from person to person, the HFS is strongly encouraged to have a process in place to ensure a safe exercise environment and to keep individuals safe and enjoying exercise.

STUDY QUESTIONS

1. Discuss the individual ACSM risk factor thresholds. Specifically, how do the individual ACSM risk factor thresholds match up with the modifiable and nonmodifiable risk factors for coronary heart disease listed by the AHA?
2. Given the 2007 scientific statement from the AHA as well as the "Public Health Approach" to getting our sedentary country more active, does the ACSM Risk Classification aid or hinder this concept of increasing PA? In other words, can you support the ACSM Risk Classification concept of limited diagnostic exercise testing for individuals at a low and moderate risk for CVD?
3. Diabetes is relatively stressed in the ACSM Risk Classification system for the need to conduct a diagnostic exercise test (at least having diabetes plus some complications). What are some of the complications of diabetes that justifies the use of diagnostic exercise testing in this population?

REFERENCES

1. American College of Sports Medicine. *ACSM's Guidelines for Exercise Testing and Prescription*. 9th ed. Baltimore (MD): Lippincott Williams & Wilkins; 2013.
2. American College of Sports Medicine. *ACSM's Resource Manual for Guidelines for Exercise Testing and Prescription*. 7th ed. Baltimore (MD): Lippincott Williams & Wilkins; 2013.
3. American College of Sports Medicine (L. Kaminsky, editor). *Health-Related Physical Fitness Assessment Manual*. 3rd ed. Baltimore (MD): Lippincott Williams & Wilkins; 2010.
4. American Association of Cardiovascular & Pulmonary Rehabilitation. *Guidelines for Cardiac Rehabilitation and Secondary Prevention Programs*. 4th ed. Champaign (IL): Human Kinetics; 2004.
5. American Association of Cardiovascular & Pulmonary Rehabilitation. *Guidelines for Pulmonary Rehabilitation Programs*. 3rd ed. Champaign (IL): Human Kinetics; 2004. 188 p.
6. American Diabetes Association. Diagnosis and classification of diabetes mellitus. *Diabetes Care*. 2007;30(suppl 1):S42–7.
7. Balady GJ, Chaitman B, Driscoll D, et al. American College of Sports Medicine and American Heart Association Joint Position Statement: Recommendations for cardiovascular screening staffing, and emergency procedures at health/fitness facilities. *Med Sci Sports Exer.* 1998;30:1009–18.
8. Brawner CA, Vanzant MA, Ehrman JK, et al. Guiding exercise using the talk test among patients with coronary artery disease. *J Cardiopulm Rehabil*. 2006;26(2):72, 5; quiz 76–7.
9. Buchner DM. Physical activity to prevent or reverse disability in sedentary older adults. *Am J Prev Med*. 2003;25(3 suppl 2):214–5.

10. Cardiovascular Risk Reduction Guidelines in Adults: Cholesterol Guideline Update (ATP IV) Hypertension Guideline Update (JNC 8) Obesity Guideline Update (Obesity 2) Integrated Cardiovascular Risk Reduction Guideline: Timeline for release of updated guidelines [Internet]. Bethesda (MD): National Heart, Lung and Blood Institute, National Institutes of Health; [cited 2011 July 7]. Available from: http://www.nhlbi.nih.gov/guidelines/cvd_adult/background.htm
11. Chobanian AV, Bakris GL, Black HR, et al. The Seventh Report of the Joint National Committee on prevention, detection, evaluation, and treatment of high blood pressure: The JNC 7 report. *JAMA*. 2003;289(19):2560–72.
12. de Oliveira Lux LG, de Albuquerque Maranhao Neto G, de Tarso Veras Farinatti P. Validity of the physical activity readiness questionnaire (PAR-Q) in elder subjects. *Rer Brasileira de Cine Desempenho Hum*. 2007;9(4):366–71.
13. Expert Panel on the Identification Evaluation and Treatment of Overweight and Obesity in Adults. Executive summary of the clinical guidelines on the identification, evaluation, and treatment of overweight and obesity in adults. *Arch Intern Med*. 1998;158(17):1855–67. Available from: http://www.ajcn.org/cgi/reprint/68/4/899
14. Fletcher GF, Balady GJ, Amsterdam EA, et al. Exercise standards for testing and training: A statement for healthcare professionals from the American Heart Association. *Circulation*. 2001;104(14):1694–740.
15. Garber CE, Blissmer B, Deschenes MR, et al. Quantity and quality of exercise for developing and maintaining cardiorespiratory, musculoskeletal, and neuromotor fitness in apparently healthy adults: Guidance for prescribing exercise. *Med Sci Sports Exer.* 2011;43(7):1334–59.
16. Gibbons RJ, Balady GJ, Bricker JT, et al. ACC/AHA 2002 guideline update for exercise testing: Summary article. A report of the American College of Cardiology/American Heart Association Task Force on Practice Guidelines (Committee to Update the 1997 Exercise Testing Guidelines). *J Am Coll Cardiol*. 2002;40(8):1531–40.
17. Giri S, Thompson PD, Kiernan FJ, et al. Clinical and angiographic characteristics of exertion-related acute myocardial infarction. *JAMA*. 1999;282(18):1731–6.
18. Haskell WL, Lee IM, Pate RR, et al. Physical activity and public health: Updated recommendation for adults from the American College of Sports Medicine and the American Heart Association. *Circulation*. 2007;116(9):1081–93.
19. Jamnik VK, Gledhill N, Shephard RJ. Revised clearance for participation in physical activity: Greater screening responsibility for qualified university-educated fitness professionals. *Appl Physiol Nut Metab.* 2007;32:1191–7.
20. Kern KB, Halperin HR, Field J. New guidelines for cardiopulmonary resuscitation and emergency cardiac care: Changes in the management of cardiac arrest. *JAMA*. 2001;285(10):1267–9.
21. Lahav D, Leshno M, Brezis M. Is an exercise tolerance test indicated before beginning regular exercise? A decision analysis. *J Gen Intern Med*. 2009;24(8):934–8.
22. Maron BJ, Araujo CG, Thompson PD, et al. Recommendations for preparticipation screening and the assessment of cardiovascular disease in masters athletes: An advisory for healthcare professionals from the working groups of the World Heart Federation, the International Federation of Sports Medicine, and the American Heart Association Committee on Exercise, Cardiac Rehabilitation, and Prevention. *Circulation*. 2001;103(2):327–34.
23. Maron BJ, Thompson PD, Puffer JC, et al. Cardiovascular preparticipation screening of competitive athletes. A statement for health professionals from the Sudden Death Committee (clinical cardiology) and Congenital Cardiac Defects Committee (cardiovascular disease in the young), American Heart Association. *Circulation*. 1996;94(4):850–6.
24. Mittleman MA, Maclure M, Tofler GH, Sherwood JB, Goldberg RJ, Muller JE. Triggering of acute myocardial infarction by heavy physical exertion. Protection against triggering by regular exertion. Determinants of Myocardial Infarction Onset Study Investigators. *N Engl J Med*. 1993;329(23):1677–83.
25. Myers J, Arena R, Franklin B, et al. Recommendations for clinical exercise laboratories: A scientific statement from the American Heart Association. *Circulation*. 2009;119(24):3144–61.
26. National Cholesterol Education Program (NCEP) Expert Panel on Detection, Evaluation, and Treatment of High Blood Cholesterol in Adults (Adult Treatment Panel III). Third Report of the National Cholesterol Education Program (NCEP) Expert Panel on Detection, Evaluation, and Treatment of High Blood Cholesterol in Adults (Adult Treatment Panel III) final report. *Circulation*. 2002;106(25):3143–421.
27. Pate RR, M Pratt, SN Blair, et al. Physical activity and public health. A recommendation from the Centers for Disease Control and Prevention and the American College of Sports Medicine. *JAMA*. 1995;273(5):402–7.
28. Persinger R, Foster C, Gibson M, Fater DC, Porcari JP. Consistency of the talk test for exercise prescription. *Med Sci Sports Exerc.* 2004;36(9):1632–6.
29. Rodgers GP, Ayanian JZ, Balady G, et al. American College of Cardiology/American Heart Association Clinical Competence Statement on Stress Testing. A Report of the American College of Cardiology/American Heart Association/American College of Physicians-American Society of Internal Medicine Task Force on Clinical Competence. *Circulation*. 2000;102(14):1726–38.
30. Siscovick DS, Weiss NS, Fletcher RH, Lasky T. The incidence of primary cardiac arrest during vigorous exercise. *N Engl J Med*. 1984;311(14):874–7.
31. Shephard RJ, Thomas S, Weller I. The Canadian Home Fitness Test. 1991 update. *Sports Med*. 1991;11(6):358–66.
32. Stedman. *Stedman's Medical Dictionary for the Health Professions and Nursing.* 5th ed. Baltimore (MD): Lippincott Williams & Wilkins; 2005.
33. Thompson PD. Cardiovascular complications of vigorous physical activity. *Arch Int Med*. 1996;156(20):2297–302.
34. Thompson PD, Buchner D, Pina IL, et al. Exercise and physical activity in the prevention and treatment of atherosclerotic cardiovascular disease: A statement from the Council on Clinical Cardiology (Subcommittee on Exercise, Rehabilitation, and Prevention) and the Council on Nutrition, Physical Activity, and Metabolism (Subcommittee on Physical Activity). *Circulation*. 2003;107(24):3109–16.
35. Thompson PD, Franklin BA, Balady GJ, et al. Exercise and acute cardiovascular events placing the risks into perspective: A scientific statement from the American Heart Association Council on Nutrition, Physical Activity, and Metabolism and the Council on Clinical Cardiology. *Circulation*. 2007;115(17):2358–68.
36. U.S. Preventive Services Task Force. Screening for coronary heart disease: Recommendation statement. *Ann Intern Med*. 2004;140(7):569–72.

37. Physical Activity Guidelines Advisory Committee. Department of Health and Human Services, 2008. Available from: http://www.health.gov/paguidelines/committeereport.aspx (Accessed: 10/18/2011)
38. Physical Activity and Health: A Report of the Surgeon General. Atlanta (GA): US Department of Health and Human Services, Centers for Disease Control and Prevention, National Center for Chronic Disease Prevention and Health Promotion; 1996.
39. Williams MA. Exercise testing in cardiac rehabilitation. Exercise prescription and beyond. *Cardiol Clin.* 2001;19(3):415–31.
40. Willich SN, Lewis M, Lowel H, Arntz HR, Schubert F, Schroder R. Physical exertion as a trigger of acute myocardial infarction. Triggers and Mechanisms of Myocardial Infarction Study Group. *N Engl J Med.* 1993; 329(23):1684–90.

PART
II

Assessments and Exercise Programming for Apparently Healthy Participants

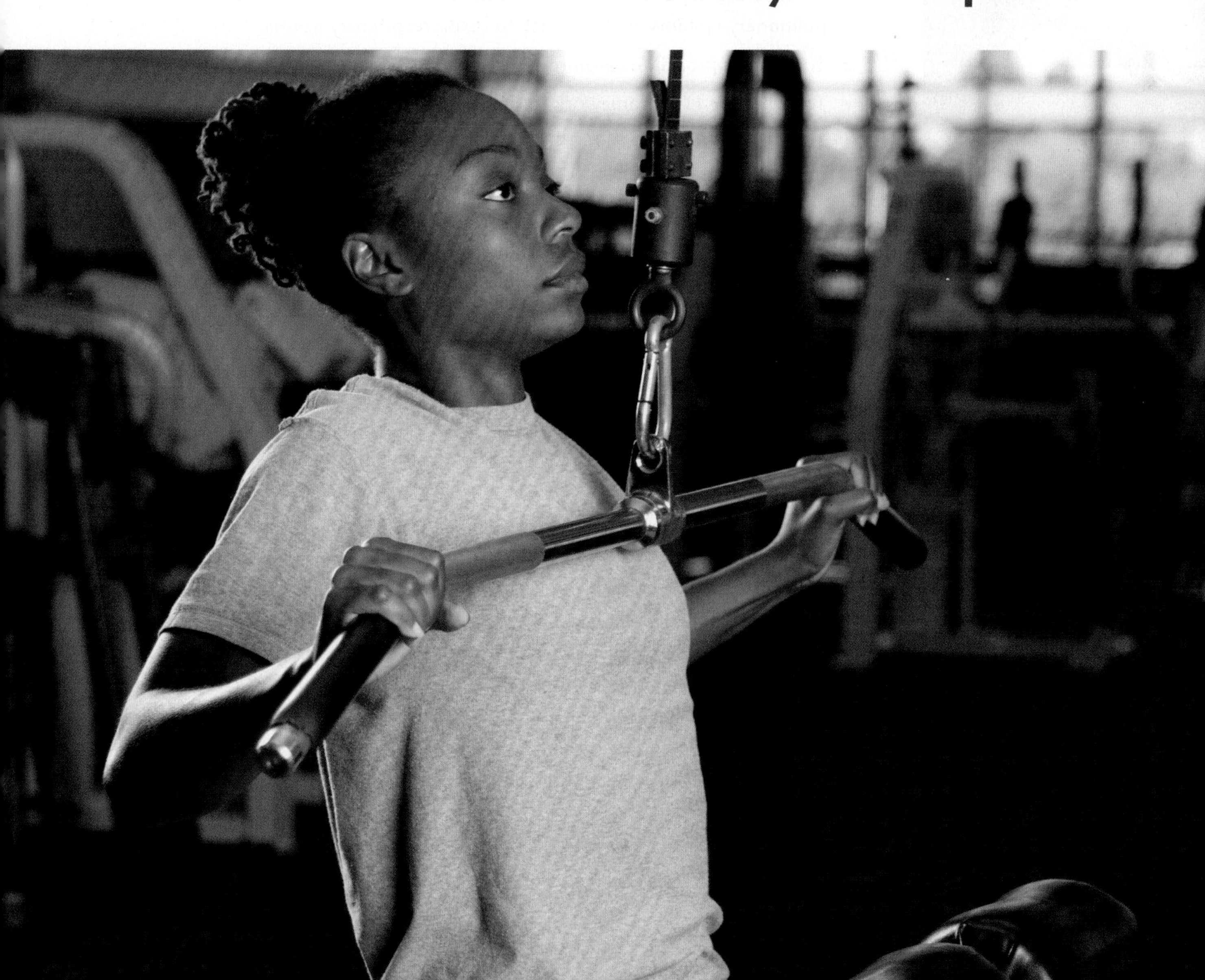

CHAPTER

3 Cardiorespiratory Fitness Assessments and Exercise Programming for Apparently Healthy Participants

Jessica Meendering • Charles Fountaine

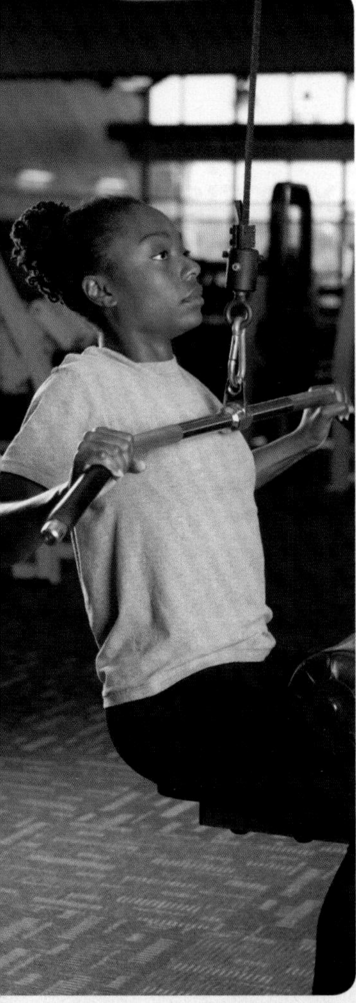

CHAPTER OBJECTIVES

- To understand basic anatomy and physiology of the cardiovascular and pulmonary systems as they relate to cardiorespiratory fitness.
- To select appropriate cardiorespiratory fitness assessments.
- To utilize the FITT framework to develop cardiorespiratory fitness.
- To understand how the effect of environment, medications, and musculoskeletal injuries may contraindicate some individuals ability to exercise.

Cardiorespiratory fitness (CRF) may be defined as the ability of the circulatory and respiratory systems to supply oxygen to the muscles to perform dynamic physical activity (12, 81). CRF is strongly associated with increased health benefits (12), and it has been well established that individuals who do moderate- or vigorous-intensity aerobic physical activity have significantly lower risk of cardiovascular disease than inactive people (81). A dose-response relationship exists between aerobic fitness and health outcomes, as increased levels of CRF are associated with numerous positive health outcomes and reductions in chronic disease and all-cause mortality (8, 12).

Therefore, the principal role of the health fitness specialist (HFS) is to provide the development and maintenance of CRF to clientele. To provide safe, evidence-based instruction, the HFS needs a firm science foundation in the physiology of the cardiovascular and pulmonary systems. Once this groundwork has been established, the HFS can then begin the art of individualized exercise prescription.

BASIC ANATOMY AND PHYSIOLOGY OF THE CARDIOVASCULAR AND PULMONARY SYSTEMS AS THEY RELATE TO CRF

Goal of the Cardiovascular and Respiratory Systems

The cardiovascular and respiratory systems work in synchrony to provide oxygen and remove waste from the body. The respiratory system supports gas exchange, promoting the movement of oxygen and carbon dioxide from the environment into the blood and from the blood back into the environment. The cardiovascular system is responsible for the delivery of oxygenated blood and nutrients to the cell to make energy in the form of adenosine triphosphate (ATP). The cardiovascular system is also responsible for the removal of "waste" from the cell, so it can be transported to its appropriate destination for elimination or recycling (see Fig. 3.1).

Anatomy and Physiology of the Cardiovascular and Respiratory Systems

The main components of the cardiovascular system are the heart and vasculature. The heart is a four-chambered muscular pump, composed of the right and left atria (upper chambers) and the right and left ventricles (lower chambers). Specifically, the right ventricle is responsible for pumping deoxygenated blood to the lungs for oxygen loading and carbon dioxide unloading. After gas exchange occurs in the pulmonary circulation, blood returns to the left side of the heart. The left ventricle is then responsible for generating the force necessary to drive the blood out of its chamber and through the vasculature. The right and left atria act to provide support to their respective ventricles, serving as a reservoir of blood that eventually moves into the ventricles. The vasculature consists of arteries, arterioles, capillaries, venules, and veins; they can be thought of as a series of tubes that branch and become smaller in diameter as they move away from the heart (Fig. 3.1).

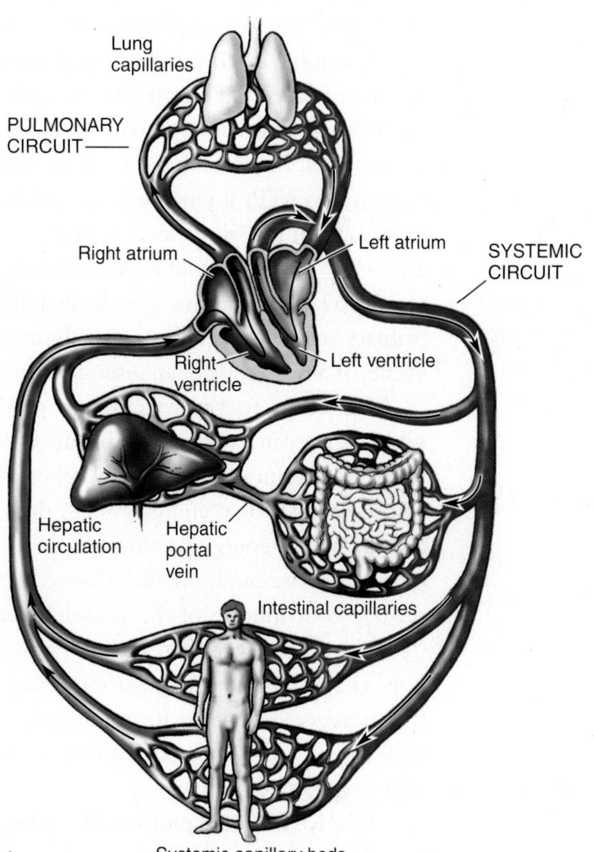

FIGURE 3.1. Schematic representation of the integration between the cardiovascular system and the respiratory system. (Reproduced from Swain D, editor. *ACSM's Resource Manual for Guidelines for Exercise Testing and Prescription*. 7th ed. Baltimore (MD): Lippincott Williams & Wilkins; 2014.)

In the systemic circulation, the arteries and arterioles carry oxygenated blood, whereas in the pulmonary circulation, the arteries and arterioles carry "deoxygenated blood," or blood that contains less oxygen than arterial blood. As the vasculature is more distal from the heart, arteries branch into smaller arterioles, which in turn branch and merge with the capillaries. The capillary is the smallest and most numerous of the blood vessels and is the location of gas and nutrient exchange. Deoxygenated blood and metabolic byproducts move out of capillaries into venules, which consolidate into veins as they move closer to the heart. Veins are responsible for delivering the deoxygenated blood back to the right side of the heart, where the cycle then repeats endlessly.

ATP Production

ATP is an energy-bearing molecule composed of carbon, hydrogen, nitrogen, oxygen, and phosphorus atoms, and is found in all living cells. Nervous transmission, muscle contractions, formation of nucleic acids, and many other energy-consuming reactions of metabolism are possible because of the energy in ATP molecules.

Cells break down the food we eat with the ultimate goal of producing ATP, which is the cellular form of energy used within the body to fuel work. Muscle cells are very limited in the amount of ATP they can store. To support muscle contraction during continuous exercise, cells must continuously create ATP at a rate equal to ATP use through a combination of three primary metabolic systems: creatine phosphate (CP), anaerobic glycolysis, and the oxidative system.

The most immediate source of ATP is the CP system. Small amounts of CP are stored within each cell, and one CP donates a phosphate group to adenosine diphosphate (ADP) to create one ATP, or a simple one-to-one trade-off. This simplicity allows for the rapid production of ATP within the cell; however, this production is short-lived. Because of this, the CP system can provide ATP to fuel work only during short-intense bouts of exercise, owing to the limited storage capacity of CP within each cell. Therefore, the CP system is the primary source of ATP during very short, intense movements, such as discus throw, shot put, and high jump, and any maximal-intensity exercise lasting less than approximately 10 seconds.

Anaerobic glycolysis is the next most immediate energy source, and consists of a metabolic pathway that breaks down carbohydrates (glucose or glycogen) into pyruvate. The bond energy produced from the breakdown of glucose and glycogen is used to phosphorylate ADP and create ATP. The net energy yield for anaerobic glycolysis, without further oxidation through the subsequent oxidative systems, is two ATPs if glucose is the substrate and three ATPs if glycogen is the substrate. When oxygen is available in the mitochondria of the cell, pyruvate continues to be broken down to acetyl CoA and enters the oxidative system. Alternatively, in the absence of adequate oxygen supply, pyruvate is converted to lactic acid, which gradually builds up in muscle cells and the blood. Anaerobic glycolysis is the primary source of ATP during medium-duration, intense exercise, such as the 200-m and 400-m sprint events or any exercise of an intensity that cannot be continued for more than approximately 90 seconds.

Anaerobic energy systems can produce ATP quickly, but they are limited in the duration for which they can continue to produce ATP. For longer-duration exercise or low-intensity exercise regardless of duration, the body relies most heavily on the oxidative metabolic energy systems. The aerobic or oxidative energy system does not contribute much energy at the onset of exercise, but is able to sustain energy production for a longer duration. As exercise intensity decreases, allowing for longer exercise duration, the relative contribution of the anaerobic energy systems decreases and the relative contribution of the aerobic energy systems increases (Fig. 3.2).

The oxidative system includes two metabolic pathways: the Krebs cycle and the electron transport chain. Unlike the anaerobic energy systems mentioned above, the oxidative systems require the presence of oxygen to produce ATP, which takes place in the mitochondria of the cell. This is why the mitochondria are known as the "powerhouse of the cell," as that is where the majority of ATP is generated.

The Krebs cycle requires the presence of glucose, proteins, or fats. These macronutrients are broken down through a series of chemical reactions with their subsequent energy collected and used

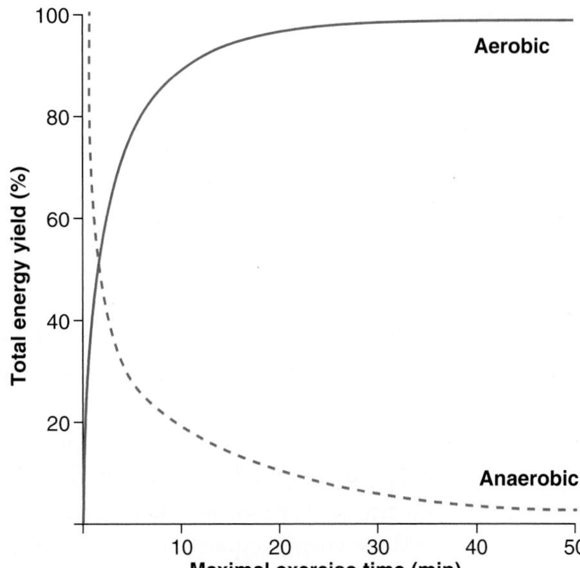

FIGURE 3.2. Relative contribution of the anaerobic and aerobic energy systems based on duration of exercise. (Reproduced from Swain D, editor. *ACSM's Resource Manual for Guidelines for Exercise Testing and Prescription*. 7th ed. Baltimore (MD): Lippincott Williams & Wilkins; 2014.)

to create ATP independently and within the electron transport chain. This oxidative system is the primary source of ATP used during low-to-moderate intensity aerobic exercise lasting longer than 1 to 2 minutes all the way up to long distance endurance events.

The anaerobic and aerobic energy systems work together to create ATP to fuel exercise. The ATP stored within the muscle cell will be used during the first few seconds of exercise onset. As stored ATP decreases, the contribution of ATP production via the CP system increases. Subsequently, as the stores of CP are reduced, anaerobic glycolysis becomes the primary contributing energy system to ATP creation. Aerobic ATP production becomes the primary fuel source in exercise lasting more than approximately 100 seconds. Figure 3.3 depicts the relative contribution of each source for exercise lasting between 1 and 160 seconds. Although the contribution of energy production differs on the basis of intensity and duration of exercise within the CP system, anaerobic glycolysis, and the oxidative systems, all of these primary metabolic pathways work in synchrony to produce the energy required to sustain the biological work of the human body.

The HFS should be familiar with the metabolic pathways used to create energy in the body and the link between the oxidative metabolic pathways, the cardiovascular system, and the respiratory system. Within this context, anaerobic metabolism can be called upon even during long-duration exercise, particularly when using interval training consisting of intermittent high-intensity bouts.

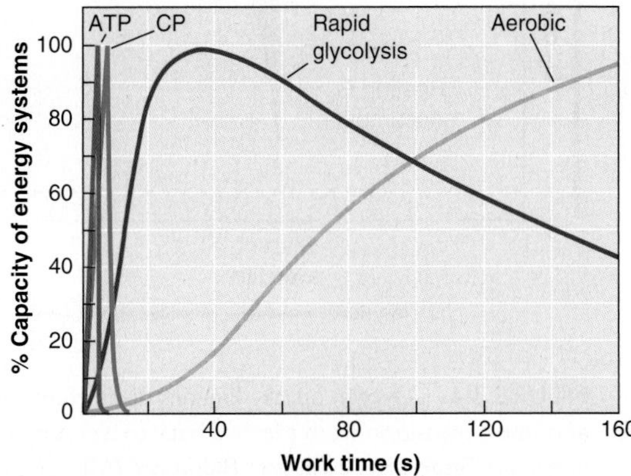

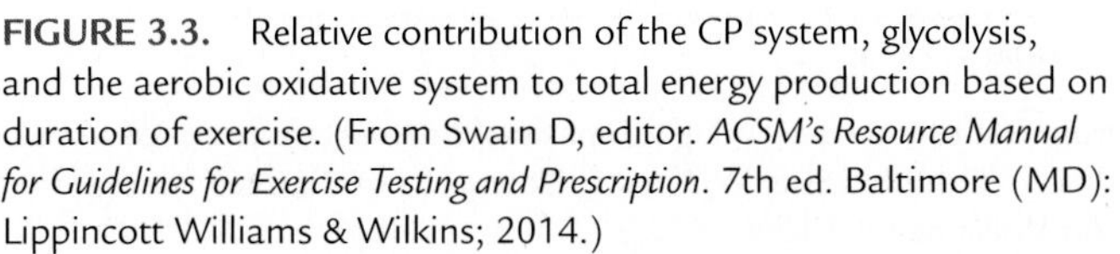

FIGURE 3.3. Relative contribution of the CP system, glycolysis, and the aerobic oxidative system to total energy production based on duration of exercise. (From Swain D, editor. *ACSM's Resource Manual for Guidelines for Exercise Testing and Prescription*. 7th ed. Baltimore (MD): Lippincott Williams & Wilkins; 2014.)

OVERVIEW OF CARDIORESPIRATORY RESPONSES TO ACUTE GRADED EXERCISE OF CONDITIONED AND UNCONDITIONED PARTICIPANTS

Oxygen Uptake Kinetics during Submaximal Single-Intensity Exercise

As discussed in the previous section, oxygen is required to create ATP via the oxidative energy system. As workload increases, so does the energy requirement, and more oxygen is required to make ATP. Therefore, the volume of oxygen the body consumes ($\dot{V}O_2$) is proportional to workload. Upon the transition from rest to submaximal exercise, $\dot{V}O_2$ increases and reaches a steady state in 1 to 4 minutes (69). Steady state is the point at which $\dot{V}O_2$ plateaus during submaximal aerobic exercise, and energy production via the aerobic energy systems is equal to the energy required to perform the set intensity of work. Prior to steady state, $\dot{V}O_2$ is lower than required to create adequate energy for the given task via the oxidative energy systems. This period of inadequate oxygen consumption has been termed *the oxygen deficit* (59). During this period, the anaerobic energy systems are responsible for providing the energy to make up for the difference between the energy produced via the aerobic energy systems and the energy required to perform the work required (35). The time required to reach steady state is influenced by the training state and the magnitude of the increase in exercise intensity (43, 69). Aerobic exercise training decreases the time required to reach steady state, thus reducing the oxygen deficit that has to be "paid back" during steady state exercise and recovery. This is beneficial because less ATP production will be required, and therefore less anaerobic byproducts from the anaerobic energy systems at the start of exercise and upon transition to a higher workload of exercise (43, 69).

After cessation of exercise, $\dot{V}O_2$ remains elevated because of the increased work associated with the resynthesis of ATP and CP within muscle cells, lactate removal, and elevated body temperature, hormones, heart rate (HR), and respiratory rate (38). This elevation in $\dot{V}O_2$ after exercise was first called *oxygen debt* (45), but is now commonly referred to as *excess postexercise oxygen consumption* (EPOC). Figure 3.4 provides a visual representation of the oxygen uptake kinetics upon transition from rest to exercise and depicts oxygen deficit, steady state, and EPOC.

Oxygen Uptake Kinetics during Graded Intensity Exercise

Graded exercise testing is used in many settings to determine baseline fitness and relevant health risks. Typically, the HFS will use either maximal or submaximal graded exercise testing

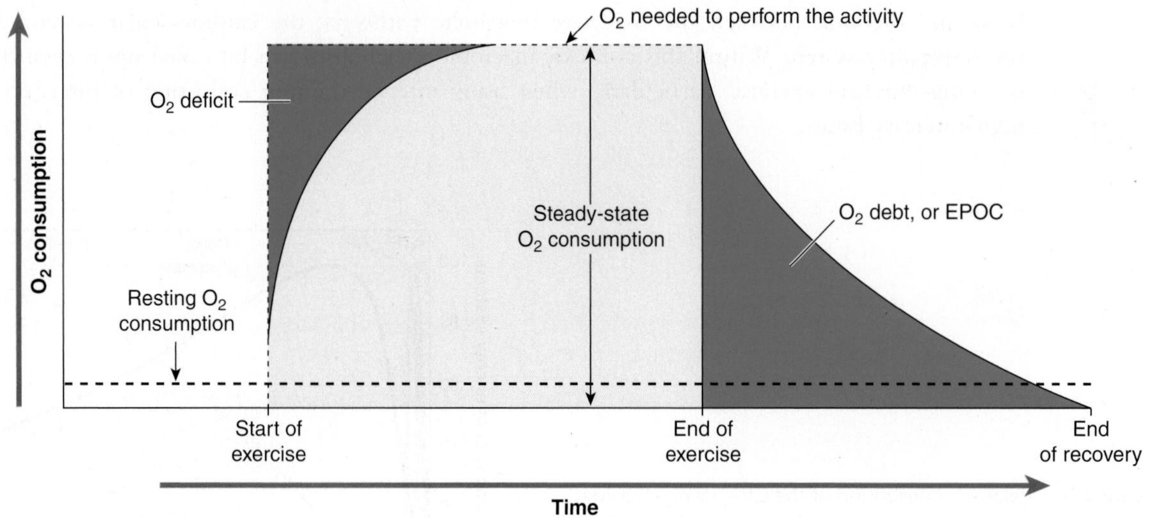

FIGURE 3.4. Oxygen uptake kinetics upon transition from rest to exercise, during submaximal single-intensity exercise, and upon transition from exercise back to a resting condition. (From Kraemer W, Fleck S, Deschenes M. *Exercise Physiology: Integrating Theory and Application*. Baltimore (MD): Lippincott Williams & Wilkins; 2012.)

to determine baseline fitness, which can be compared at future time points for assessing fitness improvements. It is important for the HFS conducting graded exercise tests to be well aware of the normal and abnormal hemodynamic response to incremental exercise, as described in the sections that follow.

During incremental exercise, VO_2 increases slowly within the first few minutes of exercise and eventually reaches a steady state at each submaximal exercise intensity. Steady state $\dot{V}O_2$ continues to increase linearly as workload increases (Fig. 3.5) until $\dot{V}O_{2max}$ is reached. Maximal $\dot{V}O_2$ is the highest volume of oxygen the body can consume. It is often used as an indicator of aerobic fitness and endurance exercise performance because a higher $\dot{V}O_{2max}$ indicates a greater capacity to create ATP via oxidative energy production and a greater ability to supply the energy required to support higher-intensity exercise workloads.

The Fick equation can be used to determine $\dot{V}O_{2max}$. The Fick principle states that $\dot{V}O_{2max} = HR_{max} \times SV_{max} \times a\text{-}\dot{V}O_2$ difference max, where $\dot{V}O_2$ = oxygen consumption ($mL \cdot kg^{-1} \cdot min^{-1}$), HR = heart rate (bpm), SV = stroke volume ($mL \cdot beat^{-1}$), and $a\text{-}\dot{V}O_2$ difference = arteriovenous oxygen difference. This equation demonstrates that $\dot{V}O_{2max}$ is dictated by maximal cardiac output ($SV_{max} \times HR_{max}$) and maximal arteriovenous oxygen difference.

Arteriovenous Oxygen Difference Response to Graded Intensity Exercise

The arteriovenous oxygen ($a\text{-}\dot{V}O_2$) difference reflects the difference in oxygen content between the arterial and the venous blood. The $a\text{-}\dot{V}O_2$ difference provides a measure of the amount of oxygen taken up by the working muscles from the arterial blood. Resting oxygen content is approximately 20 $mL \cdot dL^{-1}$ in arterial blood and 15 $mL \cdot dL^{-1}$ in venous blood, yielding an $a\text{-}\dot{V}O_2$ of about 5 $mL \cdot dL^{-1}$. During exercise, venous oxygen content decreases as a result of the increased consumption of oxygen by the working muscles, thus resulting in an increase in $a\text{-}\dot{V}O_2$ difference with increasing exercise intensity.

HR, SV, and Cardiac Output Responses to Graded Intensity Exercise

Heart rate increases linearly with increasing workload until heart rate maximum is reached, which is also typically the point of exercise maximum. Although maximal HR declines with age (20), trained athletes have lower resting HRs throughout the lifespan. Training itself has little impact on maximal HR. However, training can decrease an individual's HR at a given submaximal workload from pre- to postaerobic exercise training as a sign of increased fitness. SV is the volume of blood the heart ejects with each beat. Similar to HR, SV increases with workload, but only up to approximately 40% to 60% of $\dot{V}O_{2max}$ in the general population (18, 46). Beyond 40% to 60% of $\dot{V}O_{2max}$, SV has been shown to decrease slightly in sedentary individuals (28, 44), while continuing to increase beyond 40% to 60% of $\dot{V}O_{2max}$ in highly trained individuals (40, 87). As SV increases with training, resting HR tends to decrease, as more blood being pumped per beat allows the heart to beat less often at rest.

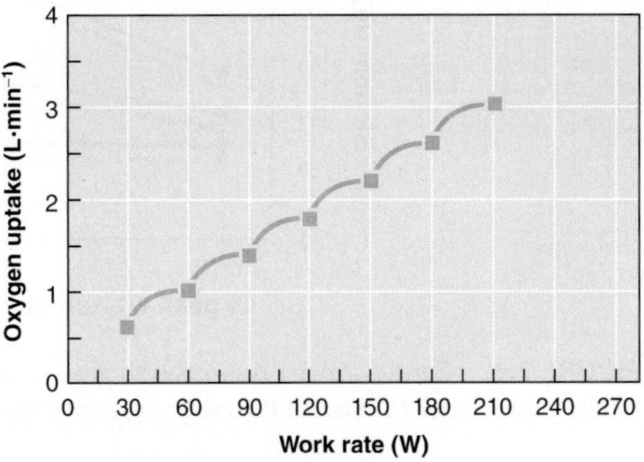

FIGURE 3.5. Relationship between oxygen uptake and workload during graded intensity exercise. (From Swain D, editor. *ACSM's Resource Manual for Guidelines for Exercise Testing and Prescription*. 7th ed. Baltimore (MD): Lippincott Williams & Wilkins; 2014.)

Cardiac output is the product of SV and HR and is also a measure of blood pumped per minute. Cardiac output increases steadily during graded intensity exercise because of the linear rise in HR and curvilinear rise in SV. However, increases in cardiac output beyond ~50% of $\dot{V}O_{2max}$ are primarily mediated by increases in HR in untrained individuals, whereas trained individuals have the capacity to increase cardiac output via increases mostly in HR and to a smaller extent in SV with increased exercise intensity (20). See Figure 3.6 for a visual comparison of HR, SV, and cardiac output responses to graded exercise intensity between trained and untrained individuals.

Pulmonary Ventilation Response to Graded Intensity Exercise

Pulmonary ventilation is the volume of air inhaled and exhaled per minute. It is calculated by multiplying the frequency of breathing by the volume of air moved per breath (tidal volume). Pulmonary ventilation increases linearly with work rate until 50% to 80% of $\dot{V}O_{2max}$, at which point it reaches the ventilatory threshold and ventilation begins to increase exponentially (82). Ventilatory threshold has been used as an indicator of performance and training intensity; trained subjects can reach higher workloads than untrained subjects before reaching their ventilatory threshold (32).

Blood Pressure Response to Graded Intensity Exercise

Blood pressure (BP) is proportional to the product of cardiac output and total peripheral resistance (TPR) (the overall resistance to blood flow by the blood vessels). Systolic blood pressure (SBP) is the pressure in the arteries during ventricular contraction, or systole, and is heavily influenced by

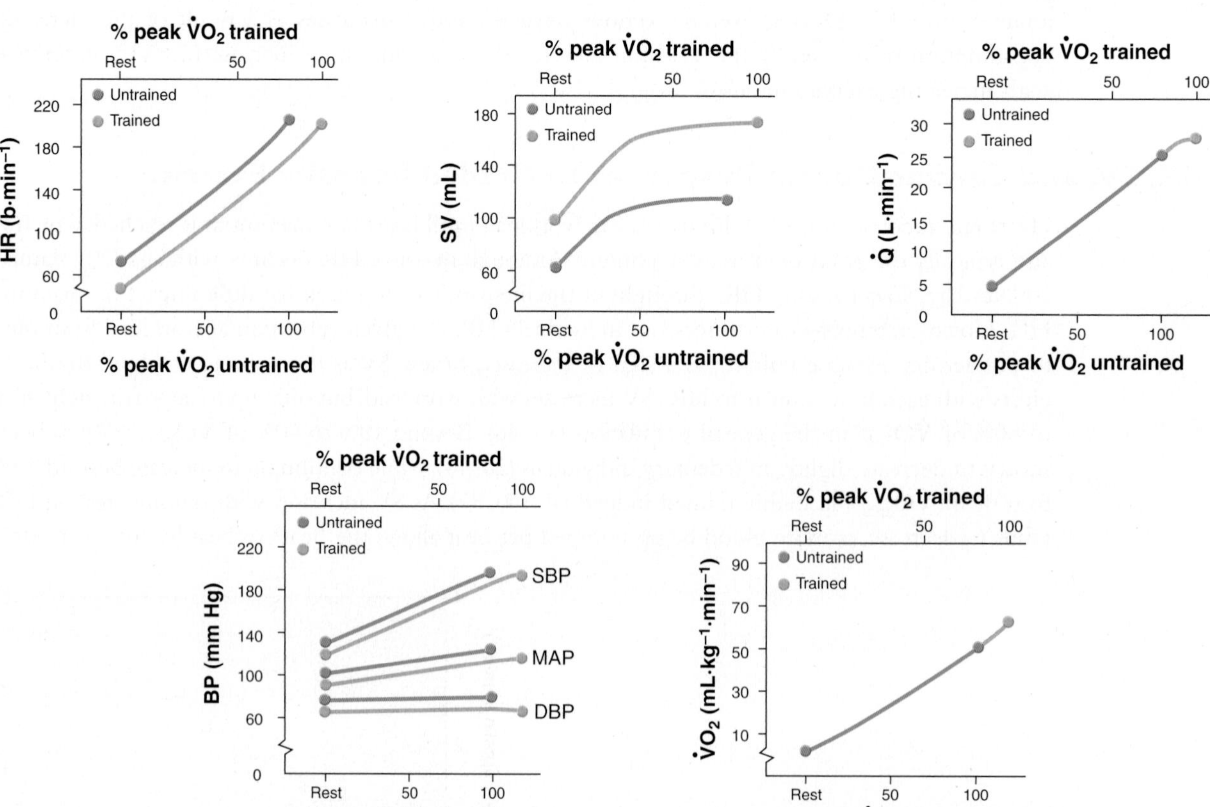

FIGURE 3.6. Cardiovascular responses to graded intensity exercise in trained and untrained individuals. (From Kraemer W, Fleck S, Deschenes M. *Exercise Physiology: Integrating Theory and Application*. Baltimore (MD): Lippincott Williams & Wilkins; 2012.)

changes in cardiac output. Thus, just as cardiac output increases linearly with increasing workload, so does SBP. Diastolic blood pressure (DBP) is the pressure in the arteries when the heart is relaxed, or diastole, and is heavily influenced by TPR. During dynamic, large muscle mass exercise, vascular beds within active muscle vasodilate, decreasing resistance within these blood vessels. In contrast, blood vessels in less metabolically active tissues constrict, increasing resistance within these blood vessels. TPR is determined by the systemic resistance throughout the entire vasculature and is thus determined by the relative proportion of the vasculature that has undergone vasodilation versus vasoconstriction during exercise. During graded exercise, TPR may drop slightly because of the large muscle vasodilation. As a result of this and the contrasting increase in cardiac output, DBP remains relatively stable (72). SBP, however, will increase linearly with exercise intensity.

Mean arterial pressure (MAP) is the average BP in the arterial system over one complete cardiac cycle (MAP = DBP + 0.33 [SBP–DBP]). MAP is not a critical value to assess during regular exercise, and instead is more commonly used in a clinical or diagnostic setting. However, it is worth noting that as a result of training, SBP, DBP, and MAP are all reduced slightly at submaximal workloads (52). See Figure 3.6 for a visual comparison of the BP responses to graded exercise intensity between trained and untrained individuals.

In summary, the HFS should understand that HR, pulmonary ventilation, a-$\dot{V}O_2$ difference, SV, cardiac output, SBP, and mean arterial BP increase during graded intensity exercise, while DBP remains stable or decreases slightly during aerobic type exercise. These cardiovascular and pulmonary adaptations support greater oxygen uptake to allow for the increase in aerobic energy production required during exercise.

MEASURING BP AND HR BEFORE, DURING, AND AFTER GRADED EXERCISE

BP and HR Assessment

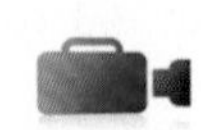

Visit thePoint to watch video 3.1 about blood pressure management.

To determine whether clients have an appropriate cardiovascular response to graded exercise, the HFS should assess BP and HR before, during, and after exercise. (See previous section for a description of the expected HR and BP response to graded intensity exercise.) Prior to exercise, BP and HR should be assessed while resting in the exercise position that will subsequently be used for exercise testing. HR can be accessed via multiple techniques, such as radial and carotid pulse palpation, auscultation with a stethoscope, or the use of a reliable HR monitor. If using pulse palpation, the pulse should be counted for a minimum of 15 seconds and multiplied by four to calculate HR in units of beats per minute (bpm). Counting HR for less than 15 seconds reduces the accuracy and reliability of this technique. If the pulse palpation technique is to be used during and after exercise to assess HR, palpation of the radial artery may be a superior choice to the carotid artery because of the possibility of activating the carotid baroreceptors and inducing a reduction in HR, SV, TPR, and MAP (9). BP is typically assessed via brachial artery auscultation. To obtain accurate and reliable BP readings, the HFS should practice standard BP assessment techniques as specified in the box titled "How to Assess Resting Blood Pressure" (66, 79).

During graded exercise testing, BP and HR should be assessed at each exercise intensity. For some tests, it is important for HR to reach a steady state before advancing, and therefore, HR should be assessed at least two times at each stage to ensure that it is appropriate to move to the next workload. Generally, this is done at the end of each of the last 2 minutes of each exercise stage. BP should also be assessed during the last minute of each exercise stage. Taking accurate HR and BP assessments during exercise is a skill that requires significant practice by the HFS in order to be completed accurately and in a timely manner while the client continues to exercise. When performing exercise HR and BP assessments, the HFS needs to ensure that the clients arm is relaxed, at heart level, and not touching any exercise equipment. After completion of exercise, BP and HR should be assessed for a minimum of 5 minutes of recovery or until each become stable (9).

HOW TO Assess Resting Blood Pressure

1. Patients should be seated quietly for at least 5 min in a chair with back support (rather than on an examination table) with their feet on the floor and their arm supported at heart level. Patients should refrain from smoking cigarettes or ingesting caffeine for at least 30 min preceding the measurement.
2. Measuring supine and standing values may be indicated under special circumstances.
3. Wrap cuff firmly around upper arm at heart level; align cuff with brachial artery.
4. The appropriate cuff size must be used to ensure accurate measurement. The bladder within the cuff should encircle at least 80% of the upper arm. Many adults require a large adult cuff.
5. Place stethoscope chest piece below the antecubital space over the brachial artery. Bell and diaphragm side of chest piece seem to be equally effective in assessing BP (15).
6. Quickly inflate cuff pressure to 20 mm Hg above first Korotkoff sound.
7. Slowly release pressure at rate equal to 2 to 5 mm Hg · s^{-1}.
8. SBP is the point at which the first of two or more Korotkoff sounds is heard (phase 1), and DBP is the point before the disappearance of Korotkoff sounds (phase 5).
9. At least two measurements should be made (minimum of 1 min apart), and the average should be taken.
10. BP should be measured in both arms during the first examination. Higher pressure should be used when there is consistent interarm difference.
11. Provide to patients, verbally and in writing, their specific BP numbers and BP goals.

Modified from American College of Sports Medicine. *ACSM's Guidelines for Exercise Testing and Prescription.* 9th ed. Philadelphia (PA): Lippincott Williams & Wilkins; 2014. For additional, more detailed recommendations, see American College of Sports Medicine. *ACSM's Health Related Physical Fitness Assessment Manual.* 3rd ed. Philadelphia (PA): Lippincott Williams & Wilkins; 2009.

Rate Pressure Product

In addition to checking for appropriate cardiovascular responses, the HFS can use these data to calculate an individual's "rate pressure product" (RPP). RPP, also referred to as double product, is the product of HR and SBP that occur concomitantly, and serves as an estimate of myocardial oxygen demand ($M\dot{V}O_2$) (RPP = HR × SBP). At rest, the heart consumes approximately 70% of the oxygen delivered to the cardiac muscle. During exercise, the cardiac muscle performs more work because of increased HR and increased contractility, and thus, $M\dot{V}O_2$ increases during exercise in direct proportion to exercise intensity (11). Therefore, if HR and SBP are lower at a given submaximal exercise intensity, the $M\dot{V}O_2$ will be lower, indicating increased fitness. The RPP can be useful to the HFS when performing exercise testing or prescribing exercise to clients with cardiovascular disease who have been medically cleared for exercise (10).

SELECTING APPROPRIATE CRF ASSESSMENTS FOR HEALTHY POPULATIONS, INCLUDING PREGNANT WOMEN

CRF Assessments Benefits

CRF is an umbrella term that serves as an indicator of the functional capacity of the heart, lungs, blood vessels, and muscles to work in synchrony to support dynamic, large muscle mass exercise (10). CRF assessment is regularly performed in both healthy and clinical populations. In clinical

TABLE 3.1 CARDIORESPIRATORY FITNESS ASSESSMENTS

Cardiorespiratory Fitness Assessment Techniques

Type of Test	Intensity	Specific Test Protocols	Major Equipment Needed
Maximal oxygen uptake $\dot{V}O_{2max}$	Maximal	Open circuit spirometry during graded exercise test to volitional fatigue (1)	Treadmill, cycle ergometer, arm ergometer, etc.
Submaximal oxygen uptake	Submaximal	Astrand-Ryhming Cycle Ergometer Test (16) YMCA Cycle Ergometer Test (86)	Cycle ergometer Cycle ergometer
Step tests	Maximal or submaximal	Queens College/McArdle Step Test (58) Harvard Step Test (22) Astrand-Ryhming Step Test (16)	Aerobic step or specific height bench, metronome
Field tests	Maximal or submaximal	Rockport Walk (51) 12-Minute Walk/Run Test (30, 31) 1.5-Mile Run Test (10)	Level walking/running surface

populations, CRF testing is used for screening, diagnosis, and prognosis of medical conditions. CRF testing is also used in both clinical and healthy populations to gain insight into the most appropriate frequency, intensity, duration, and mode of exercise to prescribe when creating individualized exercise programs, and as a motivational tool to help track progress and continually set obtainable, short-term goals (11).

Types of CRF Assessments

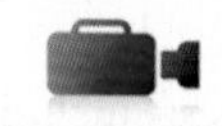

Visit thePoint to watch video 3.2 about determining the correct seat height on a cycle ergometer.

CRF can be assessed through a variety of step tests, field tests, and submaximal $\dot{V}O_2$ prediction tests. The wide variety of well-respected and widely used CRF tests allows the HFS the opportunity to select an assessment that provides the desired physiological informational while adhering to the needs of the client and the resources available. Table 3.1 provides an organizational chart of the most popular CRF tests for your reference. A detailed description of the most popular cardiorespiratory testing protocols can be found in the *ACSM Health-Related Physical Fitness Assessment Manual* (10), and additional references are listed in the table below.

Exercise	Advantages	Disadvantages
Walking	Does not require expensive equipment, special skill, or special facilities. Can be done indoors or outdoors (53)	Potential safety concerns of walking environment (67)
Jogging/running	Easily accessible and large caloric expenditure; promotes bone health	Increased injury risk because of higher impact, environmental concerns
Bicycling	Reduced impact on bones and joints	Cost of bicycle, weather, safety of cycling environment
Swimming	Buoyancy provides great alternative for individuals with joint pain	Skill level needed; chlorinated pool may aggravate respiratory conditions, and warm moist air may benefit asthmatics
Aerobic machines	Multiple options allowing exercise, regardless of weather; many provide low-impact workout option	Cost of owning machines/membership at fitness facility

The gold standard used to measure CRF is the assessment of $\dot{V}O_{2max}$ via open circuit spirometry during maximal-intensity, aerobic exercise. Open circuit spirometry requires the collection of expired air from the client during a graded intensity exercise test to maximal exertion. The volume and content of oxygen and carbon dioxide in the expired air is analyzed with a highly specific gas analyzer. These data allow for the calculation of oxygen consumption at each workload of a graded exercise test. As discussed previously, $\dot{V}O_2$ will increase linearly as workload increases until $\dot{V}O_2$ plateaus, and $\dot{V}O_{2max}$ is reached. Although assessment of $\dot{V}O_{2max}$ with gas analysis is the gold standard of CRF assessment, it requires expensive equipment, technical expertise, and maximal intensity exercise performance by the client. These requirements limit the use of $\dot{V}O_{2max}$ testing using open circuit spirometry to primarily clinical laboratory and research settings (9).

Submaximal oxygen uptake ($\dot{V}O_2$) estimates $\dot{V}O_{2max}$ from the HR response to submaximal single stage or graded exercise. Therefore, precise assessment of HR is a critical factor in determining $\dot{V}O_{2max}$, and should be a well-developed skill by the HFS. HR can easily be affected by environmental, dietary, and behavioral factors, and the HFS should do his or her best to control these factors during submaximal $\dot{V}O_2$ testing. Because submaximal testing relies on predictions, there is an increased chance of error because of a variety of factors, such as estimations on resting and maximum HR. To minimize the error of prediction, the following assumptions must be met during submaximal exercise testing: (a) steady state HR is achieved within 3 to 4 minutes at each workload, (b) HR increases linearly with work rate, (c) a consistent work rate should be maintained throughout each stage of testing, and (d) estimation/prediction of HR_{max} should be accurate (10). Unfortunately, estimation/prediction of HR_{max} is not an exact science and is highly variable. If true HR_{max} differs significantly from predicted HR_{max}, this assumption may introduce a source of error into the prediction of $\dot{V}O_{2max}$ via submaximal $\dot{V}O_2$ testing (17).

Step tests are a widely utilized form of CRF assessment because of the practicality of this technique. They are short in duration, require little equipment yet are easily portable, and allow for assessment of large groups. Various step test protocols range from submaximal to maximal, giving the HFS a wide range of choices that he or she should critically assess before determining which is most appropriate for the client. Intensity is determined by step height and step cadence. Most step tests predict $\dot{V}O_{2max}$ from recovery HR (16, 22, 58), while some step tests use steady state exercise HR to estimate CRF (57). The lower the exercise HR and the greater the rate of recovery, the higher the estimated $\dot{V}O_{2max}$.

Field tests are also widely utilized to assess CRF. The most common forms of field tests include assessment of the amount of time required to cover a set distance or assessment of the distance covered in a set amount of time. Field tests are versatile, in that they can utilize many modes of exercise, such as walking, running, cycling, and swimming. Field tests have many of the same benefits as step tests, in that they are short in duration, require little equipment, can be used for large groups, and can be performed wherever a safe, flat, known distance is available. However, field tests can be more subjective in nature, largely because of the dependency on client effort, and therefore are not as reliable as laboratory tests for assessing CRF.

Selecting the Appropriate CRF Assessment

When choosing which cardiorespiratory assessment to utilize, the HFS should consider intensity, length, and expense of the test; type and number of personnel needed; equipment and facilities needed; physician supervision needs and safety concerns; information required as a result of the assessment; required accuracy of results; appropriateness of mode of exercise; and the willingness of the participant to perform the test (10). The HFS should review the Physical Activity Readiness Questionnaire, health history, and risk assessment documents collected during the prescreening visit to help determine which assessment will be best (see Chapter 2 on prescreening and risk classification). On the basis of the client's risk classification category, the intent of the exercise test, and the other considerations, the HFS should think critically to determine whether a submaximal or maximal test is most appropriate on a case-by-case basis and to avoid a "one size fits all" approach. While maximal testing may be quite precise, it has many drawbacks, including first and foremost the increased risk of exercising to exhaustion, especially in clients presenting with any level of risk other than "low" (9). Other drawbacks to maximal testing include increased costs and time, specialized

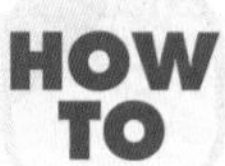

Assess CRF in Adults of Low Fitness Level: The Rockport Walking Test

Equipment Needed

1. Track or level surface
2. Stopwatch
3. HR monitor (optional)
4. Scale to measure body weight
5. Clipboard, recording sheet, and pencil
6. Calculator

Important Information and Tips

1. Although many CR fitness assessments require the individual to run/jog, these types of tests may be contraindicated for individuals with orthopedic concerns or of low fitness level. Therefore, the HFS may choose to utilize the Rockport Walking Test to assess maximal aerobic capacity.
2. The procedure for the Rockport Walking Test is as follows:
   a) Locate a level surface, preferably a track, and determine the distance or lap that is equivalent to 1 mile.
   b) After a proper warm-up, instruct the client to walk 1 mile as fast as possible, without jogging or running.
   c) Immediately after 1 mile has been completed, record the walk time in minutes.
   d) If the individual is wearing a HR monitor, record the HR achieved immediately upon reaching the 1-mile mark. If a HR monitor is not available, upon completion of the mile, take the client's pulse for 15 seconds and multiply by 4 to determine peak HR.
   e) Data may now be entered into the following formula: $\dot{V}O_{2max}$ ($mL \cdot kg^{-1} \cdot min^{-1}$) = 132.853 − (0.0769 × body weight in lb) − (0.3877 × age in yr) + (6.315 × gender [1 for men, 0 for women]) − (3.2649 × 1 mile walk time in minutes) − (0.1565 × heart rate).
   f) Data may be compared with normative tables listed in Suggested Readings.

Example

1. What is the predicted maximal aerobic capacity for a 64-year-old woman, who weighs 155 lb, completes the Rockport test in 16 minutes with a HR of 142 bpm?

$$\dot{V}O_{2max} = 132.853 - (0.0769 \times 155) - (0.3877 \times 64) + (6.315 \times 0) - (3.2649 \times 16) - (0.1565 \times 142) = 21.7\ mL \cdot kg^{-1} \cdot min^{-1}$$

2. Normative data suggest that this individual would be rated as "low average" for her age.

Reference

Kline GM, Porcari JP, Hintermeister R, et al. Estimation of $\dot{V}O_{2max}$ from a one-mile track walk, gender, age, and body weight. *Med Sci Sports Exerc.* 1987;19(3):253–9 (Ref. 51).

Suggested Reading

Morrow JR Jr, Jackson AW, Disch JG, Mood DP. *Measurement and Evaluation in Human Performance*. 4th ed. Champaign (IL): Human Kinetics; 2011 (Ref. 62).

personnel and supplies, and the discomfort of asking the client to exercise to complete exhaustion. Submaximal tests may therefore be more appropriate for many individuals and, when conducted appropriately, result in a reasonable estimate of $\dot{V}O_{2max}$ (19).

CRF in Pregnant Women

Exercise is beneficial to both mother and baby during pregnancy (6, 34), and therefore, pregnant women should be encouraged to maintain an active lifestyle during pregnancy and the postpartum period. The HFS should be aware that pregnant women are considered a special population, and thus the exercise testing and prescription guidelines for pregnant women differ slightly from the general guidelines given to nonpregnant women. The American College of Sports Medicine® (ACSM) supports the exercise guidelines for pregnancy set forth by the American College of Obstetricians and Gynecologists (6), which provide absolute and relative contraindications for exercise participation during pregnancy (6). If exercise is not contraindicated, pregnant women can follow the ACSM and Surgeon General's recommendations to accumulate a minimum of 150 minutes of moderate-intensity exercise weekly (6, 81). Exercise intensities of 60% to 70% of maximal HR or 50% to 60% of $\dot{V}O_{2max}$ (on the low end of moderate-intensity exercise) are advised for pregnant women who were not physically active before pregnancy. Women who were active before exercise can exercise at a higher workload (15). If exercise testing is warranted in a pregnant woman, maximal exercise testing should be avoided unless absolutely necessary for medical reasons. Although submaximal exercise testing is more appropriate for this population (9), there is usually little need to conduct fitness assessments in pregnant women. Special consideration should be given to the mode of exercise to ensure that the subject feels comfortable and that there is low risk of injury and falls. The HFS should also ensure that exercise testing is performed in a thermoneutral environment and during a state of adequate hydration (9). During testing, the HFS should closely monitor the pregnant woman so as not to miss any test termination signs or symptoms (6).

INTERPRETING RESULTS OF CRF ASSESSMENTS, INCLUDING DETERMINATION OF $\dot{V}O_2$ AND $\dot{V}O_{2max}$

After completing cardiopulmonary exercise assessment, the HFS should interpret the results of the assessment and share the information with his or her client. To maximize client understanding of CRF testing, individual $\dot{V}O_{2max}$ data are often compared with established criterion-referenced and normative standards. Criterion-referenced standards classify individuals into categories or groups, such as "excellent" or "needs improvement," on the basis of external criteria. In contrast, normative standards provide percentiles from data collected within a specific population. The HFS can use either type of standard when interpreting data and may find it helpful to present data to clients using both types of standards, as one may have more impact with a client on the basis of his or her perspective. Care should be taken when using normative standards to ensure that the client population and the normative standard population are similar. If there is discrepancy within the populations, normative data are not appropriate for comparisons (11). Table 3.2 provide both normative and criterion-referenced $\dot{V}O_{2max}$ data specific to age and sex.

Low CRF levels have been shown to be an independent predictor of cardiovascular disease and all-cause mortality (21, 83). The HFS should discuss this relationship with clients, as it may bring added meaning to the test results and help motivate clients to improve their CRF. Both maximal and submaximal tests can be used to evaluate CRF at a given point in time, as well as changes in CRF that result from physical activity participation (9). A higher $\dot{V}O_{2max}$, lower HR at a given intensity of submaximal exercise, or a lower recovery HR indicates an overall improvement in CRF.

TABLE 3.2 FITNESS CATEGORIES FOR MAXIMAL AEROBIC POWER FOR MEN AND WOMEN BY AGE

%		Balke Treadmill (time)	Maximal $\dot{V}O_2$ (mL·kg^{-1}·min^{-1})	12-Min Run (miles)	1.5-Mile Run (time)	Balke Treadmill (time)	Maximal $\dot{V}O_2$ (mL·kg^{-1}·min^{-1})	12-Min Run (miles)	1.5-Mile Run (time)
					Men (*n* = 15,764)				
		Age 20–29 (*n* = 2,606)				**Age 30–39 (*n* = 13,158)**			
99	Superior	32:00	61.2	2.02	8:22	30:00	58.3	1.94	8:49
95		28:31	56.2	1.88	9:10	27:11	54.3	1.82	9:31
90		27:00	54.0	1.81	9:34	26:00	52.5	1.77	9:52
85	Excellent	26:00	52.5	1.77	9:52	24:45	507	1.72	10:14
80		25:00	51.1	1.73	10:08	23:30	48.9	1.67	10:38
75		23:40	49.2	1.68	10:34	22:30	47.5	1.63	10:59
70		23:00	48.2	1.65	10:49	22:00	46.8	1.61	11:09
65	Good	22:00	46.8	1.61	11:09	21:00	45.3	1.57	11:34
60		21:15	45.7	1.58	11:27	20:20	44.4	1.55	11:49
55		21:00	45.3	1.57	11:34	20:00	43.9	1.53	11:58
50		20:00	43.9	1.53	11:58	19:00	42.4	1.49	12:25
45	Fair	19:26	43.1	1.51	12:11	18:15	41.4	1.46	12:44
40		18:50	42.2	1.49	12:29	18:00	41.0	1.45	12:53
35	Poor	18:00	41.0	1.45	12:53	17:00	39.5	1.41	13:25
30		17:30	40.3	1.43	13:08	16:15	38.5	1.38	13:48
25		17:00	39.5	1.41	13:25	15:40	37.6	1.36	14:10
20		16:00	38.1	1.37	13:58	15:00	36.7	1.33	14:33
15		15:00	36.7	1.33	14:33	14:00	35.2	1.29	15:14
10	Very poor	14:00	35.2	1.29	15:14	13:00	33.8	1.25	15:56
5		12:00	32.3	1.21	16:46	11:10	31.1	1.18	17:30
1		8:00	26.6	1.05	20:55	8:00	26.6	1.05	20:55
					Men (*n* = 25,636)				
		Age 40–49 (*n* = 16,534)				**Age 50–59 (*n* = 9,102)**			
99	Superior	29:06	57.0	1.90	9:02	27:15	54.3	1.82	9:31
95		26:16	52.9	1.79	9:47	24:00	49.7	1.69	10:27
90		25:00	51.1	1.73	10:09	22:00	46.8	1.61	11:09
85	Excellent	23:14	48.5	1.66	10:44	20:31	44.6	1.55	11:45
80		22:00	46.8	1.61	11:09	19:35	43.3	1.52	12:08
75		21:02	45.4	1.58	11:32	18:32	41.8	1.47	12.37
70		20:15	44.2	1.54	11:52	18:00	41.0	1.45	12:53

Continues

TABLE 3.2 **FITNESS CATEGORIES FOR MAXIMAL AEROBIC POWER FOR MEN AND WOMEN BY AGE** *(continued)*

%		Balke Treadmill (time)	Maximal $\dot{V}O_2$ (mL·kg^{-1}·min^{-1})	12-Min Run (miles)	1.5-Mile Run (time)	Balke Treadmill (time)	Maximal $\dot{V}O_2$ (mL·kg^{-1}·min^{-1})	12-Min Run (miles)	1.5-Mile Run (time)
65	Good	20:00	43.9	1.53	11:58	17:00	39.5	1.41	13:25
60		19:00	42.4	1.49	12:25	16:10	38.3	1.38	13:53
55		18:02	41.0	1.45	12:53	16:00	38.1	1.37	13:58
50		17:34	40.4	1.44	13:05	15:02	36.7	1.33	14:33
45	Fair	17:00	39.5	1.41	13:25	14:56	36.6	1.33	14:35
40		16:12	38.4	1.38	13:50	14:00	35.2	1.29	15:14
35	Poor	15:38	37.6	1.36	14:10	13:05	33.9	1.26	15:53
30		15:00	36.7	1.33	14:33	12:38	33.2	1.24	16:16
25		14:20	35.7	1.31	15:00	12:00	32.3	1.21	16:46
20		13:35	34.6	1.28	15:32	11:10	31.1	1.18	17:30
15		12:45	33.4	1.24	16:09	10:15	29.8	1.14	18:22
10	Very poor	11:40	31.8	1.20	17:04	9:15	28.4	1.10	19:24
5		10:00	29.4	1.13	18:39	7:30	25.8	1.03	21:40
1		7:00	25.1	1.01	22:22	4:20	21.3	0.90	27:08
		Men (*n* = 3,149)							
		Age 60–69 (*n* = 467)				**Age 70–79 (*n* = 2,682)**			
99	Superior	25:02	51.1	1.74	10:09	24:00	49.7	1.69	10:27
95		21:33	46.1	1.60	11:20	19:00	42.4	1.49	12:25
90		19:30	43.2	1.51	12:10	17:00	39.5	1.41	13:25
85	Excellent	18:00	41.0	1.45	12:53	16:00	38.1	1.37	13:57
80		17:00	39.5	1.41	13:25	14:34	36.0	1.32	14:52
75		16:00	38.1	1.37	13:58	13:25	34.4	1.27	15:38
70		15:00	36.7	1.33	14:33	12:27	33.0	1.23	16:22
65	Good	14:30	35.9	1.31	14:55	12:00	32.3	1.21	16:46
60		13:51	35.0	1.29	15:20	11:00	30.9	1.17	17:37
55		13:04	33.9	1.26	15:53	10:30	30.2	1.15	18:05
50		12:30	33.1	1.23	16:19	10:00	29.4	1.13	18:39
45	Fair	12:00	32.3	1.21	16:46	9:20	28.5	1.11	19:19
40		11:21	31.4	1.19	17:19	9:00	28.0	1.09	19:43

TABLE 3.2 **FITNESS CATEGORIES FOR MAXIMAL AEROBIC POWER FOR MEN AND WOMEN BY AGE** *(continued)*

%		Balke Treadmill (time)	Maximal $\dot{V}O_2$ (mL·kg^{-1}·min^{-1})	12-Min Run (miles)	1.5-Mile Run (time)	Balke Treadmill (time)	Maximal $\dot{V}O_2$ (mL·kg^{-1}·min^{-1})	12-Min Run (miles)	1.5-Mile Run (time)
35		10:49	30.6	1.17	17:49	8:21	27.1	1.07	20:28
30		10:00	29.4	1.13	18:39	7:38	26.0	1.04	21:28
25	Poor	9:29	28.7	1.11	19:10	7:00	25.1	1.01	22:22
20		8:37	27.4	1.08	20:13	6:00	23.7	0.97	23:55
15		7:33	25.9	1.03	21:34	5:00	22.2	0.93	25:49
10		6:20	24.1	0.99	23:27	4:00	20.8	0.89	27:55
5	Very poor	4:55	22.1	0.93	25:58	3:00	19.3	0.85	30:34
1		2:29	18.6	0.83	31:59	2:00	17.9	0.81	33:30
		Women (*n* = 5,744)							
		Age 20–29 (*n* = 1,350)				**Age 30–39 (*n* = 4,394)**			
99		27:43	55.0	1.84	9:23	26:00	52.5	1.77	9:52
95	Superior	24:24	50.2	1.71	10:20	22:06	46.9	1.62	11:08
90		22:30	47.5	1.63	10:59	20:34	44.7	1.56	11:43
85		21:00	45.3	1.57	11:34	19:03	42.5	1.50	12:23
80		20:04	44.0	1.54	11:56	18:00	41.0	1.45	12:53
75	Excellent	19:42	43.4	1.52	12:07	17:30	40.3	1.43	13:08
70		18:06	41.1	1.46	12:51	16:30	38.8	1.39	13:41
65		17:45	40.6	1.44	13:01	16:00	38.1	1.37	13:58
60		17:00	39.5	1.41	13:25	15:02	36.7	1.33	14:33
55	Good	16:00	38.1	1.37	13:58	15:00	36.7	1.33	14:33
50		15:30	37.4	1.35	14:15	14:00	35.2	1.29	15:14
45	Fair	15:00	36.7	1.33	14:33	13:30	34.5	1.27	15:35
40		14:11	35.5	1.30	15:05	13:00	33.8	1.25	15:56
35		13:36	34.6	1.27	15:32	12:03	32.4	1.21	16:43
30		13:00	33.8	1.25	15:56	12:00	32.3	1.21	16:46
25	Poor	12:04	32.4	1.22	16:43	11:00	30.9	1.17	17:38
20		11:30	31.6	1.19	17:11	10:20	29.9	1.15	18:18
15		10:42	30.5	1.16	17:53	9:39	28.9	1.12	19:01
10		10:00	29.4	1.13	18:39	8:36	27.4	1.08	20:13
5	Very poor	7:54	26.4	1.05	21:05	7:16	25.5	1.02	21:57
1		5:14	22.6	0.94	25:17	5:20	22.7	0.94	25:10

Continues

TABLE 3.2 FITNESS CATEGORIES FOR MAXIMAL AEROBIC POWER FOR MEN AND WOMEN BY AGE *(continued)*

%		Balke Treadmill (time)	Maximal $\dot{V}O_2$ (mL·kg^{-1}·min^{-1})	12-Min Run (miles)	1.5-Mile Run (time)	Balke Treadmill (time)	Maximal $\dot{V}O_2$ (mL·kg^{-1}·min^{-1})	12-Min Run (miles)	1.5-Mile Run (time)
		Women (n = 7,937)							
		Age 40–49 (n = 4,834)				**Age 50–59 (n = 3,103)**			
99	Superior	25:00	51.1	1.74	10:09	21:00	45.3	1.57	11:34
95		20:56	45.2	1.57	11:35	17:16	39.9	1.42	13:16
90		19:00	42.4	1.49	12:25	16:00	38.1	1.37	13:58
85	Excellent	17:20	40.0	1.43	13:14	15:00	36.7	1.33	14:33
80		16:34	38.9	1.40	13:38	14:00	35.2	1.29	15:14
75		16:00	38.1	1.37	13:58	13:15	34.1	1.26	15:47
70		15:00	36.7	1.33	14:33	12:23	32.9	1.23	16:26
65	Good	14:14	35.6	1.30	15:03	12:00	32.3	1.21	16:46
60		13:56	35.1	1.29	15:17	11:23	31.4	1.19	17:19
55		13:02	33.8	1.25	15:56	11:00	30.9	1.17	17:38
50		12:39	33.3	1.24	16:13	10:30	30.2	1.15	18:05
45	Fair	12:00	32.3	1.21	16:46	10:00	29.4	1.13	18:39
40		11:30	31.6	1.19	17:11	9:30	28.7	1.11	19:10
35	Poor	11:00	30.9	1.17	17:38	9:00	28.0	1.09	19:43
30		10:10	29.7	1.14	18:26	8:30	27.3	1.07	20:17
25		10:00	29.4	1.13	18:39	8:00	26.6	1.05	20:55
20		9:00	28.0	1.09	19:43	7:15	25.5	1.02	21:57
15		8:07	26.7	1.06	20:49	6:40	24.6	1.00	22:53
10	Very poor	7:21	25.6	1.03	21:52	6:00	23.7	0.97	23:55
5		6:17	24.1	0.98	23:27	4:48	21.9	0.92	26:15
1		4:00	20.8	0.89	27:55	3:00	19.3	0.85	30:34
		Women (n = 1,297)							
		Age 60–69 (n = 1,088)				**Age 70–79 (n = 209)**			
99	Superior	19:00	42.4	1.49	12:25	19:00	42.4	1.49	12:25
95		15:09	36.9	1.34	14:28	15:00	36.7	1.33	14:33
90		13:33	34.6	1.27	15:32	12:50	33.5	1.25	16:06
85	Excellent	12:28	33.0	1.23	16:22	11:46	32.0	1.20	16:57
80		12:00	32.3	1.21	16:46	10:30	30.2	1.15	18:05
75		11:04	31.0	1.18	17:34	10:00	29.4	1.13	18:39
70		10:30	30.2	1.15	18:05	9:15	28.4	1.10	19:24

TABLE 3.2 **FITNESS CATEGORIES FOR MAXIMAL AEROBIC POWER FOR MEN AND WOMEN BY AGE** *(continued)*

%		Balke Treadmill (time)	Maximal $\dot{V}O_2$ (mL·kg^{-1}·min^{-1})	12-Min Run (miles)	1.5-Mile Run (time)	Balke Treadmill (time)	Maximal $\dot{V}O_2$ (mL·kg^{-1}·min^{-1})	12-Min Run (miles)	1.5-Mile Run (time)
65	Good	10:00	29.4	1.13	18:39	8:43	27.6	1.08	20:02
60		9:44	29.1	1.12	18:52	8:00	26.6	1.05	20:54
55		9:11	28.3	1.10	19:29	7:37	26.0	1.04	21:45
50		8:40	27.5	1.08	20:08	7:00	25.1	1.01	22:22
45	Fair	8:15	26.9	1.06	20:38	6:39	24.6	1.00	22:54
40		8:00	26.6	1.05	20:55	6:05	23.8	0.98	23:47
35	Poor	7:14	25.4	1.02	22:03	5:28	22.9	0.95	24:54
30		6:52	24.9	1.01	22:34	5:00	22.2	0.93	25:49
25		6:21	24.2	0.99	23:20	4:45	21.9	0.92	26:15
20		6:00	23.7	0.97	23:55	4:16	21.2	0.90	27:17
15		5:25	22.8	0.95	25:02	4:00	20.8	0.89	27:55
10	Very poor	4:40	21.7	0.92	26:32	3:00	19.3	0.85	30:34
5		3:30	20.1	0.87	29:06	2:00	17.9	0.81	33:32
1		2:10	18.1	0.82	33:05	1:00	16.4	0.77	37:26

Adapted with permission from The Cooper Institute, Dallas, Texas. For more information: www.cooperinstitute.org.

METABOLIC CALCULATIONS AS THEY RELATE TO CARDIORESPIRATORY EXERCISE PROGRAMMING

Metabolic calculations can be a tremendous asset to the HFS. A HFS can use these calculations to determine calorie expenditure for clients interested in weight control, along with helping other clients reach daily and weekly goals for exercise.

Energy Units and Conversion Factors

Energy can be presented using many different terms in the field of exercise physiology, such as absolute oxygen consumption (L·min^{-1} or mL·min^{-1}), relative oxygen consumption (mL·kg^{-1}·min^{-1}), metabolic equivalents (METs), and kilocalories. The HFS should possess a firm understanding of the different terms used to express energy expenditure to allow for easy conversion of data from one term to another.

Oxygen consumption refers to the rate at which oxygen is consumed by the body. It can be expressed in absolute (L·min^{-1}) or relative (mL·kg^{-1}·min^{-1}) terms. Absolute oxygen consumption is the raw volume of oxygen consumed by the body, whereas relative oxygen consumption is the volume of oxygen consumed relative to body weight and can serve as a useful measure of fitness between individuals.

METs present the energy cost of exercise in a simple format that can be easily used by the general public to gauge exercise intensity. One MET is equal to the relative oxygen consumption at rest, which is approximately 3.5 mL·kg^{-1}·minute^{-1}. Using METs as energy cost units allows for the energy cost of exercise to be presented in multiples of rest. For example, if an individual is working at an energy cost of 10 METs, he or she is completing approximately 10 times the amount of work and using 10 times the amount of energy of that at rest. The compendium of physical activity provides a list of the energy cost for different forms of physical activity using METs (2–4). In addition, METs can be used to calculate energy expenditure over time ($[\text{MET} \times \text{kg} \times 3.5]/200 = \text{kcal}\cdot\text{min}^{-1}$).

Kilocalorie is an estimate of energy cost that can be related directly to physical activity and exercise, and the HFS can calculate the number of kilocalories expended during an exercise bout if oxygen consumption is measured or estimated using previously mentioned methods. The HFS can then estimate weight gain, loss, or maintenance, depending on a client's goal, remembering that 3,500 kcal equals 1 lb of fat.

As a HFS, understanding the conversion of energy between units is crucial. The flow chart in Figure 3.7 provides a visual tool to help the HFS understand the link between energy units and serves as a helpful guide when practicing unit conversions.

ACSM Metabolic Formula

Although open circuit spirometry is the gold standard technique used to assess oxygen consumption and estimate energy cost during exercise, it is not accessible and/or feasible in all applications. The ACSM provides metabolic formula (9) to allow the HFS an alternative method of energy cost estimation for popular modes of physical activity. The metabolic formula calculates gross energy

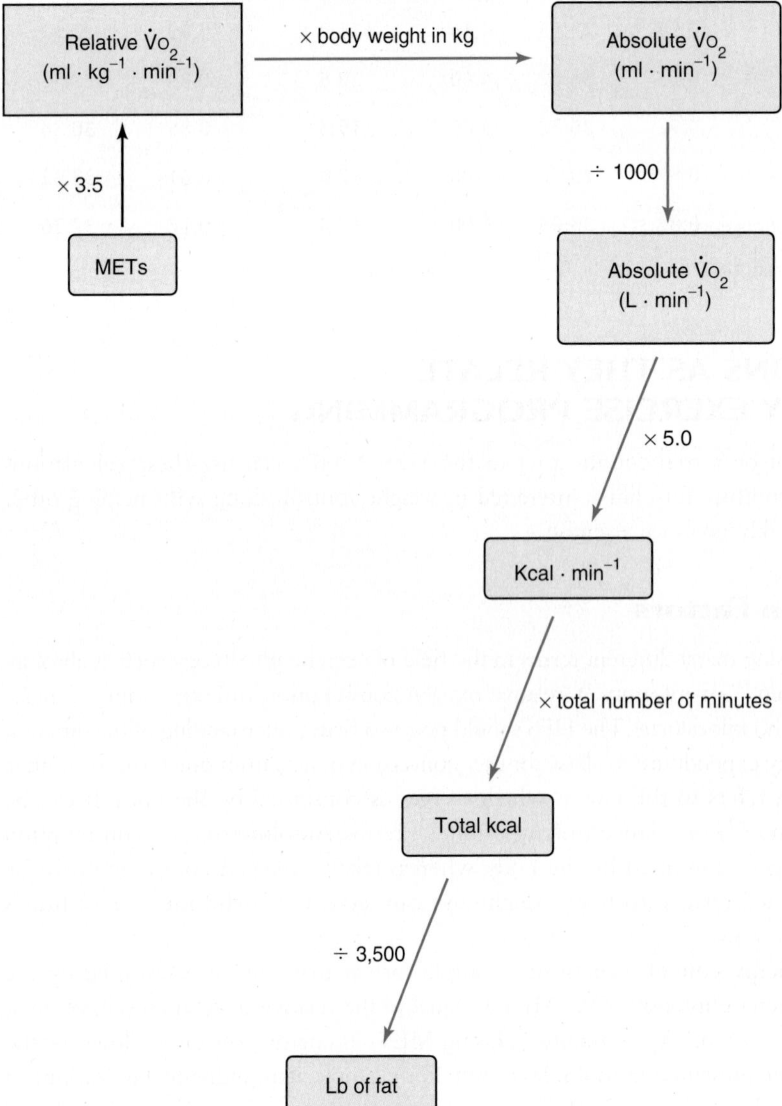

FIGURE 3.7. The energy equivalency chart: the seven energy expressions. (From Bibi KW, editor. *ACSM's Certification Review*. 3rd ed. Baltimore (MD): Lippincott Williams & Wilkins; 2010.)

TABLE 3.3 METABOLIC CALCULATIONS FOR THE ESTIMATION OF ENERGY EXPENDITURE ($\dot{V}O_2$ [ML·KG^{-1}·MIN^{-1}]) DURING COMMON PHYSICAL ACTIVITIES

	Sum These Components			
Activity	Resting Component	Horizontal Component	Vertical Component/ Resistance Component	Limitations
Walking	3.5	0.1 × speed[a]	1.8 × speed[a] × grade[b]	Most accurate for speeds of 1.9 to 3.7 min·h^{-1} (50–100 m·min^{-1})
Running	3.5	0.2 × speed[a]	0.9 × speed[a] × grade[b]	Most accurate for speeds >5 min·h^{-1} (134 m·min^{-1})
Stepping	3.5	0.2 × steps·min^{-1}	1.33 × (1.8 × step height[c] × steps·min^{-1})	Most accurate for stepping rates of 12–30 steps·min^{-1}
Leg cycling	3.5	3.5	(1.8 × work rate[d])/ body mass[e]	Most accurate for work rates of 300–1,200 kg·m·min^{-1}(50–200 W)
Arm cycling	3.5		(3 × work rate[d])/body mass[e]	Most accurate for work rates between 150–750 kg·m·min^{-1} (25–125 W)

[a]Speed in m·min^{-1}.
[b]Grade is percentage grade expressed in decimal format (*e.g.*, 10% = 0.10).
[c]Step height in meter.
Multiply by the following conversion factors:
lb to kg: 0.454; in to cm: 2.54; ft to m: 0.3048; m to km: 1.609; min·h^{-1} to m·min^{-1}: 26.8; kg·m·min^{-1} to W: 0.164; W to kg·m·min^{-1}: 6.12; $\dot{V}O_{2max}$ L·min^{-1} to kcal·min^{-1}: 4.9; $\dot{V}O_{2max}$ mL·kg^{-1}·min^{-1} to MET: 3.5
[d]Work rate in kilogram meters per minute (kg·m·min^{-1}) is calculated as resistance (kg) × distance per revolution of flywheel × pedal frequency per minute. Note: Distance per revolution is 6 m for Monark leg ergometer, 3 m for the Tunturi and BodyGuard ergometers, and 2.4 m for Monark arm ergometer.
[e]Body mass in kg.
Adapted from American College of Sports Medicine. *ACSM's Resource Manual for Guidelines for Exercise Testing and Prescription*. 5th ed. Philadelphia (PA): Lippincott Williams & Wilkins; 2006.

expenditure, which refers to the sum of energy used at rest and during exercise (Table 3.3). In contrast, net energy expenditure refers to the energy cost of exercise that exceeds the energy required to support the body at rest (net $\dot{V}O_2$) = gross $\dot{V}O_2$)–resting $\dot{V}O_2$). Thus, the energy costs calculated from the metabolic formula will represent the amount of energy required to complete the exercise task, including the energy required to support resting energy requirements. After energy cost is estimated, the conversion factors discussed above can be used to convert $\dot{V}O_2$ into the appropriate energy expression required for application purposes, such as weight loss or weight gain goals.

Examples

Tracy, a 58-kg woman, would like to begin an exercise program.

1. You advise Tracy to walk at 3.0 mph on a treadmill at 10% grade. What is her $\dot{V}O_2$?
   Walking $\dot{V}O_2$ mL·kg^{-1}·minute^{-1} = (0.1 × speed) + (1.8 × speed × fractional grade) + 3.5 mL·kg^{-1}·minute^{-1}
   3.0 mph × 26.8 = 80.4 m·minute^{-1}
   10% grade = 0.10
   Walking $\dot{V}O_2$ mL·kg^{-1}·minute^{-1} = (0.1 × 80.4) + (1.8 × 80.4 × 0.10) + 3.5 mL·kg^{-1}·minute^{-1}
   Walking $\dot{V}O_2$ mL·kg^{-1}·minute^{-1} = 26 mL·kg^{-1}·minute^{-1}
2. How many METs is this exercise intensity?
   METs = $\dot{V}O_2$ mL·kg^{-1}·minute^{-1}/3.5
   METs = 26 mL·kg^{-1}·minute^{-1}/3.5
   METs = 7.432

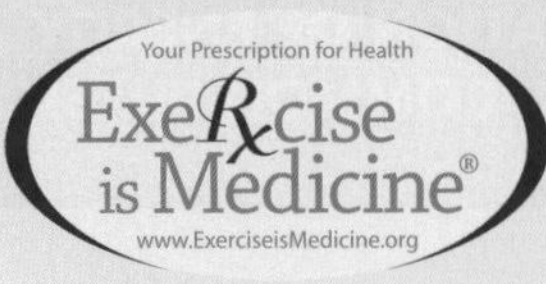

EXERCISE IS MEDICINE CONNECTION

Morris JN, Heady JA, Raffle PAB, Roberts CG, Parks JW. Coronary heart disease and physical activity of work. *Lancet.* 1953;265(6795):1053–7.

Famed British epidemiologist Dr. Jeremy Morris was one of the pioneers in helping establish a link between physical activity and coronary heart disease (CHD). In his landmark 1953 study (61), Morris and colleagues compared the incidence of CHD between conductors and drivers in London transport employees. Morris' main findings showed that the physically active conductors, whose job duties required climbing the stairs of London's fabled double-decker buses, had a different pattern of CHD from that of the bus drivers, who were sedentary for the majority of their workday. The physically active conductors had lower rates of CHD than the bus drivers, displayed symptoms of CHD at a much later age than the drivers, which were less severe, and had a substantially lower mortality rate of fatal myocardial infarction. Morris' findings that physical activity was protective against CHD were met with heavy skepticism from the prevailing conventional wisdom of the day, yet Morris pressed on, replicating his findings in future studies of postal workers and civil servants, consistently demonstrating the protective effects of regular physical activity and exercise in work and/or recreational pursuits. Dr. Morris' work also lends credence to the hazards of sedentary behavior, which have come under increased focus with the advent of inactivity physiology research. Thanks to the efforts of Dr. Morris, the HFS can enthusiastically educate clients that Exercise is Medicine.

3. Tracy decides that she would rather ride a stationary bicycle. What would be the equivalent work rate on the cycle ergometer?
   Leg cycling $\dot{V}O_{2max}$ mL·kg^{-1}·minute^{-1} = (1.8 × work rate/body weight) + (3.5) + (3.5 mL·kg^{-1}·minute^{-1})
   26 mL·kg^{-1}·minute^{-1} = (1.8 × work rate/58) + (3.5) + (3.5 mL·kg^{-1}·minute^{-1})
   19 mL·kg^{-1}·minute^{-1} = (1.8 × work rate/58)
   612 kg·m·minute^{-1} = work rate
4. If Tracy exercises as prescribed for 30 minutes, 5 days·week^{-1}, for 5 weeks, how much fat mass weight will Tracy lose? (Assume that her caloric intake stays consistent.)
   30 minutes·day^{-1} × 5 days·week^{-1} = 150 minutes·week^{-1}
   150 minutes·week^{-1} × 5 weeks = 750 total minutes
   $\dot{V}O_2$ = 26 mL·kg^{-1}·minute^{-1}
   26 mL·kg^{-1}·minute^{-1} × 58 kg = 1,450 mL·minute^{-1}
   1,450 mL·minute^{-1}/1,000 = 1.450 L·minute^{-1}
   1.450 L·minute^{-1} × 5 kcal = 7.25 kcal·minute^{-1}
   7.25 kcal·minute^{-1} × 750 minutes = 5,437.5 kcal
   5,437.5/3,500 = 1.55 lb of fat

FITT FRAMEWORK FOR THE DEVELOPMENT OF CRF IN APPARENTLY HEALTHY PEOPLE

The acronym FITT (F = frequency, I = intensity, T = time or duration, and T= type or mode) provides the framework to establish an exercise prescription in healthy individuals (Table 3.4). Given the wide array of fitness levels the HFS may encounter, the FITT principle may be customized to meet the unique goals and needs of the individual.

The CRF components of the FITT principle have been adopted from the most recent recommendations from the ACSM, American Heart Association, and the *2008 Physical Activity Guidelines for Americans.*

TABLE 3.4 AEROBIC (CARDIOVASCULAR ENDURANCE) EXERCISE EVIDENCE-BASED RECOMMENDATIONS

FITT-VP	Evidence-Based Recommendation
Frequency	• ≥5 d·wk^{-1} of moderate exercise, or ≥3 d·wk^{-1} of vigorous exercise, or a combination of moderate and vigorous exercise on ≥3 to 5 d·wk^{-1} is recommended.
Intensity	• Moderate and/or vigorous intensity is recommended for most adults. • Light- to moderate-intensity exercise may be beneficial in deconditioned persons.
Time	• 30–60 min·d^{-1} of purposeful moderate exercise, or 20–60 min·d^{-1} of vigorous exercise, or a combination of moderate and vigorous exercise per day is recommended for most adults. • <20 min of exercise per day can be beneficial, especially in previously sedentary persons.
Type	• Regular, purposeful exercise that involves major muscle groups and is continuous and rhythmic in nature is recommended.
Volume	• A target volume of ≥500 to 1,000 MET-min·wk^{-1} is recommended. • Increasing pedometer step counts by ≥2,000 steps·d^{-1} to reach a daily step count ≥7,000 steps·d^{-1} is beneficial. • Exercising below these volumes may still be beneficial for persons unable or unwilling to reach this amount of exercise.
Pattern	• Exercise may be performed in one (continuous) session per day, or in multiple sessions of ≥10 min, to accumulate the desired duration and volume of exercise per day. • Exercise bouts of <10 min may yield favorable adaptations in very deconditioned individuals
Progression	• A gradual progression of exercise volume by adjusting exercise duration, frequency, and/or intensity is reasonable until the desired exercise goal (maintenance) is attained. • This approach may enhance adherence and reduce risks of musculoskeletal injury and adverse coronary heart disease events.

Adapted from Garber CE, Blissmer B, Deschenes MR, et al. American College of Sports Medicine Position Stand. The quantity and quality of exercise for developing and maintaining cardiorespiratory, musculoskeletal, and neuromotor fitness in apparently healthy adults: Guidance for prescribing exercise. *Med Sci Sports Exerc.* 2011;43(7):1334–59.

The evidence-based recommendations for CRF following the FITT principle are as follows (9, 12, 42, 81):

Frequency

Moderate-intensity aerobic exercise should be done at least 5 days·week^{-1}, *or* vigorous-intensity aerobic exercise done at least 3 days·week^{-1}, *or* a combination of moderate- and vigorous-intensity aerobic exercise done at least 3 to 5 days·week^{-1}.

Intensity

A combination of moderate- (40%–59% $\dot{V}O_2R$) and/or vigorous-intensity (60%–84% $\dot{V}O_2R$) exercise is recommended for most healthy individuals. Intensity may be prescribed using multiple methods such as, but not limited to, HR reserve, rating of perceived exertion (RPE), percentage $\dot{V}O_{2max}$, and percentage of age-predicted maximal HR.

Time

For substantial health benefits, individuals should accrue at least 150 minutes·week^{-1} of moderate-intensity exercise *or* 75 minutes·week^{-1} of vigorous-intensity exercise *or* an equivalent combination of moderate and vigorous aerobic exercise. For additional and more substantial health benefits, moderate-intensity exercise may be increased to at least 300 minutes·week^{-1}, *or* vigorous-intensity exercise may be increased to at least 150 min·week^{-1}, *or* an equivalent combination of moderate and vigorous physical activity.

Type

All types of physical activity are beneficial as long as they are of sufficient intensity and duration. Rhythmic, continuous exercise that involves major muscle groups is the most typical choice; however, for more advanced individuals, intermittent exercise such as interval training or stop-and-go sports may be used to accumulate the recommended frequency, intensity, and time needed for CRF.

Inherent within the FITT framework are the following principles of training that the HFS must consider when prescribing cardiorespiratory exercise:

Progressive Overload

The overload principle is at the foundation of all exercise prescription. To improve CRF, the individual must exercise at a level greater than accustomed to induce adaptation. The HFS can implement the overload principle by manipulating the frequency, intensity, or time of the exercise prescription. For example, if a HFS is working with a client who typically runs on a treadmill at 75% maximal HR, for 30 minutes, 3 days·week^{-1}, the overload principle may be adhered to by increasing the intensity of the run to 80% of maximal HR, increasing the time spent running to 40 minutes, or increasing running to 4 days·week^{-1}. It is important for the HFS to understand that all variables should not be increased simultaneously, as small incremental progression allows the body to adapt, which is key to reducing the risk of overuse injuries (80).

Reversibility

The principle of reversibility can be viewed as the opposite of the overload principle. Commonly referred to as the "use it or lose it" principle, the reversibility principle dictates that once cardiorespiratory training is decreased or stopped for a significant period, previous improvements will reverse and decrease, and the body will readjust to the demands of the reduced physiological stimuli (68). Hard-earned gains in CRF can be lost if the training stimulus is removed, and the HFS should be aware that prior gains made with clients who have taken long breaks from training will necessitate readjusting previous exercise prescriptions.

Individual Differences

The principle of individual differences states that all individuals will not respond similarly to a given training stimulus (58). The HFS will encounter a wide range of individuals of varying age and fitness levels, each of whom will demonstrate varied responses to a given exercise stimulus. Within an exercise prescription for CRF, the HFS will encounter high and low responders because of the large genetic component that affects the degree of potential change in $\dot{V}O_{2max}$ (85). The variation in fitness levels necessitates a personalized exercise prescription based on the unique needs of the individual.

Specificity of Training

The specificity principle, also known as the SAID principle (specific adaptations to imposed demands), is dependent on the type and mode of exercise. The specificity principle states that specific exercise elicits specific adaptations, creating specific training effects (58). For example, if a HFS is working with a client who wishes to improve his or her time in an upcoming half-marathon, the principle of specificity dictates that in order to improve, the HFS needs to select a training stimulus specific to the activity in question. Thus, running would be the appropriate mode to select, as activities such as cycling or swimming do not train the specific muscles and movement patterns needed to complete a half-marathon.

SAFE AND EFFECTIVE EXERCISES DESIGNED TO ENHANCE CRF

As discussed in the introduction to the FITT framework, when designing an exercise program to develop CRF, the type of exercise that is generally prescribed to improve health and fitness is rhythmic and continuous and uses large muscle groups (9). Given the nearly unlimited number of ways to be physically active, there is no shortage of exercise options for the HFS to choose from when prescribing physical activity to enhance CRF. Exercise options can be viewed on a continuum, ranging from the relatively simple, such as brisk walking, to much more complex and vigorous, such as repeat 400-m interval sprints approaching 100% $\dot{V}O_{2max}$. Although the options to improve CRF may seem overwhelming at times, the ACSM has created a classification scheme to help the HFS make an appropriate exercise selection that matches the fitness level and unique interests of the clientele an HFS may be serving (9). Cardiovascular endurance exercises may be divided into four categories (Table 3.5):

Type A: endurance exercises requiring minimal skill or physical fitness to perform, such as walking or water aerobics
Type B: vigorous-intensity endurance exercises requiring minimal skill, such as running or spinning
Type C: endurance activities requiring skill to perform, such as cross-country skiing or in-line skating
Type D: recreational sports, such as tennis or basketball

Subsequently, the HFS can modify any activity from the four categories to best accommodate the skill level, physical fitness stage, and personal preferences of the individual or groups the HFS may be serving.

An additional method of classifying cardiorespiratory exercise that may be useful to the HFS is by weight-bearing or non–weight-bearing activities. Weight-bearing activities cause muscles and bones to work against gravity, such as jogging or aerobic dance, versus non–weight-bearing activities in which the stress on the bones, joints, and muscles is lessened, such as in cycling or swimming. Although some weight-bearing physical activity is important for bone health (24), many individuals may have orthopedic limitations that may necessitate the need to choose more nonimpact physical activity options. In addition, low-impact physical activity has a third or less of the injury risk of higher impact activities (81). The table below highlights five of the most popular exercise modalities (64) and the advantages and disadvantages of each.

TABLE 3.5 MODES OF AEROBIC (CARDIORESPIRATORY ENDURANCE) EXERCISES TO IMPROVE PHYSICAL FITNESS

Exercise Group	Exercise Description	Recommended for	Examples
A	Endurance activities requiring minimal skill or physical fitness to perform	All adults	Walking, leisurely cycling, aqua-aerobics, slow dancing
B	Vigorous intensity endurance activities requiring minimal skill	Adults (as per the preparticipation screening guidelines in Chapter 2) who are habitually physically active and/or at least average physical fitness	Jogging, running, rowing, aerobics, spinning, elliptical exercise, stepping exercise, fast dancing
C	Endurance activities requiring skill to perform	Adults with acquired skill and/or at least average physical fitness levels	Swimming, cross-country skiing, skating
D	Recreational sports	Adults with a regular exercise program and at least average physical fitness	Racquet sports, basketball, soccer, downhill skiing, hiking

Adapted from Armstrong LE, Brubaker PH, Whaley MH, Otto RM, American College of Sports Medicine. *ACSM's Guidelines for Exercise Testing and Prescription.* 7th ed. Baltimore (MD): Lippincott Williams & Wilkins; 2005. 366 p.

DETERMINING EXERCISE INTENSITY

The HFS has multiple options to determine the appropriate exercise intensity when prescribing physical activity to improve CRF. Options range from direct measurements in clinical or laboratory settings to more subjective ratings based on feelings of exertion or fatigue. The precision needed to determine exercise intensity will be dependent on the unique conditions, needs, and preferences of the clientele the HFS may be serving. The HFS may consider using any of the following methods to determine exercise intensity:

Heart Rate Reserve Method

The heart rate reserve (HRR), or Karvonen method, requires the HFS to determine the resting HR and maximum HR of the client. Resting HR is optimally measured in the morning while the client is in bed before rising (58), whereas maximum HR is best measured during a progressive maximal exercise test, but can also be estimated via age-predicted formulas (9). The HRR is the difference between maximum HR and resting HR. Target HR will be determined by considering the habitual physical activity, exercise level, and goals of the client (9). To assign a target HR, use the following formula:

$$\text{Target HR} = [(\text{Maximum HR}-\text{resting HR}) \times \%\ \text{intensity desired}] + \text{Resting HR}$$

For example, if your client has a maximum HR of 200 bpm and a resting HR of 60 bpm, and wishes to exercise at 65% to 75% of HRR, the HR range would be 151 to 165 bpm:

$[(200–60) \times 65\%] + 60 = \text{Target HR of } 151 \text{ bpm}$
$[(200–60) \times 75\%] + 60 = \text{Target HR of } 165 \text{ bpm}$

Peak HR Method

The peak HR method requires the HFS to determine the client's maximal HR. This may be accomplished from direct measurement, such as a $\dot{V}O_{2max}$ treadmill test, or maximum HR may be estimated from age-predicted formulas. Common estimation equations that the HFS may consider include the following:

- Maximum HR = 220 − age in years
- Maximum HR = 207 − (0.7 × age in years) (52)
- Maximum HR = 200 − (0.5 × age in years) (60)
- Maximum HR = 208 − (0.7 × age in years) (77)
- Maximum HR = 206.9 − (0.67 × age in years) (39).

The HFS should be aware that each of the above equations might overestimate maximum HR in certain populations, while underestimating in others (9). The HFS is advised to use maximal HR estimations only as a guide and to realize that estimates may not be accurate for certain individuals. Once maximal HR has been determined, the HFS may assign a target HR by following the formula:

$$\text{Target HR} = \text{Maximum HR} \times \%\ \text{intensity desired}$$

For example, if a client is 40 years old and has a selected workload of 85% of maximum HR, and the HFS chooses the equation Maximum HR = 206.9 – (0.67 × age) to estimate maximum HR, the calculations would be as follows:

$$206.9 - (0.67 \times 40) = \text{Estimated maximum HR of } 180 \text{ bpm}$$
$$180 \times 85\% = \text{Target HR of } 153 \text{ bpm}$$

Peak $\dot{V}O_2$ Method

The peak $\dot{V}O_2$ method may be used if the HFS has measured or estimated the $\dot{V}O_{2max}$ of the client in a laboratory or field setting. However, one should be cautious when assigning workload on the basis of estimated $\dot{V}O_{2max}$ because of the expected error in extrapolating HR (*e.g.*, 220–age = standard deviation of 12–15 bpm) (9). Once the $\dot{V}O_{2max}$ has been determined, the formula below may be followed:

$$\text{Target } \dot{V}O_2 = \dot{V}O_{2max} \times \% \text{ intensity desired}$$

For example, a HFS working with an individual with a measured $\dot{V}O_{2max}$ of 60 mL·kg^{-1}·minute^{-1}, with an exercise prescription of 90% maximum, would calculate the target $\dot{V}O_2$ as follows:

$$60 \times 90\% = \text{Target } \dot{V}O_{2max} \text{ of } 54 \text{ mL·kg}^{-1}\text{·min}^{-1}$$

Peak METs Method

In some instances, the HFS may choose the peak MET method to guide intensity. Whereas $\dot{V}O_{2max}$ is a relative measure of intensity, METs provide an absolute measure, allowing the intensity of various physical activity options to be compared with each other. Resources such as the Compendium of Physical Activity (2–4) feature extensive MET listings for a wide array physical activity options. Since 1 MET is equivalent to 3.5 mL·kg^{-1}·minute^{-1}, an individual's peak MET level can be determined simply by dividing one's measured or estimated $\dot{V}O_{2max}$ by 3.5. For example, an individual with a $\dot{V}O_{2max}$ of 35 would have a peak MET level of 10 METs. Once an individual's peak MET has been determined, the HFS can prescribe exercise at an appropriate workload by using a target MET level. The formula for determining target METs is as follows (11):

$$\text{Target METs} = (\% \text{ intensity desired}) [(\dot{V}O_{2max} \text{ in METs}) - 1] + 1$$

For example, for an individual with a $\dot{V}O_{2max}$ of 35 mL·kg^{-1}·minute^{-1} and who wants to exercise at an intensity of 70% the target METs can be calculated as follows:

Step 1: $\dot{V}O_{2max}$ in METs = 35 mL·kg^{-1}·minute^{-1}/3.5 mL·kg^{-1}·minute^{-1} = 10 METs
Step 2: Target METs = (0.70) (10 − 1) + 1
Step 3: Target METs = (0.70) (9) + 1
Step 4: Target METs = 6.3 + 1 = 7.3 METs

Thus, the HFS could select activities from the compendium of physical activities that correspond with a MET level between 7.0 and 7.5.

$\dot{V}O_2$ Reserve Method

The $\dot{V}O_2$ reserve ($\dot{V}O_2R$) method may be used when the HFS has directly measured or estimated the client's $\dot{V}O_{2max}$ and resting $\dot{V}O_2$ in a laboratory setting. The $\dot{V}O_2R$ is the difference between $\dot{V}O_{2max}$ and resting $\dot{V}O_2$. Target $\dot{V}O_2R$ will be dependent on the goals of the client:

$$\text{Target } \dot{V}O_2R = [(\dot{V}O_{2max} - \dot{V}O_{2rest}) \times \text{intensity desired}] + \dot{V}O_{2rest}$$

For example, for a client with a $\dot{V}O_{2max}$ of 35 mL·kg^{-1}·minute^{-1}, a resting $\dot{V}O_2$ of 3.5 mL·kg^{-1}·minute^{-1}, and a selected workload of 60% $\dot{V}O_2R$, the calculation would be as follows:

$$[(35\text{–}3.5) \times 60\%] + 3.5 = \text{Target } \dot{V}O_2R \text{ of } 22.4 \text{ mL·kg}^{-1}\text{·min}^{-1}$$

Talk Test Method

The talk test is a simple and convenient method to determine exercise intensity, especially for individuals who may be unaccustomed to physical activity. The talk test is a subjective measure of relative intensity, which helps differentiate between moderate and vigorous physical activity. If an individual is able to talk, but not sing, the physical activity is considered moderate. However, once the intensity of the activity increases to a point at which an individual is not able to say more than a few words without pausing for breath, the intensity would be considered vigorous (25, 81). Once comfortable speech is no longer possible, the vigorousness of the exercise may be outside the range for the individual to sustain, and the HFS can instruct the client to stop or reduce the level of effort.

Perceived Exertion Method

The perceived exertion method is another subjective rating of how hard one may be working. Perceived exertion is most commonly measured through Borg's RPE Scale, which ranges from 6 to 20, 6 meaning no exertion at all, and 20 meaning maximal exertion (25). The RPE range of 11 to 16 is recommended to improve CRF (7).

An additional perceived exertion scale for the HFS to be familiar with is Borg's Category Ratio Scale, commonly abbreviated as CR-10. The CR-10 uses a scale of 0 to 10, in which sitting is 0 and the highest level of effort possible is 10 (81). A CR-10 range of 5 to 8 corresponds with moderate (CR 5–6) and vigorous (CR 7–8) intensity physical activity.

ABNORMAL RESPONSES TO EXERCISE

Increases in HR, SBP, and ventilation, from rest, are normal responses to cardiorespiratory exercise in healthy individuals. Although the benefits and overall safety of cardiorespiratory exercise have been well established (9, 12), the HFS should be aware of potential abnormal responses to exercise that may necessitate the termination of exercise session and possibly require medical assistance. The "How to Read the Signs: Stopping an Exercise Test" provides general indications for stopping an exercise session (9). The HFS should consider that individuals who are detrained, returning from injury, or unaccustomed to physical activity may have a very low tolerance and capacity for exercise, and thus in addition to the general indications highlighted in the box below, the HFS should be judicious in the design of initial exercise prescriptions and communicate with his or her clients at all times.

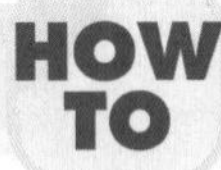

Read the Signs: Stopping an Exercise Test

The following lists general indications the HFS should watch for when giving an exercise test; being able to recognize these will avoid injury or problems.

- Onset of angina or angina-like symptoms
- Drop in SBP of ≥10 mm Hg with an increase in work rate, or if SBP decreases below the value obtained in the same position before testing
- Excessive rise in BP: SBP >250 mm Hg and/or DBP >115 mm Hg
- Shortness of breath, wheezing, leg cramps, or claudication
- Signs of poor perfusion: light-headedness, confusion, ataxia, pallor, cyanosis, nausea, or cold and clammy skin
- Failure of HR to increase with increased exercise intensity
- Noticeable change in heart rhythm by palpation or auscultation
- Participant requests to stop
- Physical or verbal manifestations of severe fatigue
- Failure of the testing equipment

*Assumes that testing is nondiagnostic and is being performed without direct physician involvement or electrocardiogram monitoring.

CONTRAINDICATIONS TO CARDIOVASCULAR TRAINING EXERCISES

The HFS will undoubtedly encounter individuals with physical or clinical limitations in which the risks of exercise testing and subsequent prescription may outweigh any potential benefits (9). Individuals with cardiac, respiratory, metabolic, or musculoskeletal disorders should be supervised by clinically trained personnel when beginning an exercise program (see Chapter 7 for more details on these populations). A thorough preexercise screening, obtaining informed consent, and review of medical history are necessary for the HFS to identify potential contraindications and to ensure the safety of the client (9). Chapter 2 provides greater detail on properly assessing risk factors along with Chapter 34, "Exercise Prescription and Medical Considerations" in *ACSM's Resource Manual for Guidelines for Exercise Testing and Prescription* (11). However, it is inevitable that the HFS will encounter apparently healthy clients who develop chest pain, breathing difficulty, musculoskeletal distress, or other worrisome symptoms during an exercise session. The HFS should immediately stop exercise, ensure client safety, and then refer the client to the appropriate health care professional.

EFFECT OF COMMON MEDICATIONS ON CARDIORESPIRATORY EXERCISE

It is not uncommon for the HFS to work with clients who may be taking prescribed and over-the-counter (OTC) medications. Whereas it is never the role of the HFS to administer, prescribe, or educate clients on the use or effects of medications (29), it is important for the HFS to understand the potential complex interactions of medication and exercise (63). Medications may alter HR, BP, and/or exercise capacity (9), and therefore clients taking medication should be strongly encouraged to communicate any changes in medication routines to the HFS (29). Please refer to Chapter 7 for the effect common OTC and prescription medications have on exercise.

SIGNS AND SYMPTOMS OF COMMON MUSCULOSKELETAL INJURIES ASSOCIATED WITH CR EXERCISE

Although a properly designed CRF prescription results in minimal risk (80), the HFS should be aware of the signs and symptoms of common musculoskeletal injuries associated with exercise (48).

- Exquisite point tenderness
- Pain that persists even when the body part is at rest
- Joint pain
- Pain that does not go away after warming up
- Swelling or discoloration
- Increased pain with weight-bearing activities or with active movements
- Changes in normal bodily functions

Previous research suggests that the amount of physical activity performed by an individual is directly related to the risk of musculoskeletal injury (80). The risk of injury is directly related to the increase in the amount of physical activity performed (80), and thus the chance for musculoskeletal injury increases as the individual performs exercise at greater levels of frequency and intensity (48). The individuals with whom the HFS may work will come from varied backgrounds, presenting a wide array of potential intrinsic and extrinsic risk factors that may predispose clients to injury (8). Common risk factors that the HFS may encounter are listed as follows (modified from Ref. 88):

Intrinsic Risk Factors
History of previous injury
Inadequate fitness or conditioning

Body composition
Bony alignment abnormalities
Strength or flexibility imbalances
Joint or ligamentous laxity
Predisposing musculoskeletal disease

Extrinsic Risk Factors
Excessive load on the body
Type of movement
Speed of movement
Number of repetitions
Footwear
Surface
Training errors
Excessive distances
Fast progression
High intensity
Running on hills
Poor technique
Fatigue
Adverse environmental conditions
Air quality
Darkness
Heat or cold
High humidity
Altitude
Wind
Worn or faulty equipment

Once the HFS has addressed potential risks, strategies to minimize injury may be employed, especially in at-risk individuals. The HFS should consider the age, level of fitness, and prior experience of potential clients when individualizing exercise prescriptions (81). It is recommended that the HFS use an intensity relative to a client's fitness level to usher in a desired level of effort, while slowly increasing the duration and frequency of physical activity before increasing intensity (81). Previous research suggests that the injury risk is increased in individuals who run, participate in sports, and engage in more than 1.25 hours·week^{-1} of physical activity (47). Therefore, when working with clients who may fit this profile, the HFS should take steps to minimize potential risk via proper assessment, client education, and exercise program design. In addition, the HFS should closely monitor increases in physical activity, especially in previously sedentary individuals, as the larger the overload to one's baseline physical activity, the greater the chance of injury (80).

EFFECTS OF HEAT, COLD, OR HIGH ALTITUDE ON THE PHYSIOLOGIC RESPONSE TO EXERCISE

Hot, cold, and high-altitude environments alter the typical physiological response to exercise. These extreme environments have the ability to stress our physiological systems to their maximal capacity and may negatively impact exercise performance before acclimatization (76). The HFS should be aware of the major challenges of exercise in hot, cold, and/or high-altitude environments and the impact of these environments on the physiological response to exercise.

Heat Stress

Hot environments reduce the body's ability to dissipate heat and thus promote an increase in core body temperature. In an effort to maintain a neutral body temperature when exposed to a hot environment, sweat rate and skin blood flow increase to promote heat loss (50). Although critical for heat dissipation, increased sweat rates and skin blood flow challenge the capacity of the cardiovascular system and may be the primary performance limiting factors during exercise in a hot environment (27). Increased sweat rates can cause a reduction in plasma volume and increase the risk of dehydration (73). Furthermore, increased sweat rates may lead to a decrease in SV, which then prompts an increase in HR to maintain cardiac output at submaximal workloads. This "HR drift," or elevated HR at submaximal loads, can decrease performance dramatically in a hot environment. Increased blood flow to the skin circulation comes at the expense of reduced blood flow to the working muscle (72). In addition to these primary cardiovascular limiting factors, other physiological changes occur during exercise in the heat that may contribute to reduced performance capacity, such as diminished central nervous system function and increased muscle glycogen utilization (27). The HFS should expect higher HR values at a given workload during exercise in the heat compared with exercise in a thermoneutral environment. HR may not reach a steady state during prolonged, submaximal intensity exercise because of the increased sweat rate, leading to cardiovascular drift. During CV drift, HR climbs over time, thereby decreasing overall performance (37, 49). Staying well hydrated during exercise may help attenuate CV drift.

Cold Stress

Exercise in a cold environment facilitates heat loss produced during exercise. However, long duration exercise events in a cold environment increase the risk of hypothermia. If core temperature is challenged, the body attempts to increase heat production and limit heat loss via shivering and vasoconstriction of blood vessels in the skin (27). Individuals with greater subcutaneous fat mass have an advantage at limiting heat loss in cold environments, as their thicker subcutaneous fat layer acts as form of insulation or barrier between the warm blood and the cold environment (74). The HR and cardiac output responses to exercise in a cold environment are similar to those of a thermoneutral environment (36); however, respiratory rate is higher at a given submaximal intensity and $\dot{V}O_{2max}$ may be slightly lower. The primary barrier to maximal performance in a cold environment may simply be the extra work associated with wearing bulky clothing during exercise. Bulky clothing increases the energy cost of exercise because of the extra weight of the clothing, alterations in movement resulting in augmented extraneous work, and increased friction as layers of clothing slide against each other during exercise (65, 78). Overall, the effect on $\dot{V}O_{2max}$ in a cold environment is negligible compared with that in a hot environment.

Altitude

Barometric pressure decreases with ascent to altitude. The partial pressure of oxygen (PO_2) is equal to the product of barometric pressure and the percentage of oxygen in the air. For example, the partial pressure at sea level is 760 mm Hg and the percentage of oxygen in dry air is 20.93%. Thus, the PO_2 at sea level is approximately 159 mm Hg ($PO_2 = 760 \times .2093$). If, however, you are at an altitude at which barometric pressure is only 550 mm Hg, the PO_2 now decreases to 115 mm Hg ($PO_2 = 760 \times .2093$). It is a common misconception that the "thin air" at altitude has less oxygen than the air at sea level; the percentage of oxygen in the air remains the same at all elevations in the stratosphere. It is the change in barometric pressure that causes the PO_2 to decrease at altitude and reduces our ability to provide oxygen to working muscles. In response to lower PO_2 at altitude, pulmonary ventilation increases. During the initial days of high-altitude exposure, SV decreases (5, 71) yet HR increases (41) to a greater extent, causing an increase in cardiac output at a given submaximal exercise intensity (84). There is typically no change noted in BP (71). Other changes that could affect performance when transferring to altitude include weight loss (70) and sleep disturbances (84). To stay at the same relative intensity of exercise (*e.g.*, submaximal HR), unacclimatized individuals will have to reduce the absolute intensity of exercise at a higher altitude because of the greater difficulty of doing exercise at the higher altitude. The time it takes to become acclimatized to altitude varies greatly between individuals and also depends on the local altitude. It is best for the HFS to assume that there will need to be a significant reduction in intensity and duration of exercise during the initial days of altitude adjustment, but that over time, exercise should become more comfortable.

ACCLIMATIZATION WHEN EXERCISING IN A HOT, COLD, OR HIGH-ALTITUDE ENVIRONMENT

Acclimatization is the process of physiological adaptation that occurs in response to changes in the natural environment. Acclimation is a related term, but refers to the process of physiological adaptation that occurs in response to experimentally induced changes in climate, such as an environmental chamber in a research laboratory (27). Both acclimatization and acclimation can improve exercise performance in extreme environments.

Heat acclimatization has been shown to elicit many favorable physiological responses that may improve exercise performance in a hot environment (13, 14, 26), such as lower core body temperature, lower skin temperature, higher sweat rate, higher plasma volume, lower HR at a specific workload, lower perception of effort, and improved conservation of sodium. As a whole, these physiological adaptations improve heat dissipation from the body to the environment and limit cardiovascular strain.

In general, heat acclimatization requires gradual exposure to exercise in the heat on consecutive days. In order for complete adaptation to occur, 2 to 4 hours of moderate- to high-intensity exercise in a hot environment for 10 consecutive days is suggested (56). Partial acclimation to the heat can also be completed by training athletes wearing additional layers of clothing in a cool environment (33). Although the acclimation benefits of this technique will never reach the magnitude of true acclimatization, it may serve a purpose when the alternative choice is no acclimation. The first few days of exercise in a hot or humid environment should be light in intensity with frequent rest periods provided. The intensity of exercise should gradually build to the length and intensity desired for performance. The benefits of acclimation decrease after only days of exposure to another climate (54) and completely dissipate after approximately 2 to 3 weeks (14). Thus, acclimatization to the heat occurs annually in individuals living in areas where there is a wide variation in climate across the course of the year.

Cold acclimatization causes the shivering threshold to be reset to a lower mean skin temperature. This is a positive adaptation as it suggests cold acclimatization enhances the ability to maintain heat production through means besides shivering (23). In addition, cold acclimatization has also been shown to improve maintenance of hand and feet temperatures (75), potentially attenuating the loss of dexterity that normally accompanies cold extremities.

Altitude acclimatization requires adjusting to the lower PO_2. The lower PO_2 at altitude stimulates the production of additional red blood cells (erythropoiesis) to increase the oxygen-carrying capacity of the blood. Within hours of ascent to altitude, the kidneys increase the release of the hormone erythropoietin to stimulate erythropoiesis, but this process takes time and the full benefits of erythropoiesis may not take effect for 4 or more weeks (27). After the oxygen-carrying capacity of the blood is restored via erythropoiesis, the HR, SV, cardiac output, and pulmonary ventilation responses to exercise revert back to more typical conditions. Today, many endurance athletes use altitude training to improve their athletic performance by practicing the "live high, train low" strategy (55), which is a unique strategy of gaining the benefits of high altitude acclimatization ("live high") and the maintenance of high-intensity training at sea level ("train low") to occur in synchrony. After returning to sea level, the benefits of altitude acclimatization have been shown to last up to 3 weeks (55).

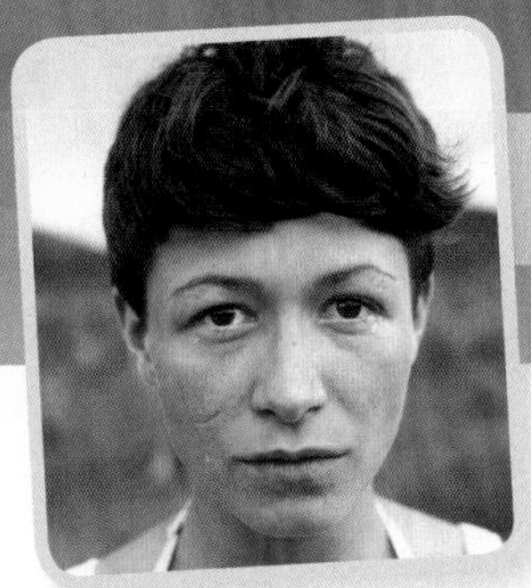

The Case of Sylvia

Submitted by **Leah Hantman, BS, ACSM-HFS, Franklin, MA, and Sarah Burnham, BS, ACSM-HFS, Somers, CT**

Sylvia is a 35-year-old single college professor who is challenged by adhering to a regular exercise routine. She needs variety to stay motivated. Teaching Sylvia about ways to use intensity and duration as a means of providing variety increased her ability to stay active. Sylvia's goal was to run the local Hot Chocolate 5K road race without walking.

Physical Data

Resting BP: 109/77 mm Hg
Resting HR: 78 bpm
Weight: 163 lb
Height: 66 in
Body mass index: 26.34 $kg \cdot m^{-2}$
Body fat percentage measured by calipers: 33.4
Cardio respiratory fitness measured by submaximal bike test: $\dot{V}O_{2max}$: 21.3 $mL \cdot kg^{-1} \cdot min^{-1}$
ACSM Risk Classification (1): Low

Psychosocial Assessment Data (2)

Sylvia viewed wellness as having the energy to complete her daily tasks and enough extra energy for extracurricular activities as well. Wellness for Sylvia involved feeling well rested, relaxed, and energetic. The most important thing to Sylvia when making her journey toward wellness was to increase her stamina to run a 5K race without stopping. She believed that by keeping a picture of her healthy self in mind and reminding herself that this journey is doing something truly good for herself and those she loves, she can overcome any obstacles. One of the biggest obstacles that Sylvia faced was time management. She was afraid that she would feel overwhelmed or tired and want to give up completely. She also got bored very quickly. Sylvia was very aware that she had control over her schedule and that she could use her stubborn nature to stick to a goal. Sylvia liked gadgets as a mechanism to help her stay on track. She also had a strong social support network of friends who were willing to help her reach her goals.

Sylvia's Program

Cardiorespiratory

Cardio will be done 3 days a week — 1 day interval and 2 days of free cardio like a group exercise class or a jog.

Interval

F: 1 day a week
I: 3 minutes HR_{max} 70% to 90% and RPE is 12 to 15 out of 20 (breath should be elevated and carrying on a conversation very difficult); 2 minutes of active recovery HR_{max} 50% to 60% and RPE is at 6 to 10 (can carry on a conversation and breathing is easier)
T: 30 to 45 minutes with warm-up and cool-down
T: intervals, cardio drills and plyometrics

continues

***The Case of Sylvia* cont.**

Free Cardio

F: 2 days a week
I: 60% to 80% HR_{max} and RPE 10 to 12
T: Goal of continual movement of 45 to 60 minutes by week 10
T: Jogging either outside or on a treadmill, a cardio group exercise class such as Zumba

Progression for Sylvia included a basic couch to 5K running program that included a progression of walk/runs to slow jog/runs to jog/runs to running at 60% to 80% HR_{max} for 45 minutes. It also incorporated hill workouts.

Muscular Fitness

F: 2 days a week
I: Reach muscle fatigue by 10 to 12 reps
T: 30 minutes or however long it takes to get through one set
T: Free weights, medicine balls, body weight, and machines

At first a workload of 70% intensity was suggested, but proved to be too high to start. Given Sylvia's $\dot{V}O_2$ of 21 $mL \cdot kg^{-1} \cdot minute^{-1}$ and her goals, interval training was suggested to burn calories and increase endurance while allowing Sylvia to ebb in and out of her comfort zone. Short bursts of high-intensity exercise (65%–85% of maximum HR) followed by lower-intensity recovery periods (50%–65% of maximum HR) proved to be more effective.

These target values of % HR_{max} provided a means of quantifying exercise intensity to optimize training results. If the optimal training intensity is 60% to 80% $\dot{V}O_{2max}$, then, according to the ACSM, the corresponding optimal training HR is 70% to 85% maximum HR (1). The theory of specific adaptations to imposed demands (SAID) and the 10% rule were applied throughout the program to ensure steady progression, avoid overtraining, and maintain self-efficacy in performance.

Sylvia completed the Hot Chocolate Run in just over 37 minutes. Her e-mail after the race showed the importance of using HR and RPE as useful feedback for training.

After the Race

Sylvia sent an e-mail after the race:

"I just wanted to thank you for your help over the last few weeks. I finished the Hot Chocolate Run faster than I anticipated. I think calibrating my RPE against my actual heart rate on Friday was HUGELY helpful. I ran further than I probably would have without stopping because I knew I was in a good workout range. When I did stop to walk (which I only did a few times), I timed myself, knowing from Friday's cardio workout that I only needed about 2 minutes max to lower my heart rate. I even kicked out the jams a little in the home stretch, sprinting to the finish line. Thanks."

Questions

- What is $\dot{V}O_2$ and how is it significant in cardiovascular fitness?
- What physiological adaptations and mental advantages come with interval training?
- In regard to $\dot{V}O_2$, what biometric traits might be correlated with physiological effect of lower levels of cardio fitness?
- What principle governs the 10% rule?

References

1. American College of Sports Medicine. *ACSM's Guidelines for Exercise Testing and Prescription*. 9th ed. Baltimore (MD): Lippincott Williams & Wilkins; 2013.
2. Bayati M, Farzad B, Gharakhanlou R, Agha-Alinejad H. A practical model of low-volume high-intensity interval training induces performance and metabolic adaptations that resemble "all-out" sprint interval training. *J Sports Sci Med*. 2011;10(3):571–6.
3. Charkoudian N. Physiologic considerations for exercise performance in women. *Clin Chest Med*. 2004;25:247–55.
4. Mannie K. Strategies for overload and progression. *Coach Athletic Dir*. 2006;75(9):8–12.
5. Moore M, Tschannen-Moran, R. *Coaching Psychology Manual*. Baltimore (MD): Lippincott Williams & Wilkins; 2009.

SUMMARY

Assessing and prescribing exercise is both an art and science; it should be taken as a serious responsibility by the HFS. There are numerous means of assessing CRF so that the HFS can accommodate a wide range of clientele safely. Also, the FITT principle provides a framework of prescribing exercise that also allows for tremendous individual variation.

Properly assessing and prescribing exercise can play a significant role in helping individuals initiate an enjoyable exercise program. Using the most appropriate assessment and prescription techniques limits all types of risk and provides the individual with a solid foundation to begin their lifetime of physical activity.

STUDY QUESTIONS

1. Maximal oxygen uptake is commonly used as a marker of aerobic exercise capacity. Explain the science behind this concept. In other words, how is oxygen used in the body and why does a greater maximal oxygen uptake equate to greater aerobic exercise capacity?
2. Write out the Fick equation. Define each term within the Fick equation and discuss how each component of the equation changes with exercise training.
3. A 165 lb woman is walking on the treadmill at 3 mph at 2% grade for 30 minutes. Calculate the $\dot{V}O_2$, METs, and estimated caloric expenditure of this activity.
4. Using the HRR method, what is the target HR range for a 55-year-old man with a resting HR of 72 bpm, with an exercise prescription of 60% to 70% of HRR?
5. Describe your cardiorespiratory exercise options for a 55-year-old obese woman with a history of lower back, knee, and ankle pain. What exercises may be contraindicated for this person and what are some alternative choices?

REFERENCES

1. Adams GM, Beam WC. *Exercise Physiology: Laboratory Manual*. 5th ed. New York (NY): McGraw-Hill; 2008.
2. Ainsworth BE, Haskell WL, Leon AS, et al. Compendium of physical activities: classification of energy costs of human physical activities. *Med Sci Sports Exerc*. 1993;25(1):71–80.
3. Ainsworth BE, Haskell WL, Whitt MC, et al. Compendium of physical activities: An update of activity codes and MET intensities. *Med Sci Sports Exerc*. 2000;32(9):S498–516.
4. Ainsworth BE, Haskell WL, Herrmann SD, et al. 2011 Compendium of physical activities: A second update of codes and MET values. *Med Sci Sports Exerc*. 2011;43(8):1575–81.
5. Alexander JK, Hartley LH, Modelski M, Grover RF. Reduction of stroke volume during exercise in man following ascent to 3,100 m altitude. *J Appl Physiol*. 1967;23:849–58.
6. American College of Obstetricians and Gynecologists. Exercise during pregnancy and the postpartum period. ACOG Committee Opinion No 267. *Obstet Gynecol*. 2002;99:171–73.
7. American College of Sports Medicine. *ACSM's Guidelines for Exercise Testing and Prescription*. 7th ed. Philadelphia (PA): Lippincott Williams & Wilkins; 2006.
8. American College of Sports Medicine. *ACSM's Resource Manual for Guidelines for Exercise Testing and Prescription*. 5th ed. Philadelphia (PA): Lippincott Williams & Wilkins; 2006.
9. American College of Sports Medicine. *ACSM's Guidelines for Exercise Testing and Prescription*. 9th ed. Philadelphia (PA): Lippincott Williams & Wilkins; 2013.
10. American College of Sports Medicine. *ACSM's Health Related Physical Fitness Assessment Manual*. 3rd ed. Philadelphia (PA): Lippincott Williams & Wilkins; 2009.
11. American College of Sports Medicine. *ACSM's Resource Manual for Guidelines for Exercise Testing and Prescription*. 6th ed. Philadelphia (PA): Lippincott Williams & Wilkins; 2010.
12. American College of Sports Medicine. Position Stand. Quantity and quality of exercise for developing and

maintaining cardiorespiratory, musculoskeletal, and neuromotor fitness in apparently healthy adults: Guidance for prescribing exercise. *Med Sci Sports Exerc.* 2011;43(7):1334–59.

13. Armstrong LE, Costil DL, Fink WK. Changes in body water and electrolytes during heat acclimation: Effects of dietary sodium. *Aviat Space Environ Med.* 1987;58:143–8.
14. Armstrong LE, Maresh CM. The induction and decay of heat acclimatization in trained athletes. *Sports Med.* 1991;2:302–12.
15. Artal R, O'Toole M. Guidelines of the American College of Obstetricians and Gynecologists for exercise during pregnancy and the postpartum period. *Brit J Sports Med.* 2003;37(1):6–12.
16. Astrand P-O, Ryhming I. A nomogram for calculation of aerobic capacity (physical fitness) from pulse rate during submaximal work. *J Appl Physiol.* 1954;7:218–21.
17. Astrand P-O. Aerobic work capacity in men and women with specific reference to age. *Acta Physiol Scand.* 1960;49(suppl):45–60.
18. Astrand PO, Cuddy TE, Saltin B, Stenberg J. Cardiac output during submaximal and maximal work. *J Appl Physiol.* 1964;19:268–74.
19. Astrand P-O. Principles of ergometry and their implications in sport practice. *Int J Sports Med.* 1984;5:102–5.
20. Astrand P-O, Rodahl K, Dahl HA, Stromme SB. *Textbook of Work Physiology: Physiological Bases of Exercise.* 4th ed. Champaign (IL): Human Kinetics; 2003.
21. Blair SN, Kohl HW, Barlow CE, Paffenbarger RS, Gibbons LW, Macera CA. Changes in physical fitness and all-cause mortality: A prospective study of healthy and unhealthy men. *JAMA.* 1995;273:1093–8.
22. Brouha L. The step test: A simple method of measuring physical fitness for muscular work in young men. *Res Quart Exerc Sport.* 1991;14:31–6.
23. Bruck K. Basic mechanisms in longtime thermal adaptation. In: Szelenyl Z, Szekely M, editors. *Advances in Physiological Science.* Vol. 23. Oxford (England): Pergamon Press; 1980. 263 p.
24. Centers for Disease Control and Prevention Web site [Internet]. Atlanta (GA): Centers for Disease Control and Prevention; [cited 2011 Aug 3]. Available from: http://www.cdc.gov/physicalactivity/everyone/health/index.html#StrengthenBonesMuscles
25. Centers for Disease Control and Prevention Web site [Internet]. Atlanta (GA): Centers for Disease Control and Prevention; [cited 2011 Aug 11]. Available from: http://www.cdc.gov/physicalactivity/everyone/measuring/index.html
26. Cheung SS, McLellan TM. Influence of heat acclimation, aerobic fitness, and hydration effects on tolerance during uncompensable heat stress. *J Appl Physiol.* 2000;84:1731–9.
27. Cheung SS. *Advanced Environmental Exercise Physiology.* Champaign (IL): Human Kinetics; 2010.
28. Christie J, Sheldahl LM, Tristani FE, Sagar KB, Ptacin JJ, Wann S. Determination of stroke volume and cardiac output during exercise: Comparison of two-dimensional and Doppler echocardiography, Fick oximetry, and thermodilution. *Circulation.* 1987;76:539–47.
29. Clark MA, Lucett S, Corn RJ. *NASM Essentials of Personal Fitness Training.* 3rd ed. Philadelphia (PA): Lippincott Williams & Wilkins; 2008.
30. Cooper KH. Testing and developing cardiovascular fitness within the United States Air Force. *J Occup Med.* 1968;10(11):636–9.
31. Cooper KH. A means of assessing maximal oxygen intake. Correlation between field and treadmill testing. *JAMA.* 1968;203(3):201–4.
32. Dawson B. Exercise training in sweat clothing in cool conditions to improve heat tolerance. *Sports Med.* 1994;17:233–44.
33. Davis JH. Anaerobic threshold: Review of the concept and directions for future research. *Med Sci Sports Exerc.* 1985;17:6–21.
34. Dempsey FC, Butler FL, Williams FA. No need for a pregnant pause: Physical activity may reduce the occurrence of gestational diabetes mellitus and preeclampsia. *Exerc Sports Sci Rev.* 2005;33:141–9.
35. diPrampero P, Boutellier U, Pietsch P. Oxygen deficit and stores at onset of muscular exercise in humans. *J Appl Physiol.* 1983;55:146–53.
36. Doubt TJ. Physiology of exercise in the cold. *Sport Med.* 1991;11:367–81.
37. Ekelund LG. Circulatory and respiratory adaptation during prolonged exercise of moderate intensity in the sitting position. *Acta Physiol Scand.* 1967;69:327–40.
38. Gaesser G, Brooks G. Metabolic bases of excess post exercise oxygen consumption: A review. *Med Sci Sports Exerc.* 1984;16:29–43.
39. Gellish RL, Goslin BR, Olson RE, McDonald A, Russi GD, Moudgil VK. Longitudinal modeling of the relationship between age and maximal heart rate. *Med Sci Sports Exerc.* 2007;39(5):822–9.
40. Gledhill N, Cox D, Jamnik V. Endurance athletes stroke volume does not plateau: Major advantage is diastolic function. *Med Sci Sports Exerc.* 1994;26:1116–21.
41. Grover, R, Reeves JT, Grover EB, Leathers JE. Muscular exercise in young men native to 3,100 m altitude. *J Appl Physiol.* 1967;22:555–64.
42. Haskell WL, Lee IM, Pate RR, et al. Physical activity and public health: Updated recommendation for adults from the American College of Sports Medicine and the American Heart Association. *Med Sci Sports Exerc.* 2007;39(8):1423–34.
43. Hickson RC, Bomze HA, Holloszy JO. Faster adjustment of O_2 update to the energy requirement of exercise in the trained state. *J Appl Physiol.* 1978;44(6):877–81.
44. Higginbotham MB, Morris KG, Williams RS, McHale PA, Coleman RE, Cobb FR. Regulation of stroke volume during submaximal and maximal upright exercise in normal man. *Circ Res.* 1986;58:281–91.
45. Hill A. The oxidative removal of lactic acid. *J Physiol.* 1914;48: x–xi.
46. Holmgren A, Johnson B, Sjostrand T. Circulatory data in normal subjects at rest and during exercise in recumbent position, with special reference to the stroke volume at different work intensities. *Acta Physiol Scand.* 1960;49:343–63.
47. Hootman JM, Macera CA, Ainsworth BE, Martin M, Addy CL, Blair SN. Association among physical activity level, cardiorespiratory fitness, and risk of musculoskeletal injury. *Am J Epidemiol.* 2001;154(3):251–8.
48. Howley ET, Franks BD. *Health Fitness Instructor's Handbook.* 4th ed. Champaign (IL): Human Kinetics; 2003.
49. Johnson JM, Rowell LB. Forearm and skin vascular responses to prolonged exercise in man. *J Appl Physiol.* 1975;39:920–92.
50. Kenney WL, Munce T. Aging and human temperature regulation. *J Appl Physiol.* 2003;95:2598–603.
51. Kline GM, Porcari JP, Hintermeister R, et al. Estimation of VO_{2max} from a one-mile track walk, gender, age, and body weight. *Med Sci Sports Exerc.* 1987;19(3):253–9.
52. Kraemer, WJ, Fleck SJ, Deschenes MR. *Exercise Physiology: Integrating Theory and Application.* Philadelphia (PA): Lippincott Williams & Wilkins; 2012.

53. Lee IM, Buchner DM. The importance of walking to public health. *Med Sci Sports Exerc.* 2008;40(7):S512–18.
54. Lee SMC, Williams WJ, Schneider SM. Role of skin blood flow and sweating rate in exercise thermoregulation after bed rest. *J Appl Physiol.* 2002;92:2026–34.
55. Levine BD, Stray-Gundersen J. "Living high-training low": Effect of moderate-altitude acclimatization with low-altitude training on performance. *J Appl Physiol.* 1997;83(1):102–12.
56. Lind AR, Bass DE. Optimal exposure time for development of acclimatization to heat. *Fed Proc.* 1963;22:704–8.
57. Mariz JS, Morrison JF, Peter J. A practical method of estimating an individual's maximal oxygen uptake. *Ergonomics.* 1961;4:97–122.
58. McArdle WD, Katch FI, Katch VL. *Exercise Physiology: Nutrition, Energy, and Human Performance.* 7th ed. Philadelphia (PA): Lippincott Williams & Wilkins; 2010.
59. Medbo JI, Mohn AC, Tabata I, Bahr R, Vaage O, Sejersted OM. Anaerobic capacity determined maximal accumulated O_2 deficit. *J Appl Physiol.* 1988;64: 50–60.
60. Miller WC, Wallace JP, Eggert KE. Predicting max HR and the HR-VO2 relationship for exercise prescription in obesity. *Med Sci Sports Exerc.* 1993;25(9):1077–81.
61. Morris JN, Heady JA, Raffle PAB, Roberts CG, Parks JW. Coronary heart disease and physical activity of work. *Lancet.* 1953;265(6795):1053–7.
62. Morrow JR Jr, Jackson AW, Disch JG, Mood DP. *Measurement and Evaluation in Human Performance.* 4th ed. Champaign (IL): Human Kinetics; 2011.
63. Muse T. Cardiovascular medication and your client. *IDEA Health and Fitness Association Web site* [Internet]. IDEA Fitness Journal May 2006 [cited 2011 Aug 12]. Available from: http://www.ideafit.com/files/pdf/fitness-library/cardiovascular-medication-and-your-client-0
64. National Sporting Goods Association. *2010 Participation — Ranked by Total Participation* [Internet]. 2011 [cited 2011 Aug 18]. 1 p. Available from: http://www.nsga.org/files/public/2010Participation_Ranked_by_TotalParticipation_4Web.pdf.
65. Patton JF. The effects of acute cold exposure on exercise performance. *J Appl Sport Sci Res.* 1988; 2:72–8.
66. Pickering TG, Hall JE, Appel LJ, et al. Recommendations for blood pressure measurement in humans and experimental animals: Part 1: Blood pressure measurement in humans: A statement for professionals from the Subcommittee of Professional and Public Education of the American Heart Association Council on High Blood Pressure Research. *Hypertension.* 2005;45:142–61.
67. Phillips EM, Capell J, Jonas S. Getting started as a regular exerciser. In: Jonas S, Phillips EM, editors. *Exercise is Medicine: A Clinician's Guide to Exercise Prescription.* Philadelphia (PA): Lippincott Williams & Wilkins; 2009.
68. Plowman SA, Smith DL. *Exercise Physiology for Health, Fitness, and Performance.* 3rd ed. Philadelphia (PA): Lippincott Williams & Wilkins; 2011.
69. Powers S, Dodd S, Beadle R. Oxygen update kinetics in trained athletes differing in VO_{2max}. *Eur J Appl Physiol.* 1985;54:306–8.
70. Pugh LGCE. Physiological and medical aspects of the Himalayan Scientific and Mountaineering Expedition, 1960–1961. *BMJ.* 1962; 2:621–33.
71. Reeves JT, Groves BM, Sutton JR, et al. Operation Everest II: Preservation of cardiac function at extreme altitude. *J Appl Physiol.* 1987;63:531–9.
72. Rowell LB. *Human Cardiovascular Control.* New York (NY): Oxford University Press; 1993.
73. Shirreffs SM, Armstrong LE, Cheuvront SN. Fluid and electrolyte needs for preparation and recovery from training and competition. *J Sports Sci.* 2004;22:57–63.
74. Smith RM, Hanna JM. Skinfolds and resting heat loss in cold air and water: Temperature equivalence. *J Appl Physiol.* 1975;39:93–102.
75. Stocks J, Taylor N, Tipton M, Greenleaf J. Human physiological responses to cold exposure. *Aviat Space and Environ Med.* 2004;75:444–57.
76. Suzuki Y. Human physical performance and cardiorespiratory responses to hot environments during submaximal upright cycling. *Ergonomics.* 1980;23:527–42.
77. Tanaka HK, Monahan KD, Seals DR. Age-predicted maximal heart rate revisited. *J Am Coll Cardiol.* 2001;37(1):153–6.
78. Teitlebaum A, Goldman RF. Increased energy cost with multiple clothing layers. *J Appl Physiol.* 1972;32:743–4.
79. U.S. Department of Health and Human Services. *The Seventh Report of the Joint National Committee on Prevention, Detection, Evaluation, and Treatment of High Blood Pressure (JNC7)–Complete Report.* Bethesda (MD): National Heart, Lung, and Blood Institute; 2004.
80. U.S. Department of Health and Human Services. *Physical Activity Guidelines Advisory Committee Report 2008.* Washington (DC): ODPHP Publication No. U0049; 2008.
81. U.S. Department of Health and Human Services. *2008 Physical Activity Guidelines for Americans.* Washington (DC): ODPHP Publication No. U0036; 2008.
82. Wasserman K, Whipp BJ, Koyal SN, Beaver WL. Anaerobic threshold and respiratory gas exchange during exercise. *J Appl Physiol.* 1973; 35:236–43.
83. Wei M, Kampert JB, Barlow CE, et al. Relationship between low cardiorespiratory fitness and mortality in normal-weight, overweight, and obese men. *JAMA.* 1999;282(16):1547–53.
84. West, JB. Physiology of extreme altitude. In: Fregly MJ, Blatteis CM. *Handbook of Physiology: Section 4: Environmental Physiology, Volume II.* New York (NY): Oxford University Press; 1996.
85. Wilmore JH, Costill DL, Kenney WL. *Physiology of Sport and Exercise.* 4th ed. Champaign (IL): Human Kinetics; 2008.
86. *YMCA Fitness Testing and Assessment Manual.* Champaign (IL): Human Kinetics; 1989.
87. Zhou B, Conlee RK, Jensen R, Fellingham GW, George JD, Fisher AG. Stroke volume does not plateau during graded exercise in elite male distance runners. *Med Sci Sports Exerc.* 2001;33:1849–54.
88. Renstrom P, Kannus P. Prevention of sports injuries. In: Strauss RH, editor. *Sports Medicine.* Philadelphia (PA): WB Saunders; 1992.

CHAPTER

4 Muscular Strength and Muscular Endurance Assessments and Exercise Programming for Apparently Healthy Participants

Avery Faigenbaum

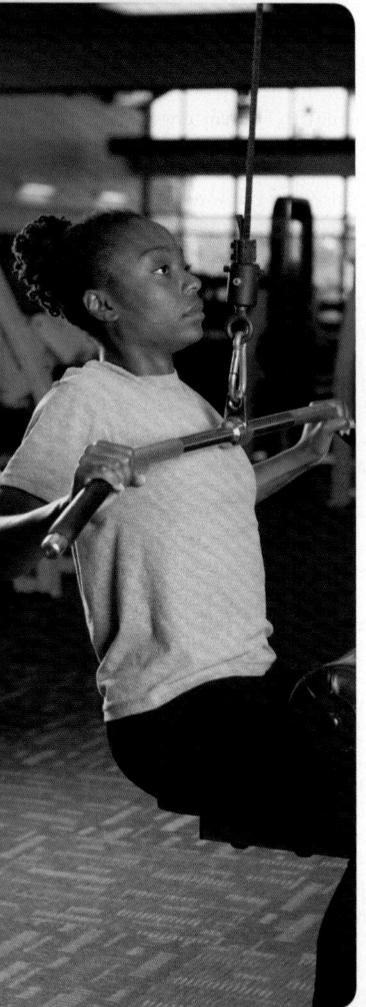

CHAPTER OBJECTIVES

- To understand the importance of muscular strength and endurance for health and fitness.
- To describe the basic structure and function of muscle.
- To explain the fundamental principles of resistance training.
- To identify resistance training program variables.
- To compare different resistance exercise modalities.
- To design resistance training programs for apparently healthy adults and individuals with medically controlled disease.

The development of muscular strength and muscular endurance is an essential component of health-related physical fitness. Since the 1980s, there has been a tremendous increase in the number of scientific publications on this topic, and resistance training has become a top 10 worldwide fitness trend (21, 48, 61). Like aerobic exercise, regular participation in a training program designed to enhance muscular strength and muscular endurance can improve the quality of life for men and women of all ages and abilities (64). The American College of Sports Medicine® (ACSM) recommends participating in a comprehensive fitness program that includes resistance exercise, and the World Health Organization now recognizes the potential benefits of muscle-strengthening activities for active adults (21, 47, 66).

In addition to enhancing all components of muscular fitness (*i.e.*, muscular strength, muscular endurance, and muscular power), regular participation in a resistance training program is associated with significantly better cardiometabolic risk profiles (27), lower risk of all-cause mortality (20), and fewer cardiovascular disease events (20). Resistance training can improve body composition as well as selected health-related biomarkers, including blood glucose levels (56) and insulin sensitivity (30). Further, an increase in lean body mass as a result of resistance training can contribute to the maintenance of, or increase in, resting or basal metabolic rate (45).

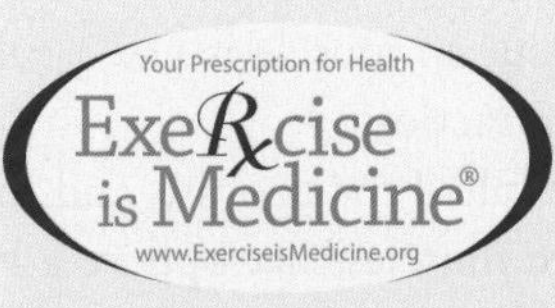

EXERCISE IS MEDICINE CONNECTION

Strength Training Can Lower Resting Blood Pressure

Cornelissen V, Fagard R, Coeckelberghs E, Vanhees L. Impact of resistance training on blood pressure and other cardiovascular risk factors. *Hypertension.* 2011;58(5):950–8.

While it has long been established that aerobics-based exercise can lower resting blood pressure (BP), there is a common misperception that resistance training does not confer the same benefit. In fact, some even discourage resistance training, particularly in middle-aged and older adults, or those with cardiovascular disease, because of misplaced fears about increases in BP. In response to this misperception, Cornelissen and colleagues performed a meta-analysis of randomized controlled trials investigating the effects of resistance training on resting BP and other cardiovascular risk factors in adults (13). All the trials lasted at least 4 weeks and included dynamic (concentric and eccentric muscle actions) or static (isometric muscle actions) resistance training. In a majority of the trials, participants in the control group were instructed not to modify their physical activity and nutrition habits. Overall, resistance training induced a significant decrease in resting BP with a mean reduction of 3.9 mm Hg in the normotensive or prehypertensive groups. The hypertensive groups also saw lowered resting BP of about the same magnitude; however, this decrease was not statistically significant. Isometric handgrip training and dynamic resistance training resulted in a decrease in BP of 13.5 and 2.8 mm Hg, respectively. In addition to the BP benefits, dynamic resistance training significantly increased $\dot{V}O_2$ peak and significantly reduced body fat percentage and plasma triglycerides. This meta-analysis suggests that both dynamic and isometric resistance training may have a beneficial effect on systolic and diastolic BP in individuals who are currently normotensive or even in prehypertensives. In addition, the clinical significance of these findings comes from large, prospective interventions, which suggest that small reductions in resting BP of 3 mm Hg can reduce the risk of coronary heart disease, stroke, and all-cause mortality (39).

Resistance training over months or years can increase bone mass and has proven to be a valuable measure for preventing, or even reversing, the loss of bone mass in people with osteoporosis (31). Importantly, regular participation in a resistance training program can contribute to an improved health-related quality of life by enhancing physical function, attenuating age-related weight gain, and enabling people to do what they enjoy while maintaining their independence (40, 42, 64).

This chapter provides a basic overview of muscle structure and function, highlights the fundamental principles of resistance exercise, and outlines program design considerations for developing, implementing, and progressing resistance training programs that are consistent with individual needs, goals, and abilities. In this chapter, the term *resistance training* (also known as *strength training*) refers to a specialized method of physical conditioning that involves the progressive use of a wide range of resistive loads and a variety of training modalities designed to enhance muscular fitness. The term *resistance training* should be distinguished from the terms *bodybuilding* and *powerlifting,* which are competitive sports.

BASIC STRUCTURE AND FUNCTION

An understanding of the basic structure and function of the muscular system is important for designing fitness programs and optimizing training adaptations. Many of the fundamental principles of resistance training discussed later in this chapter are grounded in an understanding of muscle structure and function. Although the body has more than 600 skeletal muscles that vary in shape and size, the basic purpose of skeletal muscle, especially during resistance training, is to provide force to move the joints of the body in different directions.

The smallest contractile unit within a muscle is called a sarcomere, which is made up of different proteins. A myofibril consists of many sarcomeres, and groups of myofibrils make up a single muscle fiber or muscle cell. Different types of connective tissue called fascia surround these structures and create a stable, yet flexible, environment. The connective tissue in muscle is like a rubber band that stretches and recoils to provide added force to a muscle contraction.

The muscles that are the primary movers of a joint are called the agonists and the muscles that assist in that movement are called synergists. Antagonists are muscles that oppose a movement. For example, during the biceps curl exercise, the biceps brachii and brachialis are the agonists for that movement, the brachioradialis is the synergist, and the triceps brachii is the antagonist. Only the parts of a muscle that are used during an exercise will adapt to the training stress; furthermore, different training loads stimulate different amounts of muscle. That is why it is important to understand muscle structure and be aware that different training loads recruit different muscle fibers.

Muscle Fiber Types and Recruitment

Although skeletal muscle is made up of thousands of muscle fibers, there are generally two types of muscle fibers. Type I fibers (also called slow twitch fibers) have a high oxidative capacity and a lower contractile force capability and are better for endurance activities. Type II fibers (also called fast twitch fibers) have a high glycolytic capacity and a higher contractile force capability and are better for strength and power activities. Although each muscle fiber type has various subtypes (type IIa, IIx), the ratio of type I and type II fibers in the body varies for each person and depends mainly on hereditary factors. Regular resistance training may cause a small change in fiber type composition, but these changes are primarily from one subgroup of fiber to another subgroup of fiber. Thus, resistance training will not convert type I fibers to type II fibers, but different training loads and different movement speeds can alter the involvement of different types of muscle fibers in a given movement (19).

Since muscle fibers that are not stimulated will not reap the benefits of training, it is important to understand how muscle fibers are recruited for action. Muscle fibers are innervated by a motor neuron, and this neuromuscular gathering is called a motor unit. Although each motor unit is composed of either all type I or all type II fibers, the size of a motor unit as well as the number of fibers within a motor unit varies within different muscles. The size principle of motor unit activation states that motor units are recruited from the smallest to the largest, depending on the force production demands. Smaller or low-threshold motor units (mostly type I fibers) are recruited first, and larger or high-threshold motor units (mostly type II fibers) are recruited later, depending on the demands of the exercise (see Fig. 4.1).

Training with heavy loads that can be lifted only four to six times (*e.g.*, a 4–6 repetition maximum [RM]) will activate higher-threshold motor units than training with a load that can be lifted 12 to 15 times (*e.g.*, a 12–15 RM). However, even if heavy loads are lifted, low-threshold motor units will be recruited first, and then high-threshold motor units will be activated as needed to produce the necessary force. Although exceptions exist, to recruit high-threshold motor units, specific types of resistance exercise that involve lifting heavy loads, moving lighter loads at a fast velocity, or both are needed to achieve a training effect in these muscle fibers (19). The concept of training periodization or program variation (discussed later in this chapter) is based on the principle that different training loads and power requirements recruit different types and numbers of motor units.

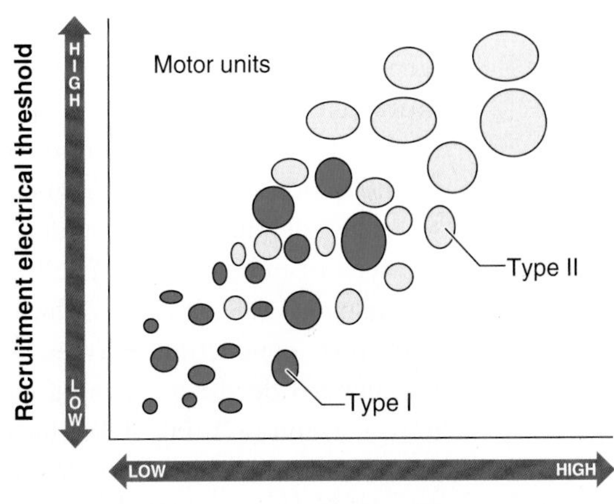

FIGURE 4.1. Size principle of motor unit recruitment. (Reproduced with permission from Baechle TR, Earle RW, editors. *Essentials of Strength Training and Conditioning*. 3rd ed. Champaign (IL): Human Kinetics; 2008. 97 p.)

Types of Muscle Action

Muscles can perform different types of muscle actions. When a weight is lifted, the involved muscles normally shorten and this is called a concentric muscle contraction, and when a weight is lowered, the involved muscles lengthen and this is called an eccentric muscle action. For example, when an individual extends the hips and knees from a parallel squat position to the standing phase, the gluteus maximus and vastus lateralis perform concentric muscle contractions (see Fig. 4.2). The gluteus maximus and vastus lateralis perform eccentric muscle action when the weight is lowered from the standing phase to the parallel squat position. If a muscle is activated but no movement at the joint

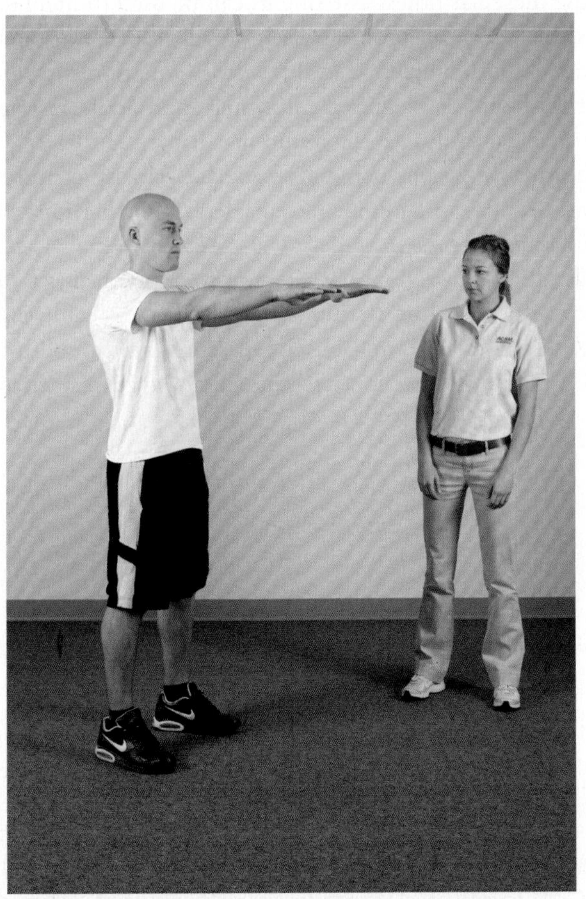

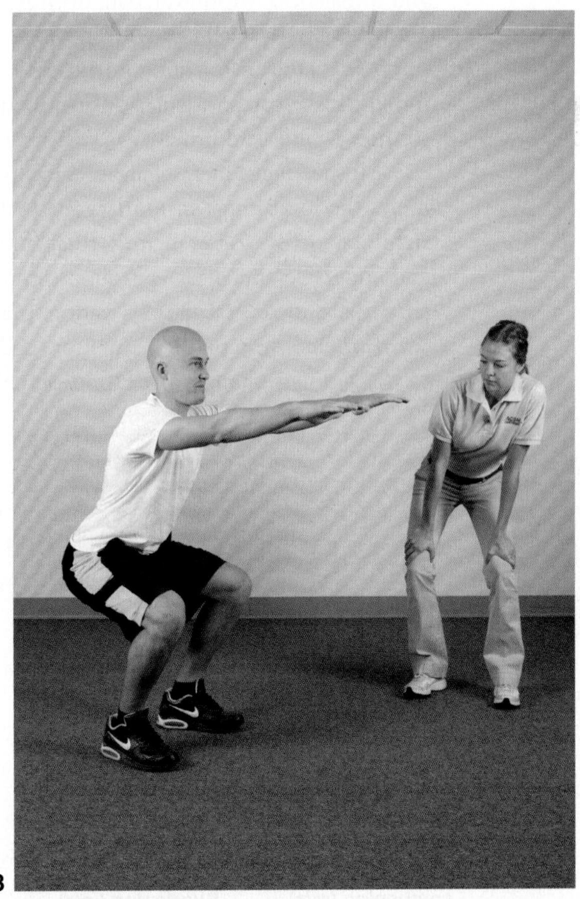

FIGURE 4.2. Squat without weights starting position **(A)** and squat position **(B)**.

takes place, the muscle action is called isometric (or static). This type of muscle action takes place during the standing phase of the squat exercise when the weight is held stationary and no visible movement occurs. Isometric muscle actions also occur when the weight is too heavy to lift any further. This typically happens during the "sticking point" of an exercise when the force produced by the muscle equals the resistance.

The amount of force produced by a muscle is dependent on a number of factors, including the type of muscle action. The highest force produced occurs during an eccentric muscle action, and maximal force produced during an isometric muscle action is greater than that seen during a concentric contraction. Further, as the velocity of movement increases, the amount of force that is generated decreases during a concentric muscle contraction and increases during an eccentric muscle action (47) (Fig. 4.3). This is an important consideration when designing resistance training programs because high force development during maximal eccentric muscle actions has been linked to muscle soreness (23). Although eccentric muscle actions are a potent stimulus for increases in muscle size and strength (16), a gradual and progressive introduction to resistance training is warranted to reduce the risk of a muscle strain. Even trained individuals who accentuate the eccentric phase of a lift can experience muscle soreness for several days after an exercise session (44). Moreover, extended periods of eccentric training with very heavy loads can result in serious complications such as rhabdomyolysis, which may harm kidney function (11).

ASSESSMENT PROTOCOLS

Muscular fitness can be assessed by a variety of laboratory and field-based measures. Results from muscular fitness tests can provide valuable information about an individual's baseline fitness and can be used to design individualized resistance training programs that target muscle weaknesses and imbalances. Moreover, data from periodic muscular fitness assessments can be used to highlight a client's progress and provide positive feedback that can promote exercise adherence. For safety purposes, adults who undergo fitness testing should complete a health history questionnaire, and individuals at cardiovascular or orthopedic risk should be identified and, when appropriate, referred to their health care provider (1). More information on this can be found in Chapter 2.

Muscular fitness tests are specific to the muscle groups being assessed, the velocity of movement, the joint range of motion (ROM), and the type of equipment available (1). Furthermore, no single test exists for evaluating total body muscular fitness, so professionals need to carefully select and supervise the most appropriate muscular fitness tests for each client. Also, individuals should participate in several familiarization/practice sessions before testing and adhere to a specific protocol (including repetition duration and ROM) to obtain a reliable fitness score that can be used to track fitness changes over time. Since an acute bout of static stretching may have adverse effects

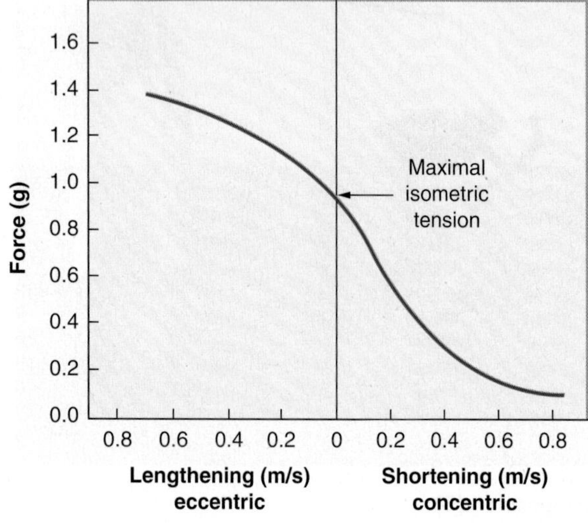

FIGURE 4.3. Force-velocity relationship. (From Ratamess N. *ACSM's Foundations of Strength Training and Conditioning*. Baltimore (MD): Lippincott Williams & Wilkins; 2012:25.)

on subsequent strength performance, large amplitude dynamic movements (also known as dynamic stretching) and test-specific activities should precede muscular fitness testing (3).

An initial assessment of muscular fitness and a change in muscular strength or muscular endurance over time can be based on the absolute value of the weight lifted or the total number of repetitions performed with proper technique. Although population-specific norms are available for most health-related muscular fitness tests, when strength comparisons are made between individuals, the values should be expressed as relative values (per kilogram of body weight). For example, a client who weighs 100 kg and lifts 75 kg on the chest press exercise has a relative strength score of 0.75 $kg \cdot kg^{-1}$, whereas a client who weighs 80 kg and lifts the same amount of weight on the same exercise has a relative strength score of 0.94 $kg \cdot kg^{-1}$. Although both clients have the same absolute strength on the chest press exercise, the lighter client has a higher measure of relative upper body strength, and this is an important consideration when comparing individual strength performance between clients.

Assessing Muscular Strength

Muscular strength is typically assessed in fitness facilities with dynamic measures that involve the movement of an external load or body part. Although isometric strength can be measured conveniently using different devices such as handgrip dynamometers, these measures are specific to the muscle group and joint angle and therefore provide limited information regarding overall muscular strength. The 1 RM, which is the heaviest weight that can be lifted only once using proper technique, is the standard muscular strength assessment (33). However, a multiple RM such as a 10 RM can also be used to assess muscular strength and provide valuable information regarding an individual's training program. For example, if a client was training with an 8 to 12 RM weight, the performance of a 10 RM strength test could provide an index of strength changes over time.

Procedures for administering 1 RM (or multiple RM) strength tests after the familiarization period and an adequate warm-up are outlined in the "how to" box. A familiarization period is particularly important for individuals with no prior resistance exercise experience because they need to learn proper exercise technique and be taught how to produce maximal effort during the test. A proper familiarization period (*e.g.*, 2 weeks of resistance training including 3–4 practice sessions for each exercise) will likely achieve appropriate familiarization and reliability for RM strength testing (33). Moreover, communication between the health fitness specialist (HFS) and the client can help determine a progression pattern of loading with reasonable accuracy. In terms of safety, properly trained spotters are needed to enhance strength testing procedures, particularly during the performance of free weight exercises such as the bench press and back squat.

Normative data for the chest press and leg press exercises are available in *ACSM's Guidelines for Exercise Testing and Prescription* (1). However, additional research is needed to provide norms for

HOW TO Assess One-Repetition Maximum (1 RM) Strength

1. Warm up for 5 to 10 min with low-intensity aerobic exercise.
2. Perform a specific warm-up with several repetitions with a light load.
3. Select an initial weight that is within the subject's perceived capacity (~50%–70% of capacity).
4. Attempt a 1 RM lift; if successful, rest approximately 3 to 5 min before the next trial.
5. Increase resistance progressively (*e.g.*, 2.5–20 kg) until the subject cannot complete the lift. A 1 RM should be obtained within four sets to avoid excessive fatigue.
6. The 1 RM is recorded as the heaviest weight lifted successfully through the full ROM with proper technique.

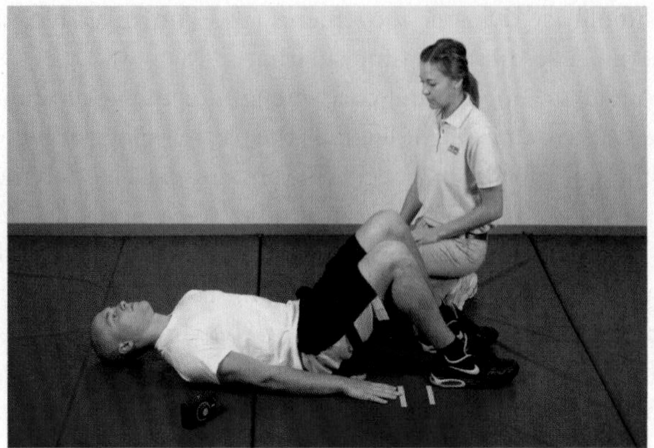
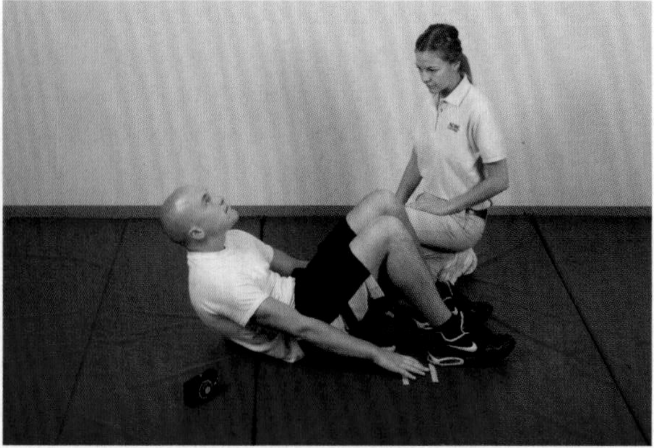

FIGURE 4.4. Starting position **(A)** and the curled up position **(B)** of the client when performing the partial curl-up test.

different exercises and different types of resistance training equipment since 1 RM performance is significantly greater on weight machines than free weights (41).

Assessing Muscular Endurance

Muscular endurance is the ability to perform repeated contractions over a period and is typically assessed with field measures such as the abdominal curl-up (Fig. 4.4) or push-up tests (Fig. 4.5). These tests can be used independently or in combination with other tests of muscular endurance to screen for muscle weaknesses and aid in the exercise prescription. For example, poor abdominal strength is thought to contribute to lower back pain, and muscles of the upper body are used in many activities of daily life (25, 40). Procedures for administering the curl-up and push-up tests are described in the "how to" boxes. Normative data for the curl-up and push-up tests are available in *ACSM's Guidelines for Exercise Testing and Prescription* (1). Of note, overweight individuals may find these tests difficult to perform, and poor results obtained during testing may discourage participation in an exercise program. HFS should carefully consider which tests are appropriate for each individual and most likely to yield beneficial information.

FUNDAMENTAL PRINCIPLES OF RESISTANCE TRAINING

Simply engaging in resistance training does not ensure that muscular fitness gains will occur. Training programs need to be based on fundamental training principles and carefully prescribed to optimize outcomes. Although factors such as initial level of fitness, heredity, age, gender, nutritional

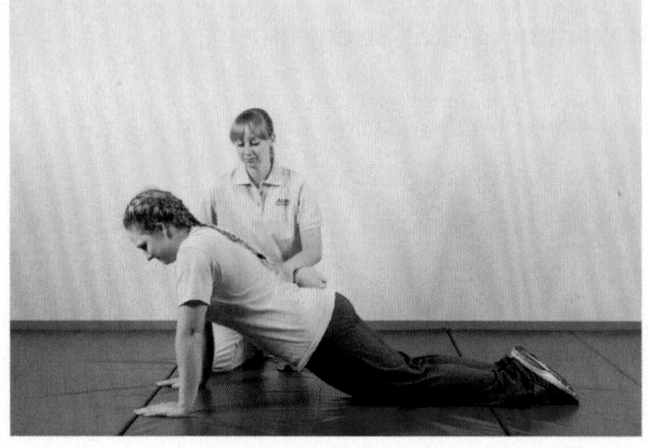
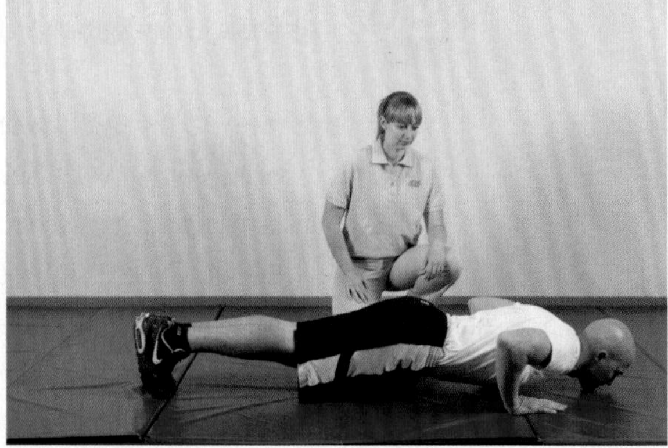

FIGURE 4.5. Proper positioning for the push-up test: **(A)** the starting position for women and **(B)** the downward position for men.

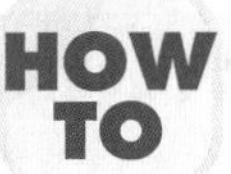

Assess Abdominal Strength and Endurance with the Curl-Up Test

1. Explain the purpose of the test to the client (to determine how many curl-ups can be completed to reflect abdominal muscular strength and endurance).
2. Explain proper breathing technique (to exhale with the effort, which occurs when curling up from the floor).
3. Two strips of masking tape are to be placed on a mat on the floor at a distance of 12 cm apart (for clients/patients younger than 45 years) or 8 cm apart (for clients/patients older than 45 years).
4. Subjects are to lie in a supine position across the tape, knees bent at 90° with feet on the floor and arms extended to their sides, such that their fingertips touch the nearest strip. This is the bottom position. To reach the top position, subjects are to flex their spines to 30°, reaching their hands forward until their fingers touch the second strip of tape.
5. A metronome is to be set at 40 beats per minute. At the first beep, the subject begins the curl-up, reaching the top position at the second beep, returning to the starting position at the third, top position at the fourth, etc.
6. Repetitions are counted each time the subject reaches the bottom position. The test is concluded either when the subject reaches 75 curl-ups or the cadence is broken.
7. Demonstrate first and provide every subject several practice repetitions prior to the start of the test.

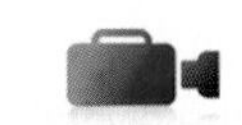

Visit thePoint to watch video 4.1, which demonstrates the partial curl-up test.

Alternatives include having the hands held across the chest with the head activating a counter when the trunk reaches a 30° position and placing the hands on the thighs and curling up until the hands reach the knee caps. Elevation of the trunk to 30° is the important aspect of the movement.

Descriptions of procedures are adapted from the American College of Sports Medicine. *ACSM's Guidelines for Exercise Testing and Prescription.* 9th ed. Baltimore (MD): Lippincott Williams & Wilkins; 2014.

status, and health habits (*e.g.*, sleep) will influence the rate and magnitude of adaptation that occurs, four fundamental principles that determine the effectiveness of all resistance training programs are (a) the principles of Progression, (b) Regularity, (c) Overload, and (d) Specificity. These basic principles can be remembered as the PROS of resistance training program design.

Principle of Progression

The principle of progression refers to the fact that the demands placed on the body must be continually and progressively increased over time to achieve long-term gains in muscular fitness. This does not mean that heavier weights should be used every workout, but rather that over time the physical stress placed on the body should gradually become more challenging to continually stimulate adaptations. Without a more challenging exercise stimulus that is consistent with individual needs, goals, and abilities, the human body has no reason to adapt any further. This principle is particularly important after the first few months of resistance training when the threshold for training-induced adaptations in conditioned individuals is higher (19).

At the start of a resistance training program, the 10 RM on the leg press might be 50 kg, which is likely an adequate stimulus to promote adaptations. But as training progresses, 10 repetitions with 50 kg would be suboptimal for stimulating gains in muscle fitness strength as 50 kg "feels easy" for 10 repetitions. If the training load is not increased at a rate that is compatible with the training-induced adaptations that are occurring, no further gains in muscular fitness will occur. A reasonable guideline for a beginner is to increase the training weight about 5% to 10% per week and decrease

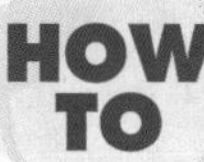

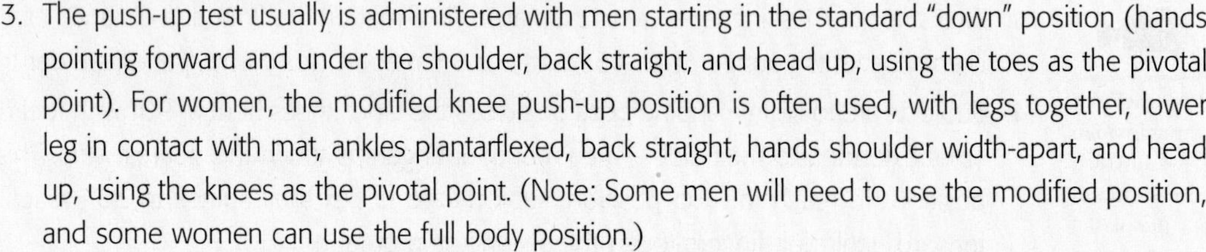

HOW TO Assess Upper Body Strength and Endurance with the Push-Up Test

1. Explain the purpose of the test to the client (to determine how many push-ups can be completed to reflect upper-body muscular strength and endurance).
2. Inform clients of proper breathing technique (to exhale with the effort, which occurs when pushing away from the floor).
3. The push-up test usually is administered with men starting in the standard "down" position (hands pointing forward and under the shoulder, back straight, and head up, using the toes as the pivotal point). For women, the modified knee push-up position is often used, with legs together, lower leg in contact with mat, ankles plantarflexed, back straight, hands shoulder width-apart, and head up, using the knees as the pivotal point. (Note: Some men will need to use the modified position, and some women can use the full body position.)
4. The subject must raise the body by straightening the elbows and return to the "down" position, until the chin touches the mat. The stomach should not touch the mat.
5. For both men and women, the subject's back must be straight at all times and the subject must push-up to a straight-arm position.
6. Demonstrate the test and allow the client to practice if desired.
7. Remind the client that the maximal number of push-ups performed consecutively without rest is counted as the score.
8. Begin the test when the client is ready. Stop the test when the client strains forcibly or is unable to maintain the appropriate exercise technique within two repetitions.

Descriptions of procedures are adapted from the American College of Sports Medicine. *ACSM's Guidelines for Exercise Testing and Prescription*. 9th ed. Baltimore (MD): Lippincott Williams & Wilkins; 2014.

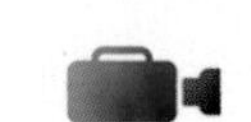

Visit thePoint to watch video 4.2, which demonstrates the push-up test for men and women.

the repetitions by 2 to 4 when a given load can be performed for the desired number of repetitions with proper exercise technique. For example, if an adult can perform 12 repetitions of the leg press exercise with proper exercise technique using 50 kg, he should increase the weight to 55 kg and decrease the repetitions to 8 if he wants to continually make gains in muscular strength. A more conservative approach would be to follow the "2 plus 2" rule. That is, once this client can perform two or more additional repetitions over the assigned repetition goal on two consecutive workouts, weight should be added to the leg press exercise during the next training session. Alternatively, he could increase the number of sets, increase the number of repetitions, or add another leg exercise to his exercise routine.

Individuals who have achieved a desired level of muscular fitness may not need to progress the training program to maintain that level of performance. However, program variation is important for exercise adherence, and experienced exercisers may benefit from periodically changing program variables to keep the training stimulus fresh and challenging. For example, altering the order of exercises or mode of resistance training can limit training plateaus.

Principle of Frequency

Resistance training must be performed regularly several times per week to make continual gains in muscular fitness. Although the optimal training frequency may depend on training status and program design, two to three training sessions per week on nonconsecutive days are reasonable for most adults. Inconsistent training will result in only modest training adaptations, and periods of inactivity will result in a loss of muscular strength and size (26, 38). The adage "use it or lose it" is appropriate for resistance exercise because training-induced adaptations cannot be stored. Although adequate recovery is needed between resistance training sessions, the principle of frequency states that long-term gains in muscular fitness will be realized only if the program is performed on a regular basis.

Principle of Overload

The overload principle is a basic tenet of all resistance training programs. The overload principle simply states that to enhance muscular fitness, the body must exercise at a level beyond that at which it is normally stressed. For example, an adult who can easily complete 10 repetitions with 20 kg while performing a chest press exercise must increase the weight, the repetitions, or the number of sets if she wants to increase her upper body strength. Otherwise, if the training stimulus is not increased beyond the level to which the muscles are accustomed, she will not maximize training adaptations even if other aspects of the training program are well designed. Overload is typically manipulated by changing the exercise intensity, duration, or frequency.

Principle of Specificity

The principle of specificity refers to the distinct adaptations that take place as a result of the training program. For example, the adaptations to resistance training are specific to the muscle actions, velocity of movement, exercise ROM, muscle groups trained, energy systems involved, and intensity and volume of training (51). The principle of specificity is often referred to as the SAID principle (which stands for specific adaptations to imposed demands). In terms of designing resistance training programs, only muscle groups that are trained will make desired adaptations in selected parameters of muscular fitness. Exercises such as the squat and leg press can be used to enhance lower body strength, but these exercises will not affect upper body strength.

In addition, the adaptations that take place in a muscle or muscle group will be as simple or as complex as the stress placed on them. For example, because basketball requires multiple-joint and multiplanar movements in the sagittal (*i.e.*, left to right), frontal (*i.e.*, front to back), and transverse (*i.e.*, upper to lower) planes, it seems prudent for basketball players to include muscle actions and complex movements that closely mimic the demands of their sport. Anatomical views of the sagittal, frontal, and transverse planes of the human body are shown in Figure 4.6. An understanding of basic biomechanics and exercise movements that take place in these planes will help HFS select exercises that are consistent with specific movement patterns, muscle actions, and joint angles that need to be trained.

It is also important that the exercises and joint ranges of motion in the training program are consistent with the demands of the target activity. Hence, the specificity principle also applies to the design of resistance training programs for individuals who want to enhance their abilities to perform activities of daily life such as stair climbing and yard work, which require multiple-joint and multiplanar movements. Observations of a sport or activity (with or without video analysis) can provide the HFS with information regarding the relevant movements and appropriate ranges of motion that are particularly important to train. The potential benefits of movement-specific resistance training are highlighted by the growing popularity of medicine balls, stability balls, and other exercise devices that are often used to enhance rotational strength, muscle power, postural control, and agility.

PROGRAM DESIGN CONSIDERATIONS

Resistance training programs should be based on a participant's health status, current fitness level, personal interests, and individual goals. By assessing the needs of each participant and applying the fundamental principles of training to the program design, safe and effective resistance training programs can be developed for each individual. Of note, the health status of each participant should be assessed

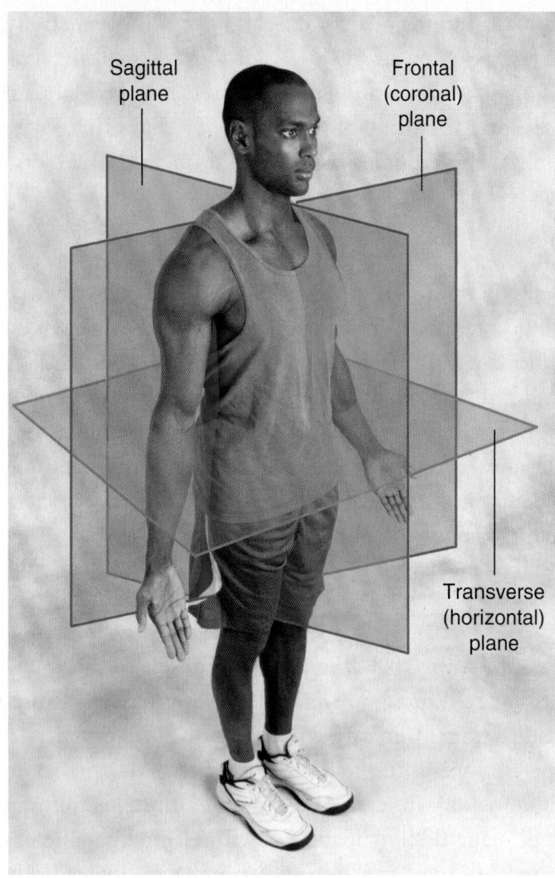

FIGURE 4.6. Anatomical planes of the human body. (From Bushman B, editor. *ACSM's Resources for the Personal Trainer.* 4th ed. Baltimore (MD): Lippincott Williams & Wilkins; 2014.)

before participating in a resistance training program because it is important to identify "at-risk" individuals who may need medical clearance and a modification of their exercise prescription (1).

An important factor to consider when designing resistance training programs is the participant's current fitness status or previous experience resistance training. Those who have the least experience resistance training tend to have a greater capacity for improvement compared with those who have been resistance training for several years. Although any reasonable resistance training program can be used to increase the muscle strength of untrained individuals, more advanced programs are needed to produce desirable adaptations in trained individuals. This is based on the observation that the potential for adaptation gradually decreases as training experience increases. Thus, as individuals gain experience with resistance training, more complex programs are needed to make continual gains in muscular fitness (19).

Types of Resistance Training

Different types of resistance training have proven to be effective for enhancing muscular fitness (8, 19, 62). Although each type of resistance exercise has advantages and disadvantages, there are several important factors to consider when selecting one type of training over another or including multiple types within a given training program. The most common types of resistance training include dynamic constant external resistance (DCER) training, variable resistance training, isokinetics, and plyometrics.

DCER Training

DCER training is the most common method of resistance training for enhancing muscular fitness. DCER describes a type of training in which the weight lifted does not change during the lifting (concentric) and lowering (eccentric) phase of an exercise. Although the term *isotonic* was traditionally used to describe this type of training, this term literally means constant (*iso*)tension (*tonic*). Because tension exerted by a muscle as it shortens varies with the mechanical advantage of the joint and the length of the muscle fibers at a particular joint angle, the term *isotonic* does not accurately describe this method of resistance exercise.

Different types of training equipment, including free weights (*e.g.*, barbells and dumbbells) and weight machines, and endless combinations of sets and repetitions can be used for DCER training. Weight machines generally limit the user to fixed planes of motion. However, they are easy to use and are ideal for isolating muscle groups. Free weights are less expensive and can be used for a wide variety of different exercises that require greater proprioception, balance, and coordination. In addition to improving health and fitness, DCER training is commonly used to enhance motor performance skills and sports performance. For example, total body weightlifting exercises such as the power clean (Fig. 4.7) and snatch are recognized as some of the most effective exercises for increasing muscle power because they require explosive movements and a more complex neural activation pattern than do traditional strength-building exercises such as the chest press or leg extension (34).

During DCER training, the weight lifted does not change throughout the ROM. Because muscle tension can vary significantly when a DCER exercise is performed, the heaviest weight that can be lifted throughout a full ROM is limited by the strength of a muscle at the weakest joint angle. As a result, DCER exercise provides enough resistance in some parts of the movement range but not enough resistance in others. For example, during the barbell bench press exercise, more weight can be lifted during the last part of the exercise than in the first part of the movement when the barbell is being pressed off the chest.

In an attempt to overcome this limitation, mechanical devices that operate through a lever arm or cam have been designed to vary the resistance throughout the exercise's ROM. These devices are known as variable resistance machines and theoretically force the muscle to contract maximally throughout the ROM by varying the resistance to match the exercise strength curve. These machines can be used to train all the major muscle groups, and by automatically changing the resistive force throughout the movement range, they provide proportionally less resistance in weaker segments of the movement and more resistance in stronger segments of the movement. Like all weight machines, variable resistance machines provide a specific movement path that makes the exercise

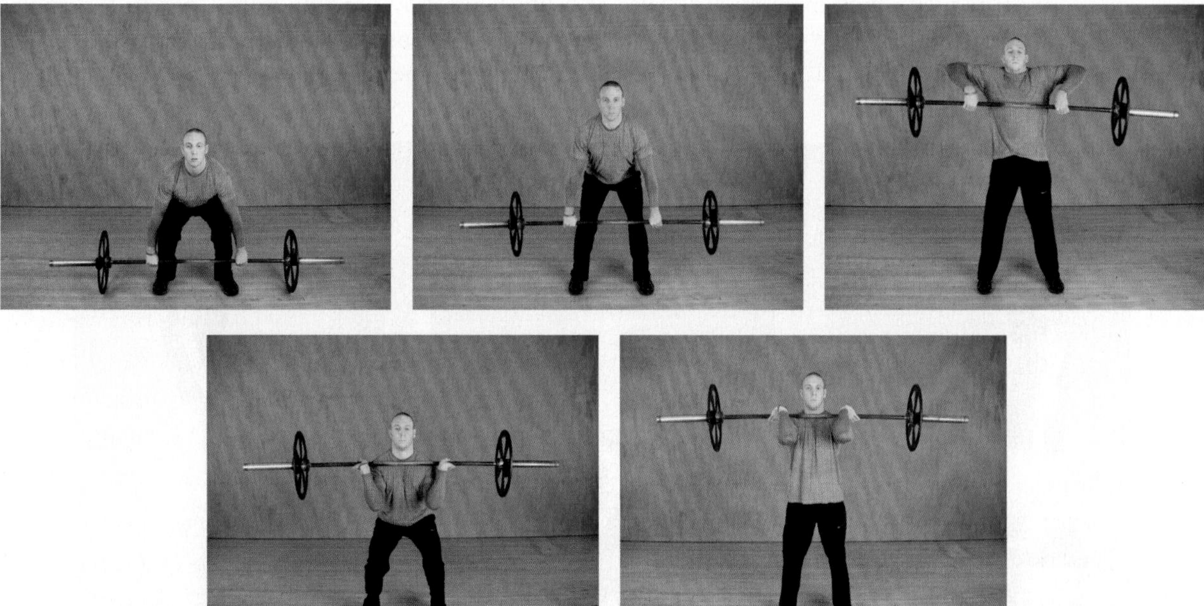

FIGURE 4.7. The clean: beginning, first pull, transition, second pull, and catch positions. (From Ratamess N. *ACSM's Foundations of Strength Training and Conditioning.* Baltimore (MD): Lippincott Williams & Wilkins; 2012:356.)

easier to perform, compared with free weight exercises, which require balance, coordination, and the involvement of stabilizing muscle groups.

Isokinetics

Isokinetic training involves dynamic muscular actions that are performed at a constant angular limb velocity. This type of training requires specialized equipment, and most isokinetic devices are designed to train only single-joint movements. Isokinetic machines generally are not used in fitness centers, but this type of training is used by physical therapists and certified athletic trainers for injury rehabilitation. Unlike other types of resistance training, the speed of movement — rather than the resistance — is controlled during isokinetic training. If the purpose of the exercise program is to increase strength at higher velocities (*e.g.*, for enhanced sports performance), performing high-speed isokinetic training appears prudent. Since data from isokinetic studies support velocity specificity (28), the best approach may be to perform isokinetic training at slow, intermediate, and fast velocities to develop increased strength and power at different movement speeds.

Plyometric Training

Plyometric training refers to a specialized method of conditioning designed to enhance neuromuscular performance (15). Unlike traditional strength-building exercises such as the bench press and squat, plyometric training is characterized by quick, powerful movements that involve a rapid stretch of a muscle (eccentric muscle action) immediately followed by a rapid shortening of the same muscle (concentric muscle action). This type of muscle action provides a physiological advantage because the muscle force generated during the concentric muscle action is potentiated by the preceding eccentric muscle action (32). Although both concentric and eccentric muscle actions are important for plyometric training, the amount of time it takes to change direction from the eccentric to the concentric phase of the movement is a critical factor in plyometric training (6). This period is called the amortization phase, which should be as short as possible (<0.1 s) to maximize training adaptations. Individuals can achieve significant gains in muscular fitness from a training program that includes plyometrics provided the exercises are sensibly progressed and performed with proper technique (10, 15).

Exercises that involve jumping, skipping, hopping, and other explosive movements with medicine balls can be considered a type of plyometric training. Although plyometric exercises are often associated with high-intensity drills such as depth jumps (*i.e.*, jumping from a box to the ground and then immediately jumping upward; Fig. 4.8), less intense activities such as double leg hops and jumping jacks can also be considered a type of plyometric exercise because every time the

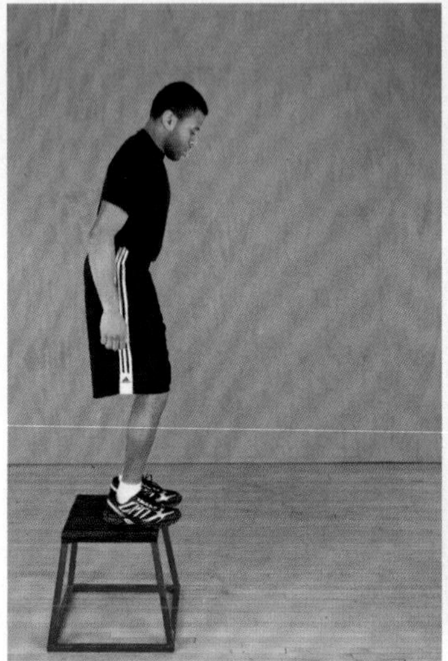
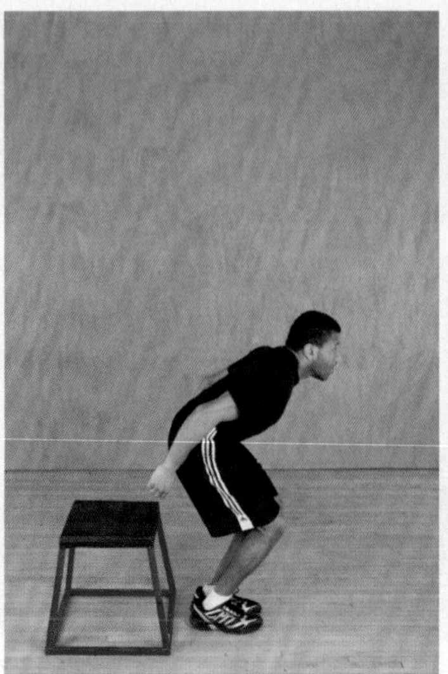
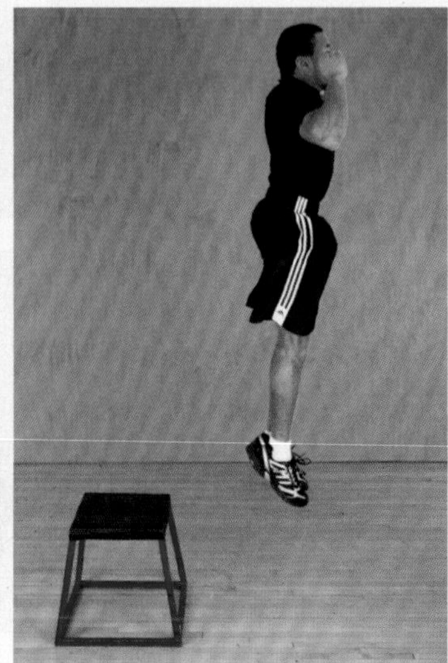

FIGURE 4.8. Depth jump. (From Ratamess N. *ACSM's Foundations of Strength Training and Conditioning.* Baltimore (MD): Lippincott Williams & Wilkins; 2012:356.)

feet hit the ground, the quadriceps go through a stretch-shortening cycle. Of practical importance, plyometric exercises can place a great amount of stress on the involved muscles, connective tissues, and joints. Therefore, this type of training needs to be carefully prescribed and progressed to reduce the likelihood of musculoskeletal injury. The importance of starting with basic movements (*e.g.*, double leg jump and freeze) or establishing an adequate baseline of strength before participating in a plyometric program should not be overlooked by the HFS.

It is reasonable for individuals to begin plyometric training with one or two sets of six to eight repetitions of lower-intensity drills and gradually progress to several sets of higher-intensity exercises over time as technical competence improves. Plyometrics are not a stand-alone fitness program and should be incorporated into a training session that includes other types of resistance training. To optimize training adaptations, performance of more than 40 repetitions per session appears to be the most beneficial plyometric training volume (15). For example, a trained individual with experience performing plyometric exercises could perform two sets of six repetitions on four different lower body movements. Other considerations for plyometric training include proper footwear and a shock absorbing landing surface (*e.g.*, suspended floor or grass playing field).

Modes of Resistance Training

Almost any mode of resistance training can be used to enhance muscular fitness provided that the fundamental principles of training are adhered to and the program is sensibly progressed over time. Some types of equipment are relatively easy to use while others require balance, coordination, and high levels of skill. A decision to use a certain mode of resistance training should be based on an individual's health status, training experience, and personal goals. The major modes of resistance training are weight machines, free weights, body weight exercises, and a broadly defined category of balls, bands, and elastic tubing.

Single-joint exercises such as the biceps curl target a specific muscle group and require less skill to perform, whereas multiple-joint exercises such as the barbell squat involve more than one joint or major muscle group and require more balance and coordination. Although both single- and multiple-joint exercises are effective for enhancing muscular fitness, multiple-joint exercises are generally considered more effective for increasing muscle strength because they involve a greater amount of muscle mass and therefore enable a heavier weight to be lifted (34). Multiple-joint exercises have also been shown to have the greatest acute metabolic and anabolic (*e.g.*, testosterone and growth hormone) hormonal response, which could have a favorable impact on the design of resistance training programs targeting improvements in muscle size and body composition (35).

Weight machines are designed to train all the major muscle groups and can be found in most fitness centers. Both single-joint (*e.g.*, leg extension) and multiple-joint (*e.g.*, leg press) exercises can be performed on weight machines, which are relatively easy to use because the exercise motion is controlled by the machine and typically occurs in only one anatomical plane. This may be particularly important to consider when designing resistance training programs for sedentary or inexperienced individuals. Weight machines are designed to fit the average male or female, although a seat pad or back pad can be used to adjust the body position of individuals who are smaller or larger. Two examples of multiple-joint exercises performed on weight machines are shown in Figures 4.9 (lat pull-down) and 4.10 (pull-up).

Free weights are also popular in fitness centers and come in a variety of shapes and sizes. Although it typically takes longer to learn proper exercise technique when using free weights compared with weight machines, there are several advantages of free weight training. For example, free weights offer a greater variety of exercises than weight machines because they can be moved in many different directions. Another important benefit of using free weights is that they require the use of additional stabilizing and assisting muscles to hold the correct body position during an exercise. Instruction on proper exercise technique, sensible starting weights, and the appropriate use of a spotter are needed to reduce the risk of an accident (29).

Total body free weight exercises, including modified cleans, pulls, and presses, can be incorporated into a training program provided that qualified instruction is available and safety measures are

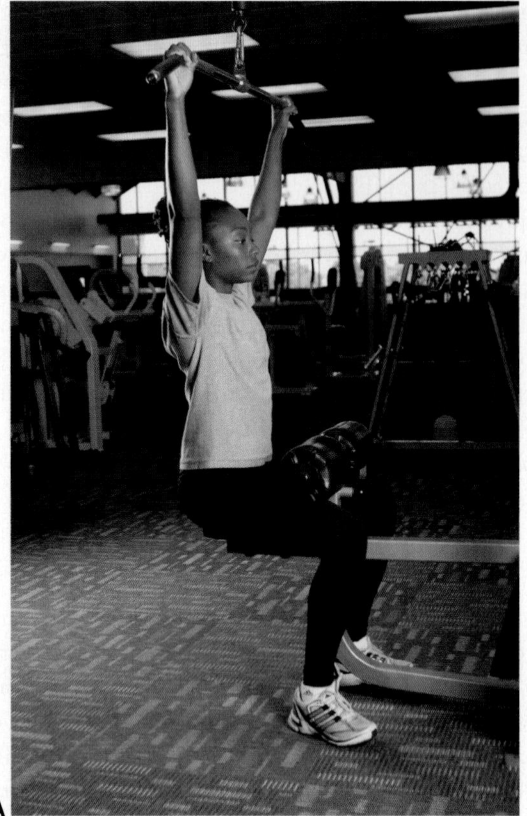

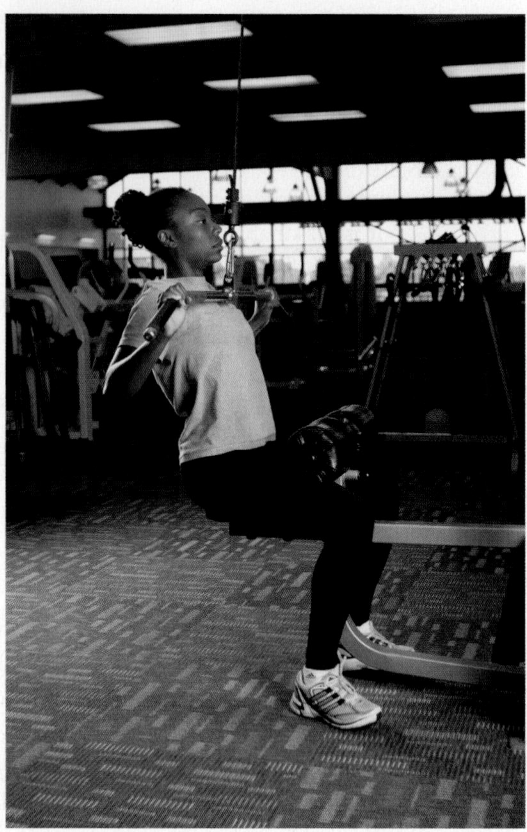

FIGURE 4.9. Pull-down: starting position **(A)** and pull-down position **(B)**.

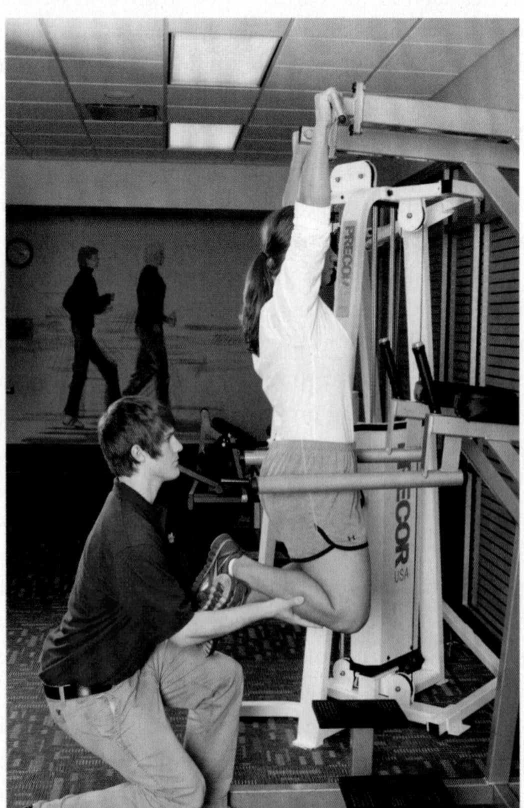

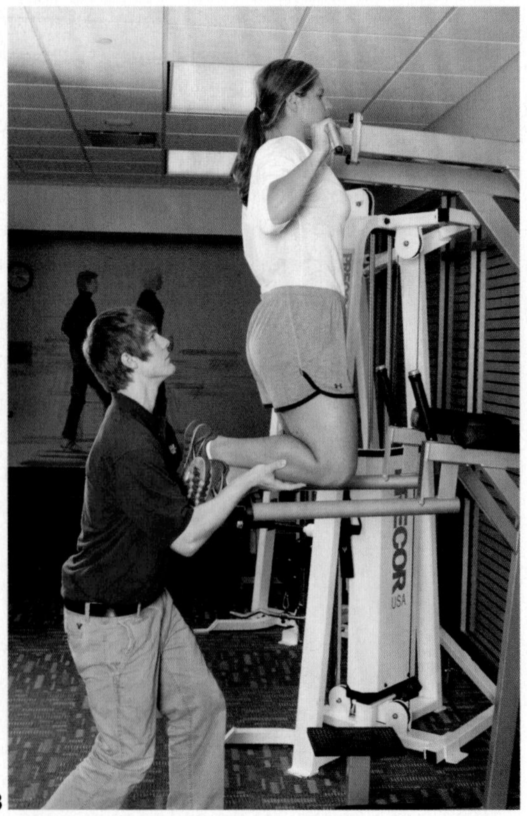

FIGURE 4.10. Assisted lat pull-up: starting position **(A)** and pull-up position **(B)**.

in place (*e.g.*, a safe lifting environment and appropriate loads) (2, 58). However, the HFS should be aware of the considerable amount of time it takes to teach advanced free weight exercises and should be knowledgeable of the progression from basic exercises (*e.g.*, front squat) to skill-transfer exercises (*e.g.*, overhead squat), and finally to weightlifting movements (*e.g.*, clean and jerk).

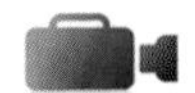

Visit thePoint to watch videos 4.3 through 4.5, which demonstrate a curl-up, a labile push-up, and a pull-up/chin-up, respectively.

Body weight exercises such as push-ups and curl-ups are some of the oldest modes of resistance training. Obviously, a major advantage of body weight training is that equipment is not needed and a variety of exercises can be performed. Conversely, a limitation of body weight training is the difficulty in adjusting the body weight to the individual's strength level. Sedentary or overweight participants may not be strong enough to perform even one repetition of a body weight exercise. In such cases, using exercise machines that allow individuals to perform body weight exercises such as pull-ups and dips by using a predetermined percentage of their body weight is desirable. These machines provide an opportunity for participants of all abilities to incorporate body weight exercises into their resistance training program and feel good about their accomplishments.

Stability balls, medicine balls, and elastic tubing are effective training modes that have been used by therapists for many years. Stability balls are lightweight, inflatable balls (about 45–75 cm in diameter) that add the elements of balance and coordination to any exercise while targeting selected muscle groups. Medicine balls come in different shapes and sizes (about 1 to >10 kg) and are an effective alternative to free weights and weight machines; Figure 4.11 shows an underhand medicine ball toss; others include the side-to-side toss, chest pass, overhead throw, back throw, vertical throw, slams, pullover pass, side toss, and front rotation throw. Resistance training with an elastic rubber cord involves performing an exercise against the force required to stretch the cord and then returning it to its unstretched state. Stability balls, medicine balls, and elastic tubing are not only relatively inexpensive, but are also being used more and more commonly as tools to enhance

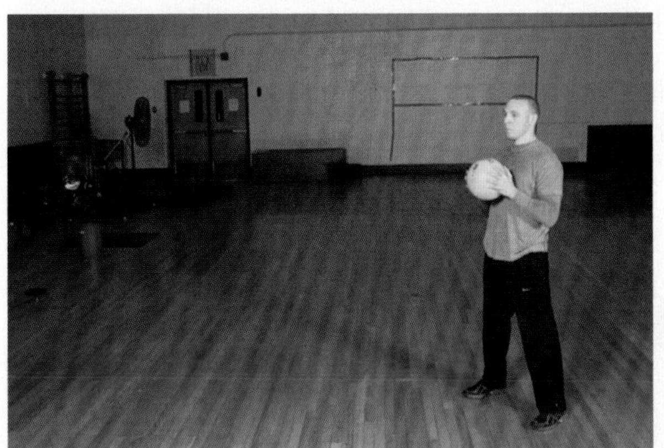

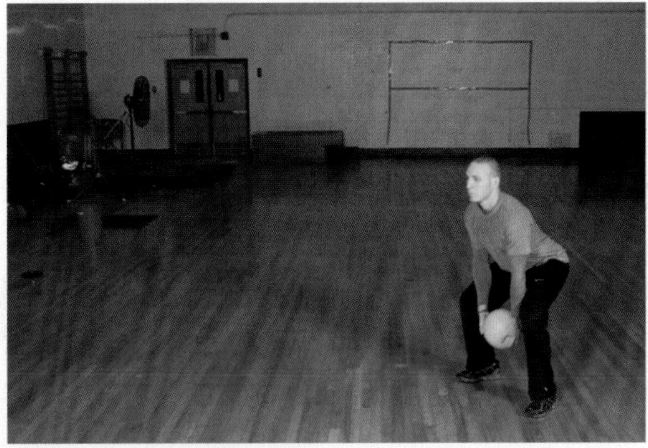

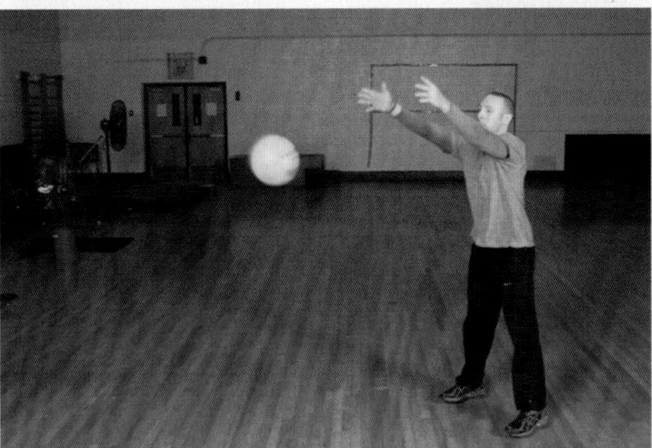

FIGURE 4.11. Underhand medicine ball toss. (From Ratamess N. *ACSM's Foundations of Strength Training and Conditioning.* Baltimore (MD): Lippincott Williams & Wilkins; 2012:363.)

TABLE 4.1 COMPARISON OF DIFFERENT MODES OF RESISTANCE TRAINING

	Weight Machines	Free Weights	Body Weight	Ball and Cords[a]
Cost	High	Low	None	Very low
Portability	Limited	Variable	Excellent	Excellent
Ease of use	Excellent	Variable	Variable	Variable
Muscle isolation	Excellent	Variable	Variable	Variable
Functionality	Limited	Excellent	Excellent	Excellent
Exercise variety	Limited	Excellent	Excellent	Excellent
Space requirements	High	Variable	Low	Low

[a]Medicine balls, stability balls, and elastic cords.

strength, muscular endurance, and power. In addition, exercises performed with balls and tubing can be proprioceptively challenging, which carries added benefit. Table 4.1 summarizes the advantages and disadvantages of different modes of resistance training.

Safety Concerns

Although all resistance training activities have some degree of medical risk, the chance of injury can be reduced by following established training guidelines and safety procedures. In addition, due to interindividual variability in the response to resistance training (17), an HFS needs to monitor the ability of all participants to tolerate the stress of strength and conditioning programs. Without proper supervision and instruction, injuries that require medical attention can happen.

In an evaluation of resistance training–related injuries presenting to emergency departments in the United States, researchers reported that men suffered more trunk injuries than women, whereas women had more accidental injuries compared with men (46). Figure 4.12 illustrates the percentage

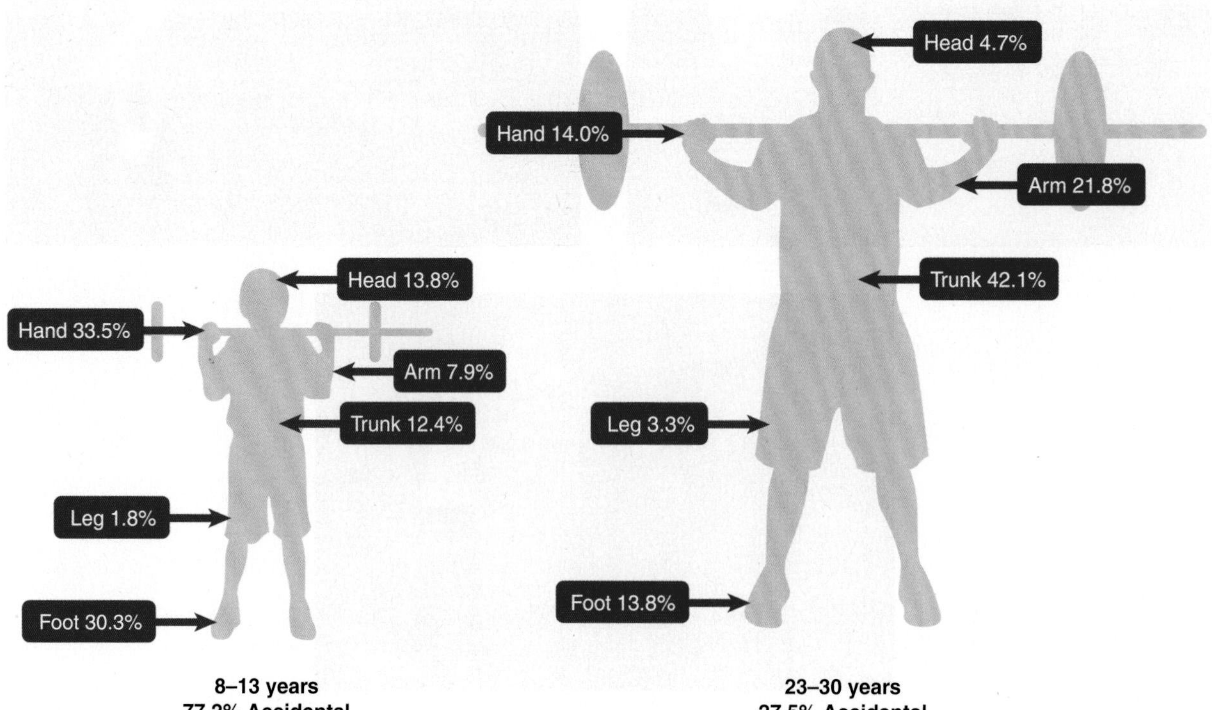

FIGURE 4.12. Resistance training-related injuries presenting to US emergency rooms.

TABLE 4.2 MODIFIABLE RISK FACTORS ASSOCIATED WITH RESISTANCE TRAINING INJURIES THAT CAN BE REDUCED (OR ELIMINATED) WITH QUALIFIED SUPERVISION AND INSTRUCTION

Risk Factor	Modification by Qualified HFS
Health-related concern	Communicate with treating clinician and modify program
Unsafe exercise environment	Adequate training space and proper equipment layout
Improper use of equipment	Clear instruction on exercise technique and training
Excessive load and volume	Gradual progression of training program
Poor trunk control	Targeted resistance exercises for core musculature
Muscle imbalances	Include agonist and antagonist exercises for selected muscle groups
Inadequate recuperation	Modify training program and consider lifestyle factors such as proper nutrition and adequate sleep

of resistance training–related injuries at each body part for men and women between the ages of 14 and 30 years who presented to US emergency departments.

Although there have not been any prospective trials that have focused specifically on measures to prevent resistance training–related injuries, an HFS who understands resistance training guidelines and acknowledges individual differences should provide supervision and instruction. This is particularly important for beginners who need to receive instruction on proper exercise technique as well as basic education on resistance training procedures (*e.g.*, weight room etiquette, appropriate spotting procedures, and the proper storage of equipment). All exercises should be performed in a controlled manner using proper breathing techniques avoiding the Valsalva maneuver. Modifiable risk factors associated with resistance training injuries that can be reduced or eliminated with qualified supervision and instruction are outlined in Table 4.2.

HFSs should be able to correctly perform the exercises they prescribe and should be able to modify exercise form and technique if necessary. When working in a fitness facility, the staff should be attentive and should try to position themselves with a clear view of the training center so that they can have quick access to individuals who need assistance. The resistance training area should be well lit and large enough to handle the number of individuals exercising in the facility at any given time. The facility should be clean, and the equipment should be well maintained.

In addition, HFSs are responsible for enforcing safety rules (*e.g.*, proper footwear and safe storage of weights) and ensuring that individuals are training effectively. Not only can HFSs enhance the safety of resistance training, but evidence indicates that HFSs who develop and directly supervise personalized programs can help clients maximize strength gains (43). Several studies have found that resistance exercise under the close supervision of a qualified HFS results in the self-selection of higher-resistance exercise intensities and greater strength gains following training as compared with resistance exercise without professional guidance and instruction (22, 49).

RESISTANCE TRAINING PROGRAM VARIABLES

Despite various claims about the best resistance training program, there is not one *optimal* combination of sets, repetitions, and exercises that will promote long-term adaptations in muscular fitness for all individuals. Rather, many program variables need to be systematically altered over time to achieve desirable outcomes (48). Clearly, resistance training programs need to be individualized and based on one's health history, training experience, and personal goals.

The program variables that should be considered when designing a resistance training program include: (a) choice of exercise, (b) order of exercise, (c) resistance used, (d) training volume (total number of sets and repetitions), (e) rest intervals between sets and exercises, (f) repetition velocity, and (g) training frequency (34). By varying one or more of these program variables, a limitless number of resistance training programs can be designed. But since individuals will respond differently to the same resistance training program, sound decisions must be made on the basis of an understanding of resistance exercise, individual needs, and personal goals. Table 4.3 summarizes ACSM's FITT principles for resistance training for apparently healthy adults (1).

Choice of Exercise

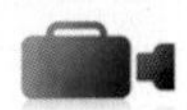

Visit thePoint to watch videos 4.6 through 4.10, which demonstrate a wood chop, squats, lunges, and a dumbbell bench press.

A limitless number of exercises can be used to enhance muscular fitness. It is important to select exercises that are appropriate for an individual's exercise technique experience and training goals. Also, the choice of exercises should promote muscle balance across joints and between opposing muscle groups (*e.g.*, quadriceps and hamstrings). Exercises generally can be classified as single-joint (*i.e.*, body-part specific) or multiple-joint (*i.e.*, structural). Although single-joint exercises that isolate muscle groups can be incorporated into a resistance training program, it is important to eventually include multiple-joint exercises to promote the coordinated use of multiple-joint movements (21).

Exercises can also be classified as closed kinetic chain or open kinetic chain. Closed kinetic chain exercises are those in which the distal joint segment is stationary (*e.g.*, squat), whereas open chain exercises are those in which the terminal joint is free to move (*e.g.*, leg extension). Closed kinetic chain exercises more closely mimic everyday activities and include more functional movement patterns (14).

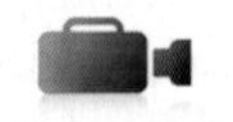

Visit thePoint to watch videos 4.11 and 4.12, which demonstrate plank and a side bridge, respectively.

Another important issue regarding the choice of exercise is the inclusion of exercises for lumbopelvic hip complex, which is commonly referred to as the core musculature (65). Strengthening the abdominals, hip, and low back enhances body control and may also reduce the risk of injury during athletic events and activities of daily life (5, 37). If individuals lack proper postural control during the

TABLE 4.3 SUMMARY OF ACSM'S FITT PRINCIPLES FOR RESISTANCE TRAINING

Frequency	Resistance train 2–3 nonconsecutive days per week
Intensity	Sedentary persons should start resistance training with 40%–50% 1 RM Intermediate exercises should use 60%–70% 1 RM to improve muscular strength Experienced exercisers can use heavier loads (≥80% 1 RM) to improve muscular strength Lighter loads (<50% 1 RM) and shorter rest periods between sets should be used to improve muscular endurance
Time	No specific resistance training duration has been identified
Type	Include multiple-joint exercises for the major muscle groups Target agonist and antagonist muscle groups to avoid muscle imbalances Different types of equipment and body weight exercises can be used
Repetitions	8–12 repetitions are recommended to improve muscular strength 15–20 repetitions are recommended to improve muscular endurance
Sets	2–4 sets are recommended to improve strength and power A single set can be effective for novices
Pattern	A rest interval of 2–3 min between each set is effective A rest of 48 h between sessions is recommended
Progression	A gradual progression of greater resistance, repetitions, and frequency is recommended

Adapted with permission from Pescatello L, editor. *ACSM's Guidelines for Exercise Testing and Prescription*. 9th ed. Baltimore (MD): Lippincott Williams & Wilkins; 2014 (1).

performance of a resistance exercise, they will not be able to transfer energy efficiently to the distal segments and will be more susceptible to an injury. Thus, prehabilitation exercises for the core musculature should be included in resistance training programs. That is, exercises that may be prescribed for the rehabilitation of an injury should be prescribed beforehand as a preventive health measure.

Exercises such as abdominal curl-ups and back extensions are useful, but they only train muscles that control trunk flexion and extension. Multidirectional exercises that involve rotational movements and diagonal patterns performed with one's own body weight or a medicine ball can be effective in strengthening the core musculature. In addition, research has indicated that the progressive introduction of greater instability during resistance training with devices such as stability balls might have application for reducing lower back pain, increasing joint stability, and enhancing core muscle activation (4). Depending on the needs and goals of the individual, other prehabilitation exercises (*e.g.*, internal and external rotation for the rotator cuff musculature) can be incorporated into the training session. For example, researchers reported that 4 to 8 weeks of prehabilitation resistance training before total knee arthroplasty improved strength and function in older adults with severe osteoarthritis (60).

Order of Exercise

There are many ways to arrange the sequence of exercises in a training session. Traditionally, beginners perform total body workouts that involve multiple exercises stressing all major muscle groups each session. In this type of workout, large muscle group exercises should be performed before smaller muscle group exercises and multiple-joint exercises should be performed before single-joint exercises. Following this exercise order will allow heavier weights to be used on the multiple-joint exercises because fatigue will be less of a factor. It is also helpful to perform more challenging exercises earlier in the workout when the neuromuscular system is less fatigued. Thus, power exercises such as plyometrics and weightlifting movements should be performed before more traditional strength exercises such as a back squat or bench so that an individual can train for maximal power without undue fatigue (2).

Individuals with resistance training experience may modify their training programs by performing a split routine program. For example, they could perform upper body exercises only during one workout and lower body exercises only during the following workout. Although different training programs are effective for enhancing muscular strength and performance, individual goals, time available for training, and personal preference should determine the exercise program that is used.

Resistance Load Used

One of the most important variables in the design of a resistance training program is the amount of resistance used for an exercise. Gains in muscular fitness are influenced by the amount of weight lifted, which is highly dependent on other program variables such as exercise order, training volume, repetition speed, and rest interval length (34). In an investigation that examined changes in muscle size and muscle composition in response to resistance exercise with light and heavy loads, the adaptive changes in muscle were significantly smaller after nonexhaustive light load training than after heavy-load training (24). These data as well as other reports demonstrate that adaptations to resistance training are linked to the intensity of the training program (48, 57). Thus, to maximize gains in muscle strength and performance, it is recommended that training sets be performed to muscle fatigue but not to exhaustion using the appropriate resistance (21).

The use of RM loads is a relatively simple method to prescribe resistance training intensity. Research studies suggest that RM loads of 6 or less have the greatest effect on developing muscle strength, whereas RM loads of 20 or more have the greatest effect on developing local muscular endurance (9, 48). Although novices can make significant gains in muscle strength with lighter loads, individuals with resistance training experience need to train periodically with heavier loads (48).

Accordingly, repetitions ranging between 8 and 12 (~60%–80% 1 RM) are commonly used to enhance muscular fitness in novice to intermediate exercises (21). Experienced exercisers may train at intensities greater than 80% 1 RM to achieve the desired gains in muscle strength (21). Using lighter weights (*e.g.*, <50% 1 RM; 15–20 repetitions) will have less effect on muscular strength but more effect on muscular endurance. Since each repetition zone (*e.g.*, 3–6, 8–12, or 15–20) has its advantages, the best approach may be to systematically vary the resistance used to avoid training plateaus and optimize training adaptations (48). Furthermore, consistent training at high intensities (*e.g.*, ≥80% 1 RM) increases the risk of overtraining.

A percentage of an individual's 1 RM can also be used to determine the resistance training intensity. If the 1 RM on the leg press exercise is 100 kg, a training intensity of 60% would be 60 kg. It is reasonable for beginners to use a resistance training intensity of approximately 50% to 60% 1 RM because they are mostly improving motor performance at this stage, and proper exercise technique is of paramount importance. As individuals get stronger and gain training experience, heavier resistances will be needed to make continual gains in muscular strength and performance. Meta-analytical procedures have found that 60% of 1 RM and 80% of 1 RM produced the largest strength increases in untrained and training adults, respectively (52). Obviously, this method of prescribing resistance exercise requires the frequent evaluation of the 1 RM. In many cases, this is not realistic because of the time required to perform 1 RM testing correctly on different exercises. Furthermore, maximal resistance testing for small muscle group assistance exercises is not typically performed.

The HFS should be knowledgeable about the relationship between the percentage of the 1 RM and the number of repetitions that can be performed. In general, most individuals can perform about 10 repetitions using 75% of their 1 RM. However, the number of repetitions that can be performed at a given percentage of the 1 RM varies with the amount of muscle mass required to perform the exercise. For example, research has shown that at a given percentage of the 1 RM, adults can perform more repetitions on a large muscle group exercise such as the back squat compared with a smaller muscle group exercise such as the arm curl (55). Therefore, prescribing a resistance training intensity of 70% of 1 RM on all exercises warrants additional consideration because at 70% of 1 RM, an individual may be able to perform 20 or more repetitions on a large muscle group exercise, which may not be ideal for enhancing muscular strength. If a percentage of the 1 RM is used for prescribing resistance exercises, the prescribed percentage of the 1 RM for each exercise may need to be changed to maintain a desired training range (*e.g.*, 8–10 RM).

Training Volume

The number of exercises performed per session, the repetitions performed per set, and the number of sets performed per exercise all influence the training volume (48). Although there has been some debate regarding resistance training volume over the past few years, it is important to remember that every training session does not need to be characterized by the same number of sets, repetitions, and exercises. The ACSM recommends that apparently healthy adults should train each muscle group for two to four sets to achieve muscular fitness goals (1). For example, the chest muscles can be trained with four sets of the bench press or two sets of the bench press and two sets of dumbbell flys.

Although untrained individuals can respond favorably to single set training, meta-analytical data have shown that multiple set training is more effective than single set training for strength enhancement in untrained and in trained populations (36, 52, 53). However, program variation characterized by periods of low-volume training can provide needed recovery for individuals who have been participating in a high-volume training program for a prolonged period. Since recovery is an integral part of any training program, high-volume training needs to be balanced with low-volume sessions to facilitate recovery. In addition, low-volume sessions provide a learning opportunity for the fitness professional to reinforce proper exercise technique on specific movement patterns.

Rest Intervals between Sets

The length of the rest period between sets will influence energy recovery and the training adaptations that take place (50, 63). For example, if the primary goal of the program is to maximize gains in muscular strength, heavier weights and longer rest intervals (*e.g.*, 2–3 min) are required, whereas if the goal is muscular endurance, lighter weights and shorter rest periods (*e.g.*, <1 min) are required (48). As previously noted with other program variables, the same rest interval does not need to be used for all exercises. In addition, fatigue resulting from a previous exercise should be considered when prescribing the rest interval if maximal gains in muscular strength are desired.

Repetition Velocity

The velocity or cadence at which a resistance exercise is performed can affect the adaptations to a training program because gains in muscular fitness are specific to the training velocity. For example, fast-velocity plyometric training or weightlifting exercises are more likely to enhance speed and power than slower-velocity resistance exercise on a weight machine (12). In any case, beginners need to learn how to perform each exercise correctly and develop an adequate level of strength before optimal gains in power performance are realized. As individuals improve muscular strength and gain experience performing higher-velocity movements, heavier loads or more complex exercises may be used to optimize training adaptations. It is likely that the performance of different training velocities and the integration of numerous training techniques may provide the most effective training stimulus (12).

Training Frequency

A resistance training frequency of two to three times per week on nonconsecutive days is recommended for beginners (21). This training frequency will allow for adequate recovery between sessions (48–72 h) and has proven to be effective for enhancing muscular fitness (52). However, trained individuals who perform more advanced programs may need a longer period of recovery time between sessions. Factors such as the training volume, training intensity, exercise selection, nutritional intake, and sleep habits may influence one's ability to recover from and adapt to the training program. For example, trained individuals who perform a split routine may resistance train four times a week, but they train each muscle group only twice a week. Although an increase in training experience does not necessitate an increase in training frequency, a higher training frequency does allow for greater specialization characterized by more exercises and a higher weekly training volume.

Periodization

Periodization is a concept that refers to the systematic variation in training program design. Since it is impossible to continually improve at the same rate over long-term training, properly varying the training variables can limit training plateaus, maximize performance gains, and reduce the likelihood of overtraining (18). The underlying concept of periodization is based on Selye's general adaptation syndrome, which proposes that after a certain period, adaptations to a new stimulus will no longer take place unless the stimulus is altered (54). In essence, periodization is a process whereby an HFS regularly changes the training stimulus to keep it effective. Although the concept of periodization has been part of resistance training program design for many years, our understanding of the benefits of periodized training programs compared with nonperiodized programs for long-term progression has recently been explored in the literature (7, 18).

The concept of periodization is not just for elite athletes, but also for individuals with different levels of training experience who want to enhance their health and fitness. By periodically varying program variables such as the choice of exercise, training resistance, number of sets, rest periods between sets, or any combination of the above, long-term performance gains will be optimized and the risk of "overuse" injuries may be reduced (48). Moreover, it is reasonable to suggest that individuals who participate in well-designed programs and continue to improve their health and fitness may be more likely to adhere to an exercise program for the long term.

For example, if a trained individual's lower body routine typically consists of the leg press, leg extension, and leg curl exercises, performing the back squat and dumbbell lunge exercises on alternate workout days will likely increase the effectiveness of the training program and reduce the likelihood of staleness and boredom. Furthermore, varying the training weights, number of sets, and/or rest interval between sets can help prevent training plateaus, which are not uncommon among fitness enthusiasts. Many times, a strength plateau can be avoided by periodically varying the exercises or varying the training intensity and training volume to allow for ample recover. In the long term, program variation with adequate recovery will allow an individual to make even greater gains because the body will be challenged to adapt to even greater demands (48).

The general concept of periodization is to prioritize training goals and then develop a long-term plan that varies throughout the year. In general, the year is divided into specific training cycles (*e.g.*, a macrocycle, a mesocycle, and a microcycle), with each cycle having a specific goal (*e.g.*, hypertrophy, strength, or power). The classic periodization model is referred to as a linear model because the volume and intensity of training gradually change over time (59). For example, at the start of a macrocycle, the training volume may be high and the training intensity may be low. As the year progresses, the volume is decreased as the intensity of training increases. Although this type of training originally was designed for athletes who attempted to peak for a specific competition, it can be modified by an HFS for enhancing health and fitness. For example, individuals who routinely perform the same combination of sets and repetitions on all exercises will benefit from gradually increasing the weight and decreasing the number of repetitions as strength improves.

A second model of periodization is referred to as an undulating (nonlinear) model because of the daily fluctuations in training volume and intensity. For example, on the major exercises, a trained individual may perform two or three sets with 8 to 10 RM loads on Monday, three or four sets with 4 to 6 RM loads on Wednesday, and one or two sets with 12 to 15 RM loads on Friday. Whereas the heavy training days will maximally activate the trained musculature, selected muscle fibers will not be maximally taxed on light and moderate training days. By alternating training volume and intensity, the participant can minimize the risk of overtraining and maximize the potential for strength enhancement (7).

GENERAL RECOMMENDATIONS

Resistance training has the potential to offer unique benefits to men and women of all ages and abilities. Regular participation in a progressive resistance training program can enhance muscular fitness and improve an individual's health status. However, the design of resistance training programs can be complex, and program variables including the choice of exercise, order of exercise, training intensity, training volume, repetition velocity, and rest period between sets and exercises need to be systematically varied over time to optimize gains in muscle fitness and performance. In addition, resistance training programs need to be individualized and consistent with personal goals to maximize outcomes and exercise adherence. Ultimately, knowledge of muscle structure and function along with an understanding of resistance training principles will determine the effectiveness of the training program.

In addition to understanding the science of resistance exercise, HFSs need to appreciate the art of prescribing exercise. Resistance training programs need to be individualized and consistent with personal needs, goals, and abilities. A key factor for safe and effective resistance training is proper program design that includes exercise instruction, sensible progression, and periodic evaluations to assess progress toward training goals. This requires effective leadership, realistic goal setting, and a solid understanding of training-induced adaptations that take place in both beginners and experienced exercisers.

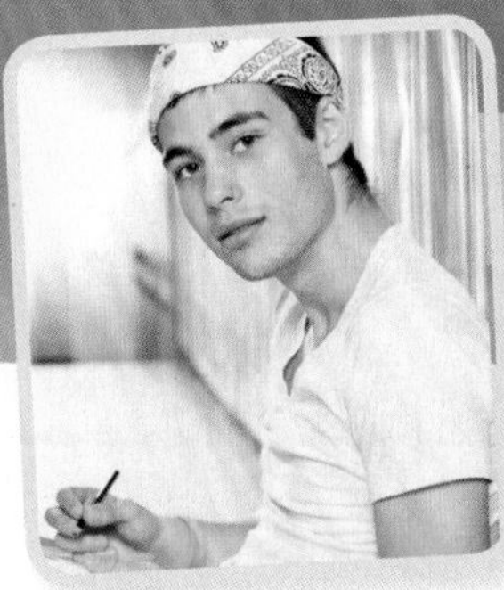

The Case of Jeremy

Submitted by: **Benjamin Gleason, ACSM-HFS, NSCA-CSCS, US Air Force, Niceville, FL**

Jeremy is a former high school athlete, now 23 years old and apparently healthy.

Narrative

Jeremy's body composition is within normal ranges, as are his BP and heart rate. He cites no family history of disease. He works out in the local gym for four sessions per week and spends 1 to 2 hours per session. This has been his primary mode of regular exercise since high school, and he plays recreational sports in the local city league in his free time. He wishes to continue his current exercise pattern, but has come to see you to discuss some issues he's been having lately. He casually complains to you during his fitness screening that he suffers mild knee pain and low back pain during and after his workouts. On observing him in a gym session, you notice that when he performs the squat, he rounds his back and places most of his weight on the balls of his feet. He also rounds his back slightly when he performs the deadlift and hyperextends his spine at the end of the lift. During standing overhead pressing movements, he leans back to force out a few extra reps. He has been suffering from mild pain in his knees and back for some time now, and says his high school sports coach used to tell him "No pain, no gain!" when he brought it up from time to time several years ago. He asks you if this pain is normal and says he doesn't want to sound like a wimp to the other guys in the gym. His typical weight program involves three or four sets of 6 to 12 repetitions on every exercise, and he performs at least three exercises for each body part in his program. Mondays he does chest and triceps, Tuesday he does legs, Thursday he does back and biceps, and Friday he does shoulders. He includes some light cardio on a stationary bike or a treadmill after most workouts.

Analysis

Jeremy's workout program is a typical one used by many bodybuilders, but his attention to detail on form leaves much to be desired. Apparently, he was not taught the proper exercise technique by his coach in high school or the fitness center staff, and Jeremy has developed some movement pattern disorders. To reduce the likelihood of knee and back pain during the squat and deadlift, he should keep the majority of his bodyweight on his heels as he descends and rises throughout the ROM and keep his back in the neutral position. It will take time to break old habits, and Jeremy will need to use a lighter load to learn proper technique on these free weight exercises. Jeremy should visit a medical professional to address any possible injuries beyond the minor pain he experiences during exercise. His habits of hyperextending his back at the top of the deadlift and arching his back to get more reps on overhead presses are likely contributors to his back pain and serve no practical advantage in resistance training as they are high-risk methods. A deadlift is complete when the lifter returns to the standing position only and not beyond (hyperextension). The posterior chain musculature (low back, gluteals, hamstrings) requires considerable attention in an effective training program, and the correct initiation of movement is imperative to reduce the risk of injury and produce the desired performance effects.

Questions

- Discuss Jeremy's tendency to round his back during deadlifts and how it may be causing his low back pain.
- Why is knee pain common in individuals who squat in an anterior-dominant manner?
- Provide at least three exercises to address Jeremy's apparent posterior chain deficiency.
- Suggest two core stability exercises that may help Jeremy hold spinal stability better.

continues

The Case of Jeremy cont.

References

Bird S, Barrington-Higgs S. Exploring the deadlift. *Strength Cond J.* 2010;32(2):46–51.

Chiu L. A teaching progression for squatting exercises. *Strength Cond J.* 2011;33(2):46–54.

Gamble P. An integrated approach to training core stability. *Strength Cond J.* 2007;29(1):58–68.

McGill S. *Low Back Disorders, Evidence-based Prevention and Rehabilitation.* Champaign (IL): Human Kinetics; 2002.

VSUMMARY

In this chapter, the benefits and importance of muscular strength and endurance for health and fitness were described. An overview of the basic structure and function of the muscle was also provided. Fundamental principles relating to resistance training for health and fitness were reviewed. The primary variables of a resistance training program were described. The role of the HFS in designing a resistance program for apparently healthy adults and individuals with controlled disease was discussed. Tools for developing an individualized resistance training program from assessment to implementation to evaluation were provided.

STUDY QUESTIONS

1. Describe the size principle of motor unit recruitment and explain its practical application to resistance exercise program design.
2. Discuss four fundamental principles that determine the effectiveness of resistance training programs.
3. Compare and contrast three different modes of resistance training and discuss the advantages and disadvantages of each method.
4. List and describe program variables that should be considered when designing a resistance training program.
5. Design a resistance training program for an untrained healthy adult and include recommendations for participant safety, program progression, and exercise adherence.

REFERENCES

1. American College of Sports Medicine. *ACSM's Guidelines for Exercise Testing and Prescription.* 9th ed. Baltimore (MD): Lippincott Williams & Wilkins; 2013.
2. Baechle T, Earle R. *Essentials of Strength Training and Conditioning.* Champaign (IL): Human Kinetics; 2008. p. 381–412.
3. Behm DG, Chaouachi A. A review of the acute effects of static and dynamic stretching on performance. *Eur J Appl Physiol.* 2011;111(11):2633–51. Epub 2011 Mar 4.
4. Behm DG, Drinkwater EJ, Willardson JM, Cowley PM. The role of instability rehabilitation resistance training for the core musculature. *Strength Cond J.* 2011;33:72–81.
5. Bihdanna T, Hewett T, Reeves P, Goldberg B, Cholewicki J. Deficits in neuromuscular control of the trunk. *Am J Sports Med.* 2007;35:1123–30.
6. Bobbert M, Huijing P, Van Ingen Schenau G. Drop jumping I. The influence of jumping technique on the biomechanics of jumping. *Med Sci Sports Exerc.* 1987;19:332–8.

7. Bompa T, Haff G. *Periodization — Theory and Methodology of Training*. Champaign (IL): Human Kinetics; 2009.
8. Brown L, editor. *Strength Training*. Champaign (IL): Human Kinetics; 2007.
9. Campos GE, Luecke TJ, Wendeln HK, et al. Muscular adaptations in response to three different resistance-training regimens: Specificity of repetition maximum training zones. *Eur J Appl Physiol*. 2002;88:50–60.
10. Chu D. *Jumping into Plyometrics*. Champaign (IL): Juman Kinetics; 1998.
11. Clarkson P. Exertional rhabdomyolysis and acute renal failure in marathon runners. *Sports Med*. 2007;37:361–3.
12. Cormie P, McGuigan MR, Newtown RU. Developing maximal neuromuscular power: Part 2 — training considerations for improving maximal power production. *Sports Med*. 2011;41:125–146.
13. Cornelissen V, Fagard R, Coeckelberghs E, Vanhees L. Impact of resistance training on blood pressure and other cardiovascular risk factors. *Hypertension*. 2011;58:950–8.
14. Davies G. The need for critical thinking in rehabilitation. *J Sport Rehabil*. 1995;4:1–22.
15. de Villarreal E, Requena B, Newton R. Does plyometric training improve strength performance? A meta-analysis. *J Sci Med Sport*. 2010;13:51.
16. Dudley G, Tesch P, Miller B, Buchanan P. Importance of eccentric actions in performance adaptations to resistance training. *Aviat Space Envir Med*. 1991;62:543–50.
17. Erskine R, Jones D, Williams A, Stewart C, Degens H. Inter-individual variability in the adaptation of human muscle specific tension to progressive resistance training. *Eur J Appl Physiol*. 2010;110:1117–25.
18. Fleck S. Periodized resistance training: A critical review. *J Strength Cond Res*. 1999;13:82–9.
19. Fleck S, Kraemer W. *Designing Resistance Training Programs*. Champaign (IL): Human Kinetics; 2004.
20. Gale C, Martyn C, Cooper C, Sayer A. Grip strength, body composition and mortality. *Int J Epidemiol*. 2007;36:228–35.
21. Garber C, Ewing C, Blissmer B, Deschenes M. American College of Sports Medicine Position Stand. The quantity and quality of exercise for developing and maintaining cardiorespiratory, musculoskeletal, and neuromotor fitness in apparently healthy adults: Guidance for prescribing exercise. *Med Sci Sports Exerc*. 2011;43.
22. Gentil P, Bottaro M. Influence of supervision ratio on muscle adaptations to resistance training in nontrained subjects. *J Strength Cond Res*. 2010;24:639–43.
23. Hamlin M, Quigley B. Quadriceps concentric and eccentric exercise 2: Differences in muscle strength, fatigue and EMG activity in eccentrically-exercised sore and non-sore muscles. *J Sci Med Sport*. 2001;4:104–15.
24. Holm L, Reitelseder S, Pedersen T, et al. Changes in muscle size and MHC composition in response to resistance exercise with heavy and light loading intensity. *J Appl Physiol*. 2008;105:1454–61.
25. Jackson AW, Morrow JR Jr, Brill PA, Kohl HW, Gordon NF, Blair SN. Relations of sit-up and sit-and reach to low back pain in adults. *J Orthop Sports Phys Ther*. 1998;27:22–6.
26. Jespersen J, Nedergaard A, Andersen L, Schjerling P, Andersen J. Myostatin expression during human muscle hypertrophy and subsequent atrophy: Increase myostatin with detraining. *Scand J Med Sci Sports*. 2011;21:213–23.
27. Jurca R, LaMonte M, Barlow C, Kampert J, Church T, Blair S. Association of muscular strength with incidence of metabolic syndrome in men. *Med Sci Sports Exerc*. 2005;37:1849–55.
28. Kanehisa H, Miyashita M. Specificity of velocity in strength training. *Eur J Appl Physiol*. 1983;52:104–6.
29. Kerr Z, Collins C, Comstock R. Epidemiology of weight training-related injuries presenting to United States emergency departments, 1990 to 2007. *Am J Sports Med*. 2010;38:765–71.
30. Klimcakova E, Polak J, Moro C, et al. Dynamic strength training improves insulin sensitivity without altering plasma levels and gene expression of adipokines in subcutaneous adipose tissue in obese men. *J Clin Endocrinol Metab*. 2006;91:5107–12.
31. Kohrt W, Bloomfield S, Little K, Nelson M, Yingling V. American College of Sports Medicine position stand: Physical activity and bone health. *Med Sci Sports Exerc*. 2004;36:1985–96.
32. Komi P. Stretch shortening cycle: A powerful model to study normal and fatigued muscle. *J Biomech*. 2000;33: 1197–206.
33. Kraemer W, Ratamess N, Fry A, French D. Strength training: Development and evaluation of methodology. In: Maud P, Foster C, editors. *Physiological Assessment of Human Fitness*. Champaign (IL): Human Kinetics; 2006. p. 119–50.
34. Kraemer WJ, Ratamess NA. Fundamentals of resistance training: Progression and exercise prescription. *Med Sci Sports Exerc*. 2004;36:674–88.
35. Kraemer WJ, Ratamess NA. Hormonal responses and adaptations to resistance exercise and training. *Sports Med*. 2005;35:339–61.
36. Krieger J. Single versus multiple sets of resistance exercise: A meta-regression. *J Strength Cond Res*. 2009;23:1890–901.
37. Leetun D, Ireland M, Wilson J, Ballantyne B, Davis I. Core stability measures as risk factors for lower extremity injuries in athletes. *Med Sci Sports Exerc*. 2004;36:926–34.
38. Lemmer JT, Hurlbut DE, Martel GF, et al. Age and gender responses to strength training and detraining. *Med Sci Sports Exerc*. 2000;32:1505–12.
39. Lewington S, Clarke R, Qizilbash N, Peto R, Collins R. Age specific relevance of usual blood pressure to vascular mortality: A meta analysis of individual data for one million adults in 61 prospective studies. *Lancet*. 2002;360:1903–13.
40. Liu C, Latham N. Progressive resistance strength training for improving physical function in older adults. *Cochrane Database Syst Rev*. 2009;(3):CD002759.
41. Lyons T, McLester J, Arnett S, Thoma M. Specificity of training modalities on upper body one repetition maximum performance: Free weights vs. Hammer strength equipment. *J Strength Cond Res*. 2010;24:2984–8.
42. Mason C, Brien S, Craig C, Gauvin L, Katzmarzyk P. Musculoskeletal fitness and weight gain in Canada. *Med Sci Sports Exerc*. 2007;39:38–43.
43. Mazzette S, Kraemer W, Volek J, et al. The influence of direct supervision of resistance training on strength performance. *Med Sci Sports Exerc*. 2000;32:1175–84.
44. Newton M, Morgan G, Sacco P, Chapman D, Nosaka K. Comparison of responses to strenuous eccentric exercise of the elbow flexors between resistance-trained and untrained men. *J Strength Cond Res*. 2008;22:597–607.
45. Pratley R, Nicklas B, Rubin M, et al. Strength training increases resting metabolic rate and norepinephrine levels in healthy 50- to 65-yr-old men. *J Appl Physiol*. 1994;76:133–7.
46. Quatman C, Myer G, Khoury J, Wall E, Hewett T. Sex differences in "weightlifting" injuries presenting to United States Emergency Rooms. *J Strength Cond Res*. 2009;23:2061–7.
47. Ratamess N. *ACSM's Foundations of Strength Training and Conditioning*. Philadelphia (PA): Lippincott Williams & Wilkins; 2012.

48. Ratamess N, Alvar B, Evetoch T, et al. Progression models in resistance training in healthy adults. *Med Sci Sports Exerc.* 2009;41:687–708.
49. Ratamess NA, Faigenbaum AD, Hoffman JR, Kang J. Self-selected resistance training intensity in healthy women: The influence of a personal trainer. *J Strength Cond Res.* 2008;22:103–11.
50. Ratamess NA, Falvo MJ, Mangine GT, Hoffman JR, Faigenbaum AD, Kang J. The effect of rest interval length on metabolic responses to the bench press exercise. *Eur J Appl Physiol.* 2007;100:1–17.
51. Reilly T, Morris T, Whyte G. The specificity of training prescription and physiological assessment: A review. *J Sport Sci.* 2009;27:575–89.
52. Rhea M, Alavar B, Burkett LN, Ball S. A meta-analysis to determine the dose response for strength development. *Med Sci Sports Exerc.* 2003;35:456–64.
53. Rhea M, Alvar B, Burkett L. Single vs multiple sets for strength: A meta-analysis to address the controversy. *Res Q Exerc Sport.* 2002;73:485–8.
54. Selye H. *The Stress of Life.* New York (NY): McGraw Hill; 1956.
55. Shimano T, Kraemer W, Spiering B, et al. Relationship between the number of repetitions and selected percentages of one repetition maximum in free weight exercises in trained and untrained men. *J Strength Cond Res.* 2006;20:819–23.
56. Sillanpää E, Laaksonen D, Häkkinen A, et al. Body composition, fitness and metabolic health during strength and endurance training and their combination in middle-aged and older women. *Eur J Appl Physiol.* 2009;106:285–96.
57. Steib S, Schoene D, Pfeifer K. Dose-response relationship of resistance training in older adults: A meta-analysis. *Med Sci Sports Exerc.* 2009;42:902–14.
58. Stone M, Fry A, Richie M, Stoessel-Ross L, Marsit J. Injury potential and safety aspects of weightlifting movements. *Strength Cond J.* 1994;16:15–21.
59. Stone MH, O'Bryant H, Garhammer J. A hypothetical model of strength training. *J Appl Strength Cond Res.* 1981;5:35–50.
60. Swank A, Kachelman J, Bibeau W, et al. Prehabilitation before total knee arthroplasty increases strength and function in older adults with severe osteoarthritis. *J Strength Cond Res.* 2011;25:318–25.
61. Thompson W. Worldwide survey of fitness trends for 2011. *ACSM's Health Fitness J.* 2010;14:8–17.
62. Westcott W. *Building Strength and Stamina.* Champaign (IL): Human Kinetics; 2003.
63. Willardson J. A brief review: Factors affecting the length of the rest interval between resistance exercise sets. *J Strength Cond Res.* 2006;20:978–84.
64. Williams MA, Haskell WL, Ades PA, et al. Resistance exercise in individuals with and without cardiovascular disease: 2007 update. *Circulation.* 2007;116:572–84.
65. Wilson J, Dougherty C, Ireland M, Davis I. Core stability and its relationship to lower extremity function and injury. *J Am Acad Orthop Surg.* 2005;13:316–25.
66. World Health Organization. *Global Recommendations on Physical Activity for Health.* Geneva (Switzerland): WHO Press; 2010.

CHAPTER

5 Flexibility Assessments and Exercise Programming for Apparently Healthy Participants

Meir Magal • Chris Eschbach

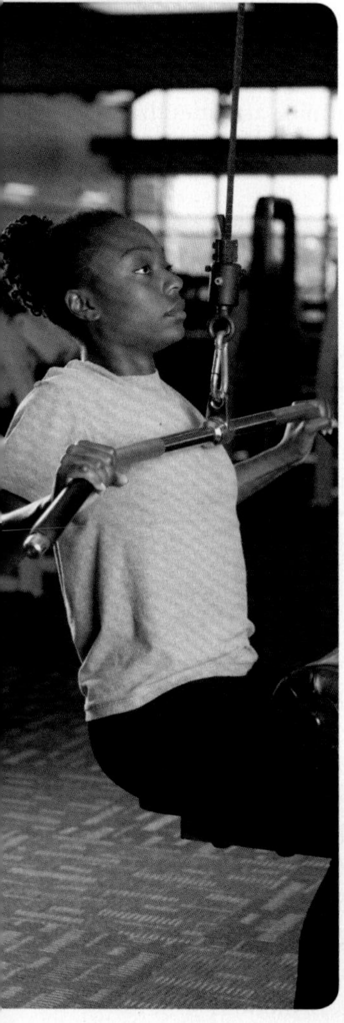

CHAPTER OBJECTIVES

- To understand the context of flexibility as it relates to health and wellness.
- To describe the basic anatomy and physiology of the musculoskeletal system related to flexibility.
- To differentiate modes of range of motion exercises and their strengths and weaknesses.
- To select appropriate assessment protocols for flexibility and analyze the results of those assessments.
- To formulate appropriate programs for development of whole body flexibility.

Development and maintenance of flexibility has long been a recommended component of health-related fitness (26). The President's Council on Physical Fitness and Sports was in part prompted by the report of Kraus and Hirschland (58) that American children performed poorly compared with European children in a fitness assessment, especially on flexibility. The American College of Sports Medicine® released its first position stand on cardiorespiratory and muscular fitness in 1981; however, it didn't include recommendations for flexibility exercises until 1998 (1). Similar to other components of fitness, it is important to maintain an adequate range of motion (ROM) necessary for activities of daily living. However, this increase in ROM through flexibility training does not seem to decrease the incidence of low back pain or muscle soreness (40, 85, 87, 100), and it has not been shown to improve athletic performance. In some cases, it actually has been shown to decrease performance (54, 56, 57, 106). Flexibility requirements are specific to the demands of individual activities, with some activities requiring more than average ROM at particular joints (*e.g.*, gymnastics and ballet) (29, 73).

BASIC PRINCIPLES OF FLEXIBILITY

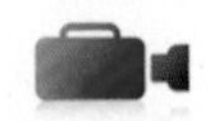

Visit thePoint to watch video 5.1, which demonstrates dynamic arm circles.

Flexibility is defined as ROM of a joint or group of joints, as per the skeletal muscles and not any external forces (41). The flexibility of any given movable joint includes both static and dynamic components. Static flexibility is the full ROM of a given joint because of external forces. It can be achieved by the use of gravitational force, a partner, or specific exercise equipment (3). In contrast, dynamic flexibility is the full ROM of a given joint achieved by the voluntary use of skeletal muscles in combination with external forces (93). Although it is recognized that dynamic flexibility is greater than static flexibility for a given joint, the two may be independent of each other (45). Each movable joint has its own anatomical structure that helps define the ROM for which that joint can move. Because of this joint specificity, the ROM of one particular joint may not predict the ROM of other joints, although individuals participating in a full-body ROM program or performing activities that move several joints through their full ROM will generally have a greater full-body flexibility (33).

Factors Affecting Flexibility

ROM of a given joint is determined by several factors, including muscle properties, physical activity and exercise, anatomical structure, age, and gender.

Muscle properties: The inherent properties of muscle tissue play a major role in the ROM of a given joint. Skeletal muscles, when stretched, exhibit both viscous and elastic properties (viscoelastic properties), which allow them to extend through the process of creep and stress relaxation (80). In addition, research has suggested that the viscoelastic properties of skeletal muscle may be altered and lead to an increase in ROM by either an external thermal modality (*i.e.*, heat pad) or a physically active warm-up (81, 91, 92, 97). Nevertheless, this finding is not well documented in humans, and therefore, more research is needed to further validate these findings (32, 33).

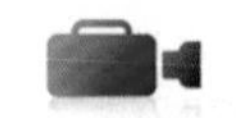

Visit thePoint to watch video 5.2, which demonstrates the soldier walk.

Physical activity and exercise: Both single and multiple bouts of physical activity can lead to greater flexibility of the affected joints, primarily by moving joints through a fuller ROM during exercise than would normally occur (27, 44, 88). In addition, resistance training programs that incorporate full ROM exercises may also increase flexibility of the affected joints (61, 98), assuming both agonist and antagonist muscle(s) around the joint are being trained (13). For instance, pull-ups or chin-ups move the shoulder through a ROM not normally done in day-to-day activities, thereby increasing shoulder ROM. Further, athletes who regularly perform ROM exercise, during aerobic, resistance, or flexibility exercise, improve performance, at least in part, through an enhanced level of flexibility (46, 52, 107). Nonetheless, discrepancies exist in the level of flexibility necessary for a variety of activities (29), such as athletes in the same sport but at different competitive levels (collegiate vs. professional) (96) and athletes in the same sport but in a different position (28, 84). Further, there is also a difference in the level of flexibility between dominant and nondominant limbs in athletes who participate in sports that involve bilateral asymmetrical motions such as tennis and baseball (23, 64).

Anatomical structures: The ROM of a given joint is influenced by its structure and the anatomical structures surrounding it. Freely moveable joints (synovial) may be classified into one of six groups, each with a specific permissible plane or planes of movement (Fig. 5.1) (33, 105). Further, joint flexibility is not affected equally by connective tissues around joints. Johns and Wright (1962) demonstrated that relative contributions of various soft tissues to joint stiffness are as follows: joint capsule (47%), muscles (41%), tendons (10%), and the skin (2%) (50). In addition, soft tissue bulk including muscle and subcutaneous fat tissues may affect joint flexibility because of potential movement restriction (17, 105).

Age and gender: Several studies have examined the relationship between the degree of flexibility within a given joint relative to age and gender. These studies have demonstrated that with aging, there is a reduction in collagen solubility, which may lead to increases in tendon rigidity and therefore reduction in ROM (82). This reduction may be further exacerbated by age-related conditions such as degenerative joint disease and decreased levels of physical activity (43, 82). Normative data collected on thousands of men and women at the Cooper Institute show that women

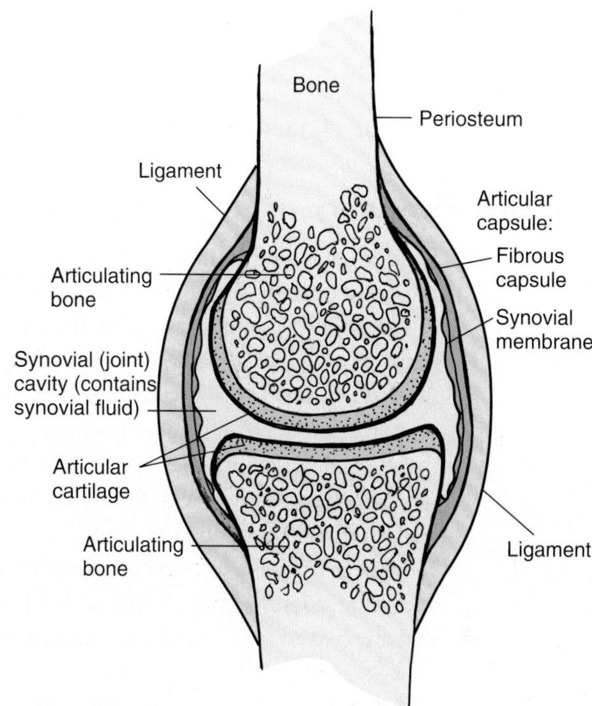

FIGURE 5.1. Classification of synovial joints. (From Bushman B, editor. *ACSM's Resources for the Personal Trainer*. 4th ed. Baltimore (MD): Lippincott Williams & Wilkins; 2014.)

consistently have greater ROM across almost all measured joints compared with men (48). Some of the reasons for increased female flexibility include smaller muscles and wider hips (62) and differences in hormonal levels (86). A study by Park et al. (86) has demonstrated that changes in estradiol and progesterone levels during ovulation led to a greater degree of knee joint laxity. Furthermore, it was also demonstrated that women have a more compliant Achilles tendon, resulting in greater ankle flexibility and lower muscle stiffness (51).

MODES OF FLEXIBILITY TRAINING

There are four types of flexibility training modes. Three of these modes — static, ballistic, and proprioceptive neuromuscular facilitation (PNF) — are considered "traditional" flexibility training modes (94). Dynamic flexibility training, however, is becoming more common, especially as part of the warm-up routine (32, 68). Of all the different modes, static flexibility training can be further subdivided into three categories: (a) slow and constant stretch with a partner (passive); (b) slow and constant stretch without any assistance, or "self-stretching"; and (c) slow and constant stretch against a stationary object (isometric) (100).

Static Flexibility

Static stretching is the most commonly used flexibility protocol of all (100), and regardless of the type of static stretching, each involves a slow and constant motion that is held in the final position, or point of mild discomfort, for 15 to 30 seconds (1). To achieve optimal degree of ROM, it is recommended to repeat each exercise no more than four times, since there are only minimal gains with additional repetitions (99). The advantage of using this method involves both relaxing and concurrent elongation of the stretched muscle without stimulation of a stretch reflex (80). Several studies have demonstrated that static stretching can lead to both short- and long-term gains in flexibility (4, 5, 22, 69) through a decrease in muscle/tendon stiffness and viscoelastic stress relaxation (65, 66). Although many researchers and practitioners view static stretching as effective and beneficial (4, 5,

22, 80) (Fig. 5.2), others have raised concerns. Since static stretching is slow and controlled, it does not provide an increase in muscle temperature and blood flow redistribution that is needed before and after exercise, respectively (71, 95). In addition, the view that static stretching may improve performance is equivocal, with several studies reporting an increase (46, 52, 107), several reporting a decrease (7, 18, 69), and others reporting no changes (103, 109) in performance.

Ballistic Flexibility

Ballistic stretching involves rapid and bouncing-like movements in which the resultant momentum of the body or body segments is used to extend the affected joint through the full ROM (33). This type of stretching technique, as opposed to static stretching and PNF, is no longer advocated (59, 102) to improve a joint's ROM. Ballistic stretching is used by some athletes and coaches to increase the blood flow to the muscle prior to competition or practice. Owing to the nature of the movements, this type of stretching produces a rapid and high degree of tension inside the muscle, which may potentially lead to muscle and tendon injuries (80, 81, 94). The risk of injury may be further exacerbated by a myotatic reflex, which is common with this mode of stretching (33). However, the hypothesis that ballistic stretching leads to muscle or connective tissue injury has never been supported by the scientific literature (77, 103). In respect of the effectiveness of this technique and when compared with static stretching, ballistic stretching does not provide any added benefit (5, 42, 63). Thus, it is recommended to use techniques that are viewed as safer and may potentially be more effective such as static stretching and PNF (32).

Proprioceptive Neuromuscular Facilitation

Proprioceptive neuromuscular facilitation (PNF) is a collection of stretching techniques combining passive stretch with isometric and concentric muscle actions designed to use the autogenic and reciprocal inhibition responses of the Golgi tendon organs (GTOs) (32, 33). It is hypothesized that through the responses of the GTO, the muscle and tendon are able to elongate and achieve greater ROM (32). However, it has been recently suggested that the effectiveness of PNF technique is mediated via increased pain tolerance rather than mechanoreceptors input (9). PNF stretching (Fig. 5.3) was first developed to help physical therapists treat patients with neuromuscular paralysis and later adopted for use by athletes as a technique to increase ROM (93).

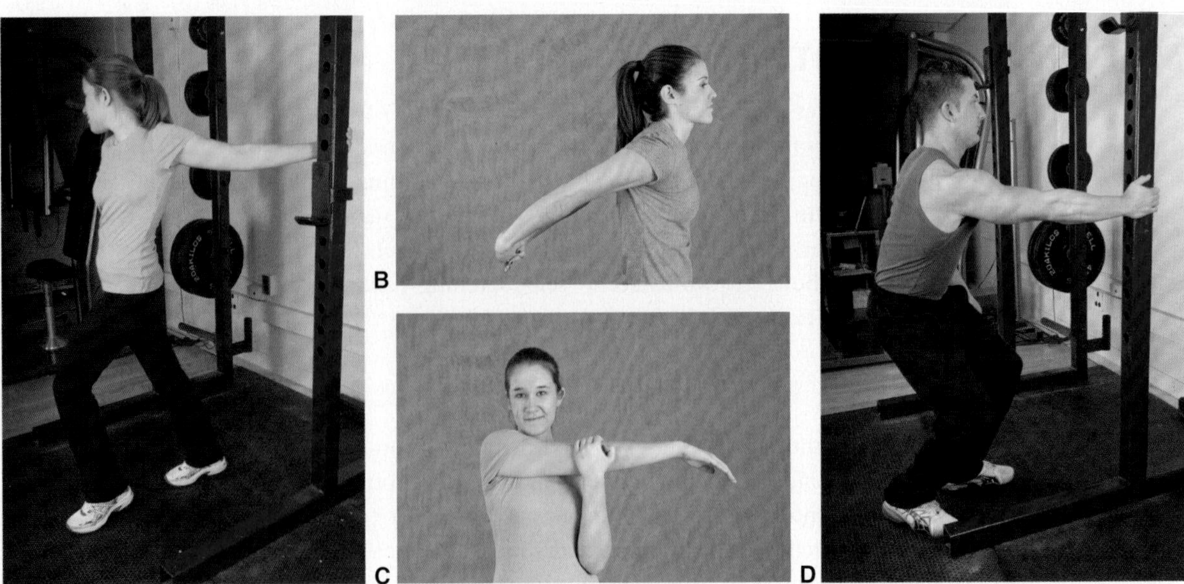

FIGURE 5.2. Examples of static stretches: (**A**) pectoral wall stretch, (**B**) posterior shoulder hyperextension, (**C**) anterior cross-arm stretch, and (**D**) lat stretch. (From Ratamess N. *ACSM's Foundations of Strength Training and Conditioning*. Baltimore (MD): Lippincott Williams & Wilkins; 2012.)

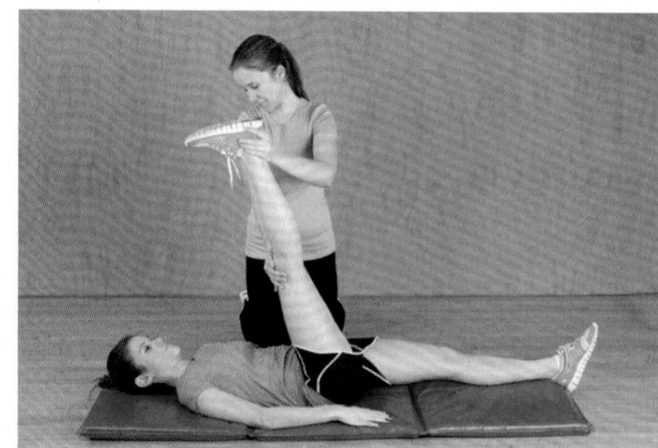

FIGURE 5.3. PNF stretching. (From Ratamess N. *ACSM's Foundations of Strength Training and Conditioning*. Baltimore (MD): Lippincott Williams & Wilkins; 2012:171.)

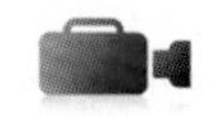

Visit thePoint to watch video 5.3, which demonstrates PNF stretching.

There are three types of PNF stretching techniques: (a) hold-relax, (b) contract-relax, and (c) hold-relax with agonist contraction (11, 14, 75, 98). Each technique comprises three phases: (a) a passive prestretch, (b) passive stretch, and (c) contractions (3). When PNF is compared with other stretching techniques with respect to effectiveness of improving ROM, the data are inconsistent. Some studies have demonstrated that PNF is superior to both static and ballistic stretching techniques (42, 90, 104), whereas others have found no difference (10, 14, 30, 63). Despite the wide support that the PNF technique has among researchers and practitioners, it has been pointed out that there are some limitations such as the need for a trained partner and the potentially high risk for musculature injury (16, 39).

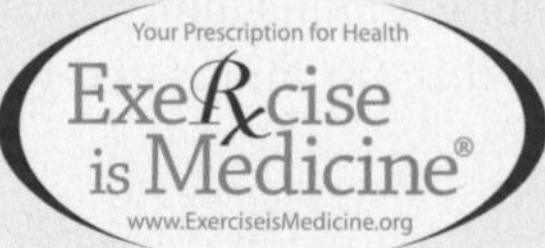

EXERCISE IS MEDICINE CONNECTION

Williams K, Christiaan A, Steinberg L, et al. Evaluation of the effectiveness and efficacy of Iyengar yoga therapy on chronic low back pain. *Spine*. 2009:34(19);2066–76.

Yoga has been used for more than 5,000 years around the world as a means of health improvement, with well-documented studies showing increased in flexibility and ROM, a key aspect of health-related fitness. Yoga's use has increased dramatically as a popular exercise modality in the United States in the recent past.

In addition to the benefits to flexibility, yoga has often been used to ease pain and dysfunction associated with chronic low back pain (CLBP), a serious medical problem affecting as many as 80% of all adults and a leading cause of lost work time; however, evidence to support yoga as "medicine" for treating CLBP has only recently surfaced.

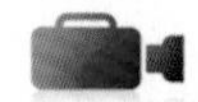

Visit thePoint to watch videos 5.4 and 5.5, which demonstrate the kneeling cat and modified cobra positions.

Williams et al. randomly assigned 90 participants to either a yoga group or a control group, with the yoga group receiving 24 weeks of biweekly yoga classes designed for CLBP. Outcomes for disability, pain, pain medication, and depression were assessed at 12 (midway), 24 (immediately after), and 48 weeks (6-month follow-up) after the start of the intervention. Outcomes included significant reductions in functional disability and pain intensity in the yoga group at the end of the 24-week intervention. There were also a significantly greater proportion of yoga participants reporting clinical improvements at both 12 and 24 weeks. In addition, depression was significantly lower in yoga participants in CLBP. Although both groups experienced a reduction in pain medication, there was no difference between groups. Even after 6-month follow-up, the yoga group still showed significantly improved functional disability, pain intensity, and depression compared with standard medical care.

In summary, appropriately designed yoga programs can be an effective treatment for reducing pain, pain medication, disability, and depression associated with CLBP.

Dynamic Flexibility

As opposed to the previously mentioned stretching techniques, dynamic flexibility uses slow and controlled, sport-specific movements that are designed to increase core temperature and enhance activity-related flexibility and balance (5, 38, 68). In view of the fact that these exercises are sport specific, there is no comprehensive list of dynamic exercises. The design of such exercises is only limited by the knowledge and resourcefulness of the coach/trainer (38). In the past few years, several studies have examined the effectiveness of dynamic flexibility in relation to the degree of flexibility and athletic performance, and the effects of preexercise static and dynamic stretches on anaerobic performance in different populations. One study has demonstrated that both static and dynamic stretches improve the ROM of the hamstring muscle, yet static stretching was more effective (5). Further, whereas some studies have demonstrated that a warm-up that included dynamic stretching was superior for improving sport performance to the one that included static stretching (72, 76, 101), others have failed to show those differences (19, 34, 103). Also related to dynamic stretching, eccentric training was recently introduced as a new technique that is designed to reduce the occurrence of injuries and improve flexibility and performance. Using this technique, the participant is instructed to resist a flexion in a given joint by eccentrically contracting the antagonist muscles during the entire ROM (79). Two studies examining this technique have demonstrated some merit when compared with static stretching (78, 79). These recent findings emphasize the controversy that surrounds the issue of the usefulness of different stretching techniques.

MUSCLE AND TENDON PROPRIOCEPTORS

There are two types of sensory organs that provide muscular dynamic and limb movement information to the central nervous system (70). These sensors, muscle spindles (see Fig. 5.4), and GTOs (see Fig. 5.5) should be considered when discussing stretching and flexibility. Muscle spindles are a collection of 3 to 10 intrafusal, specialized muscle fibers that are innervated by gamma motor

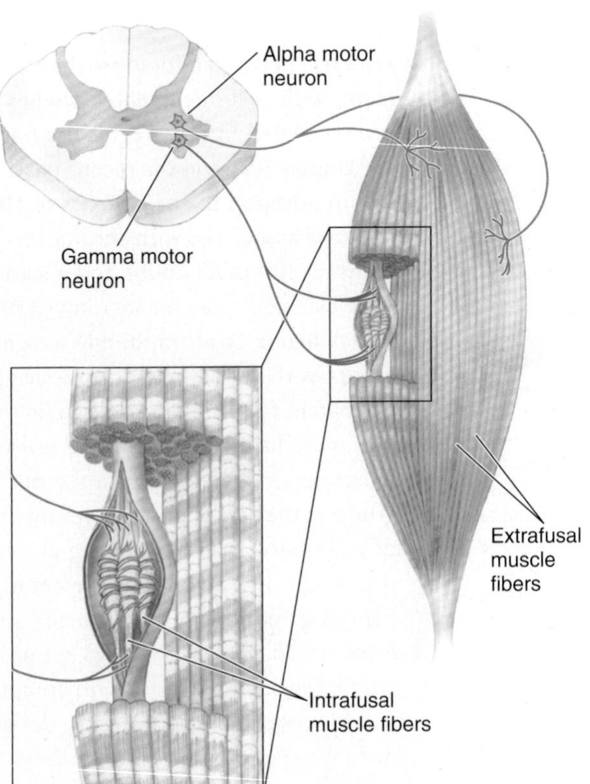

FIGURE 5.4. Structure and location of the muscle spindles. (From Bear MF, Connors BW, Parasido MA. *Neuroscience: Exploring the Brain*. 2nd ed. Philadelphia (PA): Lippincott Williams & Wilkins; 2001.)

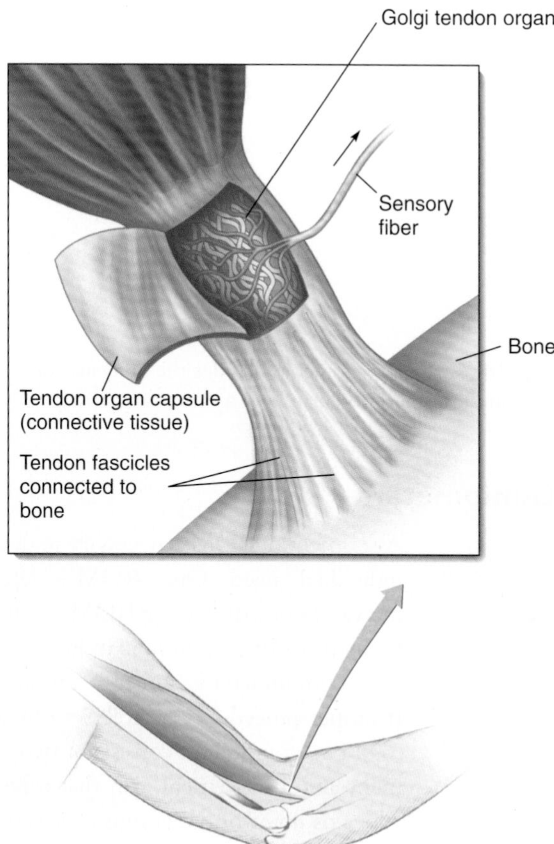

FIGURE 5.5. Structure and location of the GTO. (From Premkumar K. The Massage Connection: Anatomy and Physiology, 2nd Ed. Baltimore: Lippincott Williams and Wilkins, 2004.)

neurons and provide information about the rate of change in muscle length. The intrafusal muscle fibers run parallel to the extrafusal muscle fibers (regular muscle fibers), which are innervated by alpha motor neurons and are responsible for tension development (31, 33) (Fig. 5.4). When muscle spindles are stimulated, there is a dual response in which a rapid tension development is initiated in the stretched muscle and inhibited in the antagonist muscle. The response in the stretched muscle is known as a stretch or myotatic reflex, and the response in the antagonist muscle is known as reciprocal inhibition (14, 33, 75). These responses serve an important role in both static stretching and PNF. Since the myotatic reflex is less likely to occur in slow and controlled movements, static stretch is viewed as safer and more effective than ballistic stretch (33). During a PNF when there is an increase in tension in the antagonist muscle with a concurrent elongation of the agonist muscle, a further lengthening of the stretched muscle is thought to be mediated by reciprocal inhibition (32).

GTOs are located in the musculotendinous junction and respond to changes in muscle tension (Fig. 5.5). These organs are encapsulated in a series with 10 to 15 muscle fibers and can identify and provide a response to changes in the amount of tension (static) and the rate of tension (dynamic) development. When the GTOs are stimulated, there is a dual response in which tension development is inhibited in the contracting muscle (autogenic inhibition) and initiated in the antagonist muscles (31, 33). Similar to the muscle spindles' response, the GTO plays an important role in PNF. The active tension development in the muscle prior to a stretch elicits autogenic inhibition, which promotes further lengthening of the affected muscle (14, 32, 75).

FLEXIBILITY ASSESSMENT PROTOCOLS

Different methods and tools are used to measure ROM and flexibility. Among the most common are the use of goniometers, sit-and-reach tests, and functional movement screenings.

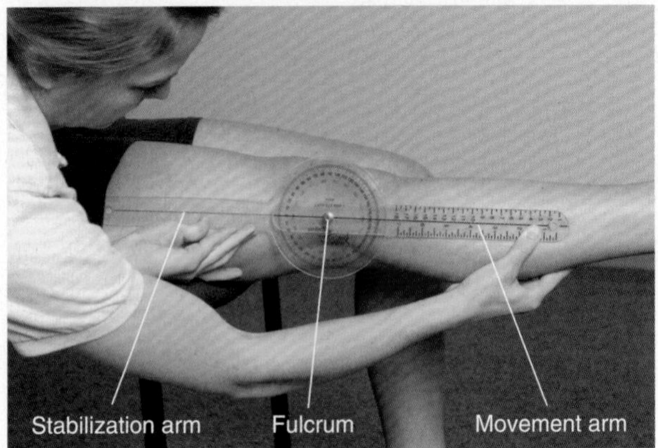

FIGURE 5.6. A goniometer includes the body axis or fulcrum, a stabilization arm, and a movement arm.

Goniometers

Assessment of ROM is necessary to determine the need for a flexibility training program relative to the individual's needs. Once ROM is determined, an appropriate program prescription with the goal of increasing or maintaining ROM can be implemented. Given that ROM is joint specific, the most useful method for determining individual joint flexibility is through the use of a goniometer (see Fig. 5.6).

A goniometer is similar to a protractor and is used to measure a joint's ROM expressed in degrees. If proper procedures are followed by an HFS, goniometer measurements are both valid and reliable (60). The goniometer consists of two arms: a stabilization arm that is fixed to the proximal body segment and a movement arm that follows the distal body segment as it is moved through its ROM. The axis point of the goniometer is placed at a predetermined anatomical landmark, generally at the joint axis of rotation. Procedures for goniometry assessment of commonly measured joints are listed below (see Table 5.1). General guidelines for proper goniometry assessment include the following:

- Before assessment, provide the client with an overview of the process.
- Demonstrate proper technique for movement of the joint being assessed.
- Instruct the client to move slowly through the proper ROM.
- During movement, ensure that the goniometer maintains proper orientation relative to predefined anatomical landmarks (it may be helpful to mark specific body segments to assure consistent placement over time).
- Measure three consecutive trials averaging the values as the final score.
- If average ROM is lesser than 50°, it is recommended that the measures fall within ±5° of the mean. If the average ROM is greater than 50°, the three measures should fall within ±10° of the mean. Measurements should continue until they meet the criteria or are otherwise considered invalid (2, 60).

Sit-and-Reach Tests

Although goniometry is the most useful method to assess joint specific ROM, the sit-and-reach test is perhaps the most commonly used assessment for flexibility in the lower back and hip joint. Although other joints in the body (including the spine and shoulder girdle) can and should be assessed for flexibility, there are a dearth of tests and norms for flexibility assessment of these joints. The sit-and-reach test may be useful to evaluate ROM of the spine and hips for effective completion of activities of daily living, although there has not been evidence demonstrating reduction in low back pain relative to ROM measured by the sit-and-reach (49). It should be noted that sit-and-reach testing may need to be modified for various subpopulations, including the young, the old, and the pregnant, although specific procedures and norms are lacking. Procedures for two different sit-and-reach tests (Fig. 5.7) are described in the box titled "How to Perform the Sit-and-Reach Test." Normative data for these sit-and-reach tests are in Tables 5.2 and 5.3.

TABLE 5.1 PROCEDURES FOR GONIOMETRY ASSESSMENT OF JOINTS COMMONLY OF CONCERN TO HEALTH AND FITNESS PROFESSIONALS

Movement	Plane of Motion	Axis of Motion	Average Range	Goniometer Position	Stabilization	Starting/Ending Body Position	
				Upper Body			
Spine							
Lumbar flexion	Sagittal	Bilateral	4-in increase	Tape measure position 1. Top point: Spinous process C7 2. Bottom point: Level to posterior superior iliac spine (PSIS)	Client is seated on floor or table with pelvis stabilized to prevent anterior/posterior tilting with legs extended	Client is in good posture with a stabilized cervical, thoracic, and lumbar spine in 0° of flexion, extension, rotation, or lateral flexion. Head is in neutral position. Client performs lumbar flexion until first sign of resistance	Extension Flexion **FIGURE 5.8.** Lumbar flexion and extension. (From Bushman B, editor. *ACSM's Resources for the Personal Trainer.* 4th ed. Baltimore (MD): Lippincott Williams & Wilkins; 2014.)
Lumbar extension	Sagittal	Bilateral	2-in difference as spine extends	Tape measure position 1. Top point: Spinous process C7 2. Bottom point: Level to PSIS	Client is seated on floor or table with pelvis stabilized to prevent anterior/posterior tilting with legs extended	Client is in good posture with a stabilized cervical, thoracic, and lumbar spine in 0° of flexion, extension, rotation, or lateral flexion. Head is in neutral position. Client performs lumbar flexion until first sign of resistance	

(continued)

TABLE 5.1 PROCEDURES FOR GONIOMETRY ASSESSMENT OF JOINTS COMMONLY OF CONCERN TO HEALTH AND FITNESS PROFESSIONALS *(continued)*

Movement	Plane of Motion	Axis of Motion	Average Range	Goniometer Position	Stabilization	Starting/Ending Body Position
Shoulder						
Glenohumeral flexion	Sagittal	Bilateral	0°–180°	1. Axis point: Lateral aspect of grater tubercle 2. Stabilization arm: Perpendicular to the floor 3. Movement arm: Align with midline of humerus and reference the lateral epicondyle	Client is in good posture with a stabilized scapula (retracted), thoracic, and lumbar spine. Stabilize scapula to prevent tilting, rotation, or elevation	Client is seated with Glenohumeral in 0° of flexion, extension, abduction, or adduction. Head is in neutral position. Palm of hand should be facing the body. Elbow should be extended completely. Client performs glenohumeral flexion until the first sign of resistance
Glenohumeral extension	Sagittal	Bilateral	0°–60°	1. Axis point: Lateral aspect of grater tubercle 2. Stabilization arm: Perpendicular to the floor 3. Movement arm: Align with midline of humerus and reference the lateral epicondyle	Client is in good posture with a stabilized scapula (retracted), thoracic, and lumbar spine. Stabilize scapula to prevent tilting, rotation, or elevation. Place towel under humerus to stabilize and align with acromion process	Client is prone on table with Glenohumeral in 0° of flexion, extension, abduction, or adduction. Head is in neutral position. Palm of hand should face the body. Elbow should be extended completely. Client performs glenohumeral extension until the first sign of resistance

FIGURE 5.9. Glenohumeral flexion and extension. (From Bushman B, editor. *ACSM's Resources for the Personal Trainer.* 4th ed. Baltimore (MD): Lippincott Williams & Wilkins; 2014.)

Glenohumeral internal rotation	Transverse	Longitudinal	0°–70°	1. Axis point: Olecranon process of the elbow 2. Stabilization arm: Perpendicular to the floor 3. Movement arm: Aligned with lateral midline of ulna and reference the ulnar styloid	Client is in good posture with a stabilized scapula (retracted), thoracic, and lumbar spine. Stabilize scapula to prevent tilting, rotation, or elevation. Place towel under humerus to stabilize and align with acromion process	Client is supine on table with humerus abducted at 90° and elbow is flexed at 90°. Elbow is at 0° of supination and pronation. Client performs glenohumeral internal rotation until the first sign of resistance	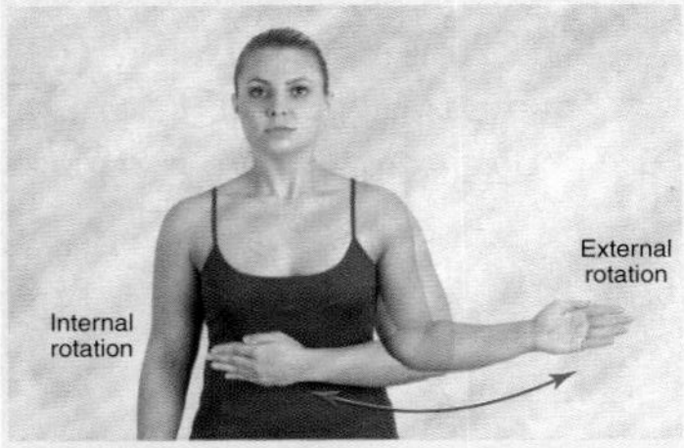 Internal rotation External rotation **FIGURE 5.10.** Glenohumeral internal rotation and external rotation. (From Bushman B, editor. *ACSM's Resources for the Personal Trainer.* 4th ed. Baltimore (MD): Lippincott Williams & Wilkins; 2014.)
Glenohumeral external rotation	Transverse	Longitudinal	0°–90°	1. Axis point: Olecranon process of the elbow 2. Stabilization arm: Perpendicular to the floor 3. Movement arm: Aligned with lateral midline of ulna and reference the ulnar styloid	Client is in good posture with a stabilized scapula (retracted), thoracic, and lumbar spine. Stabilize scapula to prevent tilting, rotation, or elevation. Place towel under humerus to stabilize and align with acromion process	Client is supine on table with humerus abducted at 90° and elbow is flexed at 90°. Elbow is at 0° of supination and pronation. Client performs glenohumeral external rotation until the first sign of resistance	

(continued)

TABLE 5.1 PROCEDURES FOR GONIOMETRY ASSESSMENT OF JOINTS COMMONLY OF CONCERN TO HEALTH AND FITNESS PROFESSIONALS *(continued)*

Movement	Plane of Motion	Axis of Motion	Average Range	Goniometer Position	Stabilization	Starting/Ending Body Position
Lower Body						
Hip						
Hip flexion (testing leg fully extended)	Sagittal	Bilateral	0°–90°	1. Axis point: Greater trochanter of the lateral thigh 2. Stabilization arm: Lateral midline of the pelvis 3. Movement arm: Lateral midline of the femur, using the lateral epicondyle as a reference	Client is in good posture with a stabilized scapula, thoracic, lumbar spine, and pelvic area. Pelvis should not rise off table. Opposite leg not being assessed should have knee flexed and foot flat on table for added stability and protection for the back	Client is supine on table with hip in 0° of flexion, extension, abduction, adduction, and rotation. Testing leg has knee fully extended. Client performs hip flexion until the first sign of resistance or until the pelvis rotates or knee breaks extension
Hip flexion (testing knee flexed 90° and hip flexed 90°)	Sagittal	Bilateral	0°–120°	1. Axis point: Greater trochanter of the lateral thigh 2. Stabilization arm: Lateral midline of the pelvis 3. Movement arm: Lateral midline of the femur, using the lateral epicondyle as a reference	Client is in good posture with a stabilized scapula, thoracic, lumbar spine, and pelvic area. Pelvis should not rise off table. Opposite leg not being assessed should have knee flexed and foot flat on table for added stability and protection for the back	Client is supine on table with knee flexed at 90° and hip flexed at 90°, and hip is in 0° of abduction, adduction, and rotation. Knee is flexed to reduce contraction of hamstrings. Client performs hip flexion until the first sign of resistance or until the pelvis rotates
Hip extension (testing leg fully extended)	Sagittal	Bilateral	0°–30°	1. Axis point: Greater trochanter of the lateral thigh 2. Stabilization arm: Lateral midline of the pelvis 3. Movement arm: Lateral midline of the femur, using the lateral epicondyle as a reference	Client is in good posture with a stabilized scapula, thoracic, lumbar spine, and pelvic area. Pelvis should not rise off table. Opposite leg not being assessed should have leg fully extended on table for added stability	Client is prone on table with hip in 0° of flexion, extension, abduction, adduction, and rotation. Testing leg has knee fully extended. Client performs hip extension until the first sign of resistance or until the pelvis rotates

FIGURE 5.11. Hip flexion with the testing leg fully extended **(A)** and with the testing knee and hip both flexed 90° **(B)**; hip extension with the testing leg fully extended **(C)**. (**A** and **C** from Bushman B, editor. *ACSM's Resources for the Personal Trainer.* 4th ed. Baltimore (MD): Lippincott Williams & Wilkins; 2014. **B** from Kaminsky L. *ACSM's Health-Related Physical Fitness Assessment Manual.* 4th ed. Baltimore (MD): Lippincott Williams & Wilkins; 2014.)

Hip abduction	Frontal	Anterior/ posterior	0°–45°	1. Axis point: Locate anterior superior iliac spine (ASIS) 2. Stabilization arm: Imaginary line connecting axis point ASIS to other ASIS 3. Movement arm: Anterior midline of the femur, using the midline of the patella as a reference	Client is in good posture with a stabilized scapula, thoracic, lumbar spine, and pelvic area. Stabilize for lateral trunk flexion on both sides	Client is supine on table with hip in 0° of flexion, extension, and rotation. Testing leg has knee fully extended. Client performs hip abduction until the first sign of resistance or lateral trunk flexion occurs on either side	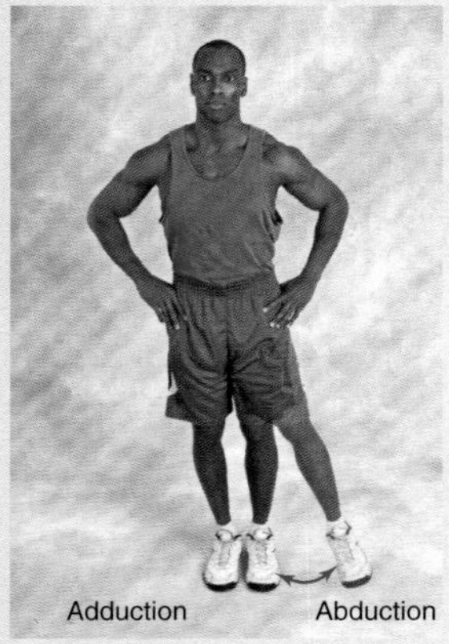 **FIGURE 5.12.** Hip adduction and abduction. (From Bushman B, editor. *ACSM's Resources for the Personal Trainer*. 4th ed. Baltimore (MD): Lippincott Williams & Wilkins; 2014.)
Hip adduction	Frontal	Anterior/ posterior	0°–30°	1. Axis point: Located at the ASIS 2. Stabilization arm: Imaginary horizontal line connecting axis point ASIS to other ASIS 3. Movement arm: Anterior midline of the femur, using the midline of the patella as a reference	Client is in good posture with a stabilized scapula, thoracic, lumbar spine, and pelvic area. Opposite leg not being tested should be abducted fully to allow for testing hip to be assessed	Client is supine on table with hip in 0° of flexion, extension, and rotation. Testing leg has knee fully extended. Client performs hip adduction until the first sign of resistance or lateral trunk flexion or pelvic rotation occurs	

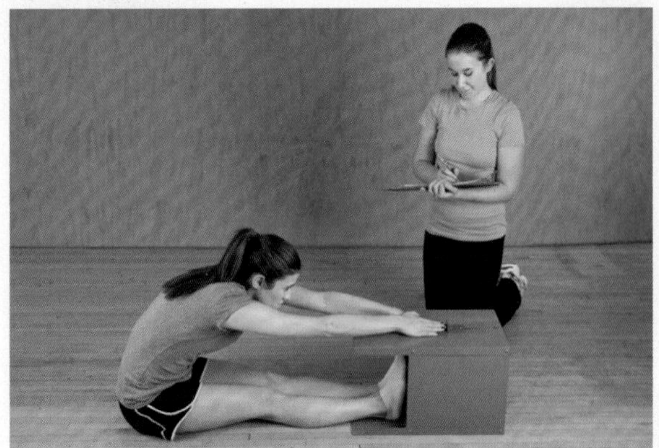

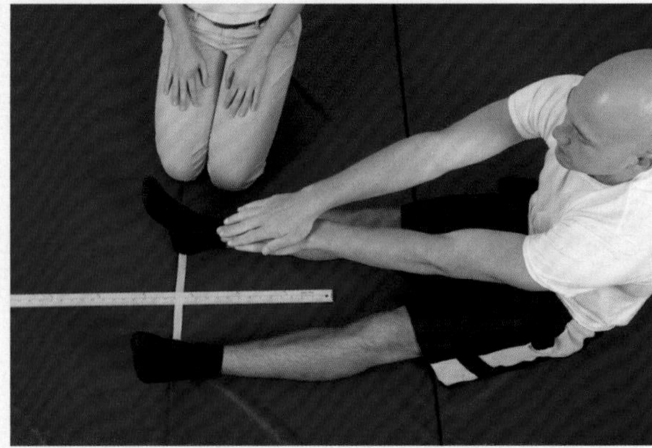

FIGURE 5.7. Sit-and-reach tests. **A.** Test using a sit-and-reach box. (From Ratamess N. *ACSM's Foundations of Strength Training and Conditioning*. Baltimore (MD): Lippincott Williams & Wilkins; 2012.) **B.** The YMCA sit-and-reach test.

Functional Movement Screenings

The assessment of compensatory movement patterns via dynamic movements to assess individuals for potential weakness and imbalances in strength, flexibility, and motor control has gained popularity in recent years. These assessments strive to examine overall movement patterns, recognize irregularities, and prescribe corrective exercises, with the hope of reducing the chance of injury.

These dynamic movement assessments rely on both qualitative and quantitative observations during specific movement patterns to make prescription recommendations. Commonly, the use of functional movement screening (FMS) includes seven tests that are scored using a rank order scale. The seven tests are the squat, hurdle step, lunge, shoulder mobility, active straight leg raise, push-up, and rotary stability (15). Research has demonstrated the use of these screenings is capable of predicting individuals at risk for injury in military officers, professional football players, firefighters,

TABLE 5.2 FITNESS CATEGORIES FOR TRUNK FORWARD FLEXION USING A SIT-AND-REACH BOX (CM)[a] BY AGE AND SEX

	Age (yr)									
	20–29		30–39		40–49		50–59		60–69	
Category	M	W	M	W	M	W	M	W	M	W
Excellent	40	41	38	41	35	38	35	39	33	35
Very good	39	40	37	40	34	37	34	38	32	34
	34	37	33	36	29	34	28	33	25	31
Good	33	36	32	35	28	33	27	32	24	30
	30	33	28	32	24	30	24	30	20	27
Fair	29	32	27	31	23	29	23	29	19	26
	25	28	23	27	18	25	16	25	15	23
Needs improvement	24	27	22	26	17	24	15	24	14	22

[a]These norms are based on a sit-and-reach box in which the "zero" point is set at 26 cm. When using a box in which the zero point is set at 23 cm, subtract 3 cm from each value in this table.

M, men; *W*, women.

Reprinted with permission from Dalrymple KJ, Davis SE, Dwyer GB, Moir GL. Effect of static and dynamic stretching on vertical jump performance in collegiate women volleyball players. *J Strength Cond Res. 2010;24(1):149–55. Copyright © 2003*. Used with permission from the Canadian Society for Exercise Physiology www.csep.ca

TABLE 5.3 **FITNESS CATEGORIES FOR THE YMCA SIT-AND-REACH TEST (IN) BY AGE AND SEX**

		Age (yr)											
		18–25		26–35		36–45		46–55		56–65		>65	
Percentile	**Category**	M	W	M	W	M	W	M	W	M	W	M	W
90	Well above average	22	24	21	23	21	22	19	21	17	20	17	20
80	Above average	20	22	19	21	19	21	17	20	15	19	15	18
70		19	21	17	20	17	19	15	18	13	17	13	17
60	Average	18	20	17	20	16	18	14	17	13	16	12	17
50		17	19	15	19	15	17	13	16	11	15	10	15
40	Below average	15	18	14	17	13	16	11	14	9	14	9	14
30		14	17	13	16	13	15	10	14	9	13	8	13
20	Well below average	13	16	11	15	11	14	9	12	7	11	7	11
10		11	14	9	13	7	12	6	10	5	9	4	9

M, men; W, women.

Adapted with permission from (111).

and female college athletes (8, 12, 53, 83). Individuals who have undergone training to understand the techniques of dynamic assessment have been shown to have high interrater reliability, and the method can be a reliable tool for screenings (74).

FLEXIBILITY PROGRAM DESIGN

The framework for developing and maintaining whole body ROM is structured around the same underlying principles that all health-related fitness components utilize progressive overload, specificity of training, individual differences, and reversibility. The components of a health-related fitness program consisting of frequency, intensity, time, and type (FITT) are the foundation for which flexibility programs are developed. Assessment of ROM at specific joints helps determine the need for a flexibility program. Healthy individuals with inadequate ROM for particular activities should engage in a program that caters to their specific needs. Once adequate ROM is achieved, a maintenance program should be prescribed. For individuals with hypermobility in joint ROM, there does not seem to be a benefit of participation in a flexibility training program (29, 54, 56, 57, 106).

The principle of progressive overload in the context of flexibility demonstrates that for ROM to improve, it must be stressed beyond its normal range. This may be accomplished by completing the flexibility exercises recommended below or by participating in activities that elicit greater ROM in targeted joints. The principle of overload for flexibility training may be applied by increasing frequency (sessions per day or week), intensity (point of stretch), and/or time for each session. Individual differences as it relates to neuromuscular function and structure should be taken into consideration in the design of a flexibility program. Progression with increasing ROM is dependent on those individual differences and factors that affect flexibility as discussed. The principle of reversibility should also be considered with respect to flexibility training like other modes of exercise. Feland et al. (25) demonstrated that flexibility gains are lost within 4 to 8 weeks of ceasing flexibility exercises.

After assessment of flexibility, a training program may be necessary to increase or maintain ROM relative to individual goals. To improve ROM, two to three training sessions per week for at

HOW TO Perform the Sit-And-Reach Test

Pretest: Before testing, the participant should remove his or her shoes and perform a short warm-up of approximately 5-minute moderate aerobic activity followed by a few select flexibility exercises. It is also recommended that the participant refrain from fast, jerky movements.

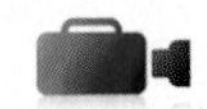

Visit thePoint to watch video 5.6, which explains how to perform the YMCA sit and reach test.

For the Canadian Trunk Forward Flexion test, the client sits without shoes and the soles of the feet flat against the flexometer (sit-and-reach box) at the 26-cm mark. Inner edges of the soles are placed within 2 cm of the measuring scale. For the YMCA sit-and-reach test, a yardstick is placed on the floor and tape is placed across it at a right angle to the 15-in mark. The participant sits with the yardstick between the legs, with legs extended at right angles to the taped line on the floor. Heels of the feet should touch the edge of the taped line and be about 10 to 12 in apart. (Note the zero point at the foot/box interface and use the appropriate norms.)

The participant should slowly reach forward with both hands as far as possible, holding this position approximately 2 seconds. Be sure that the participant keeps the hands parallel and does not lead with one hand. Fingertips can be overlapped and should be in contact with the measuring portion or yardstick of the sit-and-reach box.

The score is the most distant point (in centimeters or inches) reached with the fingertips. The best of two trials should be recorded. To assist with the best attempt, the participant should exhale and drop the head between the arms when reaching (and otherwise breath normally, never holding breath). Testers should ensure that the knees of the participant stay extended; however, the participant's knees should not be pressed down. Norms for the Canadian test are presented below (Table 5.2). Note that these norms use a sit-and-reach box in which the zero point is set at the 26-cm mark. If you are using a box in which the zero point is set at 23 cm (*e.g.*, FitnessGram), subtract 3 cm from each value in this table. The norms for the YMCA test are presented below (see Table 5.3).

Source: *YMCA Fitness Testing and Assessment Manual*. 4th ed. Chicago (IL):YMCA of the USA. p. 158–60 (108).

least 3 to 4 weeks may be required (20, 21, 25). During each of the training sessions, each exercise should include two to four repetitions in which the stretch is held between 10 and 30 seconds, with 30 to 60 seconds in older individuals, with a goal of accumulating 60 seconds of stretch across two to four repetitions (89, 102). Increasing the duration of each repetition beyond 30 to 60 seconds does not seem to lead to improved ROM benefits except perhaps in an elderly population (6, 25). Generally, joints of the neck, shoulders, upper and lower back, pelvis, hips, and legs will need to be trained as it relates to daily activity and performance (99). Flexibility training should be conducted when a muscle is warm and therefore should be completed after an aerobic warm-up of at least 5 minutes and some general flexibility exercises. Also, testing may occur subsequent to cardiovascular or strength sessions. Since some researchers have demonstrated that acute preexercise flexibility training may have negative effects on ensuing performance, postexercise flexibility training may be more beneficial (54, 56, 57, 106). The intensity of the flexibility training is dependent on the individual, but it is recommended that a given stretch will be held to the point of mild discomfort. The duration of the training session may vary on the basis of the mode of the flexibility exercise. Static ROM training session should be at minimum 10 minutes, and if PNF stretching is being employed, a 6-second contraction followed by a 10- to 30-second assisted stretch is recommended (1). The mode of the flexibility program should depend on the individual and available equipment. Generally, increased ROM has been demonstrated in all modes of flexibility training (67, 110). Table 5.4 lists some static stretches for the major muscle groups.

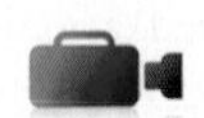

Visit thePoint to watch videos 5.7 and 5.8, which demonstrate pendulum leg swings and dynamic hip rotation, respectively.

TABLE 5.4 STATIC STRETCHES FOR THE MAJOR MUSCLE GROUPS

Stretch	Muscle Involved	Starting Position	Description
			Upper Body
Neck			
Flexion or stretching extensors? (Fig. 5.13A)	• Obliquus capitis superior Rectus capitis superior major Rectus capitis superior minor Obliquus capitis inferior Semispinalis capitis Splenius cervicis Longissimus capitis Levator scapulae	Standing or sitting	Starting with the superior segments, slowly flex your cervical spine so that your chin moves toward your chest. Maintain your chest and shoulders in a static position
Extension or stretching flexors? (Fig. 5.13A)	• Longus capitis Longus colli sternohyoid Omohyoid Platysma	Standing or sitting	Place both hands behind your neck so that your fingers are just below your occiput and along the upper vertebrae on both sides. Carefully look back and up, extending your cervical spine while supporting your head and neck with your hands
Lateral bending (Fig. 5.13B)	• Upper trapezius Anterior, middle, and posterior scalene Sternocleidomastoid Splenius capitis	Standing or sitting	Take your right hand and reach over the top of your head, placing it palm down on your head so that your middle two fingers touch your left ear. Carefully, pull your head directly toward the right side, being careful not to let your head move forward or back. Repeat to the left
Rotation (Fig. 5.13C)	• Sternocleidomastoid Longissimus capitis Splenius capitis Obliquus capitis inferior	Standing or sitting	Use your left hand to reach behind your back and pull your right forearm gently inferiorly and toward the left, depressing your right shoulder. Carefully turn your head toward the left. Repeat toward the right

FIGURE 5.13. Neck extension **(A)**, flexion **(B)**, lateral flexion **(C)**, and rotation **(D)**. (From Ratamess N. *ACSM's Foundations of Strength Training and Conditioning*. Baltimore (MD): Lippincott Williams & Wilkins; 2012:49.)

(continued)

TABLE 5.4 STATIC STRETCHES FOR THE MAJOR MUSCLE GROUPS *(continued)*

Stretch	Muscle Involved	Starting Position	Description	
Shoulder				
Extension or stretching flexors?	• Pectoralis major Anterior deltoid Long head of biceps brachii Coracobrachialis	Standing	Lock your hands together behind back with elbows only slightly flexed. Lift interlocked hands up behind your back, extending your shoulders. No need to bend your back forward!	
Flexion or stretching extensors?	• Latissimus dorsi Teres major Posterior deltoid Long head of the triceps brachii Rhomboid major and minor through their action on the scapula	Standing in front of a chair	Place both hands on the back of a chair or object of similar height. Then carefully bend at the waist until arms are straightened overhead with a roughly 90° angle at the waist. Be careful to keep your lower back straight, allowing the forward bend to come from flexion at the hips	
Abduction abductors?	• Middle deltoid Supraspinatus Upper trapezius through its action in superiorly rotating the scapula (a necessary and integral motion in abducting the shoulder)	Standing	Reach your right hand behind your back. Grasp your right forearm with your left hand. Adduct your right arm by carefully pulling it toward the left until a gentle stretch is felt at the right shoulder. Then slowly lean your head toward the left, increasing the stretch at both your right shoulder and your upper trapezius. Repeat toward the right	Abduction Adduction **FIGURE 5.14.** Shoulder abduction and adduction. (From Bushman B, editor. *ACSM's Resources for the Personal Trainer*. 4th ed. Baltimore (MD): Lippincott Williams & Wilkins; 2014.)
Abduction abductors?	• Pectoralis major Latissimus dorsi Teres major Rhomboids major and minor via their action on the scapula	Standing	Extend your right arm overhead, palm facing to the left. Reach your entire arm directly toward the left and continue with left side-bending of your torso. Repeat to the right leading with your left hand	

Horizontal adduction adductors	• Anterior deltoid Sternal portion of pectoralis major Coracobrachialis	Standing	Abduct arms to shoulder level with palms facing upward. Horizontally abduct both shoulders, keeping them at shoulder level. You may use a doorway to help assist with this movement. Ideally, both sides can be stretched simultaneously (as the tension from one side stabilizes the origin on the other side); however, this is not necessary, and effective stretches can be performed unilaterally	 **FIGURE 5.15.** Shoulder horizontal adduction and horizontal abduction. (From Bushman B, editor. *ACSM's Resources for the Personal Trainer*. 4th ed. Baltimore (MD): Lippincott Williams & Wilkins; 2014.)
Horizontal adduction adductors	• Posterior deltoid Teres minor Infraspinatus Upper and middle trapezius Rhomboid major and minor via their attachment to the scapula	Standing	To stretch your left shoulder horizontal abductors, grasp the posterior aspect of your left elbow with your right hand. Horizontally adduct your left shoulder by pulling your left elbow horizontally across toward your right shoulder just beneath the chin. Repeat with the right	
Internal rotation rotators	• Subscapularis Latissimus dorsi Pectoralis major Teres major Anterior deltoid	Standing in a doorway, right arm at your side, elbow flexed to 90°, and palm facing forward against the doorframe	To stretch your right shoulder internal rotators, keep your right elbow at your side and right hand against the door frame, then carefully turn your body toward the left until you feel a gentle stretch. Repeat for your left shoulder	
External rotation Rotators	• Infraspinatus Teres minor Posterior deltoid	Standing	Internally rotate your left shoulder by placing your left hand behind your back with the palm facing posteriorly. Place the palm of your right hand over the anterior aspect of your left shoulder. Back into a doorway with the posterior surface of the left elbow against the door jam. While maintaining firm support of the anterior shoulder with the left palm and hand (do not let the shoulder push forward), carefully move your entire body backward, forcing the elbow forward, until an easy stretch is felt in your left shoulder. Repeat on the opposite side to stretch your right shoulder	

(continued)

TABLE 5.4 STATIC STRETCHES FOR THE MAJOR MUSCLE GROUPS *(continued)*

Stretch	Muscle Involved	Starting Position	Description	
Elbow				
Flexion flexors	• Long and short heads of the biceps brachii Brachialis Brachioradialis	Standing	Clasp your hands together behind your lower back, extend your elbows completely, and then externally rotate your arms so that your palms are facing your buttocks. Now extend both shoulders by lifting the hands up and away from your buttocks	**FIGURE 5.16.** Elbow flexion and extension. (From Bushman B, editor. *ACSM's Resources for the Personal Trainer*. 4th ed. Baltimore (MD): Lippincott Williams & Wilkins; 2014.)
Extension extensors	• Long, medial, and middle heads of the triceps brachii Anconeus	Standing	Extend your right arm overhead and flex your elbow maximally. Place the palm of your left hand against your right forearm just distal to the elbow, with your fingers curving over your right elbow. Squeeze your elbow joint to keep it maximally flexed, and then slowly pull it posteriorly and medially. Repeat with the left arm	
Supination supinators	• Supinator Biceps brachii	Standing with arms relaxed at sides	To stretch the supinators of your right arm, flex your right elbow slightly and pronate your right forearm so that the palm is facing down. Using your left hand, grasp your right forearm just proximal to your wrist. Pronate your right forearm while externally rotating your right humerus. Repeat with the left forearm	**FIGURE 5.17.** Elbow supination and pronation. (From Bushman B, editor. *ACSM's Resources for the Personal Trainer*. 4th ed. Baltimore (MD): Lippincott Williams & Wilkins; 2014.)
Pronation pronators	• Pronator teres Pronator quadratus	Standing	To stretch the pronators of your right forearm, extend your right elbow and supinate your right hand. With your left hand, grasp your right forearm just proximal to the wrist. Using your left hand, rotate your right wrist externally, further supinating your right forearm. Be sure to keep your upper arm from externally rotating as well – this may require an active contraction of the shoulder internal rotators. Repeat with the left forearm	

Wrist and Hand				
Extension extensors	• Extensor carpi radialis Extensor digitorum Extensor indicis Extensor digiti minimi Extensor carpi radialis Extensor pollicis longus Extensor pollicis brevis	Sitting or standing	To stretch the extensors of your left arm and hand, extend your left arm out in front of you with your elbow extended, forearm pronated. Flex your left wrist and then attempt to flex fingers 2–5 into a fist. Repeat on the right arm	FIGURE 5.18. Wrist extension and flexion. (From Bushman B, editor. *ACSM's Resources for the Personal Trainer*. 4th ed. Baltimore (MD): Lippincott Williams & Wilkins; 2014.)
Flexion flexors	• Flexor carpi radialis Flexor digitorum profundus Flexor digitorum superficialis Palmaris longus Flexor pollicis longusFlexor carpi ulnaris	Sitting or standing	To stretch the flexors of your left wrist and hand, extend your left arm out in front of you with your elbow extended and palm supinated. Use your right hand to extend the fingers and the wrist of your left hand by carefully pulling the fingers back toward you. Repeat with the right	
Fingers				
Flexion and adduction flexors and adductors	• Umbricales Interossei (plantar adductors, dorsal abductors) Flexor pollicis brevis Abductor pollicis brevis Abductor pollicis longus Flexor digiti minimi Opponens pollicis Opponens digiti minimi	Sitting or standing with upper arms at sides, elbows flexed, and palms together	Place your hands together in front of you, matching your palms and fingers as if you are about to pray. With elbows flexed and wrists and fingers extended, elevate both elbows by flexing both shoulders, while lowering both hands extending the wrists. Keep palms together and finger matched. Now maximally abduct all fingers	FIGURE 5.19. Finger flexion and adduction. (From Armiger P, Martyn M. *Stretching for Functional Flexibility*. Baltimore (MD): Lippincott Williams & Wilkins; 2009.)

(continued)

TABLE 5.4 STATIC STRETCHES FOR THE MAJOR MUSCLE GROUPS *(continued)*

Stretch	Muscle Involved	Starting Position	Description
Trunk			
Extension extensors (Fig. 5.20A)	• Multifidus Spinalis thoracis Longissimus thoracis Iliocostalis thoracis Quadratus lumborum Erector spinae	Lying on the floor, supine	Bring both of your knees up to your chest flexing both hips. Using your arms and hands, pull both of your knees closer to your chest. Continue pulling until your buttocks are off the floor, flexing your mid and lower spine. You may carefully flex your cervical and upper thoracic spine by pulling your head up toward your knees
Flexion flexors (Fig. 5.20A)	• Rectus abdominis External oblique Internal oblique	Lying on the floor, prone, with elbows flexed and palms on the floor just beneath the shoulders	Slowly attempt to press your chest and shoulders up and forward while taking care not to extend your head and neck. Your hip bones (ASIS) should remain in contact with the floor
Lateral flexors bending (Fig. 5.20B)	• Internal oblique External oblique Iliocostalis lumborum Multifidus Quadratus lumborum	Lying on the floor on your left side	To stretch the lateral flexors on your left side, laterally flex your torso toward the right by pressing up with your left arm and hand. Be sure to bend directly sideways, staying in the frontal plane. Repeat on the right side
Rotation (Fig. 5.20C)	• Internal and external oblique Rotators Semispinalis Multifidus	Sitting on the floor with both legs extended	Straighten your spine and then step your left foot over and place it on the right side of your right knee. Now rotate your upper body and head toward the left, placing your right elbow against the lateral side of your left knee. Continue turning to the left by applying pressure against your left knee with your right elbow. Repeat on the opposite side

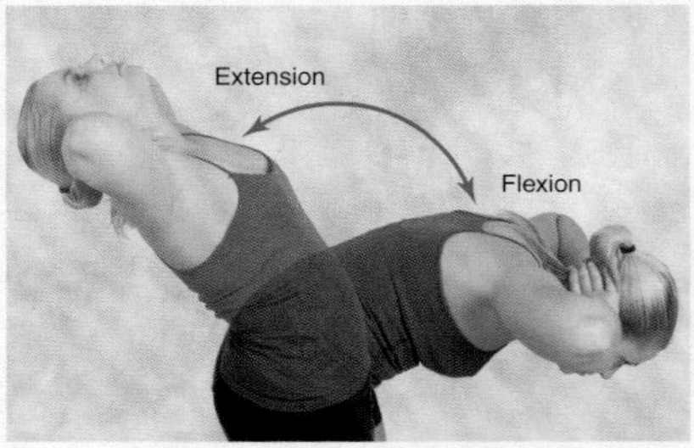

A
Extension
Flexion

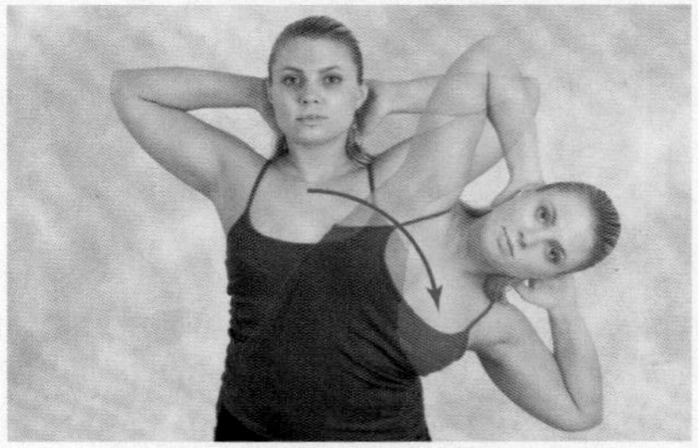

B

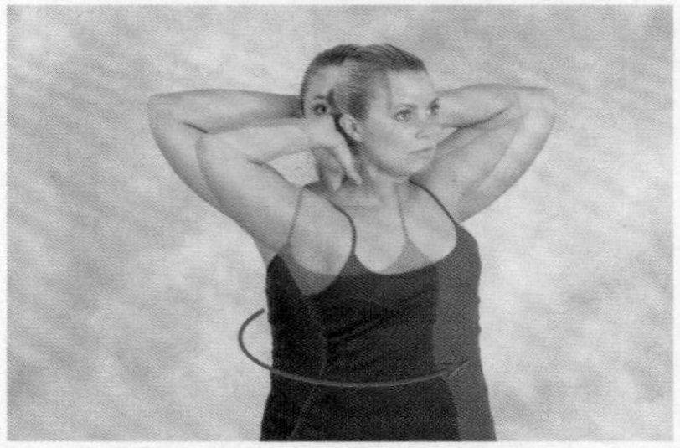

C

FIGURE 5.20. **A.** Trunk extension and flexion. **B.** Trunk lateral flexion. **C.** Trunk rotation. (From Bushman B, editor. *ACSM's Resources for the Personal Trainer.* 4th ed. Baltimore (MD): Lippincott Williams & Wilkins; 2014.)

Lower Body

Hip

Flexors	• Psoas major and minorIliacus Rectus femoris Sartorius Tensor fasciae latae	Standing	To stretch the hip flexors on your right side, first step forward about 2 ft with your left foot. While keeping your torso and hips facing forward, move your upper body and hips anteriorly over your left foot by flexing your left knee and allowing a relaxed flexion in your right knee and ankle. You may allow your right heel to come off the floor. Contract your abdominals to keep your lower back from extending. Repeat on your left side	FIGURE 5.21. Hip flexion and extension. (From Bushman B, editor. *ACSM's Resources for the Personal Trainer.* 4th ed. Baltimore (MD): Lippincott Williams & Wilkins; 2014.)
Extensors	• Gluteus maximus Hamstrings Semimembranosus Semitendinosus Long head of biceps femoris	Lying supine	To stretch the hip extensors on your left side, grasp your left knee with your right hand. Using your right arm and hand, pull your left knee up and across your torso toward your right shoulder, flexing and adducting your left hip. While keeping your knee in this position, actively extend your left knee to add stretch to the hamstrings, which also extend the hip. Repeat on the opposite side	
Adductors	• Adductor magnus Adductor longus Adductor brevis Pectineus Gracilis	Lying on the floor with knees extended and legs abducted	Using the abductors of your hips, abduct your legs to their end range. You may assist this stretch by placing the medial borders of your feet against a wall. As you achieve a stretching sensation, you can scoot your feet slightly farther apart on the wall	
Abductors	• Gluteus medius Gluteus minimus Tensor fasciae latae	Standing	To stretch your left hip abductors, step forward and toward the left with your right foot so that your right foot rests just ahead and to the left of your left foot. Using your left hand, reach overhead and toward the right. Continue bending toward the right with your upper body	

(continued)

TABLE 5.4 STATIC STRETCHES FOR THE MAJOR MUSCLE GROUPS *(continued)*

Stretch	Muscle Involved	Starting Position	Description	
Internal rotators	• Anterior fibers of the gluteus medius Hip adductors and medial hamstrings (semimembranosus and semitendinosus)	Lying supine, with the left knee flexed to 90°	To stretch the internal rotators of your left hip, place the ankle of your left leg on top of and across the right thigh, making sure that the lateral lower left leg is lying on top of the right femur. Now, place your left hand on your left knee and carefully press it toward the floor, taking care not to let your hips twist. Repeat on the right	External rotation Internal rotation **FIGURE 5.22.** Hip internal rotation and external rotation. (From Bushman B, editor. *ACSM's Resources for the Personal Trainer.* 4th ed. Baltimore (MD): Lippincott Williams & Wilkins; 2014.)
External rotators	• Piriformis Gluteus maximus Posterior fibers of gluteus medius Inferior and superior gemelli Obturator internus and externus Quadratus femoris	Lying on the floor, supine	To stretch the external rotators of your left hip, flex your left hip to just above 90°. Next, adduct your left hip by pulling your left knee over toward the right by pulling with your right hand. You may allow your left hip/buttock to come slightly off the floor. Repeat for the right hip	
Knee				
Flexors	• Semimembranosus Semitendinosus Long and short heads of biceps femoris Popliteus Gastrocnemius	Standing	To stretch the knee flexors of your left leg, stand facing a chair so that you can comfortably straighten your leg and place your heel on top of the chair. Choose a chair or similar object that will allow you to keep your spine straight once you have lifted your leg onto it. (Note: many people will have to choose a lower surface.) Carefully lean forward while keeping your spine straight	Flexion Extension **FIGURE 5.23.** Knee flexion and extension. (From Bushman B, editor. *ACSM's Resources for the Personal Trainer.* 4th ed. Baltimore (MD): Lippincott Williams & Wilkins; 2014.)
Extensors	• Rectus femoris Vastus intermedius Vastus lateralis Vastus medialis	Standing on your left leg, holding onto a chair or other object with your left hand for support	To stretch the extensors of the right knee, flex your right knee and grab your right shin just proximal to the ankle with your right hand. Tighten your abdominals and concentrate on not allowing your back to arch (extend). Now pull your right ankle posteriorly and then superiorly toward your buttock. Repeat for the left knee	

Ankle and Foot

Extensors (dorsiflexors)	• Anterior tibialis Extensor digitorum longus Extensor digitorum brevis Extensor hallicis longus Extensor hallicis brevis Peroneus tertius	Standing	To stretch the extensors of the right ankle, foot, and toes, flex the right knee and plantar flex the foot and toes. Place the dorsum of your right foot and toes on the floor about 18 in behind you. Slowly bend your left knee, applying a gentle stretch to your right ankle, foot, and toes, bending them further into plantar flexion. Repeat on the left	Dorsiflexion Plantar flexion **FIGURE 5.24.** Ankle dorsiflexion and plantarflexion. (From Bushman B, editor. *ACSM's Resources for the Personal Trainer.* 4th ed. Baltimore (MD): Lippincott Williams & Wilkins; 2014.)
Flexors (plantarflexors)	• Gastrocnemius Soleus Peroneus brevis Posterior tibialis Flexor digitorum longus Flexor digitorum brevis Flexor hallicis longus Flexor hallicis brevis	Standing	To stretch the flexors of the ankle, foot, and toes of your right leg, step forward about 18 in with your left foot. Flex both knees while keeping your right heel on the ground. Maintain a neutral-to-high right arch (this may require a slight external rotation of your right tibia). You may move slightly forward over your left foot. Repeat to stretch the left ankle, foot, and toes	
Invertors	• Tibialis posterior Tibialis anterior Flexor digitorum longus Flexor hallicis longus	Seated with your left ankle supported across your right knee	To stretch the invertors of the left foot, use your right hand to dorsiflex the toes of your left foot and then continue to push your left forefoot into dorsiflexion and eversion (sole of the foot away from you). Repeat for the right foot	Inversion and adduction (supination) Eversion and abduction (pronation) **FIGURE 5.25.** Ankle inversion and eversion. (From Bushman B, editor. *ACSM's Resources for the Personal Trainer.* 4th ed. Baltimore (MD): Lippincott Williams & Wilkins; 2014.)
Evertors	• Peroneus longus, brevis, and Tertius Extensor digitorum longus	Standing	To stretch the evertors of your right footstep, place your right foot on top of your left foot. Now carefully align your right foot to roll over onto its outside edge. Next. bend carefully bend your right knee, moving it forward. Repeat for the left foot.	

(continued)

TABLE 5.4 STATIC STRETCHES FOR THE MAJOR MUSCLE GROUPS *(continued)*

Stretch	Muscle Involved	Starting Position	Description	
Toes				
Extensors	• Extensor digitorum longus Extensor digitorum brevis Extensor hallicis longus Extensor hallicis brevis Extensor digiti minimi	Seated with left ankle crossed over your right knee	To stretch the extensors of your left foot and toes, place your right hand over the dorsal surface of the toes of your left foot. Carefully flex all 5 toes toward dorsal surface of your foot. Repeat for the right foot	A B **FIGURE 5.26.** Toe extension **(A)** and flexion **(B)**. (From Armiger P, Martyn M. *Stretching for Functional Flexibility*. Baltimore (MD): Lippincott Williams & Wilkins; 2009.)
Flexors	• Flexor digitorum longus Flexor digitorum brevis Flexor hallicis longus Flexor hallicis brevis Flexor digiti minimi brevis	Seated with your left ankle crossed over the right knee	To stretch the toe flexors of your left foot, grasp the toes of your left foot with the fingers and palm of your right hand. Extend all 5 toes and dorsiflex your ankle by pushing the toes toward the shin and allowing the ankle to dorsiflex. Repeat for your right foot	

Numerous examinations have reported no link between ROM training and prevention of low back pain, injury, or postexercise muscle soreness (35, 40, 85, 87, 100). In addition, individuals with ROM imbalances may be at an increased risk for injury during activity (55) and therefore benefit from ROM exercises. This benefit, however, may be limited to those with ROM imbalances and not be effective as a simple means of injury prevention. Further, there has been recent research suggesting a link between antibiotics and musculotendinous injuries. Individuals who are using fluoroquinolone antibiotics are at an increased risk for tendon rupture and joint and muscle damage and therefore should approach flexibility exercises with extreme caution (24, 47).

OVERALL ROM RECOMMENDATIONS

To determine appropriate program design, one must differentiate between flexibility training with the sole purpose of increasing ROM (often using static stretching) and flexibility exercises with the primary purpose of preparing for fitness training or sport-specific training. The former may be necessary for someone who has limited ROM due to genetics or disuse because of injury or lack of activity. The latter is generally part of a dynamic warm-up prior to more intense or skill-dependent exercise and therefore allows for better preparation (37, 100). However, ROM warm-up activities that do not include a dynamic component (and therefore do not tend to increase body temperature, blood flow, etc.) have not shown a benefit to performance or reduction in injury rate during subsequent activity (40, 56, 57, 85, 87, 100, 106).

Acute beneficial effects from static flexibility exercise as it relates to performance are not well supported. Preactivity static flexibility training has been shown to decrease strength, sprint performance, endurance performance, and efficiency because it relates to energy expenditure and power output (54–57, 106). With the demonstrated detrimental effects of static stretching, it is therefore recommended that preactivity ROM be dynamic and/or that flexibility programming occur postactivity or during the training session. Dynamic exercise during the warm-up period with the purpose of increasing body temperature and blood flow will naturally increase ROM during the activity. To date, there is not sufficient evidence to advocate against routine flexibility exercises, especially those following, or separate from, other exercise sessions (6), as chronic increases in ROM have yielded conflicting results related to injury prevention and performance. In addition, some research has demonstrated a reduction of overuse injuries among individuals with increased flexibility (36), whereas others demonstrate that typical muscle stretching programs do not produce a reduction in exercise-related injuries (87). Perhaps the most prudent recommendation to the health professional is to assess individual client needs and requirements and determine the ROM necessary for desired activity. Initial assessment of joint-specific ROM to determine client status would be the first step in the development of a program. If the client is in need of increased ROM, it would be prudent to implement a flexibility training program as previously described. A client with adequate or hyper ROM may be placed on a maintenance program or focus on other areas of health-related fitness until time for reassessment.

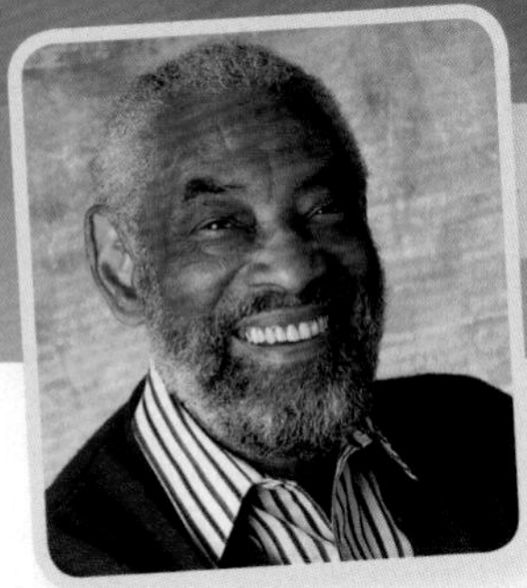

The Case of Allen

Submitted by: **Stephanie Marie Otto, PHD, HFS, Assistant Professor, Gustavus Adolphu College, St. Peter, MN**

Allen is a retired Navy officer who experienced tightening in his chest and dizziness during a recent walk.

Narrative

Allen retired from the Navy 10 years ago and is currently not working. He spends his days gardening and playing with his four grandchildren. Every morning, he walks along the beach for 20 minutes, and he regularly engages in strength-training activities from his Navy days, but he never has done much flexibility exercise. Allen has played bingo twice a week at the local bingo hall for the past year, but his wife complains because he comes home smelling of smoke. During a recent walk, Allen experienced tightness in his chest and dizziness. He is concerned and not sure what to do. He cannot believe he might be at risk for cardiovascular disease. He comes to you for advice and guidance. After your some preliminary testing and information gathering, you discover that Allen's blood pressure is 160/88, and he also revealed to you that his father past away from a heart attack at the age of 53. His total cholesterol is 190 mg·dL^{-1}, low-density lipoprotein is 149, and high-density lipoprotein is 43. Allen is 58 years old and his body mass index is 23 kg·m^{-2}. Allen came in a year ago for an assessment, and his results were as follows.

Aerobic fitness ($\dot{V}O_{2max}$): 40.3 mL·kg^{-1}·min^{-1} (no chest pain reported during this exercise test)
Upper body strength (bench press weight ratio): 0.98
Leg strength (leg press weight ratio): 1.97
Push-ups: 32
Curl-ups: 28
YMCA sit-and-reach: 4 in
Skinfold: 19.1%

Allen is worried about his experience during his last walk and comes to you for advice about his current activity participation and lifestyle. He cannot understand how this could be happening to him since he has been active for most of his life and worked hard to control his weight.

Goals

Goal 1: Improve flexibility
Goal 2: Understand what may have been causing the chest pain and dizziness during his last walk
Goal 3: Maintain current weight.

Questions

- Given the information above, identify the risk factors and determine the risk stratification for Allen.
- How would you proceed after this initial conversation with Allen?
- Assuming Allen is cleared for exercise, how would you plan for his next session with you?
- What other lifestyle factors would you want to discuss with Allen that are contributing to his risk of developing cardiovascular disease?
- Assuming Allen is cleared for exercise, and considering his goals, what would you recommend as an activity plan?

References

American College of Sports Medicine. *ACSM's Guidelines for Exercise Testing and Prescription*. 8th ed. Philadelphia (PA): Lippincott Williams & Wilkins; 2010.

Neiman D. *Exercise Testing and Prescription: A Health Related Approach*. 7th ed. New York (NY): McGraw Hill; 2011.

Garber CE, Blissmer B, Deschenes MR, et al. Quantity and quality of exercise for developing and maintaining cardiorespiratory, musculoskeletal, and neuromotor fitness in apparently healthy adults: Guidance for prescribing exercise. *Med Sci Sports Exerc*. 2011;43(7):1334–59.

SUMMARY

Development and maintenance of flexibility is one of the five components of health-related fitness, and maintaining an adequate ROM is important for activities of daily living. Nevertheless, controversy exists in regard to the overall benefits of flexibility training for injury prevention or sport performance. Since flexibility training involves multiple modes, the HFS can choose which is best for each client and implement these as part of a dynamic warm-up or during the cool-down phase of exercise. Many different methods and tools are used to assess ROM and flexibility. Among the most common are the use of goniometers for the measurement of ROM, sit-and-reach tests for the measurement of distance, and FMS for the measurement of irregular movement patterns. Overall flexibility exercise prescription depends on the mode of the exercise and should be set on the basis of established ACSM guidelines.

STUDY QUESTIONS

1. Characterize the various modes of flexibility training, including the advantages and disadvantages of each.
2. Differentiate between the two types of sensory organs that provide muscular dynamic and limb movement information to the central nervous system with respect to location and function.
3. Design a sample static flexibility exercise prescription based on the FITT principle.
4. Assess the controversy that surrounds the need for flexibility training with respect to health and athletic performance.

REFERENCES

1. American College of Sports Medicine Position Stand. The recommended quantity and quality of exercise for developing and maintaining cardiorespiratory and muscular fitness, and flexibility in healthy adults. *Med Sci Sports Exerc.* 1998;30(6):975–91.
2. American Medical Association. *Guides to the Evaluation of Permanent Impairment.* 4th ed. Chicago (IL): American Medical Association; 1993. xxii, 613 p.
3. Baechle TR, Earle RW, editors. *Essentials of Strength Training and Conditioning.* 3rd ed. Champaign (IL): National Strength & Conditioning Association (U.S.), Human Kinetics; 2008. p. 296–305.
4. Bandy WD, Irion JM. The effect of time on static stretch on the flexibility of the hamstring muscles. *Phys Ther.* 1994;74(9):845–50; discussion 50–2.
5. Bandy WD, Irion JM, Briggler M. The effect of static stretch and dynamic range of motion training on the flexibility of the hamstring muscles. *J Orthop Sports Phys Ther.* 1998;27(4):295–300.
6. Bandy WD, Irion JM, Briggler M. The effect of time and frequency of static stretching on flexibility of the hamstring muscles. *Phys Ther.* 1997;77(10):1090–6.
7. Behm DG, Bambury A, Cahill F, Power K. Effect of acute static stretching on force, balance, reaction time, and movement time. *Med Sci Sports Exerc.* 2004;36(8):1397–402.
8. Burton SL. *Performance and Injury Predictability during Firefighter Candidate Training.* Blacksburg (VA): Virginia Polytechnic Institute and State University; 2006.
9. Chalmers G. Re-examination of the possible role of Golgi tendon organ and muscle spindle reflexes in proprioceptive neuromuscular facilitation muscle stretching. *Sports Biomech.* 2004;3(1):159–83.
10. Chen CH, Nosaka K, Chen HL, Lin MJ, Tseng KW, Chen TC. Effects of flexibility training on eccentric exercise-induced muscle damage. *Med Sci Sports Exerc.* 2011;43(3):491–500.
11. Cherry DB. Review of physical therapy alternatives for reducing muscle contracture. *Phys Ther.* 1980;60(7):877–81.
12. Chorba RS, Chorba DJ, Bouillon LE, Overmyer CA, Landis JA. Use of a functional movement screening tool to determine injury risk in female collegiate athletes. *N Am J Sports Phys Ther.* 2010;5(2):47–54.
13. Church JB, Wiggins MS, Moode FM, Crist R. Effect of warm-up and flexibility treatments on vertical jump performance. *J Strength Cond Res.* 2001;15(3):332–6.

14. Condon SM, Hutton RS. Soleus muscle electromyographic activity and ankle dorsiflexion range of motion during four stretching procedures. *Phys Ther.* 1987;67(1):24–30.
15. Cook G. *Movement: Functional Movement Systems.* West Sussex (UK): Lotus Publishing; 2011. p. 74–85.
16. Cornelius WL. Flexibility exercise: Effective practices. *Natl Str Cond Assoc J.* 1989;11(6):61–2.
17. Cornelius WL, Hinson MM. The relationship between isometric contractions of hip extensors and subsequent flexibility in males. *J Sports Med Phys Fitness.* 1980;20(1):75–80.
18. Cramer JT, Housh TJ, Weir JP, Johnson GO, Coburn JW, Beck TW. The acute effects of static stretching on peak torque, mean power output, electromyography, and mechanomyography. *Eur J Appl Physiol.* 2005;93(5–6):530–9.
19. Dalrymple KJ, Davis SE, Dwyer GB, Moir GL. Effect of static and dynamic stretching on vertical jump performance in collegiate women volleyball players. *J Strength Cond Res.* 2010;24(1):149–55.
20. de Weijer VC, Gorniak GC, Shamus E. The effect of static stretch and warm-up exercise on hamstring length over the course of 24 hours. *J Orthop Sports Phys Ther.* 2003;33(12):727–33.
21. Decoster LC, Cleland J, Altieri C, Russell P. The effects of hamstring stretching on range of motion: A systematic literature review. *J Orthop Sports Phys Ther.* 2005;35(6):377–87.
22. Depino GM, Webright WG, Arnold BL. Duration of maintained hamstring flexibility after cessation of an acute static stretching protocol. *J Athl Train.* 2000;35(1):56–9.
23. Ellenbecker TS, Roetert EP, Piorkowski PA, Schulz DA. Glenohumeral joint internal and external rotation range of motion in elite junior tennis players. *J Orthop Sports Phys Ther.* 1996;24(6):336–41.
24. FDA Requests Boxed Warnings on Fluoroquinolone Antimicrobial Drugs Seeks to Strengthen Warnings Concerning Increased Risk of Tendinitis and Tendon Rupture [Internet]. Silver Spring (MD): United States Food and Drugs Administration; [cited 2011 May 20]. Available from: http://www.fda.gov
25. Feland JB, Myrer JW, Schulthies SS, Fellingham GW, Measom GW. The effect of duration of stretching of the hamstring muscle group for increasing range of motion in people aged 65 years or older. *Phys Ther.* 2001;81(5):1110–7.
26. Friedrich LJ. *A Treatise on Gymnastics.* Northampton (MA): Simeon and Butler; 1828. p. 1–7.
27. Getchell B. *Physical Fitness: A Way of Life.* 2d ed. New York (NY): Wiley; 1979. xv, 352 p.
28. Gleim GW. The profiling of professional football players. *Clin Sports Med.* 1984;3(1):185–97.
29. Gleim GW, McHugh MP. Flexibility and its effects on sports injury and performance. *Sports Med.* 1997;24(5):289–99.
30. Godges JJ, Macrae H, Longdon C, Tinberg C, Macrae PG. The effects of two stretching procedures on hip range of motion and gait economy. *J Orthop Sports Phys Ther.* 1989;10(9):350–7.
31. Guyton AC, Hall JE. *Textbook of Medical Physiology.* 11th ed. Philadelphia (PA): Elsevier Saunders; 2006. xxxv, 1116 p.
32. Haff GG. Roundtable discussion: Flexibility training. *Strength Cond.* 2006;28(2):64–85.
33. Hall SJ. *Basic Biomechanics.* 5th ed. Boston (MA): McGraw-Hill; 2007. xvi, 544 p.
34. Handrakis JP, Southard VN, Abreu JM, et al. Static stretching does not impair performance in active middle-aged adults. *J Strength Cond Res.* 2010;24(3):825–30.
35. Hart L. Effect of stretching on sport injury risk: A review. *Clin J Sport Med.* 2005;15(2):113.
36. Hartig DE, Henderson JM. Increasing hamstring flexibility decreases lower extremity overuse injuries in military basic trainees. *Am J Sports Med.* 1999;27(2):173–6.
37. Harvey L, Herbert R, Crosbie J. Does stretching induce lasting increases in joint ROM? A systematic review. *Physiother Res Int.* 2002;7(1):1–13.
38. Hedrick A. Dynamic flexibility training. *Strength Cond.* 2000;22(5):33–8.
39. Hedrick A. Flexibility: Flexibility and the conditioning program. *Natl Str Cond Assoc J.* 1993;15(4):62–7.
40. Herbert RD, Gabriel M. Effects of stretching before and after exercising on muscle soreness and risk of injury: Systematic review. *BMJ.* 2002;325(7362):468.
41. Holt J, Holt LE, Pelhan TW. Flexibility redefined. In: Bauer T, editor. *XIIIth International Symposium for Biomechanics in Sport.* Ontario (Canada): Lakehead University; 1996. p. 170–4.
42. Holt LE, Travis TM, Okita T. Comparative study of three stretching techniques. *Percept Mot Skills.* 1970;31(2):611–6.
43. Houck JC, De Hesse C, Jacob R. The effect of ageing upon collagen metabolism. *Symp Soc Exp Biol.* 1967;21:403–25.
44. Hubley CL, Kozey JW, Stanish WD. The effects of static stretching exercises and stationary cycling on range of motion at the hip joint. *J Orthop Sports Phys Ther.* 1984;6(2):104–9.
45. Hunter DG, Spriggs J. Investigation into the relationship between the passive flexibility and active stiffness of the ankle plantar-flexor muscles. *Clin Biomech (Bristol, Avon).* 2000;15(8):600–6.
46. Hunter JP, Marshall RN. Effects of power and flexibility training on vertical jump technique. *Med Sci Sports Exerc.* 2002;34(3):478–86.
47. Huston KA. Achilles tendinitis and tendon rupture due to fluoroquinolone antibiotics. *N Engl J Med.* 1994;331(11):748.
48. The Cooper Institute. *Physical Fitness Assessments and Norms.* Dallas (TX): The Cooper Institute; 2005. p. 29–30.
49. Jackson AW, Morrow JR Jr, Brill PA, Kohl HW 3rd, Gordon NF, Blair SN. Relations of sit-up and sit-and-reach tests to low back pain in adults. *J Orthop Sports Phys Ther.* 1998;27(1):22–6.
50. Johns RJ, Wright V. Relative importance of various tissues in joint stiffness. *J Appl Physiol.* 1962;17(5):824–8.
51. Kato E, Toshiaki O, Kentaro C, et al. Musculotendinous factors influencing difference in ankle joint flexibility between men and women. *Int J Sport Health Sci.* 2005;3:218–25.
52. Kerrigan DC, Xenopoulos-Oddsson A, Sullivan MJ, Lelas JJ, Riley PO. Effect of a hip flexor-stretching program on gait in the elderly. *Arch Phys Med Rehabil.* 2003;84(1):1–6.
53. Kiesel K, Plisky PJ, Voight ML. Can serious injury in professional football be predicted by a preseason functional movement screen? *N Am J Sports Phys Ther.* 2007;2(3):147–58.
54. Kistler BM, Walsh MS, Horn TS, Cox RH. The acute effects of static stretching on the sprint performance of collegiate men in the 60- and 100-m dash after a dynamic warm-up. *J Strength Cond Res.* 2010;24(9):2280–4.
55. Knapik JJ, Bauman CL, Jones BH, Harris JM, Vaughan L. Preseason strength and flexibility imbalances associated with athletic injuries in female collegiate athletes. *Am J Sports Med.* 1991;19(1):76–81.
56. Knudson D, Noffal G. Time course of stretch-induced isometric strength deficits. *Eur J Appl Physiol.* 2005;94(3):348–51.

57. Knudson DV, Noffal GJ, Bahamonde RE, Bauer JA, Blackwell JR. Stretching has no effect on tennis serve performance. *J Strength Cond Res.* 2004;18(3):654–6.
58. Kraus H, Hirschland R. Minimum muscular fitness tests in school children. *Res Q.* 1954;25:178–88.
59. Lamontagne A, Malouin F, Richards CL. Viscoelastic behavior of plantar flexor muscle-tendon unit at rest. *J Orthop Sports Phys Ther.* 1997;26(5):244–52.
60. Lea RD, Gerhardt JJ. Range-of-motion measurements. *J Bone Joint Surg Am.* 1995;77(5):784–98.
61. Leighton JR. A study of the effect of progressive weight training on flexibility. *J Assoc Phys Ment Rehabil.* 1964;18:101–4 PASSIM.
62. Liguori G, Carroll-Cobb S. *FitWell: Questions and Answers.* New York (NY): McGraw Hill; 2011.
63. Lucas RC, Koslow R. Comparative study of static, dynamic, and proprioceptive neuromuscular facilitation stretching techniques on flexibility. *Percept Mot Skills.* 1984;58(2):615–8.
64. Magnusson SP, Gleim GW, Nicholas JA. Shoulder weakness in professional baseball pitchers. *Med Sci Sports Exerc.* 1994;26(1):5–9.
65. Magnusson SP, Simonsen EB, Aagaard P, Sorensen H, Kjaer M. A mechanism for altered flexibility in human skeletal muscle. *J Physiol.* 1996;497(Pt 1):291–8.
66. Magnusson SP, Simonsen EB, Dyhre-Poulsen P, Aagaard P, Mohr T, Kjaer M. Viscoelastic stress relaxation during static stretch in human skeletal muscle in the absence of EMG activity. *Scand J Med Sci Sports.* 1996;6(6):323–8.
67. Mahieu NN, McNair P, De Muynck M, et al. Effect of static and ballistic stretching on the muscle-tendon tissue properties. *Med Sci Sports Exerc.* 2007;39(3):494–501.
68. Mann DP, Jones MT. Guidelines to the implementation of a dynamic stretching program. *Strength Cond J.* 1999;21(6):53–55.
69. Marek SM, Cramer JT, Fincher AL, et al. Acute effects of static and proprioceptive neuromuscular facilitation stretching on muscle strength and power output. *J Athl Train.* 2005;40(2):94–103.
70. McArdle WD, Katch FI, Katch VL. *Exercise Physiology: Energy, Nutrition, and Human Performance.* 6th ed. Philadelphia (PA): Lippincott Williams & Wilkins; 2007. 1068, I-41 p.
71. McGlynn GH, Laughlin NT, Rowe V. Effect of electromyographic feedback and static stretching on artificially induced muscle soreness. *Am J Phys Med.* 1979;58(3):139–48.
72. McMillian DJ, Moore JH, Hatler BS, Taylor DC. Dynamic vs. static-stretching warm up: The effect on power and agility performance. *J Strength Cond Res.* 2006;20(3):492–9.
73. McNeal JR, Sands WA. Stretching for performance enhancement. *Curr Sports Med Rep.* 2006;5(3):141–6.
74. Minick KI, Kiesel KB, Burton L, Taylor A, Plisky P, Butler RJ. Interrater reliability of the functional movement screen. *J Strength Cond Res.* 2010;24(2):479–86.
75. Moore MA, Hutton RS. Electromyographic investigation of muscle stretching techniques. *Med Sci Sports Exerc.* 1980;12(5):322–9.
76. Needham RA, Morse CI, Degens H. The acute effect of different warm-up protocols on anaerobic performance in elite youth soccer players. *J Strength Cond Res.* 2009;23(9):2614–20.
77. Nelson AG, Kokkonen J. Acute ballistic muscle stretching inhibits maximal strength performance. *Res Q Exerc Sport.* 2001;72(4):415–9.
78. Nelson RT. A comparison of the immediate effects of eccentric training vs static stretch on hamstring flexibility in high school and college athletes. *N Am J Sports Phys Ther.* 2006;1(2):56–61.
79. Nelson RT, Bandy WD. Eccentric training and static stretching improve hamstring flexibility of high school males. *J Athl Train.* 2004;39(3):254–8.
80. Noakes T. *Lore of Running.* 4th ed. Champaign (IL): Human Kinetics; 2003. xi, 931 p.
81. Noonan TJ, Best TM, Seaber AV, Garrett WE Jr. Thermal effects on skeletal muscle tensile behavior. *Am J Sports Med.* 1993;21(4):517–22.
82. O'Brien M. Functional anatomy and physiology of tendons. *Clin Sports Med.* 1992;11(3):505–20.
83. O'Connor FG, Deuster PA, Davis J, Pappas CG, Knapik JJ. Functional movement screening: Predicting injuries in officer candidates. *Med Sci Sports Exerc.* 2011;43(12):2224–30.
84. Oberg B, Ekstrand J, Moller M, Gillquist J. Muscle strength and flexibility in different positions of soccer players. *Int J Sports Med.* 1984;5(4):213–6.
85. Park DY, Chou L. Stretching for prevention of Achilles tendon injuries: A review of the literature. *Foot Ankle Int.* 2006;27(12):1086–95.
86. Park SK, Stefanyshyn DJ, Loitz-Ramage B, Hart DA, Ronsky JL. Changing hormone levels during the menstrual cycle affect knee laxity and stiffness in healthy female subjects. *Am J Sports Med.* 2009;37(3):588–98.
87. Pope RP, Herbert RD, Kirwan JD, Graham BJ. A randomized trial of preexercise stretching for prevention of lower-limb injury. *Med Sci Sports Exerc.* 2000;32(2):271–7.
88. Raab DM, Agre JC, McAdam M, Smith EL. Light resistance and stretching exercise in elderly women: effect upon flexibility. *Arch Phys Med Rehabil.* 1988;69(4):268–72.
89. Roberts JM, Wilson K. Effect of stretching duration on active and passive range of motion in the lower extremity. *Br J Sports Med.* 1999;33(4):259–63.
90. Sady SP, Wortman M, Blanke D. Flexibility training: Ballistic, static or proprioceptive neuromuscular facilitation? *Arch Phys Med Rehabil.* 1982;63(6):261–3.
91. Safran MR, Garrett WE Jr, Seaber AV, Glisson RR, Ribbeck BM. The role of warmup in muscular injury prevention. *Am J Sports Med.* 1988;16(2):123–9.
92. Sawyer PC, Uhl TL, Mattacola CG, Johnson DL, Yates JW. Effects of moist heat on hamstring flexibility and muscle temperature. *J Strength Cond Res.* 2003;17(2):285–90.
93. Shellock FG, Prentice WE. Warming-up and stretching for improved physical performance and prevention of sports-related injuries. *Sports Med.* 1985;2(4):267–78.
94. Shrier I. Does stretching improve performance? A systematic and critical review of the literature. *Clin J Sport Med.* 2004;14(5):267–73.
95. Smith LL, Brunetz MH, Chenier TC, et al. The effects of static and ballistic stretching on delayed onset muscle soreness and creatine kinase. *Res Q Exerc Sport.* 1993;64(1):103–7.
96. Sprague HA. Relationship of certain physical measurements to swimming speed. *Res Q.* 1976;47(4):810–4.
97. Strickler T, Malone T, Garrett WE. The effects of passive warming on muscle injury. *Am J Sports Med.* 1990;18(2):141–5.
98. Tanigawa MC. Comparison of the hold-relax procedure and passive mobilization on increasing muscle length. *Phys Ther.* 1972;52(7):725–35.
99. Taylor DC, Dalton JD Jr, Seaber AV, Garrett WE Jr. Viscoelastic properties of muscle-tendon units. The biomechanical effects of stretching. *Am J Sports Med.* 1990;18(3):300–9.

100. Thacker SB, Gilchrist J, Stroup DF, Kimsey CD Jr. The impact of stretching on sports injury risk: A systematic review of the literature. *Med Sci Sports Exerc.* 2004;36(3):371–8.
101. Thompsen AG, Kackley T, Palumbo MA, Faigenbaum AD. Acute effects of different warm-up protocols with and without a weighted vest on jumping performance in athletic women. *J Strength Cond Res.* 2007;21(1):52–6.
102. Thompson WR. *ACSM's Guidelines for Exercise Testing and Prescription.* 8th ed. Philadelphia (PA): Lippincott Williams & Wilkins; 2009. xxi, 380 p.
103. Unick J, Kieffer HS, Cheesman W, Feeney A. The acute effects of static and ballistic stretching on vertical jump performance in trained women. *J Strength Cond Res.* 2005;19(1):206–12.
104. Wallin D, Ekblom B, Grahn R, Nordenborg T. Improvement of muscle flexibility. A comparison between two techniques. *Am J Sports Med.* 1985;13(4):263–8.
105. Watkins J. *Structure and Function of the Musculoskeletal System.* 2nd ed. Champaign (IL): Human Kinetics; 2010. 96 p.
106. Wilson JM, Hornbuckle LM, Kim JS, et al. Effects of static stretching on energy cost and running endurance performance. *J Strength Cond Res.* 2010;24(9):2274–9.
107. Worrell TW, Smith TL, Winegardner J. Effect of hamstring stretching on hamstring muscle performance. *J Orthop Sports Phys Ther.* 1994;20(3):154–9.
108. YMCA of the USA. *YMCA Fitness Testing and Assessment Manual.* 4th ed. Champaign (IL): Human Kinetics; 2000. p. 158–60.
109. Young W, Clothier P, Otago L, Bruce L, Liddell D. Acute effects of static stretching on hip flexor and quadriceps flexibility, range of motion and foot speed in kicking a football. *J Sci Med Sport.* 2004;7(1):23–31.
110. Yuktasira B, Kayab F. Investigation into the long-term effects of static and PNF stretching exercises on range of motion and jump performance. *J Body Mov Ther.* 2009;13(1):11–21.

CHAPTER

6 Body Composition and Weight Management

Katrina DuBose • Deb Reibe • Sarah Henes

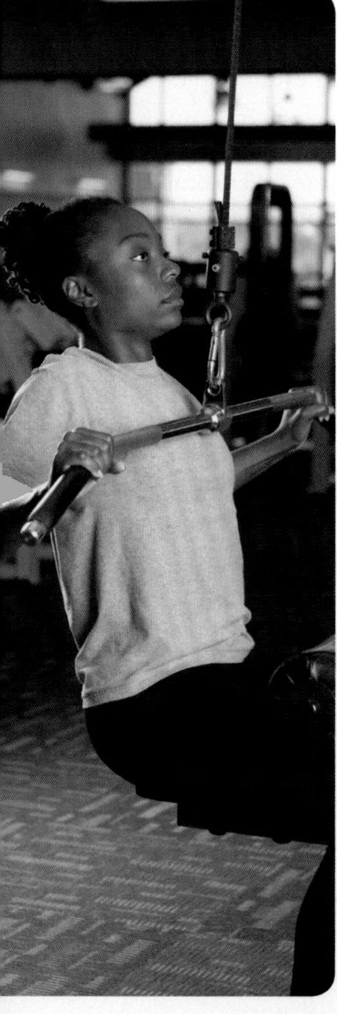

CHAPTER OBJECTIVES

- To understand and apply the various methods for assessing body composition.
- To evaluate body composition assessment as related to patient population and BMI status.
- To understand the key nutrition messages and concepts of both the MyPlate and the MyPyramid, as described by the 2010 USDA Dietary Guidelines.
- To understand and apply the ACSM's metabolic calculations.

The prevalence of overweight and obesity has been increasing in the United States and in developed countries around the world. Recent estimates indicate that approximately 68% of the US population are classified as overweight or obese (body mass index [BMI] ≥25 kg·m^{-2}), with approximately 34% classified as obese (BMI ≥30 kg·m^{-2}) and 6% as severely obese (BMI ≥40 kg·m^{-2}) (13). Population studies suggest that obesity rates have been relatively stable since 2003, but the prevalence of extreme obesity continues to increase (13, 39, 40). Obesity rates among children have tripled since the 1980s and are now at 17% (41). The prevalence of obesity varies by racial and ethnic groups, with higher rates found in African American, Hispanic, and Mexican American populations compared with non-Hispanic Whites (13).

Overweight and obesity are characterized by high amounts of body fat in relation to overall lean body mass and are linked to numerous chronic diseases, including hypertension, cardiorespiratory disease, dyslipidemia, Type 2 diabetes, some cancers, sleep apnea, arthritis, and other musculoskeletal problems (50). Several medical conditions exist that promote weight gain (*e.g.*, Cushing syndrome); however, these conditions are uncommon. In most individuals, overweight and obesity are the result of excess caloric consumption and/or inadequate energy expenditure.

Obesity is associated with premature mortality from cardiorespiratory disease and other diseases such as cancer (50). Central (abdominal) obesity is associated with the metabolic syndrome, a clustering of metabolic factors that increase the risk of cardiorespiratory disease (36). Other comorbidities associated with obesity such as Type 2 diabetes, dyslipidemia, and hypertension, as well as poor dietary habits and a sedentary lifestyle, also increase the risk of cardiorespiratory disease.

Body composition is an important component of health-related physical fitness. It is important for the health fitness specialist (HFS) to understand how to properly measure body composition, make sound weight loss goals, and formulate exercise and nutritional recommendations for weight loss and weight management. This chapter will discuss the different methods for measuring body composition, review American College of Sports Medicine® (ACSM) exercise guidelines for weight loss, and provide sound physical activity and nutritional information regarding weight management.

MEASURING BODY COMPOSITION

Anthropometric Methods

Anthropometrics are a set of noninvasive, quantitative techniques for determining body size by measuring, recording, and analyzing specific dimensions of the body, such as height, weight, and body circumference.

Height and Weight

Height is measured using a wall-mounted stadiometer or measuring rod attached to a balance beam scale. Instruct the clients to remove their shoes and hair ornaments, stand straight with their heels together, and look straight ahead. Before taking the measurement, ask that the client take a deep breath and hold it. Record the height in either inches or centimeters.

Weight is measured using a calibrated balance beam or electronic scale. Clients should wear only light clothing. Instruct clients to remove their shoes, empty their pockets, void if necessary, and stand in the center of the platform with weight distributed evenly on both feet. Record the weight in either pounds or kilograms.

Body Mass Index

Body mass index (BMI) is a measure of weight in relation to a person's height. It is calculated by dividing body weight in kilograms by height in meters squared (refer to the How to Calculate BMI box) or can be determined with a BMI table (Table 6.1).

BMI is used to classify individuals as underweight (<18.5 $kg \cdot m^{-2}$), normal weight (18.5–24.9 $kg \cdot m^{-2}$), overweight (25.0–29.9 $kg \cdot m^{-2}$), or obese (≥30 $kg \cdot m^{-2}$) (13) and to identify individuals at risk for obesity-related diseases (Table 6.2). For most individuals, obesity-related health problems increase with a BMI ≥25 $kg \cdot m^2$. A BMI ≥30 $kg \cdot m^2$ is associated with hypertension, dyslipidemia, coronary heart disease, and mortality (52). BMI can be used to classify children and adolescents as overweight or obese using the standard BMI formula along with a BMI for age growth chart provided by the Centers for Disease Control and Prevention (9). In children and adolescents, overweight is defined as the 85th to <95th percentile of BMI for age and sex, whereas obesity is defined as ≥95th percentile for age and sex.

HOW TO Calculate BMI

The following example can be used to learn how to calculate BMI. An individual weighing 150 lb (or 68.18 kg [divide weight in pounds by 2.2]), standing 66-in tall (or 1.68 m tall [multiply height in inches by 0.0254]) has a BMI of:

$$\begin{aligned} \text{BMI} &= \text{weight (kg)/height (m}^2) \\ &= 68.18 \text{ kg}/(1.68 \text{ m})^2 \\ &= 68.18/2.82 \\ &= 24.2 \text{ kg·m}^{-2} \end{aligned}$$

Another formula eliminates the need to convert pounds and inches to kilograms and meters. Using the same example:

$$\begin{aligned} \text{BMI} &= (\text{weight [lb]/height [in}^2]) \times 704.5 \\ &= (150 \text{ lb}/66 \text{ in}^2) \times 704.5 \\ &= (0.0344352) \times 704.5 \\ &= 24.2 \text{ kg·m}^{-2} \end{aligned}$$

TABLE 6.1 BMI CHART

BMI ($kg \cdot m^{-2}$)	19	20	21	22	23	24	25	26	27	28	29	30	35	40
Height (in)							**Weight (lb)**							
58	91	96	100	105	110	115	119	124	129	134	138	143	167	191
59	94	99	104	109	114	119	124	128	133	138	143	148	173	198
60	97	102	107	112	118	123	128	133	138	143	148	153	179	204
61	100	106	111	116	122	127	132	137	143	148	153	158	185	211
62	104	109	115	120	126	131	136	142	147	153	158	164	191	218
63	107	113	118	124	130	135	141	146	152	158	163	169	197	225
64	110	116	122	128	134	140	145	151	157	163	169	174	204	232
65	114	120	126	132	138	144	150	156	162	168	174	180	210	240
66	118	124	130	136	142	148	155	161	167	173	179	186	216	247
67	121	127	134	140	146	153	159	166	172	178	185	191	223	255
68	125	131	138	144	151	158	164	171	177	184	190	197	230	262
69	128	135	142	149	155	162	169	176	182	189	196	203	236	270
70	132	139	146	153	160	167	174	181	188	195	202	207	243	278
71	136	143	150	157	165	172	179	186	193	200	208	215	250	286
72	140	147	154	162	169	177	184	191	199	206	213	221	258	294
73	144	151	159	166	174	182	189	197	204	212	219	227	265	302
74	148	155	163	171	179	186	194	202	210	218	225	233	272	311
75	152	160	168	176	184	192	200	208	216	224	232	240	279	319
76	156	164	172	180	189	197	205	213	221	230	238	246	287	328

Source: Adapted from U.S. Department of Health & Human Services, National Health, Lung, and Blood Institute, People Science Health, Body Mass Index Table 1. 2012 http://www.nhlbi.nih.gov/guidelines/obesity/bmi_tbl.htm

TABLE 6.2 CLASSIFICATION OF DISEASE RISK BASED ON BMI AND WAIST CIRCUMFERENCE (50)

		Disease Risk[a] Relative to Normal	
		Waist Circumference	
		Men ≤102 cm	Men >102 cm
Weight	BMI	Women ≤88 cm	Women >88 cm
Underweight	<18.5	—	—
Normal	18.5–24.9	—	—
Overweight	25.0–29.9	Increased	High
Obesity			
Class I	30.0–34.9	High	Very high
Class II	35.0–39.9	Very high	Very high
Class III	≥40	Extremely high	Extremely high

[a]Disease risk for Type 2 diabetes, hypertension, and cardiovascular disease. Dashes (—) indicate that no additional risk at these levels of BMI was assigned. Increased waist circumference can also be a marker for increased risk even in persons of normal weight.

BMI does not differentiate between fat and fat-free mass, so it is not a true measure of body fatness. Limitations of using BMI to classify individuals as normal, overweight, or obese must be recognized. Individuals with high levels of muscle mass can be misclassified as overweight or, in extreme cases, obese (*e.g.*, elite body builder). BMI can underestimate body fat in persons who have lost muscle mass (*e.g.*, older adults). High BMI in very short individuals (under 5 ft) may not reflect fatness. Despite these limitations, BMI is a very useful measurement, particularly when assessing large groups of people, because of its convenience and low cost. When possible, an HFS should use clinical judgment when assessing individual clients and use BMI with other measures of body composition for a more complete profile of an individual. It is possible to predict percentage body fat from BMI, but this is not recommended because of the high margin of error associated with this technique (±5% fat) (12).

Circumference Measures

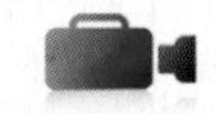

Visit thePoint to watch video 6.0 about using tape to measure waist circumference.

Circumference measures are a beneficial adjunct to other anthropometric measures. They are easily understood by clients and can be used with extremely obese individuals, particularly when skinfold thicknesses are too large for standard skinfold calipers. Circumference measures can be used to determine body fat distribution, an important predictor of the health risks of obesity. Central obesity (also referred to as abdominal or android obesity) is associated with a higher risk of cardiometabolic diseases compared with gynoid obesity, which is characterized by a greater proportion of fat distributed on hips and thighs (43). The standard circumference sites are described in Table 6.3 and shown in Fig. 6.1.

Body fat distribution can be determined using the waist-to-hip ratio (WHR). This assessment helps the HFS identify individuals with higher amounts of abdominal fat. To determine the WHR, divide the circumference of the waist by the circumference of the hips (buttocks/hips; Table 6.3). If a female client has a waist circumference of 31 in and a hip circumference of 42 in, her WHR is 35/42 = 0.83. Health risks increase as WHR increases, and standards for risk vary with age and sex (see Table 6.4).

Waist circumference alone can be used as an indicator of health risk because it reflects the level of abdominal obesity (7). Health risks are high when the waist circumference is ≥35 in (88 cm) for women and 40 in (102 cm) for men. Further, waist circumference can be used with BMI to more precisely classify disease risk (see Table 6.2).

TABLE 6.3 STANDARDIZED DESCRIPTION OF CIRCUMFERENCE SITES (1, 2)

Site	Location Description
Abdomen	With the subject standing upright and relaxed, a horizontal measure taken at the greatest anterior extension of the abdomen, usually at the level of the umbilicus
Arm	With the subject standing erect and arms hanging freely at the sides with hands facing the thigh, a horizontal measure is taken midway between the acromion and the olecranon processes
Buttocks/hips	With the subject standing erect and feet together, a horizontal measure is taken at the maximal circumference of buttocks. This measure is used for the hip measure in a waist/hip measure
Calf	With the subject standing erect (feet apart ~20 cm), a horizontal measure taken at the level of the maximum circumference between the knee and the ankle, perpendicular to the long axis
Forearm	With the subject standing, arms hanging downward but slightly away from the trunk and palms facing anteriorly, a measure is taken perpendicular to the long axis at the maximal circumference
Hips/thigh	With the subject standing, legs slightly apart (~10 cm), a horizontal measure is taken at the maximal circumference of the hip/proximal thigh, just below the gluteal fold
Mid-thigh	With the subject standing and one foot on a bench so the knee is flexed at 90°, a measure is taken midway between the inguinal crease and the proximal border of the patella, perpendicular to the long axis
Waist	With the subject standing, arms at the sides, feet together, and abdomen relaxed, a horizontal measure is taken at the narrowest part of the torso (above the umbilicus and below the xiphoid process). The National Obesity Task Force (NOTF) suggests obtaining a horizontal measure directly above the iliac crest as a method to enhance standardization. Unfortunately, current formulae are not predicated on the NOTF suggested site

Percentage Body Fat Methods

Anthropometric measurements provide important information about the relationship between obesity and health, but do not provide precise estimates of body composition. Body composition is the relative proportion of fat and fat-free tissue in the body. Determining body composition, or percentage body fat, helps the HFS: (a) identify individuals with high and low levels of body fat that are associated with increased health risks; (b) design appropriate exercise prescriptions; (c) formulate dietary recommendations; (d) assess the progress of a client in response to a weight management program; and (e) estimate weight loss goals. Body composition can be measured using various techniques that vary in terms of accuracy, cost, and complexity. The more common body composition measurements that are used in health/fitness settings include skinfolds and bioelectrical impedance. Laboratory measures include underwater weighing, plethysmography, and dual-energy X-ray absorptiometry (DEXA).

Tables 6.5 and 6.6 provide percentile values for percentage body fat in men and women, respectively. Experts have not agreed on an exact percentage body fat value associated with optimal health risk; however, a range of 10% to 22% for men and 20% to 32% for women is considered satisfactory for health (30).

Skinfold Measurements

Skinfold measurements are used to determine the amount of subcutaneous fat, that is, the fat located directly below the skin. Skinfold measures can be used to determine body composition and correlate

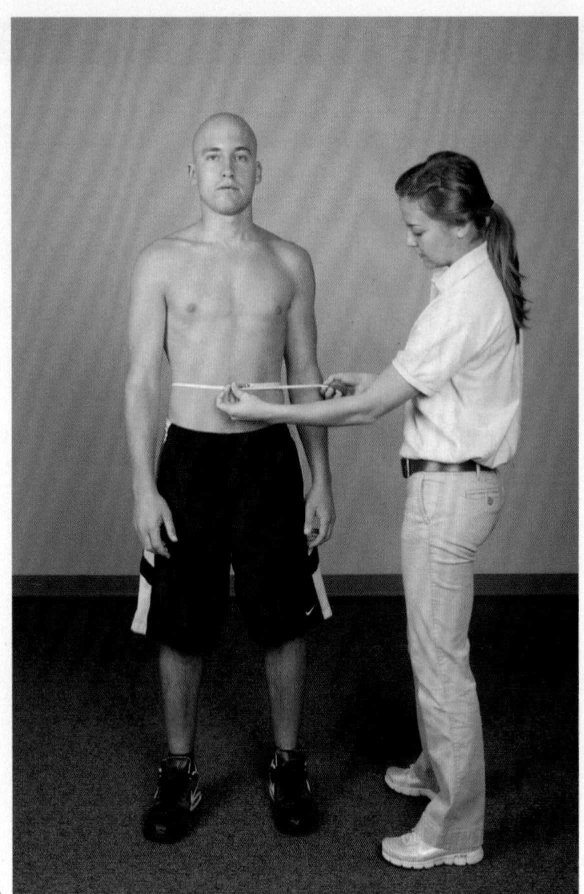

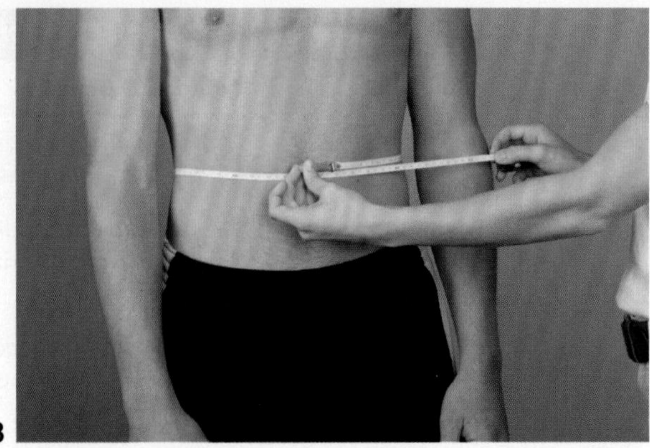

FIGURE 6.1. Measuring waist circumference. The waist is measured at the smallest circumference above the umbilicus (usually 1–2 in).

well with body composition determined by underwater weighing and DEXA. This technique is based on the assumptions that (a) approximately one-third of total body fat is located subcutaneously and (b) the amount of subcutaneous fat is proportional to total body fat (2). However, these assumptions vary with sex, age, and ethnicity, which introduce some error into the prediction of percentage body fat from skinfold measurements. Other factors that may contribute to measurement

TABLE 6.4 HIP TO WAIST RATIO NORMS FOR MEN AND WOMEN (4)

Age	Low Risk	Moderate Risk	High Risk
	Men (yr)		
20–29	<0.83	0.83–0.88	>0.88
30–39	<0.84	0.84–0.91	>0.91
40–49	<0.88	0.88–0.95	>0.95
50–59	<0.90	0.90–0.96	>0.96
60–69	<0.91	0.91–0.98	>0.98
	Women (yr)		
20–29	<0.71	0.71–0.77	>0.77
30–39	<0.72	0.72–0.78	>0.78
40–49	<0.73	0.73–0.79	>0.79
50–59	<0.74	0.74–0.81	>0.81
60–69	<0.76	0.76–0.83	>0.83

TABLE 6.5 BODY COMPOSITION (% BODY FAT) FOR MEN

	Age						
% Body Fat	20–29	30–39	40–49	50–59	60–69	70–79	
99	4.2	7.0	9.2	10.9	11.5	13.6	
95	6.3	9.9	12.8	14.4	15.5	15.2	VL[a]
90	7.9	11.9	14.9	16.7	17.6	17.8	
85	9.2	13.3	16.3	18.0	18.8	19.2	
80	10.5	14.5	17.4	19.1	19.7	20.4	E
75	11.5	15.5	18.4	19.9	20.6	21.1	
70	12.7	16.5	19.1	20.7	21.3	21.6	
65	13.9	17.4	19.9	21.3	22.0	22.5	
60	14.8	18.2	20.6	22.1	22.6	23.1	G
55	15.8	19.0	21.3	22.7	23.2	23.7	
50	16.6	19.7	21.9	23.2	23.7	24.1	
45	17.4	20.4	22.6	23.9	24.4	24.4	
40	18.6	21.3	23.4	24.6	25.2	24.8	F
35	19.6	22.1	24.1	25.3	26.0	25.4	
30	20.6	23.0	24.8	26.0	26.7	26.0	
25	21.9	23.9	25.7	26.8	27.5	26.7	
20	23.1	24.9	26.6	27.8	28.4	27.6	P
15	24.6	26.2	27.7	28.9	29.4	28.9	
10	26.3	27.8	29.2	30.3	30.9	30.4	
5	28.9	30.2	31.2	32.5	32.9	32.4	
1	33.3	34.3	35.0	36.4	36.8	35.5	VP
n =	1,826	8,373	10,442	6,079	1,836	301	

Total n = 28,857.
Norms are based on Cooper Clinic patients.
[a]Very lean – No less than 3% body fat is recommended for males.
VL, very lean; E, excellent; G, good; F, fair; P, poor; VP, very poor.
Reprinted with permission from The Cooper Institute, Dallas, Texas. For more information: www.cooperinstitute.org.

TABLE 6.6 FITNESS CATEGORIES FOR BODY COMPOSITION (% BODY FAT) FOR WOMEN BY AGE

		A (yr)					
% Body Fat		20–29	30–39	40–49	50–59	60–69	70–79
99	Very lean*	9.8	11.0	12.6	14.6	13.9	14.6
95		13.6	14.0	15.6	17.2	17.7	16.6
90	Excellent	14.8	15.6	17.2	19.4	19.8	20.3
85		15.8	16.6	18.6	20.9	21.4	23.0
80		16.5	17.4	19.8	22.5	23.2	24.0
75	Good	17.3	18.2	20.8	23.8	24.8	25.0
70		18.0	19.1	21.9	25.1	25.9	26.2
65		18.7	20.0	22.8	26.0	27.0	27.7
60		19.4	20.8	23.8	27.0	27.9	28.6
55	Fair	20.1	21.7	24.8	27.9	28.7	29.7

(continued)

TABLE 6.6 **FITNESS CATEGORIES FOR BODY COMPOSITION (% BODY FAT) FOR WOMEN BY AGE** *(continued)*

% Body Fat		Age 20–29	30–39	40–49	50–59	60–69	70–79
50		21.0	22.6	25.6	28.8	29.8	30.4
45		21.9	23.5	26.5	29.7	30.6	31.3
40		22.7	24.6	27.6	30.4	31.3	31.8
35	Poor	23.6	25.6	28.5	31.4	32.5	32.7
30		24.5	26.7	29.6	32.5	33.3	33.9
25		25.9	27.7	30.7	33.4	34.3	35.3
20		27.1	29.1	31.9	34.5	35.4	36.0
15	Very poor	28.9	30.9	33.5	35.6	36.2	37.4
10		31.4	33.0	35.4	36.7	37.3	38.2
5		35.2	35.8	37.4	38.3	39.0	39.3
1		38.9	39.4	39.8	40.4	40.8	40.5
n =		1360	3597	3808	2366	849	136

Total *n* = 12,116
Norms are based on Cooper Clinic patients.
VL, very lean; E, excellent; G, good; F, fair; P, poor; VP, very poor.
Reprinted with permission from The Cooper Institute, Dallas, Texas. For more information: www.cooperinstitute.org

error include poor technique and/or an inexperienced evaluator, an extremely obese or extremely lean client, and an improperly calibrated caliper (tension should be set at ~12 $g \cdot m^{-2}$). The accuracy of predicting the percentage body fat from skinfolds is ±3.5%, assuming that proper technique is used when taking measures and that an appropriate regression equation is used to estimate percentage body fat (21).

Various regression equations have been developed to predict body density or percentage body fat from skinfold measurements. Table 6.8 lists generalized equations that allow calculation of body density for a wide range of individuals. Other population-specific equations that are sex-, age-, ethnicity-, fatness-, and sport-specific are available and may provide a more accurate estimate of body composition. Most regression equations determine body density, which can then be converted to percentage body fat. The following are two of the most commonly used body density regression equations (5, 47):

Brozek equation: % body fat = (495/body density) − 450
Siri equation: % body fat = (457/body density) − 414.2

Population-specific formulas for estimating percentage body fat from body density that are sex-, age-, ethnicity- and fatness-specific are also available (21).

Bioelectrical Impedance

Bioelectrical impedance analysis (BIA) is a rapid, noninvasive body composition assessment tool. In this method, a harmless electrical current is passed through the body and the impedance to that current is measured. Electrical impedance is related to the percentage of water contained in various body tissues. Lean tissue, which is composed of mostly water and electrolytes, is a good electrical conductor, whereas fat tissue, which contains much less water, acts as an impedance to the electrical current. BIA estimates total body water and relies on regression equations to estimate percentage body fat.

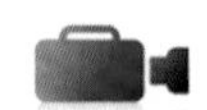

Visit thePoint to watch videos 6.1 and 6.2 about using skinfolds to measure body fat in men and women.

HOW TO Measure Skinfolds

Skinfolds are measured at standardized sites, described in Table 6.7 and shown in Fig. 6.2. The skinfold sites must be precisely located using anatomical landmarks, and the following procedures must be followed for the accurate determination of body composition (1, 6):

- Take all measurements on the right side of the client's body. The client's skin should be dry and lotion free. Do not take skinfold measurement immediately after exercise.
- Identify and mark all sites before measuring.
- Firmly grasp the skinfold (two layers of skin and subcutaneous fat) between the thumb and the index finger of your left hand, 1 cm above the site to be measured. To grasp the skinfold, place the thumb and index finger about 3 in apart on a line that is perpendicular to the long axis of the skinfold. Pull the skinfold up and away from the body.
- Keep the fold elevated while you take the measure. Keep pinching the fold with your left hand throughout the entire measurement.
- Hold the caliper in your right hand with the dial facing up. Place the jaws of the calibers perpendicular to the fold 1 cm below the fingers and halfway between the crest and the base of the fold, and release all pressure on the scissor grip while keeping the caliper perpendicular to the skinfold.
- Record the skinfold measurement to the nearest 0.5 mm, 1 to 2 seconds after releasing the scissor grip.
- Take skinfold measures in rotational order to allow time for the skinfold to regain its normal thickness.
- Take a minimum of two measurements at each site. If duplicate measurements are not within 1 or 2 mm (or 10%), retest this site.
- Calculate the average for each skinfold site. Using the client's measurements and validated skinfold equations, percentage body fat can be estimated.

TABLE 6.7 STANDARDIZED DESCRIPTIONS OF SKINFOLD SITES (1, 2)

Site	Location Description
Abdominal	Vertical fold; 2 cm to the right side of the umbilicus
Triceps	Vertical fold; on the posterior midline of the upper arm, halfway between the acromion and the olecranon processes, with the arm held freely to the side of the body
Biceps	Vertical fold; on the anterior aspect of the arm over the belly of the biceps muscle, 1 cm above the level used to mark the triceps site
Chest/pectoral	Diagonal fold; one-half the distance between the anterior axillary line and the nipple (men), or one-third of the distance between the anterior axillary line and the nipple (women)
Medial calf	Vertical fold; at the maximum circumference of the calf on the midline of its medial border
Midaxillary	Vertical fold; on the midaxillary line at the level of the xiphoid process of the sternum. An alternate method is a horizontal fold taken at the level of the xiphoid/sternal border in the midaxillary line
Subscapular	Diagonal fold (at a 45° angle); 1–2 cm below the inferior angle of the scapula
Suprailiac	Diagonal fold; in line with the natural angle of the iliac crest taken in the anterior axillary line immediately superior to the iliac crest
Thigh	Vertical fold; on the anterior midline of the thigh, midway between the proximal border of the patella and the inguinal crease (hip)

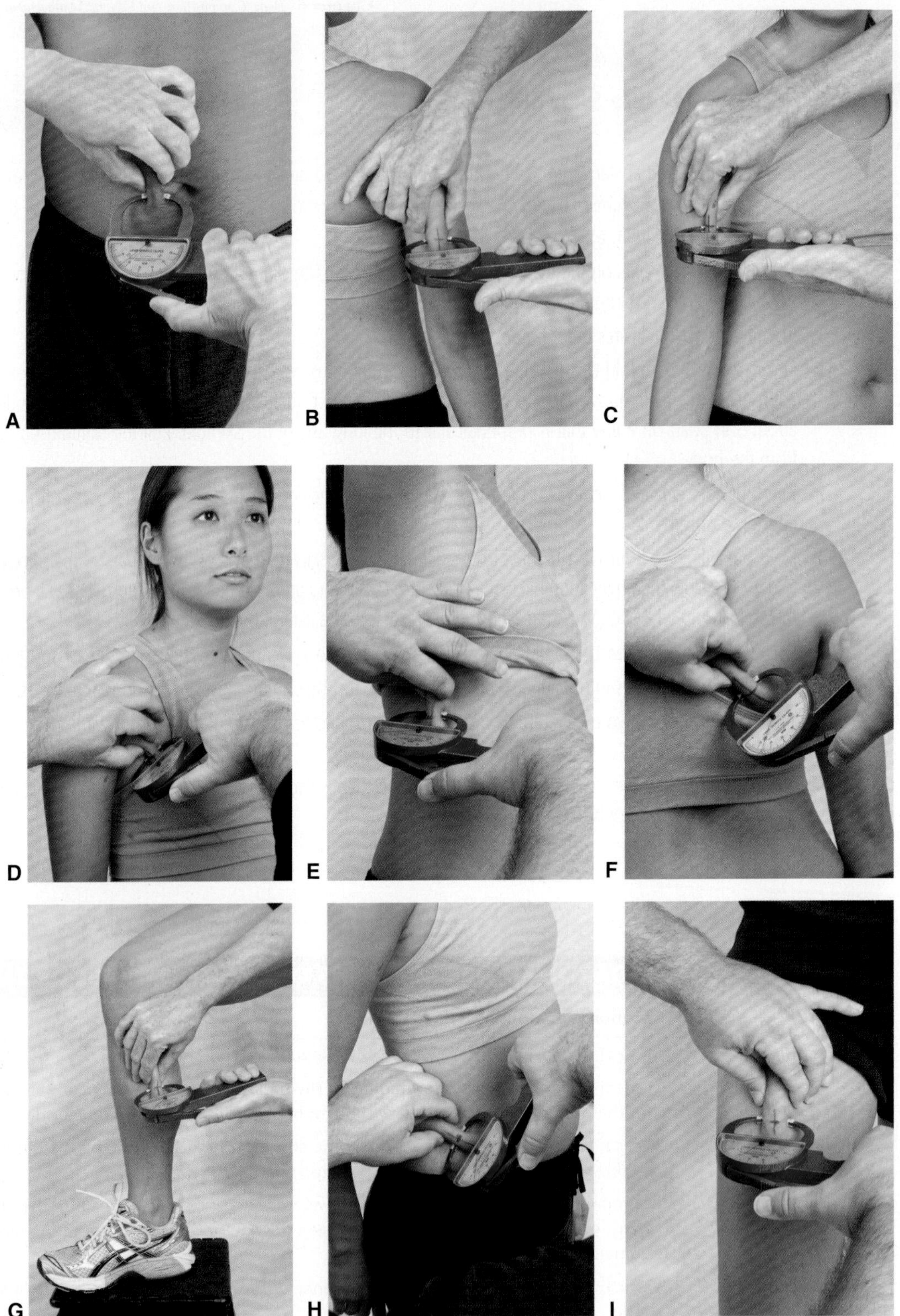

FIGURE 6.2. Common skinfold sites. **A.** Abdominal: vertical fold, 2 cm to the right side of the umbilicus. **B.** Triceps: vertical fold on the posterior midline of the upper arm, halfway between the acromion and the olecranon processes, with the arm held freely to the side of the body. **C.** Biceps: vertical fold on the anterior aspect of the arm over the belly of the biceps muscle, 1 cm above the level used to mark the triceps site. **D.** Chest: diagonal fold, one-half the distance between the anterior axillary line and the nipple (men) or one-third of the distance between the axillary line and the nipple (women). **E.** Midaxillary: vertical fold on the midaxillary line at the level of the xiphoid process of the sternum. **F.** Subscapular: diagonal fold (at a 45° angle), 1 to 2 cm below the inferior angle of the scapula. **G.** Medial calf: vertical fold at the maximum circumference of the calf on the midline of its medial border. **H.** Suprailium: diagonal fold in line with the natural angle of the iliac crest taken in the anterior axillary line immediately superior to the iliac crest. **I.** Thigh: vertical fold, on the anterior midline of the thigh, midway between the proximal border of the patella and the inguinal crease (hip). (From Bushman B, ed. *ACSM's Resources for the Personal Trainer*. 4th ed. Baltimore (MD): Lippincott Williams & Wilkins; 2014.)

TABLE 6.8 GENERALIZED SKINFOLD EQUATIONS TO DETERMINE BODY DENSITY (BD) (23, 44)

	Men	Women
Seven-site formula (chest, midaxillary, triceps, subscapular, abdomen, suprailiac, and thigh)	BD = 1.112 − 0.00043499 (sum of seven skinfolds) + 0.00000055 (sum of seven skinfolds)^2 − 0.00028826 (age) *[See 0.008 or ~3.5% fat]*	BD = 1.097 − 0.00046971 (sum of seven skinfolds) + 0.00000056 (sum of seven skinfolds)^2 − 0.00012828 (age) *[See 0.008 or ~3.8% fat]*
Three-Site Formula		
Chest, abdomen, and thigh	BD = 1.10938 − 0.0008267 (sum of three skinfolds) + 0.0000016 (sum of three skinfolds)^2 − 0.0002574 (age) *[See 0.008 or ~3.4% fat]*	NA
Chest, triceps, and subscapular	BD = 1.1125025 − 0.0013125 (sum of three skinfolds) + 0.0000055 (sum of three skinfolds)^2 − 0.000244 (age) *[See 0.008 or ~3.6% fat]*	NA
Triceps, suprailiac, and thigh	NA	BD = 1.099421 − 0.0009929 (sum of three skinfolds) + 0.0000023 (sum of three skinfolds)^2 − 0.0001392 (age) *[See 0.009 or ~3.9% fat]*
Triceps, suprailiac, and abdominal	NA	BD = 1.089733 − 0.0009245 (sum of three skinfolds) + 0.0000025 (sum of three skinfolds)^2 − 0.0000979 (age) *[See 0.009 or ~3.9% fat]*

The accuracy of predicting the percentage body fat from BIA ranges between ±2.7% and 6.3% (16). Selecting an appropriate regression equation and controlling potential sources of measurement error, particularly the client's hydration status, help keep measurement error in the lower end of this range. The following guidelines will assist in attaining an accurate prediction of percentage body fat using BIA (20):

- Complete measurements in a thermoneutral environment
- No eating or drinking within 4 hours of the test
- No exercise within 12 hours of the test
- Urinate within 30 minutes of the test
- No alcohol consumption within 48 hours of the test
- No diuretic medication within 7 days of the test (clients should not discontinue use of prescribed diuretic medication unless approved by their personal physician)
- Avoid taking measurements prior to menstruation to avoid the possible effects of water retention in women
- Use the same BIA analyzer when measuring change in a client's body composition over time

Laboratory Methods for Measuring Body Composition

There are a number of sophisticated methods that you can use to determine percentage body fat. These methods tend to be more precise than the methods described above, but require expensive specialized equipment that is not available in most health/fitness settings. However, the HFS should have knowledge of these advanced techniques, as they are often used as the reference that the simpler measures are compared with.

Hydrostatic (underwater) weighing (HW) is a widely used technique for determining body composition. This technique calculates body density from body volume, based on Archimedes principle, which states that the weight under water is directly proportional to the volume of water displaced by the body volume. The protocol requires that a person be weighed on land and underwater. The densities of muscle and bone are higher than the density of water, while fat is less dense than water. A person with high levels of muscle and bone will be heavier in water compared with a person with higher levels of fat. HW has a standard error of the estimate of ±2.7% body fat (31).

Air displacement plethysmography (ADP) also measures body volume and is an alternative to HW for determining body composition. ADP has many advantages over HW, in that it is quick and noninvasive, does not require submersion in water, and accommodates children, adults, and older adults as well as individuals who are obese or disabled. There is one commercial system currently available (BOD POD, Life Measurement Instruments, Concord, CA). The accuracy of ADP is similar to that of HW (2).

DEXA uses very low current X-rays at two energy levels to measure bone mineral content, body fat, and lean soft tissue mass. This method requires an individual to lie supine on a table while being scanned from head to toe. DEXA is safe and easy to use, but the instrumentation can be very expensive. With appropriate standards and methodology, the reproducibility of DEXA is 1.7% for percentage body fat (3).

WEIGHT MANAGEMENT

The causes of obesity are complex and multifactorial and are a mixture of genetic, behavioral, physiological, geographical, economic, and social factors. The *F as in Fat report* (29) noted that the states with the highest levels of physical inactivity and the lowest levels of fruit and vegetable consumption had the highest rankings of obesity. Although many other factors contribute to an individual's body weight, a healthy diet and regular physical activity are critical for attaining and/or maintaining a healthy weight.

Weight Loss Goals

Developing realistic weight loss goals is important when working with those who are trying to lose weight. The National Heart, Lung, and Blood Institute recommend that a 5% to 10% weight reduction results in improved overall health (51).

Safe and effective weight loss should occur at a rate of 1 to 2 lb·week^{-1} (51). With this in mind, using the above example, the person would take 8.5 to 17 weeks or 2.5 to 4.25 months to reach their desired weight. Although people can lose 2 lb·week^{-1}, it is difficult to maintain this amount of weight loss consistently over time, and the time frame of 8.5 weeks or 2.5 months is most likely unrealistic for most people. Thus, it is possible to reduce a person's percentage body fat 3% to 6% in 3 to 4 months; however, it may take longer depending on the person. Depending on the weight loss goal, multiple (*i.e.*, 3–4) goals may need to be created until the person reaches the desired percentage body fat and weight.

Measuring body weight is a good method to use for weekly tracking because depending on which percentage body fat method is used, there could be a 3% to 6% error in the estimated value. Therefore, if percentage body fat was measured each week, it would be difficult to determine either whether a change has actually occurred or whether it is a reflection of measurement error. This problem does not exist with absolute weight, although it is best to measure weight at a consistent time of day. Also, a person can weigh himself or herself each week without having to see a specialist to be measured (28).

Energy Balance

The management of body weight is dependent on energy balance: energy intake (the amount of calories consumed) and energy expenditure (the amount of calories expended). To reduce body weight, energy expenditure must exceed energy intake, referred to as a negative energy balance.

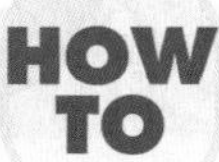

Estimate Desired Body Weight and Percentage Body Fat

Knowing a person's percentage body fat and current body weight is needed to develop weight loss goals. Below is an equation that can be used to develop a desired body weight once the person's percentage body fat is known and a desired percentage body fat has been determined.

1. Estimate percentage body fat (using one of the methods discussed earlier in this chapter)
2. Fat mass = Total body mass × (Percentage body fat/100)
3. Fat-free mass = Total body mass − Fat mass
4. Desired weight = Fat-free mass/[1 − (Desired percentage body fat/100)]

Example:

1. Percentage body fat = 31%; Total body mass = 213 lb; Desired percentage body fat = 25%
2. Fat mass = Total body mass × (Percentage body fat/100)
   = 213 × 0.31
   = 66.03 lb
3. Fat-free mass = Total body mass − Fat mass
   = 213 − 66.03
   = 146.97 lb
4. Desired weight = Fat-free mass/[1 − (Desired percentage body fat/100)]
   = 146.97/[1 − 0.25]
   = 146.97/0.75
   = 195.96 (~196 lb)

Conversely, an individual gains weight when in a positive energy balance, that is, when energy intake exceeds energy expenditure. Body weight is maintained when an individual is in energy balance — expending the same number of calories as they are consuming.

Total energy expenditure (TEE) is the total number of calories expended each day and reflects the amount of energy required to carry out all metabolic processes within the body. Examples of these metabolic processes include growth of new cells, maintaining the functions of body tissues, and providing fuel for movement of the body, including exercise. There are three components to determining TEE:

- Resting energy expenditure (REE *or* resting metabolic rate [RMR] *or* basal metabolic rate [BMR]): 60% to 70% TEE
- Thermic effect of food: 10% TEE
- Physical activity expenditure: 20% to 30% TEE

Resting energy expenditure (REE) is the largest component of TEE and is the energy required to maintain normal regulatory balance and body functions at rest. In the simplest terms, REE (sometimes referred to as BEE or basal energy expenditure) is the amount of calories a person uses if he or she was to do no activity throughout the day. There are several factors that influence REE. To some degree, everyone's "metabolism" is determined by their genes; however, there are several other factors within the individual that contribute to a person's REE, including their body composition. Lean body mass, such as skeletal muscle, has a major influence on REE. Body tissues, such as the brain, the liver, and other organs, and even fat mass contribute to one's metabolism, although fat

TABLE 6.9 **COMMON REE (KCAL · DAY^{-1}) PREDICTIVE EQUATIONS FOR ADULTS**

	Men	Women
Harris-Benedict (for adults)	66.47 + 13.75 (wt in kg) + 5 (ht in cm) − 6.8 (age in yr)	665 + 9.6 (wt in kg) + 1.8 (ht in cm) − 4.7 (age in yrs)
Mifflin-St. Jeor (for obese adults)	10 (wt in kg) + 6.3 (ht in cm) − 5 × age + 5	10 (wt in kg) + 6.3 (ht in cm) − 5 × age − 161

mass is much less metabolically active than other body tissues. A person's age, gender, and ethnicity also influence REE, primarily because of the impact on lean body mass.

Another component that contributes to a person's TEE is the thermic effect of food. Although this may account for a small percentage of a person's total metabolism, it is important to note that the act of eating and digestion of foods require energy. The most controllable of all the influences on a person's total metabolism, however, is how active he or she is. The more physically active an individual is, the greater his or her TEE.

To calculate an individual's total energy needs, REE must first be measured or calculated using predictive equations. Next an activity factor is used to calculate TEE for that individual. REE can be measured using indirect calorimetry, which measures an individual's oxygen consumption, although is not widely available. Predictive equations can also be used to estimate REE; however, predictive equations that incorporate fat-free mass provide the most accurate prediction of REE. Predictive equations take into account an individual's age, gender, height, and weight or fat-free mass. Table 6.9 provides examples of commonly used predictive equations for adults.

In determining an individual's energy needs, a physical activity factor needs to be included in the prediction equation. The Institute of Medicine (IOM) has developed a physical activity level (PAL) that takes into account TEE and BEE, independent of gender (17).

Low active: PA $= 1.4 < \text{PAL} < 1.6$
Active: PA $= 1.6 < \text{PAL} < 1.9$
Very active: PA $= 1.9 < \text{PAL} < 2.5$

Although a true baseline PAL would be 1.0, it is not practical that any one individual would not expend any energy over and above what is necessary for survival; therefore, the "low active" range, otherwise known as sedentary, is 40% to 60% above baseline. Similarly, for those persons who are "very active," their PAL is at least 100% above baseline.

When calculating energy needs for weight loss, first determine REE with either indirect calorimetry or the appropriate predictive equation. Then multiply this by the appropriate activity factor. Table 6.10 shows daily energy needs for various population groups.

Following is an example for determining TEE prediction for a 35-year-old man, who is 6 ft 0 in, weighs 180 lb, and is low active. Using the Harris–Benedict equation, the calculated REE would be (15):

$$\begin{aligned}\text{REE (kcal·day}^{-1}) &= 66.47 + 13.75 \text{ (wt in kg)} + 5 \text{ (ht in cm)} - 6.8 \text{ (age in yr)}\\ &= (66.47 + 13.75\ (81.82) + 5\ (182.9) - 6.8\ (35)\\ &= 1{,}869 \text{ kcal·day}^{-1}\end{aligned}$$

$$\begin{aligned}\text{TEE} &= \text{(REE)} \times \text{(PAL)}\\ &= (1{,}869) \times (1.5) = 2{,}803 \text{ kcal}\\ &= 2{,}803 \text{ kcal}\end{aligned}$$

As previously mentioned, the recommended rate of weight loss in adults is 1 to 2 lb·week^{-1}, which is equal to a daily caloric deficit of 500 to 1,000 calories. In the above example, the individual

TABLE 6.10 ESTIMATED CALORIE NEEDS PER DAY BY AGE, GENDER, AND PAL (18)

		PAL		
Gender	**Age**	**Sedentary**	**Moderately Active**	**Active**
Female	2–3	1,000–1,200	1,000–1,4000	1,000–1,400
	4–8	1,200–1,400	1,400–1,600	1,400–1,800
	9–13	1,400–1,600	1,600–2,000	1,800–2,200
	14–18	1,800	2,000	2,400
	19–30	1,800–2,000	2,000–2,200	2,400
	31–50	1,800	2,000	2,200
	51+	1,600	1,800	2,000–2,200
Male	2–3	1,000–1,200	1,000–1,400	1,000–1,400
	4–8	1,200–1,400	1,400–1,600	1,600–2,000
	9–13	1,600–2,000	1,800–2,200	2,000–2,600
	14–18	2,000–2,400	2,400–2,800	2,800–3,200
	19–30	2,400–2,600	2,600–2,800	3,000
	31–50	2,200–2,400	2,400–2,600	2,800–3,000
	51+	2,000–2,200	2,200–2,400	2,400–2,800

needs about 2,800 calories a day to maintain his weight at a low activity level. To achieve 1 lb of weight loss per week, this person's caloric requirements would be approximately 2,300 calories per day, or a 500 calorie daily deficit. It should be noted that it is not recommended for an individual to consume less than 1,200 calories a day unless medically indicated, as this low-calorie intake is not likely to meet basic nutrient needs.

TREATMENT OF OBESITY THROUGH EXERCISE

ACSM Position Stand

In 2009, ACSM developed a position stand on appropriate physical activity interventions for weight loss and prevention of weight gain in adults (11). Regarding weight loss, the combination of diet and moderate-to-vigorous physical activity (MVPA) ($\geq$150 min·wk^{-1}) produces the largest weight loss compared with diet or physical activity only.

Although the exact amount of PA necessary for weight maintenance after weight loss is currently unknown, it is well established that regular MVPA is necessary to prevent weight regain after weight loss has occurred. Further, to prevent general weight gain, engaging in MVPA for at least 150 minutes a week is typically sufficient; however, the ACSM position stand indicates that engaging in more than 250 minutes a week of MVPA would result in better weight maintenance. Thus, it can be concluded that MVPA has a greater role in the prevention of weight regain and weight maintenance after weight loss has occurred rather than as a stand-alone weight loss method (11).

Weight Loss using the FITT Principle

Exercise is defined as a physical activity that is structured and repetitive, uses large muscle groups, and has the intent of changing one or more fitness components. Exercise promotes increased levels of energy expenditure, and should be done at a moderate to vigorous intensity. Types of exercise activities that work well for the overweight and obese include walking, swimming, water aerobics, jogging/walking in water, biking, and elliptical and rowing machines (48). All these activities can be done at an appropriate intensity and for a long duration without negatively impacting the knee and hip joints. Weightlifting is also important to include after an aerobic activity has been incorporated into a person's routine, as it will build lean muscle mass and slow the reduction in RMR that often occurs with weight loss and aging.

Depending on the amount of excess body weight and the aerobic fitness of the client, the FITT principle can be adjusted to meet the needs of the client. There have been numerous studies examining the amount and type of physical activity that is needed to promote and maintain weight loss (24–26). Often the person who is trying either to lose weight or to maintain weight loss will be working with a nutritionist for dietary advice. This is important as a reduction in energy consumption and an increase in energy expenditure will result in more weight loss than either method used alone. If you are working with a client who has not exercised in a long time, has never exercised, or is severely obese, initially doing exercise in 10-minute bouts at least three times a day may be necessary. The client may exercise for longer durations as their fitness level increases. This is also a good strategy to use if the client has a very busy schedule and cannot fit in one 30-minute bout.

The FITT principle for weight loss following ACSM guidelines is as follows:

Frequency: ≥5 days·week^{-1} to maximize caloric expenditure.

Intensity: Moderate- to vigorous-intensity aerobic activity should be encouraged. Initial exercise training intensity should be moderate (*i.e.*, 40% to $<60\%$ VO_2R or HRR). Eventual progression to more vigorous exercise intensity (*i.e.*, =60% VO_2R or HRR) may result in further health and physical fitness benefits.

Time: A minimum of 30 minutes·day^{-1} (*i.e.*, 150 min·wk^{-1}) progressing to 60 minutes·day^{-1} (*i.e.*, 300 min·wk^{-1}) of moderate-intensity aerobic activity. Incorporating more vigorous-intensity exercise into the total volume of exercise may provide additional health benefits. However, vigorous-intensity exercise should be encouraged in individuals who are both capable and willing to exercise at higher than moderate-intensity levels with recognition that vigorous-intensity exercise is associated with the potential for greater injuries (42). Accumulation of intermittent exercise of at least 10 minutes is an effective alternative to continuous exercise and may be a particularly useful way to initiate exercise (24).

Type: The primary mode of exercise should be aerobic physical activities that involve the large muscle groups. As part of a balanced exercise program, resistance training and flexibility exercise should be incorporated.

Demonstrating Exercises

Demonstrating exercises to clients is a critical element to program implementation. Exercise demonstration allows the client to see what has been verbally explained and also allows key aspects of the exercise to be highlighted. This is especially true with either an overweight or an obese client. Depending on the severity of obesity, it may also be necessary to identify suitable equipment. Keep in mind that some equipment has a maximum weight limit or the person may not fit or be comfortable while exercising on the equipment. Further, certain basic activities may be difficult, such as going down and getting up from the floor or bending over. Thus, specific exercises in a person's exercise program may need to be either modified or removed. All these aspects should be considered when designing an exercise program for an overweight and obese client.

General Training Principles

When designing a training program for overweight and obese clients, it may be of considerable value for the HFS to become familiar with the 2009 ACSM position stand (11). Since each person will be at a different starting point and will have different goals regarding weight loss, the 2009 position stand combined with the 2010 Dietary Guidelines for Americans will help the HFS to individualize specific weight loss plans (19).

Although there are numerous approaches to planning exercise for weight loss, the basic principles of exercise prescription are outlined in Chapter 3. In addition, Chapter 7 provides detailed

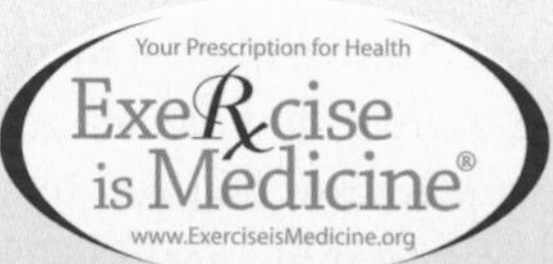

EXERCISE IS MEDICINE CONNECTION

The Look AHEAD Research Group. Long-term effects of a lifestyle intervention on weight and cardiovascular risk factors in individuals with Type 2 diabetes mellitus: Four-year results of the look AHEAD trial. *Arch Intern Med.* 2010;170:1566–75.

The Look AHEAD (Action for Health in Diabetes) group conducted a 4-year randomized clinical trial that compared the effects of a lifestyle intervention with diabetes support and education (DSE) standard care. The purpose of this study was to examine the effects the Look AHEAD trial had on weight loss and cardiovascular disease risk factors. The lifestyle intervention consisted of diet modification, physical activity, and behavior modification and was designed to produce at least a 7% weight loss at 1 year. The diet consisted of a 1,200 to 1,800 $kcal \cdot day^{-1}$ goal based on initial weight, with less than 30% of total calories from fat and at least 15% of total calories from protein. The exercise goal was to obtain at least 175 minutes of physical activity a week through walking. The behavioral strategies stressed included self-monitoring, goal setting, and problem solving. The lifestyle intervention group met with counselors weekly for the first 6 months and three times a week for the next 6 months. For years 2 to 4, they met with the counselors at least once a month. The DSE group was invited to attend three group sessions each year where diet, physical activity, or social support was discussed. Weight, aerobic fitness, blood draw, and blood pressure were measured annually, and the participants received an honorarium. Although the paper presents results for all cardiovascular disease risk factors, only the results for the weight loss and maintenance are going to be discussed. At the end of the first year, the lifestyle group lost more weight (8.6% change) than did the DSE group (1% change). Further, the lifestyle group was able to maintain the weight loss better than the DSE group over the 4-year period (4.7% vs. 1.1%, respectively; $P < .001$). When the weight loss was averaged over the 4 years, the lifestyle group lost more weight (mean change: -6.15% from initial weight) than the DSE group (mean change: -0.88% from initial weight). This is the first study to track weight loss and weight loss maintenance for such a long period. The results are very encouraging given the fact weight loss among that patients with Type 2 diabetes is very challenging. The participants in this study had an average BMI of 36.0 ± 5.6 $kg \cdot m^{-2}$, so they were considered obese. This study shows that the combination of diet, physical activity, and behavioral modification is necessary not only to promote weight loss, but also to maintain the weight loss over a long period.

information about exercise prescription in people with cardiovascular, metabolic, and pulmonary disease, many of which are often present in the overweight and obese. Most importantly, if someone is overweight, obese, and currently sedentary, the HFS needs to use caution and empathy in the early stages of an exercise program. The sedentary overweight and obese person is likely to find exercise initially uncomfortable and accompanied by soreness the following day or two (delayed onset muscle soreness or DOMS). These feelings may also bring about lower levels of self-efficacy and a lower desire to achieve the intended weight loss goals. Therefore, prescribing exercise becomes just as much art as science when working with this population.

Metabolic Equations

The ACSM metabolic equations can be used to estimate the amount of calories that will be expended during a workout or to estimate the length of time an individual has to exercise to expend a certain amount of calories. A calorie, also known as a kilocalorie (kcal), is an expression of energy intake and expenditure. It takes approximately 3,500 calories to make and store 1 lb of body weight. Below is an example of using metabolic equations to determine caloric expenditure. Either of these yields a reasonable estimate of calories expended and can be useful in setting exercise and dietary goals with a client.

These metabolic calculations yield a range of caloric expenditures that can be expected while performing the exercise. Keep in mind also that this value of $kcal \cdot min^{-1}$ includes the calories that would have been expended at rest, so this is the "gross" caloric expenditure for the 30 minutes. Refer to Chapters 3 and 7 to determine "net" caloric expenditure, or the calories strictly from the exercise.

Weight Management Myths

When working with someone who is trying to lose weight, they may ask about some common myths.

Myth #1: Fat Turns into Muscle or Vice Versa

Fat and muscle are two separate tissues in the body. It is impossible to change one type into the other. During weight loss, fat mass in the body typically decreases while the amount of muscle mass may increase if exercise is of sufficient intensity (overload principle).

Myth #2: Spot Reducing Works

It is not possible to reduce fat in a chosen region of the body. Fat reduction occurs in a somewhat random fashion and is not likely to be the same for any two persons. What will happen, however, is that if a client wants to lose fat around his or her waist and does an excessive number of core

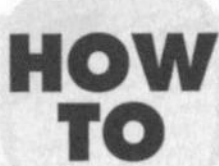

Calculate Metabolic Equations (Weight Management)

Here is an example calculating caloric expenditure using metabolic equations.

Female – height: 63 in, weight: 68 kg, BMI: 26.6 $kg \cdot m^{-2}$

Client walks on a treadmill at 3.5 mph and a 5% grade for 30 minutes.

What is the client's total caloric expenditure?

$$mph \times (26.8\ m \cdot min^{-1}) = m \cdot min^{-1}$$

$$(3.5\ mph) \times (26.8\ m \cdot min^{-1}) = 93.8\ m \cdot min^{-1}$$

$$5\%\ grade = 0.05$$

$$\dot{V}O_2\ (mL \cdot kg^{-1} \cdot min^{-1}) = (0.1 \times m \cdot min^{-1}) + (1.8 \times m \cdot min^{-1} \times grade) + 3.5$$

$$\dot{V}O_2\ (mL \cdot kg^{-1} \cdot min^{-1}) = (0.1 \times 93.8) + (1.8 \times 93.8 \times 0.05) + 3.5$$

$$\dot{V}O_2\ (mL \cdot kg^{-1} \cdot min^{-1}) = 9.38 + 8.44 + 3.5$$

$$\dot{V}O_2 = 21.32\ mL \cdot kg^{-1} \cdot min^{-1}$$

$$(mL \cdot kg^{-1} \cdot min^{-1}) \times 1{,}000/kg = \dot{V}O_2\ L \cdot min^{-1})$$

$$(21.32 \times 1{,}000)/58 = 1.24\ L \cdot min^{-1}$$

$$L \cdot min^{-1} \times 5 = kcal \cdot min^{-1}$$

Note: approximately 5 kcal are consumed for every liter of oxygen

$$1.24 \times 5 = 6.2\ kcal \cdot min^{-1}$$

$$6.2\ kcal \cdot min^{-1} \times 30\ min = 186\ kcal$$

Total caloric expenditure on treadmill = 186 kcal for 30 min.

This information can then be used to determine how many minutes, over how many days, the client will need to exercise to achieve her weight loss goals.

exercises, he or she will increase his or her core muscle mass, but not necessarily reduce the fat located around the core.

Myth #3: Gaining Weight at the Start of an Exercise Program Is from Increased Muscle

Muscle hypertrophy occurs only after 6 to 8 weeks of higher-intensity resistance training, and therefore it is highly unlikely to see any muscle gain in the first 2 months of exercise. Even beyond that point, most people will not exercise at an intensity to produce significant increases in muscle mass. Instead, what is more likely, and discouraging, is that those new to exercise may overcompensate their calorie intake, thinking their new-found exercise "allows" them to eat more, thereby increasing their overall body weight.

TREATMENT OF OBESITY THROUGH NUTRITION

One of the key messages in the 2010 Dietary Guidelines for Americans is the previously mentioned concept of energy balance (19). The guidelines encourage individuals to consume fewer calories, eat more nutrient dense foods, and be more physically active so as to achieve and maintain a healthy weight. The overall goal of the Dietary Guidelines is to help all Americans manage their weight to reduce their risk of chronic diseases such as hypertension, heart disease, and Type 2 diabetes and to promote a healthy lifestyle.

Although the Food Pyramid still remains an important concept in helping Americans recognize the importance of eating a variety of food groups, the 2010 Dietary Guidelines focus on portion control and increasing specific food groups with the "MyPlate" approach (10) (Table 6.11; Fig. 6.3). General dietary messages from the 2010 Dietary Guidelines include the following:

1. Balancing calories: enjoy your food, but eat less; avoid oversized portions.
2. Foods to increase: make half your plate fruits and vegetables; make at least half your grains whole grains; choose fat-free or low-fat (1%) milk.
3. Foods to reduce: high sodium foods such as soup, bread, and frozen meals; drink less sugary drinks such as regular sodas, sports drinks, energy drinks, and fruit drinks.

   In addition to recommending certain foods to emphasize or reduce, the Dietary Guidelines also provide recommendations for the percentage of calories from the three macronutrients — carbohydrate, protein, and fat, as shown in Table 6.12 (18).

   The 2010 Guidelines also encourage individuals to follow specific evidence-based behavioral practices in helping to monitor caloric intake and manage body weight. These behavioral-based strategies are intended to give people additional skills toward achieving their weight-related goals:
4. Focus on the total number of calories consumed.
   - Know your calorie needs.
   - Weigh yourself and adjust what and how much you eat and exercise based on your weight change over time.
5. Monitor food intake.
   - Track what you eat using a food journal or an online food planner (*i.e.*, Choosemyplate.gov SuperTracker).
   - Check calories and servings on food packages.
   - Pay attention to feelings of hunger and eat until you are satisfied not full.
   - Plan out regularly scheduled meals and snacks.
   - Limit eating while watching TV, which can result in overeating.
6. Choose smaller portions or lower-calorie options when eating out.
   - Choose a smaller size option (*i.e.*, appetizer and small plates).
   - Share larger portions or take home part of your meal.
   - Choose dishes that include vegetables (or salads with low-fat/fat-free dressing), fruits, and/or whole grains.

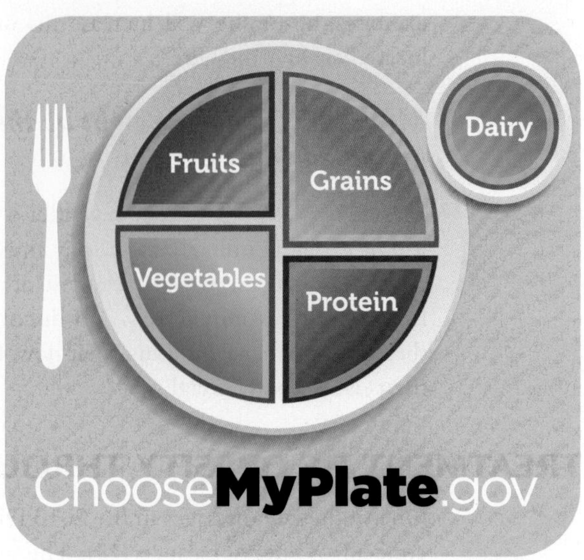

FIGURE 6.3. MyPlate: The new healthy eating guide.

- Avoid choosing foods with the words: creamy, fried, battered, or buttered.
- Keep portions of syrups, dressings, and sauces small.

7. Prepare, serve, and consume smaller portions of foods and beverages, especially those high in calories.
   - Use smaller plates.
   - Portion out small amounts of food.
   - To feel satisfied with fewer calories, replace large portions of high-calorie foods with lower-calorie foods such as vegetables and fruits (higher-fiber foods).

TABLE 6.11 **KEY RECOMMENDATIONS OF THE 2010 DIETARY GUIDELINES**

Increase fruit and vegetable intake	Fresh, frozen, and canned; if using canned vegetables, rinse off liquids stored in since this portion contains sodium
Color your plate	Eat a variety of vegetables, especially dark green, red, and orange vegetables and beans and peas
Consume at least half of all grains as whole grains	For example, buckwheat, bulgar, millet, oatmeal, quinoa, rolled oats, brown or wild rice, whole-grain barley, whole rye, and whole wheat Use the nutrition facts label to choose good or excellent sources of fiber Good sources of fiber are 10%–19% of the daily value per serving; excellent sources of dietary fiber contain 20% or more
Increase intake of fat-free (skim) or low-fat (1%) milk	Includes milk products such as milk, yogurt, cheese, or fortified soy beverages
Choose a variety of protein foods	Include seafood, lean meat and poultry, eggs, beans and peas, soy products, and unsalted nuts and seeds
Increase the amount and variety of seafood consumed	Choose seafood (*e.g.*, salmon, tuna, trout, tilapia, shrimp, crab, and oysters) in place of some meat and poultry twice a week
Replace protein foods that are higher in solid fats	Replace, for example, fried meats, bacon, sausage, with choices that are lower in solid fats and calories and/or are sources of oils
Use oils to replace solid fats when possible	Use olive, canola, corn, safflower, or sunflower oil in small amounts rather than solid fats such as butter, stick margarine, shortening, and lard
Choose foods that provide more potassium, dietary fiber, calcium, and vitamin D	These foods include vegetables, fruits, whole grains, and milk and milk products

Modified from http://www.health.gov/dietaryguidelines/dga2010/dietaryguidelines2010.pdf.

TABLE 6.12 RECOMMENDED MACRONUTRIENT PROPORTIONS BY AGE (18)

	Carbohydrate (%)	Protein (%)	Fat (%)
Young children (1–3 years)	45–65	5–20	30–40
Older children and adolescents (4–18 years)	45–65	10–30	25–35
Adults (≥19 years)	45–65	10–35	20–35

8. Eat a nutrient-dense breakfast.
9. Limit screen time, including TV, computer, and video games, to less than 2 hours a day.

TREATMENT OF OBESITY THROUGH OTHER METHODS

Different strategies exist for modifying a person's body composition and promoting weight loss. Although many of these strategies are effective, some are considered unsafe and should not be used by individuals trying to lose weight. Inappropriate weight loss methods include saunas, electric stimulators, sweat suits, vibrating belts, body wraps, overexercising, very low calorie diets, fad diets, and dietary supplements (Table 6.13).

Appropriate weight loss methods include exercise, dietary changes, behavioral strategies, and bariatric surgery. Bariatric surgery rates have increased from 7.0 to 38.6 per 100,000 adults between 1998 and 2002 (49), and current rates are estimated to be almost double that of 2002. Although this surgery is very effective at producing weight loss (46), the effects of exercise in combination with this surgery are currently unknown. Moreover, it is unknown whether the exercise prescription should be different from those who chose not to undergo the surgery (1). For many people, though, bariatric surgery is medically indicated because of severe obesity and/or comorbidities threatening their health. The HFS should recognize that weight loss is not easy, and for some people, the health risk of being overweight is such that medical care should be sought. However, for those not interested or indicated for surgery, adding a behavioral component to their exercise and diet plan may aid them in achieving their weight loss goals.

TABLE 6.13 INAPPROPRIATE WEIGHT LOSS METHODS AND CONSEQUENCES (45, 52, 53, 55, 56)

Method	Negative Consequences
Saunas	Dehydration, only lose water weight, low amount of weight loss, temporary weight loss
Vibrating belts	No weight loss
Body wraps	Small weight loss, temporary weight loss, skin irritation
Overexercising	Overuse injury, unhealthy amount of weight loss
Electric muscle stimulators	No change in body composition, bruising, and skin irritation
Sweat suits	Dehydration, only lose water weight, low amount of weight loss, temporary weight loss
Dietary supplements	Not regulated by FDA, so dosage may not be known; may have nutrient drug interactions, drug-drug interactions, and other side effects such as nausea, dizziness, and racing heart
Very low calorie diets	May not meet nutrient needs of the individual promoting deficiencies in specific nutrients (*e.g.*, calcium deficiency leads to brittle, broken bones, hip fractures); could lead to dehydration, constipation, or fatigue
Fad diets	Often "cut out" a food group, which leads to specific nutrient, vitamin, and mineral deficiencies; not sustainable for long periods; could lead to "yo-yo" dieting (*i.e.*, intervals of weight loss followed by weight gain); low carbohydrate diets do not meet body's requirement for a minimum of 130 g of carbohydrates a day; could lead to fatigue and lack of energy; could lead to dehydration and/or constipation; not recommended

Behavioral Strategies

Interventions that combine diet, physical activity, and behavior therapy are the most effective programs for weight loss and weight maintenance (50). Behavioral weight loss programs not only target dietary intake and physical activity, but also provide clients with strategies to help them make the necessary lifestyle changes. Key strategies used in behavioral weight loss programs include the following:

- Self-monitoring — keeping food or physical activity logs or monitoring body weight on a regular basis
- Goal setting — setting realistic goals for the number of minutes of exercise one will accomplish during the next week or month
- Stimulus control — modifying one's environment to enhance successful behavior change such as removing "risky" foods from the refrigerator or hanging an exercise adherence calendar in a prominent spot
- Problem solving — identifying situations that pose a problem for overeating (such as holidays) and developing a solution to eat healthy and avoid excess caloric intake

There are many additional behavioral strategies that clients can use to enhance a weight management program. See Chapter 11 for more information on behavioral strategies that can assist with weight loss goals.

Weight Loss Supplements

The HFS has a responsibility to encourage healthy weight loss, when indicated, by eating a balanced diet including adequate fruit and vegetables, limiting sugary beverages and energy-dense foods, and including regular exercise and activity. Taking this approach is considered safe and reasonable and should provide sufficient nutrition to meet daily needs. However, despite this, many different weight loss products and supplements are available to the public, often with little or no evidence to support their value. One of the most reputable resources for information on vitamins, minerals, supplements, and herbal products is the Office of Dietary Supplement (37). Although medications and drugs prescribed by a doctor are regulated by the U.S. Food and Drug Administration (FDA), supplements and herbal products are not regulated by the government in terms of efficacy, safety, dosing, and purity of the product. The FDA Web site does list updates and warnings related to supplements (both dietary and herbal) and is an important resource for HFSs and their clients (8).

The rating on effectiveness is based on available research (32). Some advertised physiological mechanisms for dietary supplements include increased energy expenditure, modified carbohydrate metabolism, decreased fat production, and blocked absorption of dietary fat. However, numerous safety concerns have been raised with some supplements (*e.g.*, ephedra, bitter orange, and chitosan), occasionally resulting in their removal from the consumer market.

People of all ages experiment with weight loss products, including caffeine and energy drinks. Although a safe upper limit has been established for adults and caffeine (250–300 mg·d^{-1}), there is no recommendation for adolescents. Therefore, as a general rule, caffeine and energy drinks should be consumed with caution, particularly in the younger/adolescent population. Many energy drinks are also high in sugar and calories, so regardless of age, the consumption of these drinks may be a source of excess calories and not "cost-effective" in terms of the benefits outweighing the risks. Side effects of energy drinks and caffeine depend on the individual's sensitivity, but may include sleeplessness, nervousness, irritability, and anxiety. Resources for additional information on supplements and herbal products can be found at the end of this chapter.

Dieting

Although many people may also experiment with "dieting" for weight loss, in general, most popular diets are to be approached with caution. Ideally, individuals interested in the current popular diet fads should first seek the advice of a Registered Dietitian or other health care professional trained in nutrition to determine the safety and effectiveness of the diet. Diets to be cautious of include those promoting low carbohydrates, excessive protein intake, or any meal pattern that eliminates or emphasizes any one particular food group. For instance, the IOM recommends at least 130 g of carbohydrate each day for all age groups (22). Thus, diets prescribing low carbohydrate intake may fall short of this requirement and likely lead to cravings. Individuals need a variety of foods from each food group to meet their needs for growth, development, and maintenance throughout the lifespan. Any client who wishes to "go on a diet" should first consider his or her optimal health/dietary needs. A more prudent approach may be to consider permanent dietary changes (such as eating more fruits and vegetables) as opposed to "going on a diet."

Medications

Table 6.14 shows the effect of common medications on weight management and their physiological action (14, 27, 33–35, 54). Many of these medications, taken for high blood pressure, seizure disorders, allergies, and so on, can actually promote weight gain. Therefore, it is important to know all the medications your client is taking, as they may inhibit your client's weight loss attempts.

NUTRITION THROUGH THE LIFESPAN

Along with regular exercise, it is important to incorporate proper daily nutrition habits to achieve and successfully maintain weight loss. However, this should not be considered a "one-time" diet, but instead a lifelong strategy of healthy eating. To solidify this point, one of the key recommendations of the 2010 Dietary Guidelines is to "manage appropriate calorie balance during each stage of life including childhood, adolescence, adulthood, pregnancy and breastfeeding, and older age" (18). Specific needs for pregnant women, children, and older adults are discussed below.

Pregnancy

During pregnancy, there are increased energy and nutrient needs to support the growth of the developing fetus. The pregnant woman needs an additional 300 calories each day to ensure that enough essential nutrients are available for both mother and baby. Although pregnant women are strongly encouraged to eat a well-rounded diet, it is also important for the pregnant women to take a vitamin specifically designed for prenatal purposes.

In addition to the increased daily need for protein, there is also an increased dietary need for folic acid and iron that is provided in a prenatal vitamin. Folic acid (a B vitamin) is important in the prevention of serious birth defects such as neural tube defect and congenital heart disease. Extra iron is needed to help support the increased blood supply needed to carry extra oxygen throughout the pregnancy. It is usually recommended that pregnant women take a prenatal vitamin as directed by her doctor, since taking higher or lower doses of a given vitamin or mineral could be harmful to the developing baby. It is also recommended that pregnant women do not take herbal or botanical supplements, since they are not FDA regulated in terms of dosage, purity, and testing. Harmful effects of herbal supplements are not yet fully known, and therefore, it is best for woman to avoid these altogether while pregnant. In addition, given that the demand for other nutrients such as calcium, protein, and carbohydrate increase during pregnancy, this is certainly not an appropriate time for a woman to go on any type of self-prescribed "diet," especially one intended for weight loss.

Children and Older Adults

The HFS should also have sufficient knowledge of the unique dietary needs of children and older adults. On the basis of the 2010 Dietary Guidelines (22), vitamin D recommendations have increased for almost all age groups, but particularly for children and older adults (≥65 years). For children and

TABLE 6.14 EFFECT OF MEDICATION ON WEIGHT MANAGEMENT AND THE ACTION ON THE BODY (14, 27, 33–35, 54)

Medication	Effect	Action
Corticosteroid		
Prednisone	Weight gain	Increased appetite/decreased ability to absorb blood glucose
Antidepressant		
Paxil	Weight gain	
Zoloft	Weight gain	
Wellbutrin	Weight loss	
Prozac	Weight loss	
Antihypertensive		
Cardura and Inderal	Weight gain	Fatigue/shortness of breath/water retention
Hormone replacement therapy/ oral contraceptives	Weight gain	
Antiseizure		
Depakote	Weight gain	
Zonegran	Weight loss	
Topamax	Weight loss	
Diabetes Medication		
Insulin	Weight gain	Weight gain: decreases resting RMR; stimulates insulin secretion; increases number of fat cells
Sulfonylureas	Weight gain	
Thiazolidinediones	Weight gain	
Glucophage	No change	
Precose	No change	
Byetta	Weight loss	
Symlin	Weight loss	
Heartburn		
Nexium	Weight gain	
Prevacid		
Antihistamine	Weight gain	Increase food intake via hypothalamic receptors and leptin regulative system
α-Blockers	Weight gain	Unknown
β-Blockers	Weight gain	Decreased RMR; increased fatigue and causes reduction in physical activity
Migraine medication	Weight gain	Increased appetite; stimulated insulin secretion
Nicotine	Weight loss (?)	Reducing appetite; increasing RMR
Caffeine	Weight loss (?)	Reducing appetite; stimulate thermogenesis; promote water loss

adolescents ages 1 to 18, the recommended dietary intake is now 600 IU, and recommendations have been increased to 800 IU for adults older than 71 years. Also in the older adult, vitamin D is particularly important in its role of promoting the absorption of calcium and in maintaining serum calcium levels, which in turn protects bone strength (39). Although sunlight is a natural source of vitamin D, it is also fortified into many foods, including dairy, breads, and cereals and can therefore be obtained rather easily in most diets.

Calcium is an important nutrient during childhood and adolescence. It is crucial for bone and teeth health at this life stage and is also important in the prevention of osteoporosis later in life. Calcium absorption declines with age, thus increasing the need of this nutrient in the older adult population. Postmenopausal women (51 years and older) tend to experience greater bone loss and decreased absorption of calcium, which increases the need in this population to 1,200 $mg \cdot day^{-1}$. Older men aged 70 years and older also have increased needs at 1,200 $mg \cdot day^{-1}$. Calcium supplements are best absorbed when doses are 500 mg or less.

In older adults, vitamin B_{12} supplementation can be important, as 10% to 30% of older individuals develop atrophic gastritis, a condition that decreases secretion of hydrochloric acid in the stomach, which in turn decreases the absorption of naturally occurring vitamin B_{12} (38). Thus, it is recommended that adults 50 years and older either take a vitamin B_{12} supplement or consume sufficient amounts of fortified foods such as breakfast cereals.

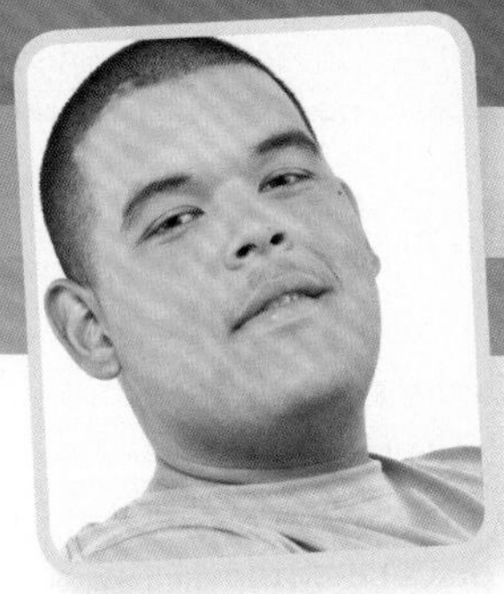

The Case of Ryan

Submitted by **Linda Vaughn, MS, MBA, ACSM-HFS, YMCA of Metropolitan Atlanta, Atlanta, GA**

Ryan, a 22-year-old, 425-lb man, presented at his local YMCA to seek help in losing weight, specifically stating, "I'm 22 years old and weigh less than the rest of my family. I've never had a date and I don't want any more male 'boobies'."

Narrative

The HFS coach informed Ryan that his goals would require at least a 2-year commitment to healthy eating and regular exercise, to which Ryan agreed. Ryan stated that he had recently lost 50 lb. He said that he lived with his grandmother while he was in college and that she consistently served southern homestyle (fried) meals, and it was hard to say "no" to her cooking; he was afraid of offending her. His affect was somewhat flat at presentation. The HFS coach used calibrated scales to verify that his body weight was 425 lb. The HFS coach then administered the Resources for Exercise Maintenance Survey (1) to determine what type of support Ryan needed. It was determined that Ryan needed specific support in his inability to tolerate discomfort, his lack of self-management skills, and his lack of social support among family members. On investigating Ryan's preferred activities, the HFS coach advised Ryan to begin walking on a treadmill for at least 20 minutes, three times a week, at an intensity of 64% to 70% of his maximum heart rate; to begin a strength training program (no more than two sets of 8 to 10 repetitions of at least eight different muscle groups); and to begin tracking his food intake. Within 3 weeks, Ryan reported a weight loss of 27 lb to his coach and revealed to his coach that he was "working out" three times a day every day and eating clif bars and salads for his meals (approximately 1,000 calories each day). The coach verified Ryan's workouts via the FitLinxx system to reflect that he was swimming at least 20 to 30 minutes a day, attending group cycling classes, step aerobics classes, Taekwondo classes, or yoga classes daily (55 min), as well as running outdoors (33–40 min). In addition, he reported to his coach that he was weight training everyday with no off-days between workouts; this was reflected in the FitLinxx system as calisthenics at an intensity of level 9 out of 10 for, on average, 45 to 60 minutes, however, not always daily. The coach advised Ryan that he needed to eat more to sustain himself at rest at his present body weight and even more to support 3 hours of workouts a day. After calculating Ryan's caloric needs for REE and his TEE, the HFS coach advised Ryan that he needed to eat more food or exercise less to avoid muscle degradation in his efforts. Ryan was resistant, stating "No one has ever told me I had to eat more, and I feel good!"

The Case of Ryan cont.

Questions

- What is the TEE for Ryan based on his current body weight and his current exercise regimen?
- What modifications should occur in Ryan's self-imposed fitness prescription?
- How can Ryan effectively deal with his grandmother's cooking?
- How can Ryan deal with his lack of familial support in his efforts to be become healthier?

Reference

Annesi JJ. *The Coach Approach: An Exercise Support Process Implementation Handbook.* 3rd ed. Atlanta, GA: YMCA of Metropolitan Atlanta; 2007.

Additional Resources

Donnelly JE, Blair SN, Jakicic JM, Manore MM, Rankin JW, Smith BK. Appropriate physical activity intervention strategies for weight loss and prevention of weight regain for adults. *Med Sci Sports Exerc.* 2009;41:459–71.

Fitness Education Network. *American College of Sports Medicine Certified Personal Trainer Workshop Course Workbook.* Fitness Education Network; 2009. 53 p.

SUMMARY

Obesity has reached epidemic levels in the United States, and determining a person's obesity status is a key part of the HFS job duties. Each HFS should be experienced in a variety of methods to measure obesity status, as different methods may be better for different individuals. While some methods are quite precise (*e.g.*, HW and DEXA), they are not very practical. Therefore, regular practice with BMI, skinfolds, circumferences, and so on is important for the HFS. Once a person's obesity status is determined, realistic weight loss or weight maintenance goals can be created. Through the 2009 ACSM position stand, the HFS has a guideline for developing exercise programs that address weight management with regard to frequency, intensity, time, and type of exercise and goals for caloric intake.

A person's nutritional needs change over time because of medical conditions, aging, pregnancy, and so on. Although working with a Registered Dietitian is ideal, the HFS should be aware of the different nutritional needs for pregnant women, children, and older adults. The 2010 dietary guidelines are a good resource for the HFS when discussing client nutritional needs. The information highlighted in this chapter will enable the HFS to fully support a client with weight management by appropriately incorporating nutrition, physical activity, and behavior modification in individual client goal setting.

STUDY QUESTIONS

1. Discuss the pros and cons of percentage body fat measurement methods in individuals with a BMI >35 kg·m^{-2}.
2. Compare and contrast the difference between the Food Guide Pyramid and the MyPlate campaign.
3. Robert walked on a treadmill at a speed 2.5 mph and a grade of 10% for 40 minutes. How many kilocalories did he expend?

REFERENCES

1. American College of Sports Medicine. *ACSM's Guidelines for Exercise Testing and Prescription*. 9th ed. Baltimore (MD): Lippincott Williams & Wilkins; 2010.
2. American College of Sports Medicine. *ACSM's Guidelines for Exercise Testing and Prescription*. 8th ed. Baltimore (MD): Lippincott Williams & Wilkins; 2010.
3. Bray GA. *A Guide to Obesity and the Metabolic Syndrome*. Boca Raton (FL): CRC Press; 2011.
4. Bray GA, Gray DS. Obesity. Part I — Pathogenesis. *West J Med*. 1988;149:429–41.
5. Brozek J, Grande F, Anderson JT, Keys A. Densitometric analysis of body composition: Revision of some quantitative assumptions. *Ann NY Acad Sci*. 1963;110:113–40.
6. Callaway CW, Chumlea WC, Bouchard C. Circumferences. In: Lohman TG, Roche AF, Martorell R, editors. *Anthropometric Standardization Reference Manual*. Champaign (IL): Human Kinetics; 1988. p. 39–54.
7. Canoy D. Distribution of body fat and risk of coronary heart disease in men and women. *Curr Opin Cardiol*. 2008;23(6):591–8.
8. http://www.fda.gov/. Accessed October 12, 2012.
9. http://www.cdc.gov/healthyweight/assessing/bmi/childrens_bmi/about_childrens_bmi.html. Accessed July 20, 2011.
10. http://www.choosemyplate.gov/. Accessed July 20, 2011.
11. Donnelly JE, Blair SN, Jakicic JM, Manore MM, Rankin JW, Smith BK. Appropriate physical activity intervention strategies for weight loss and prevention of weight regain for adults. *Med Sci Sports Exerc*. 2009;41:459–71.
12. Duren DL, RJ Sherwood, SA Czerwinski, et al. Body composition methods: Comparisons and interpretation. *J Diabetes Sci Technol*. 2008;2(6):1139–46.
13. Flegal KM, Carroll MD, Odgen CL, Curtin LR. Prevalence and trends in obesity among US adults. *JAMA*. 2010;303(3):235–41.
14. http://www.fitwoman.com/expert-advice/fitbriefings/medications-and-weight-gain. Accessed July 5, 2011.
15. Frankenfield D, Roth-Yousey L, Compher C. Comparison of predictive equations for resting metabolic rate in healthy non-obese and obese adults: A systematic review. *J Am Diet Assoc*. 2005;105(5):775–89.
16. Graves JE, Kanaley JA, Garzareooa L, Pollock ML. Anthropometry and body composition assessment. In: Maud PJ, Foster C, editors. *Physiological Assessment of Human Fitness*. 2nd ed. Champaign (IL): Human Kinetics; 2006. p. 185–225.
17. Gerrior S, WenYen J, Basiotis P. An easy approach to calculating estimated energy requirements. *Prev Chronic Dis*. 2006;3(4):A129.
18. http://www.health.gov/dietaryguidelines/dga2010/dietaryguidelines2010.pdf. Chapter 2 and Table A2-Appendix 2. Accessed July 20, 2011
19. http://www.health.gov/dietaryguidelines/dga2010/dietaryguidelines2010.pdf. Chapter 3. Accessed July 20, 2011.
20. Heyward VH. *Advanced Fitness Assessment and Exercise Prescription*. Champaign (IL): Human Kinetics; 2010.
21. Heyward VH, DR Wagner. *Applied Body Composition Assessment*. 2nd ed. Champaign (IL): Human Kinetics; 2004.
22. http://www.iom.edu/Activities/Nutrition/SummaryDRIs/~/media/Files/Activity%20Files/Nutrition/DRIs/New%20Material/5DRI%20Values%20SummaryTables%2014.pdf Accessed July 10, 20 2011.
23. Jackson AS, ML Pollock. Practical assessment of body composition. *Physician Sports Med*. 1985;13(5):76, 80, 82–90.
24. Jakicic JM, Winters C, Lang W, Wing RR. Effect of intermittent exercise and use of home exercise equipment on adherence, weight loss, and fitness in overweight women. *JAMA*. 1999;282(16):1554–60.
25. Jakicic JM, Marcus BH, Gallagher KL, Napolitano M, Lang W. Effect of exercise duration and intensity on weight loss in overweight, sedentary women: A randomized trial. *JAMA*. 2003;290:1323–30.
26. Jeffery RW, Wing RR, Sherwood NE, Tate DF. Physical activity and weight loss: Does prescribing higher physical activity goals improve outcome? *Am J Clin Nutr*. 2003;78:684–9.
27. http://www.johnshopkinshealthalerts.com/alerts/prescription_drugs/JohnsHopkinsPrescriptionsDrugsHealthAlert_656-1.html. Accessed July 5, 2011.
28. Klem ML, Wing RR, McGuire MT, Seagle HM, Hill JO. A descriptive study of individuals successful at long-term maintenance of substantial weight loss. *Am J Clin Nutr*. 1997;66:239–46.
29. Levi J, Vinter S, St. Larent R, Segal LM. *F as in Fat: How Obesity Threatens American's Future*. Washington (DC): Trust for American's Health and Robert Wood Johnson Foundation; 2010. p. 1–124. Retrieved from www.healthyamericans.org.
30. Lohman TG. Body composition methodology in sports medicine. *Physician Sports Med*. 1982;10(12):46–7.
31. Lohman TG. *Advances in Body Composition Assessment*. Champaign (IL): Human Kinetics; 1992.
32. http://www.mayoclinic.com/health/weight-loss/HQ01160. Accessed July 21, 2011.
33. http://www.mayoclinic.com/health/caffeine/HQ00369. Accessed July 5, 2011.
34. http://www.medicinenet.com/script/main/art.asp?articlekey=56339&page=1. Accessed July 5, 2011.
35. http://www.medicinenet.com/script/main/art.asp?articlekey=56339&page=2. Accessed July 5, 2011.
36. National Cholesterol Education Program (U.S.). *Third Report of the National Cholesterol Education Program (NCEP) Expert Panel on Detection, Evaluation, and Treatment of High Blood Cholesterol in Adults (Adult Treatment Panel III): Final Report*. Washington (DC): National Institutes of Health; 2002.
37. http://ods.od.nih.gov. Accessed July 21, 2011.
38. http://ods.od.nih.gov/factsheets/vitaminb12/. Accessed July 21, 2011.
39. http://ods.od.nih.gov/factsheets/vitamind/. Accessed July 21, 2011.
40. Ogden CL, Carroll MD, McDowell MA, Flegal KM. Obesity among adults in the United States — No statistically significant change since 2003–2004. *NCHS Data Brief*. 2007;(1):1–8.
41. Ogden CL, Carroll MD, Curtin LR, Lamb MM, Flegal KM. Prevalence of high body mass index in US children and adolescents, 2007–2008. *JAMA*. 2010;303(3):242–49.
42. Perri MG, Anton SD, During PE, et al. Adherence to exercise prescriptions: Effect of prescribing moderate versus high levels of intensity and frequency. *Health Psychol*. 2002;21(5):452–8.
43. Pi-Sunyer FX. The epidemiology of central fat distribution in relation to disease. *Nutr Rev*. 2004;62(7 Pt 2):S120–6.
44. Pollack ML, DH Schmidt, AS Jackson. Measurement of cardiorespiratory fitness and body composition in the clinical setting. *Compr Ther*. 1980;6(9):12–27.
45. Porcari JP, McLean KP, Foster C, Kernozek T, Crenshaw B, Swensen C. Effects of electrical muscle stimulation on

body composition, muscle strength, and physical appearance. *J Strength Cond Res*. 2002;16(2):165–72.
46. Schauer PR, Burgera B, Ikramuddin S, et al. Effect of laparoscropic Roux-en Y gastric bypass on type 2 diabetes mellitus. *Ann Surg*. 2003;238(4):467–84.
47. Siri WE. Body composition from fluid spaces and density: Analysis of methods. 1961. *Nutrition*. 1993;9(5):480–91; discussion 480, 492.
48. https://sites.google.com/site/compendiumofphysicalactivities/. Accessed November 11, 2011.
49. Smoot TM, Xu P, Hilsenrath P, Kuppersmith NC, Singh KP. Gastric bypass surgery in the United States, 1998–2002. *Am J Public Health*. 2006;96(7):1187–9.
50. U.S. Department of Health and Human Services. Public Health Service, National Institutes of Health. National Heart, Lung, and Blood Institute. Clinical Guidelines on the Identification, Evaluation, and Treatment of Overweight and Obesity in Adults. NIH publication No 98-4083. September 1998.
51. U.S. Department of Health and Human Services. Public Health Service, National Institutes of Health. National Heart, Lung, and Blood Institute. The Practical Guide: Identification, Evaluation, and Treatment of Overweight and Obesity in Adults. NIH publication No. 00-4084. October 2000.
52. http://www.webmd.com/healthy-beauty/features/body-wraps-what-to-expect. Accessed August 2, 2011.
53. http://www.weighttraining.com/faq/do-vibration-exercise-machines-work. Accessed August 2, 2011.
54. http://en.wikipedia.org/wiki/Nicotine. Accessed July 5, 2011.
55. http://www.wisegeek.com/will-a-sauna-help-me-lose-weight.htm. Accessed August 2, 2011.
56. http://online.wsj.com/article/SB10001424052748704779704574553790579199098.html. Accessed August 2, 2011.

Additional Resources for Information About Supplements and Herbal Products

http://www.consumerlab.com — This site reports results of an independent testing lab to measure active ingredients in popular supplements. Products must have within 20% of what is on the label. Some information is free. Detailed lists of products require payment.

http://www.iherb.com — The Natural Pharmacist is a trusted reference for 500 dietary supplements.

http://www.herbmed.org HerbMd information on herbals w/ evidence and warnings — Short research summaries. Promotes alternative medical treatments, but does not support outlandish claims.

http://www.uspverified.org — Has information about products that have passed the USP test. Brochures to use for a class or health fair may be available.

http://www.herbalgram.org — This site is maintained by the American Botanical Council.

Am Assoc. Clinical Endocrinologists medical guidelines for the clinical use of dietary supplements and nutraceuticals. 2003. http://guidelines.gov

http://dietary-supplements.info.nih.gov/databases/ibids.html.

The National Center for Complementary and Alternative Medicine. http://nccam.nih.gov

Fact sheets at http://ods.od.nih.gov

Center for Food Safety and Applied Nutrition, Food and Drug Administration. Dietary Supplements. http://www.cfsan.fda.gov/~dms/ds-prod.html

Food and Nutrition Information Center. National Agricultural Library/USDA, 10301 Baltimore Ave, Room 105, Beltsville MD 2005-2351. Dietary Supplements Resource List. See http://www.nal.usda.gov/fnic/etext/000015.html

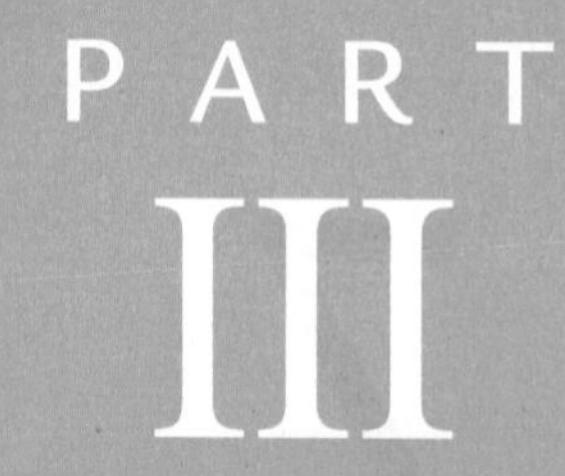

PART III

Exercise Programming for Special Populations

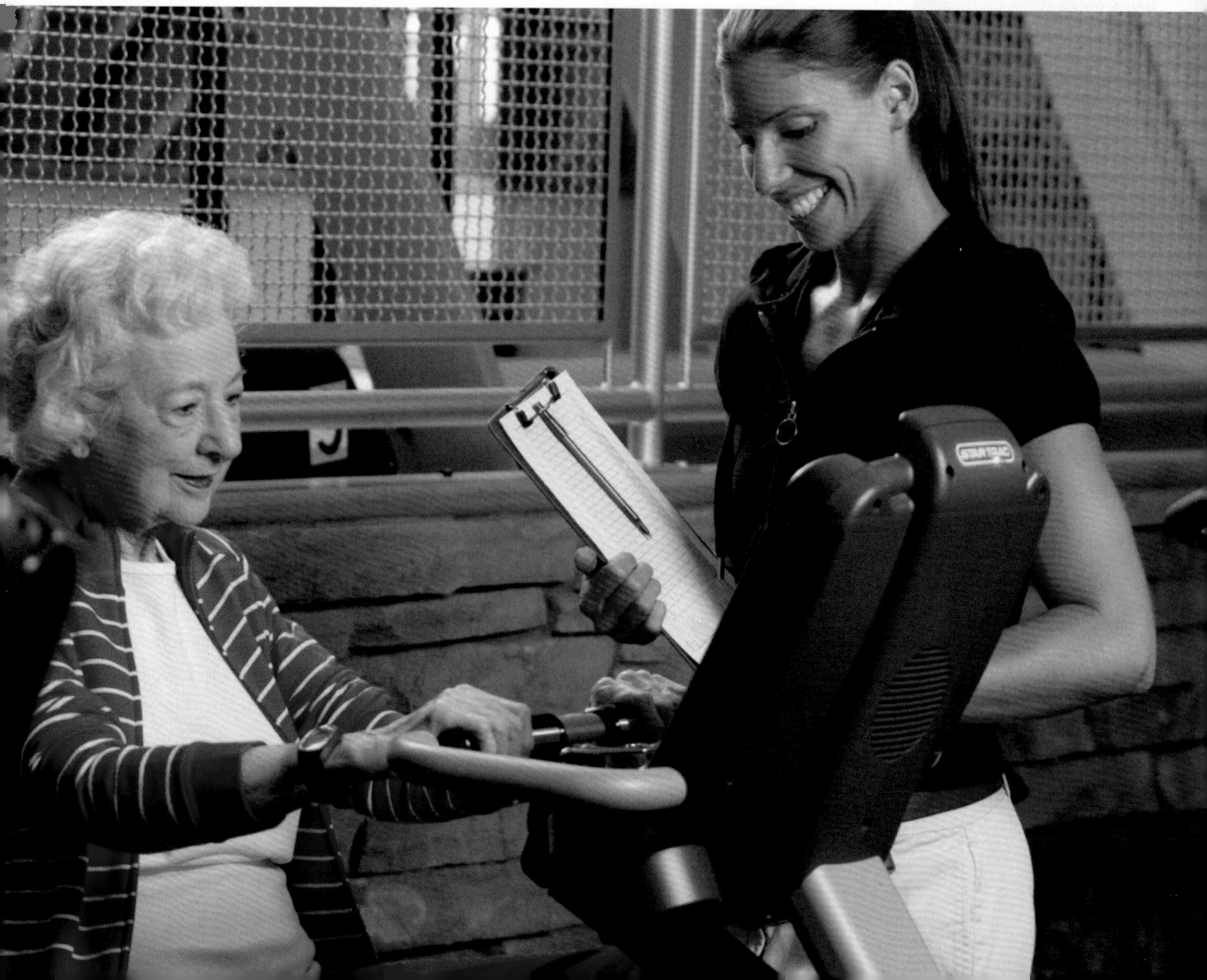

CHAPTER

7 Exercise for Individuals with Controlled Cardiovascular, Pulmonary, and Metabolic Diseases

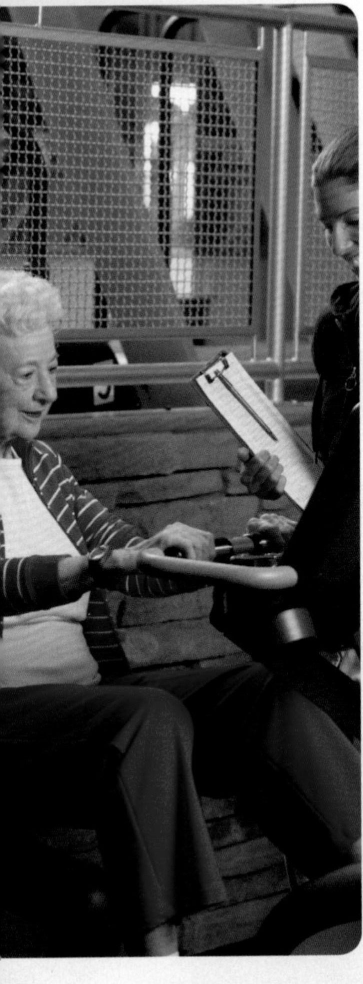

J. Larry Durstine • Keith Burns
Benjamin Gordon • Gary Liguori

CHAPTER OBJECTIVES

- To describe the pathophysiology of common cardiovascular, metabolic, and pulmonary conditions.
- To describe the role medications play in altering the exercise response in various chronic diseases.
- To explain the nuances of exercise prescription in various chronic diseases compared with apparently healthy individuals.

The Health Fitness Specialist (HFS) is responsible for developing exercise prescriptions for healthy clients and those with medically controlled diseases who are cleared by their physician for independent exercise. The role of physical activity and exercise training in primary and secondary disease prevention is well established (2, 5, 49). Developed guidelines provide recommendations regarding the amount of physical activity and exercise that offers significant health-fitness benefits. Individuals with chronic diseases often present unique and challenging exercise limitations, but physical activity and exercise should not be avoided and instead should become part of their medical management plan. Individuals with a chronic condition can experience health-fitness benefits such as reduced disease symptoms, reduced medication reliance, and aid in the restoration of mental well-being (49). Because diseases usually impose exercise limitations and restrictions, the HFS must know these limitations to ensure a safe and effective exercise prescription and just as importantly, when to refer someone back to his or her physician or to more specialized exercise training with a Clinical Exercise Specialist or Registered Clinical Exercise Physiologist. This chapter reviews disease pathology, exercise considerations and contraindications, and the process for developing a proper FITT (frequency, intensity, time, and type) plan to allow optimal physical activity and exercise programming for the client with a cardiovascular, metabolic, and pulmonary disease who has been cleared by his or her physician for independent exercise training.

PATHOPHYSIOLOGY OF COMMON CARDIOVASCULAR, METABOLIC, AND PULMONARY DISEASES

Cardiovascular Disease

Cardiovascular diseases (CVDs) account for more Americans deaths than any other disease, with nearly 650,000 total deaths annually (22). The most recent figures show the total health care cost for CVD was estimated at $316 billion dollars (22). The financial cost and prevalence, along with the associated morbidity and mortality, make it important for the HFS to understand the cardiovascular pathology and exercise measures for working with this population. A strong understanding of the disease pathology and specific exercise nuances will allow the HFS to effectively design an exercise prescription to lessen the effects of CVD and improve the client's health-fitness status and quality of life.

Coronary Heart Disease

Coronary artery disease (CAD) is one of the most prevalent types of CVD and also accounts for the most cardiovascular deaths (22). CAD is characterized by any one of several factors, including a buildup of atherosclerotic plaques, vascular remodeling, luminal stenosis, and inflammation, brought on by numerous factors, including dyslipidemia and hypertension (HTN). Central to CAD is the formation of atherosclerotic plaque in the elastic and smooth lining inside of arteries (Fig. 7.1). Plaque formations in the coronary arteries can cause an obstruction of blood flow to cardiac muscle tissue downstream of the obstruction resulting in reduced cardiac function and/or tissue death (necrosis) (45, 70). Atherosclerosis is a process where fatty streaks develop causing the artery wall to thicken while reducing luminal diameter. This is a progressive and dangerous arterial buildup of fat and fibrous plaques. The atherosclerotic process begins with a focal injury to the lining of the artery and eventually causes damage to the endothelium. The endothelium then becomes more permeable to lipids, allowing low density lipoprotein cholesterol (LDL-C) to easily move through the damaged endothelium and into the arterial intima layer. Once inside the intima, macrophages oxidize LDL-C and begin the formation of arterial foam cells. As these foam cells evolve and begin to release cholesterol into the surrounding areas of the cell, fatty streaks start to form around the initial injury site and the plaque formation process begins (72). Fatty streak formation starts a repeating cycle of repair and remodeling in the artery, during which the luminal diameter is progressively reduced until either a partial or complete impairment of blood flow occurs (53). A partial impairment of coronary artery blood flow and thus oxygen to the cardiac tissue is referred to as myocardial ischemia, whereas the complete obstruction of blood flow to the cardiac myocardial tissue is referred to as a myocardial infarction (MI) or a heart attack and results in tissue death or narcosis (45).

Myocardial ischemia is an imbalance between myocardial oxygen demand and supply. Two common types of myocardial ischemia are stable and unstable ischemia. Stable ischemia is often a result of increased oxygen demand of the heart, as seen with exercise. The impaired ability to deliver blood to the cardiac tissue during exercise starves the tissue from needed oxygen and results in chest pain known as angina and decreased exercise capacity (99). The symptoms of stable ischemia lessen as the oxygen demands of the heart decrease, or when exercise eases or ceases, allowing the coronary arteries to effectively supply the cardiac tissue with an adequate supply of blood flow and oxygen. Unstable ischemia is a more severe condition often seen with symptoms at rest during a time of little exertional stress and therefore lower oxygen demand. Individuals with unstable ischemia need to

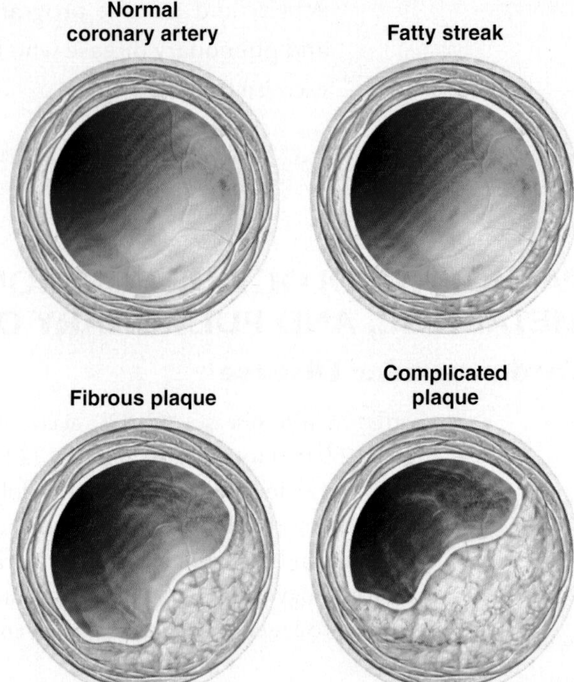

FIGURE 7.1. Depiction of the typical progression for plaque buildup in a coronary artery. The disease process begins with a normal coronary artery and the progression to fatty streak to an artery with complicated plaque. (Asset provided by Anatomical Chart Co.)

seek medical treatment immediately, as unstable ischemia may be a warning sign that a heart attack is imminent (99). In no case should this person be performing exercise or an exercise test.

Hypertension

Hypertension (HTN) is common among patients with CAD. HTN is considered the "silent killer" because its signs and symptoms often go unnoticed. The severity of HTN, however, cannot be overlooked and, if left untreated, is a major risk factor for developing multiple complications such as atherosclerosis, stroke, heart attack, chronic heart failure, kidney failure, and damage to the eyes (15).

HTN is characterized as a persistent elevation in either systolic blood pressure (SBP) (>140 mm Hg) or diastolic blood pressure (DBP) (>90 mm Hg) (90) and is separated into either primary or secondary categories. Primary HTN accounts for 90% to 95% of all cases, has no established pathology, and is thus considered idiopathic (arising spontaneously or from an obscure or unknown cause) (53, 98). Secondary HTN, which accounts for very few cases, is associated with identifiable causes such as renal disease, stress, drug-induced side effects, sleep apnea, neurologic disorders, and many others (53).

Blood pressure is regulated by two factors: cardiac output and total peripheral vascular resistance. Cardiac output (Q) is a function of heart rate (HR) and stroke volume (SV) minus the amount of blood pumped with each heart contraction ($Q = HR \times SV$). Increased peripheral resistance is the most common characteristic of primary and secondary HTN and is caused either by chronic vasoconstriction, or narrowing of the peripheral arterioles, or by vascular plaque buildup. When HTN is present, arterioles lose elasticity because of the increased presence of fibrous collagen tissue. Collagen decreases proper arteriole constriction and relaxation, which is important in normal blood flow regulation. In time, this leads to increased vascular resistance, increased blood pressure, and eventually increased atherosclerosis development (53).

Metabolic Diseases/Disorders

Metabolic diseases/disorders have varying genetic or environmental causes that alter metabolic processes. The most common of these are diabetes, hyperlipidemia, and obesity, each of which responds well to exercise therapy. If not treated properly, each can lead to various metabolic problems, including CAD.

Diabetes

Type 1 and Type 2 diabetes mellitus are defined by a decrease in the production, release and/or effectiveness, and action of insulin. Either form of diabetes results in increased blood glucose levels, a condition referred to as hyperglycemia (39). In addition, diabetes can cause vasculature damage and starves cells of needed glucose.

Type 1 diabetes is quite uncommon, found in only 5% to 10% of all patients with diabetes. It is characterized by an absolute deficiency in blood insulin release because of the destruction of pancreatic insulin secreting beta cells (33). Type 1 diabetic patients should be referred to exercise professionals with more specialized training to prescribe and monitor exercise.

The Type 2 diabetic patient has elevated glucose levels typically as a result of increasing insulin resistance. Excessive abdominal fat is a leading cause of Type 2 diabetes. The disease responds well to exercise therapy and drugs that either increase insulin sensitivity or decrease blood glucose levels.

Hyperlipidemia

Hyperlipidemia, defined as elevated blood cholesterol and triglyceride levels, is caused by a combination of genetic and/or environmental factors (37). Lipids are packaged with protein and travel through the blood as lipoproteins. Lipoproteins are classified by their density: chylomicrons, very-low density lipoproteins (VLDLs), low density lipoproteins (LDLs), and high density lipoproteins (HDLs) (79). HDL is responsible for aiding in the removal of lipids from the circulation, through reverse cholesterol transport. Hence, HDL cholesterol (HDL-C) is referred to as the "good" cholesterol. Also, if HDL-C levels are less than 40 $mg \cdot dL^{-1}$, very little reverse cholesterol transport occurs, leading to further vascular lipid accumulation and accelerated atherosclerosis rates. Excessive amounts of total blood cholesterol ($<$200 $mg \cdot dL^{-1}$) and LDL-C, or "bad" cholesterol ($<$130 $mg \cdot dL^{-1}$), are associated with increased risk of atherosclerosis and CAD.

Obesity

Obesity is defined as an excessive accumulation of body fat and is associated with a body mass index (BMI) $\geq$30 $kg \cdot m^{-2}$ (91). Although the causes of obesity are complex and multifaceted, the combination of increased caloric consumption and decreased daily physical activity are the primary contributors (32). Regardless of its genesis, obesity is associated with a multitude of comorbidities, including insulin resistance, decreased growth hormone, increased cholesterol synthesis and excretion (19), and an increased incidence of all-cause mortality (17).

Pulmonary Diseases

Most pulmonary diseases are grouped into two categories: chronic obstructive pulmonary diseases (COPDs) and chronic restrictive pulmonary diseases (CRPDs). However, patients with pulmonary disease can present a multitude of unique challenges for exercise therapy and therefore should typically be referred for more specialized care.

Chronic Obstructive Pulmonary Disease

Chronic obstructive pulmonary disease (COPD) is an umbrella term for a collection of pulmonary diseases, including chronic bronchitis, emphysema, and asthma (Fig. 7.2) (85). COPD is characterized by progressive airflow limitation associated with an abnormal inflammatory lung response that limits the lung's ability to move air during inhalation and exhalation (85). Chronic bronchitis is characterized by a cough lasting for at least 3 months (59), resulting in chronic pulmonary inflammation, which leads to damage of the bronchial lining and impeded lung function and air flow obstruction (13). Emphysema is the permanent enlargement of airspaces along with necrosis of alveolar walls (67) causing an accumulation of air in the lung tissue (53).

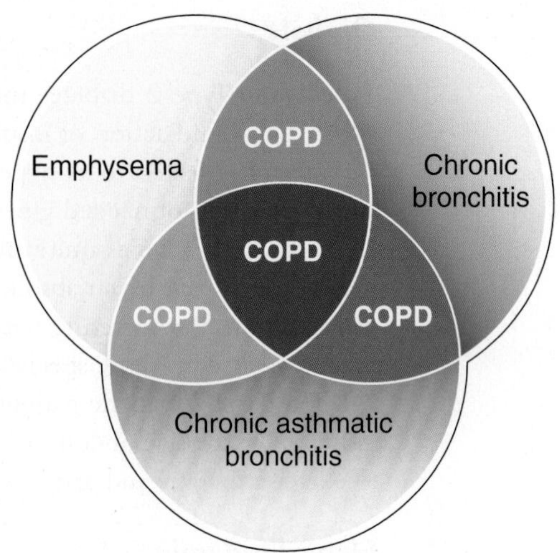

FIGURE 7.2. The relationships among emphysema, chronic bronchitis, chronic asthmatic bronchitis, and COPD. Most clients with COPD have a combination of these diseases. (From McConnell TH. *The Nature of Disease Pathology for the Health Professions*. Philadelphia (PA): Lippincott Williams & Wilkins; 2007.)

Asthma consists of both inflammation and increased smooth muscle constriction in the lungs in response to various stimuli (67). Triggers for asthma include environmental, biochemical, autonomic, immunologic, infectious, endocrine, and psychological factors (53). During an asthmatic episode, inflammatory mediators are released, causing bronchial smooth muscle spasm, edema formation, and the production of mucous resulting in vascular congestion.

Chronic Restrictive Pulmonary Disease

Chronic restrictive pulmonary disease (CRPD), also known as interstitial lung disease, is made up of a small group of diseases that cause inflammation resulting in lung tissue necrosis and decreased lung volume (67). Both COPD and CRPD clients have limited gas exchange within the lungs, frequent shortness of breath, and difficulty breathing. The HFS scope of practice does not include most aspects of pulmonary disease, given its unique physiological challenges. Therefore, other than exercise-induced asthma, and particularly in emphysema and CRPD, individuals suffering from pulmonary disease should be referred to more specialized care.

ROLE OF EXERCISE TRAINING IN MEDIATING COMMON CARDIOVASCULAR, METABOLIC, AND PULMONARY DISEASES

Exercise has been shown to have positive effects on both primary and secondary disease prevention (56). An estimated 90 million Americans are currently living with a chronic health condition, and this number is expected to rise with a rapid expansion of the older population. Even in light of the increased prevalence of disease, many people are unaware of the potential disease altering benefits that exercise can provide (55). Therefore, the HFS is in a unique position to use this knowledge for the individual and collective improvement of health through appropriately applied exercise prescriptions.

Cardiovascular

Exercise training is beneficial for individuals with a history of or at high risk for an MI (49). Exercise has been shown to decrease coronary inflammatory markers (*e.g.*, C-reactive protein and PLAC) (64), decrease stress and damage on the coronary arteries, increase new blood vessel growth (angiogenesis) and vascular regeneration, which are all likely to promote faster recovery from an MI (87). Regular exercise can also decrease blood platelet adhesiveness, fibrinogen levels, and blood viscosity, all reducing the risk of clotting and a second MI (104). In addition, regular exercise can improve self-efficacy and psychosocial well-being (49). Patients who engage in exercise after MI can restore their health to near or above pre-MI fitness status and are able to return their lives to a

EXERCISE IS MEDICINE CONNECTION

Your Prescription for Health
ExeRxcise is Medicine®
www.ExerciseisMedicine.org

Milani RV, Lavie CJ, Mehra MR. Reduction in C-reactive protein through cardiac rehabilitation and exercise training. *J Am Coll Cardiol.* 2004;6:1056–61.

Milani and colleagues (2004) conducted a study in which the effects of a 3-month formal phase II cardiac rehabilitation and exercise training program had on C-reactive protein (CRP) levels. The study consisted of two groups with the populations of both groups having diagnosed CAD. The exercise group underwent a 3-month phase II cardiac rehabilitation program and the control group did not. Patients in the exercise group received formalized exercise instruction, meeting three times a week for a duration of an hour, and were encouraged to exercise on their own (1–3 times a week) in between sessions. Patients also received individual and group counseling from a registered dietitian who stressed dietary management as recommended by the Adult Treatment Panel III guidelines and also placed special emphasis on the Mediterranean diet. Results showed people who engaged in the cardiac rehabilitation program had significant decreases in the levels of CRP and blood triglycerides and a significant increase in HDL-C. Since many of the patients in the exercise group were also taking medications, the data were analyzed to determine whether it was the medications or the exercise (or a combination) causing the reduction in CRP levels. It was found that patients taking a statin medication had significant decrease in CRP levels over the course of the rehabilitation program. Also, patients who were not taking a statin medication showed the same decreases in CRP levels as the statin users. The authors of this study reported the favorable effects of exercise training on CRP levels independent of statin therapy. This study demonstrates that therapeutic lifestyle modifications, promoted by a 3-month cardiac rehabilitation and dietary management, can produce significant improvements in CRP levels and other cardiac risk factors, such as blood lipids, and in exercise capacity which in turn can promote health and overall well-being.

Adapted from Pescatello L. *ACSM's Guidelines for Exercise Testing and Prescription*. 9th ed. Baltimore (MD): Lippincott Williams & Wilkins; 2014.

pre-MI state (50). For clients suffering from ischemia and thus at high risk, the effect of exercise can help reduce the risk of an initial MI while also raising the overall quality of life (47). Exercise has also been shown to prevent, slow, and even reverse vasculature atherosclerotic plaque development, allowing for an increase in the ischemic threshold during daily activities or exercise (16).

Endurance exercise does lower resting SBP and DBP values by 5 to 7 mm Hg (54), and for individuals at risk for developing HTN, endurance exercise is thought to slow blood pressure rise and delay HTN development (90). Although not fully understood, possible mechanisms for exercise-induced reductions in blood pressure include an alteration in renal functioning, a decrease in plasma norepinephrine levels, and an increase in circulating vasodilator substances (105).

Metabolic

Type 2 diabetic patients gain health-fitness benefits rather quickly once an exercise program is initiated. Perhaps the most beneficial aspect is the improved insulin sensitivity that is reported with exercise training (39, 96), which can result in a lower medication requirement and greater control of blood glucose levels (96). In addition, if body fat is reduced, as may occur from the indirect effect of exercise, further increases in insulin sensitivity are found (39, 96).

Dyslipidemic clients engaging in physical activity and exercise reduce postprandial lipidemia or the amount of cholesterol in their blood after a meal (46). Exercise also provides a positive benefit on other blood lipid values by lowering blood concentrations of LDL-C and increasing concentrations of HDL-C (39, 43, 100).

The role of exercise in treating obesity is most effective when used in combination with caloric restriction (48, 102). To be expected, increased exercise in an obese client promotes the loss of regional fat, especially abdominal fat deposits (19, 103), which can also result in improved psychological well-being (19). With noticeable reductions in body weight and fat, clients have a tangible result that can increase self-image and self-esteem. However, even when tangible reductions in body fat or weight do not occur, exercise participation may still produce other positive health-fitness benefits (40).

Ultimately, regular exercise yields improvement in many obesity comorbidities, including decreased fasting blood glucose levels, increased insulin sensitivity, decreased triglyceride levels, and decreased CAD risk factors (37). The HFS is expected to have an understanding of the basic mechanisms involved in these positive changes to better prescribe exercise that is meaningful to each individual client.

Pulmonary

The scientific literature is mixed as to the extent that exercise plays a role in reducing the pathologies of pulmonary diseases (88). Although exercise may not cure pulmonary diseases, it does bring a noticeable increase in quality of life (35). In fact, the overall benefit of exercise allows the pulmonary client to exercise longer at higher intensities (59).

METABOLIC CALCULATIONS AS THEY RELATE TO EXERCISE PROGRAMMING IN CONTROLLED DISEASE POPULATIONS

A "one size fits all" approach is not effective to individualized exercise prescription or programming. Rather, the successful HFS should create specific and individualized programs to meet the client's needs and health goals. The American College of Sports Medicine® (ACSM) metabolic equations are useful mathematical tools, as they help tailor caloric expenditure and exercise intensity to meet the needs of each client (3). A more in-depth look at exercise prescription can be found in Chapters 3 and 6; however, these calculations are specific to apparently healthy individuals and may not be as reliable when used expenditure in individuals with certain chronic conditions. The HFS should be able to determine "kcal" expenditure both during rest and any activity (3).

The Art and Science of Exercise Prescription

The guidelines for exercise prescription presented in this book are based on a strong foundation of scientific information. In the past 20 years, the body of scientific information regarding exercise prescription for individuals with chronic disease has increased significantly (39). Nonetheless, the application of these principles should not be completed in an exceedingly rigid and precise fashion. Rather, the procedures presented in this chapter are principles and accordingly should be utilized with flexibility and with careful attention to the contraindications, limitations, and goals of the individual. Because the physiological responses vary considerably across individuals as to exercise responses and adaptations, the HFS must be prepared to modify exercise prescriptions in accordance with these exercise responses observed in individual participants. Consequently, development and implementation of the exercise prescription in a rigid, mathematical fashion is inappropriate. One overriding objective of the exercise prescription is to promote a physically active lifestyle. Thus, the most fitting exercise prescription is the one that is successful in attaining this behavioral change. The HFS uses the basic scientific process, knows the individual client's needs, and develops and implements an appropriate exercise prescription. Chronic diseases present unique and challenging limitations for the HFS in developing an exercise program. The role of the HFS is to be aware of such limitations and use scientifically developed principles in conjunction with his or her own experiences to adapt and implement a properly designed exercise prescription that is effective in optimizing health-fitness benefits and ensures safety. Thus, the HFS must recognize that the process of making an exercise prescription is an art as well as a science.

Cardiovascular

Physical activity and exercise are advised for individuals diagnosed with CVD or having experienced some type of cardiovascular event (10). The many benefits of cardiovascular rehabilitation programming have been previously defined and include reduced disease symptoms and a reduced chance of experiencing a second cardiovascular event (10). After the completion of a cardiac rehabilitation program, the HFS can provide a setting for CVD clients to continue safe exercise with proper supervision.

Special FITT Considerations for Persons with Chronic Diseases

Clients with cardiovascular, metabolic, or pulmonary systems need to include physically activity and exercise as part of lifestyle change. The HFS needs to be diligent in using the FITT principle carefully to develop an individualized exercise program that ensures patient safety while maximizing functional capacity and developing optimal health-fitness benefits. Each component of the FITT principle is discussed below for each disease. Tables 7.1 and 7.2 present general aerobic and resistance exercise guidelines for patients diagnosed with chronic diseases, respectively.

Cardiovascular Disease

Cardiovascular disease (CVD) pathology is associated with reduced functional capacity and exercise tolerance, and in general, CVD patients have higher sedentary rates than most other individuals (56). In addition, other factors such as medications (*e.g.*, β-blockers, β-adrenergic blocking agents, central

TABLE 7.1 GENERAL AEROBIC TRAINING GUIDELINES TO BE APPLIED TO IN THE EFFECTIVE DEVELOPMENT OF EXERCISE PRESCRIPTIONS FOR THE TREATMENT OF A CHRONIC DISEASED POPULATION

Frequency ($d \cdot wk^{-1}$)	CVD: 4–7 TD1M: 3–7 TD2M: 3–7 Pulmonary: 3–5
Intensity	CVD: 40%/50%–85% HRR or RPE ~11–14 (6–20 scale) TD1M: 50%–80% HRR or RPE = 12–16 (6–20 scale) TD2M: 50%–80% HRR or RPE = 12–16 (6–20 scale) Pulmonary: Prescribed on a individual basis, based on Graded Exercise Test (GXT) with scale for dyspnea.
Time	CVD: Achieve 1,500–2,000 kcal of energy each week or 20–60 min a session TD1M: 20–60 min a session moderate Intensity (*e.g.*, 600 METs·min·wk^{-1}) TD2M: 20–60 min a session At least 150 min·wk^{-1} at moderate intensity (*e.g.*, 600 METs·min·wk^{-1}) or 90 min·wk^{-1} at vigorous intensity (*e.g.*, 540 METs·min·wk^{-1}) Pulmonary: 20–60 min a session
Type	CVD: Large dynamic muscle group exercises TD1M: Walk, bicycle, jogging, water aerobic activities TD2M: Walk, bicycle, jogging, water aerobic activities Pulmonary: Walking and cycling are most strongly recommended

TD1M, Type 1 diabetes mellitus; TD2M, Type 2 diabetes mellitus.
Information taken with permission from Cooper CB. Exercise in chronic pulmonary disease: Aerobic exercise prescription. *Med Sci Sports Exerc.* 2001;33:S671–9; Exercise Prescription for Patients with Cardiac Disease. In: Gordon NF, Thompson WR, Pescatello LS, editors. *ACSM's Guidelines for Exercise Testing and Prescription*. Philadelphia (PA): Lippincott Williams & Wilkins; 2008. p. 207–10; Exercise Prescription for Other Clinical Populations. In: Gordon NF, Thompson WR, Pescatello LS, editors. *ACSM's Guidelines for Exercise Testing and Prescription*. Philadelphia (PA): Lippincott Williams & Wilkins; 2008. p. 232–4; Schairer JR. Exercise prescription in patients with cardiovascular disease. In: Ehrman J, editor. *ACSM's Resource Manual for Guidelines for Exercise Testing and Prescription*. 6th ed. Philadelphia (PA): Lippincott Williams & Wilkins; 2010. p. 559–70; Verity L. Exercise prescription in patients with diabetes. In: Ehrman J, editor. *ACSM's Resource Manual for Guidelines for Exercise Testing and Prescription*. 6th ed. Philadelphia (PA): Lippincott Williams & Wilkins; 2010. p. 600–17.

TABLE 7.2 GENERAL RESISTANCE TRAINING GUIDELINES TO BE APPLIED TO IN THE EFFECTIVE DEVELOPMENT OF EXERCISE PRESCRIPTIONS FOR THE TREATMENT OF A CHRONIC DISEASED POPULATION

Frequency ($d \cdot wk^{-1}$)	CVD: 2–3 T1DM: 2–3 T2DM: 2–3 Pulmonary: 2–3 (4–5 $d \cdot wk^{-1}$ for respiratory muscles)
Intensity	CVD: 60%–80% 1 RM low to moderate RPE ~14–16 (6–20 scale) T1DM: 60%–80% 1 RM low to moderate RPE ~14–16 (6–20 scale) T2DM: 60%–80% 1 RM low to moderate RPE ~14–16 (6–20 scale) Pulmonary: 50%–80% 1 RM low to moderate RPE ~12–15 (6–20 scale) (possibly lower depending on severity of COPD)
Time	CVD: 8–12 exercises 2–3 sets/exercise T1DM: 8–12 exercises 2–3 sets/exercise T2DM: 8–12 exercises 2–3 sets/exercise Pulmonary: 8–12 exercises 2–3 sets/exercise
Type	CVD: elastic bands, light (1–5 lb) hand weights, light free weights with wall pulleys, and machines T1DM: All major muscle groups Upper body: 4–5 exercises Lower body: 4–5 exercises T2DM: All major muscle groups Upper body: 4–5 exercises Lower body: 4–5 exercises Pulmonary: free weights, elastic bands, body weight exercises, and machine exercises

T1DM, Type 1 diabetes mellitus; T2DM, Type 2 diabetes mellitus.
Information taken with permission from: Cooper CB. Exercise in chronic pulmonary disease: Aerobic exercise prescription. *Med Sci Sports Exerc.* 2001;33:S671–9; Exercise Prescription for Patients with Cardiac Disease. In: Gordon NF, Thompson WR, Pescatello LS, editors. *ACSM's Guidelines for Exercise Testing and Prescription*. Philadelphia (PA): Lippincott Williams & Wilkins; 2008. p. 207–10; Exercise Prescription for Other Clinical Populations. In: Gordon NF, Thompson WR, Pescatello LS, editors. *ACSM's Guidelines for Exercise Testing and Prescription*. Philadelphia (PA): Lippincott Williams & Wilkins; 2008. p. 232–4; Schairer JR. Exercise prescription in patients with cardiovascular disease. In: Ehrman J, editor. *ACSM's Resource Manual for Guidelines for Exercise Testing and Prescription*. 6th ed. Philadelphia (PA): Lippincott Williams & Wilkins; 2010. p. 559–70; Verity L. Exercise prescription in patients with diabetes. In: Ehrman J, editor. *ACSM's Resource Manual for Guidelines for Exercise Testing and Prescription*. 6th ed. Philadelphia (PA): Lippincott Williams & Wilkins; 2010. p. 600–17.

α_2 agonists, nitrates, nitroglycerin, calcium channel blockers [CCBs], cardiac glycosides, and ACE inhibitors), myocardial ischemia, intermittent claudication, and angina all impact the application of the FITT principle with CVD clients.

Exercise frequency is usually prescribed as 5 or more days each week (4). In recent years, multiple exercise episodes each day and intermittent work have also been recommended. Multiple daily physical activity or exercise episodes lasting 10 to 15 minutes and totaling 30 minutes or more each day provide numerous health benefits (4). CVD clients usually have limited functional capacities; therefore, shorter exercise episodes of 10 to 15 minutes performed two or three times each day may be useful and often result in exercise being better tolerated. In addition, intermittent work (alternating higher- and lower-intensity exercise) can also be useful (56). CVD clients making these lifestyle modifications that include physical activity and exercise may experience concerns with program adherence and motivation. The HFS has a significant role in helping facilitate the motivation and support the adherence of clients making lifestyle modifications.

Typically, exercise intensity is measured as a percentage of $\dot{V}O_2$ max, $\dot{V}O_2$ reserve, or heart rate reserve (HRR) (5); however, this may be difficult to calculate in many cases of cardiac disease (12). In these cases, rating of perceived exertion (RPE) as an alternative measurement of exercise intensity may be useful (4). Exercise intensity is always prescribed below the myocardial ischemic threshold; however any client experiencing ischemia should be exercising in the presence of someone with more specific training than the HFS.

Exercise time or duration varies with the disease severity. The overall exercise goal for cardiac clients is to progress to 60 minutes of aerobic conditioning a day. However, starting with less time may be appropriate, and increases in duration ranging from 1 to 5 minutes per session depending on exercise tolerance have been suggested (5, 56).

Resistance training also offers health-fitness benefits beyond that of aerobic conditioning alone. The FITT for resistance training is no different than in the general population; however, most cardiac patients will likely start at a low level. Therefore, potential exercise equipment for completing these exercises includes elastic bands, light (1–5 lb) hand weights, light free weights with wall pulleys, and machines.

Metabolic Disease

Type 2 diabetes should incorporate physical activity and exercise as part of its management plan (6, 7). The HFS can safely work with well-controlled Type 2 diabetic patients. If the Type 2 diabetic patient is experiencing frequent swings in the blood glucose level, they should be referred to a health care professional and encouraged to exercise under the supervision of more skilled personnel. When developing an exercise prescription for the diabetic client, it is important to consider the need to reduce overall body fat, which can be complicated if the client is taking an oral hypoglycemic agent (1, 38). The HFS must balance the appropriate exercise volume to aid in body fat reduction while not adversely effecting blood glucose levels and being aware of diabetes-related complications (101).

Being physically active and exercising 5 to 7 days a week is recommended for the Type 2 diabetic patient (1). Because weight loss is so important, special consideration is given to physical activity and exercise volume and frequency to maximize weight loss (20). Exercise intensity ranges between 50% and 80% HRR and $\dot{V}O_2$ reserve and corresponds to an RPE of 12 to 16 (1). Exercise duration begins with a daily accumulation of 20 minutes and progresses to 60 minutes of daily aerobic conditioning. As with CVD clients, multiple daily physically activity or exercise episodes of 10 minutes or more may be used as well as the use of intermittent work (lower exercise intensity mixed with higher exercise intensity). The overall goal is to obtain the health-fitness benefits associated with 150 minutes of total physical activity and exercise each week. Also additional health-fitness benefits are obtained when a goal of 300 minutes of physical activity and exercise is reached (21). Aerobic exercise that emphasizes large muscle groups using rhythmic motion is recommended, although the type of exercise chosen should reflect the individual's interest and goals.

Resistance training for diabetic clients is recommended as long as there is an absence of contraindications such as retinopathy and recent laser treatment (1). Exercise frequency and intensity recommendations are not different from those used for healthy sedentary individuals. Exercise intensity is set at 60% to 80% of 1 RM with two to three sets of 8 to 12 repetitions. Exercise duration is usually set at 8 to 10 multiple-joint exercises for all major muscle groups and is often performed in one whole body session or split into a multiple sessions (1). Exercise type or mode is based on the presence of exercise limitations and includes free weights, elastic bands, free weight exercises, and any of a variety of machines.

In addition, diabetic clients must always wear medical identification, and because diabetes slows the healing process, maintaining proper foot care to reduce foot sores and blisters is vital. With longer healing times, foot sores and blisters are more likely to become infected and result in more serious complications. Most importantly when exercising, diabetic patients must have an available source of carbohydrates. Exercising with a partner is often recommended for individuals with diabetes. Finally, exercise in the early evening should be completed with caution because exercising at this time could cause hypoglycemic conditions later in the night, possibly during sleep and could cause dire consequences (38).

Pulmonary Disease

Clients with advanced stages of COPD and CRRD are especially unique among the chronic diseases presented in this chapter (80, 84). In most cases, these clients are unlikely to ever fully vanquish their symptoms, and progressively, their functional capacity and exercise tolerance become more restricted (80). The scope of practice for the HFS does not warrant working with this population and instead encourages referral to the appropriate health care personnel.

The HFS is prepared to work with a well-controlled asthma client and should encourage him or her to perform aerobic exercise at least 3 to 5 days a week. Unfortunately, there is not a true consensus regarding the optimal intensity for aerobic training in the asthmatic client, and therefore guidelines for older adults are often used (see Chapter 9). Another technique used to guide in developing exercise intensity is the use of the dyspnea scale rating with a value in the range of 3 to 5 on a scale of 0 to 10 (58). Exercise duration recommendations for the pulmonary client are to obtain at least 20 minutes each session and, in the long term, move progressively toward 60 minutes of continuous or intermittent physical activity and aerobic conditioning.

EFFECTS OF MYOCARDIAL ISCHEMIA, MYOCARDIAL INFARCTION, AND HTN ON CARDIORESPIRATORY RESPONSES DURING EXERCISE

CVD continues to be the leading cause of death in the United States for men and women alike (108). The prevalence of CVD continues to rise even as medical technology finds new ways to improve overall survival rates (23–31). An individual who suffers an MI has likely had a significant level of ischemia as one key predisposing factor. As an MI survivor, this individual still has ischemia and limited exercise tolerance and functional capacity.

In addition to CVD, HTN is a common disorder across the US adult population with a prevalence of about one in four adults (54). Although HTN can go undetected for many years, it nonetheless possesses some medical considerations when physical activity and exercise are performed. Therefore, because of the high prevalence of CVD and HTN in the United States, the HFS must be keenly aware of these conditions, their etiology, and their likely impact on an individual's exercise and functional performance.

Myocardial Ischemia

Myocardial ischemia, or simply ischemia, indicates a shortage of oxygenated blood flow to the heart myocardium. The prevalence of ischemia in the United States is approximately 7% while the proportion of individuals suffering ischemia increases with age. Ischemia is an imbalance of oxygen supply and demand. Impaired blood supply is a result of several mechanisms: the most common being atherosclerosis, congestive heart failure (CHF), or both. Oxygen demand is elevated dramatically during physical or emotional exertion. If oxygen supply fails to match an increased demand, even briefly, then ischemia is present. If ischemia is prolonged, then viable myocardium becomes at risk for necrosis and infarction. Oftentimes, ischemia is associated with chest pain, or angina.

In a typical exercise session, myocardial oxygen demand is increased, which is met by an increased frequency and vigor of the heart pumping action. This linear relationship continues until an individual reaches maximum exercise capacity. However, in the ischemic person, maximum exercise capacity is limited by insufficient myocardial oxygen supply. If the heart is deficient such as in the case of CHF or because the arteries are partially blocked as in atherosclerosis, oxygen delivery to target muscle is impaired and exercise capacity is limited. Avoiding this "ischemic threshold" is a critical concern of the HFS in prescribing exercise.

Myocardial Infarction

An MI occurs when there is prolonged ischemia and can result in heart tissue death or necrosis (70). The ischemia duration necessary to produce an infarct varies; therefore, the HFS must design exercise prescriptions that safely avoid the ischemic threshold or the HR at which angina symptoms develop. Also, because of the loss of heart tissue with necrosis, any necrosis will negatively impact the contractile state of the heart as a pump, thus lowering ejection fraction and limiting exercise capacity and tolerance (60).

Initiating exercise in the post-MI patient is approached with caution. Because access to graded exercise test results is less common (45, 93), the "art" of exercise prescription takes on greater importance. Known benefits for clients after an MI include reducing the likelihood for a second infarct, decreasing return to work time, increasing overall functional capacity, and improving self-efficacy (51).

Although post-MI exercise is relatively safe (68), including vigorous exercise (36, 68), the HFS must understand each client's exercise limitations and myocardial oxygen supply. Therefore, only after gaining medical clearance and physician approval for independent exercise is the initiation of exercise programming appropriate. The HFS may likely work with this type of patient after the patient has completed a supervised round of cardiac rehabilitation under the guidance of the medical community.

Hypertension

Daily physical activity and exercise is often used as part of the treatment for HTN, although such programming should be implemented with caution (54, 82). Normally, a single exercise session causes a linear increase in SBP while a steady constant DBP is maintained (62, 75). In the hypertensive person, SBP changes with exercise are often curvilinear and reach excessively high levels (<250 mm Hg). This dramatic increase in arterial pressure puts undue pressure on the arterial intima, increasing the likelihood of dislodging atherosclerotic plaques and/or thrombi precipitating an MI or stroke. In addition, repeated periods of high-intensity exercise could further exacerbate endothelial damage (74, 107).

Given the potential acute and chronic concerns associated with exercise and HTN, the HFS must be aware of and follow guidelines for initiating and terminating exercise in the hypertensive client. By adhering to these standards, the hypertensive person with the guidance from the HFS can safely use regular physical activity and exercise as an important adjunct to any pharmaceutical therapy in managing blood pressure.

EXERCISE CONCERNS, PRECAUTIONS, AND CONTRAINDICATIONS RELATED TO CARDIOVASCULAR, METABOLIC, AND PULMONARY DISEASES

The information found in Table 7.3 presents the clinical indications and contraindications for cardiac rehabilitation patients (inpatient and outpatient). This information and the points summarized below are meant to help the HFS develop and implement a safe exercise prescription as discussed in this chapter.

- As with any chronic disease, the HFS must foster a safe environment that facilitates clients' understanding of their disease and exercise limitations.
- Before starting exercise, clients must have the knowledge to define angina and its treatment, identify CVD symptoms and provoking factors, and understand their exercise tolerance limits (10). By knowing this information, clients can better understand their disease, their exercise limits, and health implications while fostering safe exercise.
- A primary exercise programming goal is for the CVD client to reduce disease risk and increase the ease in completing activities of daily living. Exercise training will increase functional capacity and exercise tolerance and reduce the chance of experiencing another cardiovascular event (10).
- The early stages of the exercise prescription usually begin with the use of lower, more conservative exercise intensities. This initial exercise intensity is often set at 10 to 15 heart beats per

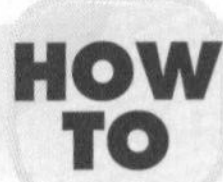

HOW TO Initiate Exercise in a CAD Patient In Lieu of a Graded Exercise Test (GXT)

Equipment Needed

1. Blood pressure monitoring equipment: stethoscope and blood pressure cuff (sphygmomanometer)
2. ECG monitoring unit (3- or 12-lead)
3. RPE chart
4. Exercise equipment (*i.e.*, treadmill, recumbent cycle, elliptical)

Important Information and Tips

1. The results of a GXT can be a valuable tool in the initiation of an exercise prescription (1). However, in certain cases, a GXT test may not have been previously administered. Yet even without the GXT results, a safe and effective exercise prescription can be developed.
2. Reasons for not performing a GXT before starting an exercise prescription include extreme deconditioning, orthopedic limitations, recent successful percutaneous intervention, or uncomplicated or stable myocardial infarction (2).
3. Since the client's response to exercise is not documented, client safety is of utmost concern and the exercise prescription should reflect this. Initiation of exercise at a low intensity, slow exercise intensity progression, and constant monitoring of physiologic symptoms help ensure client safety.

Example of an Exercise Prescription

FITT Framework for a CAD patient without a GXT (2–4).

1. Frequency: Minimum 3 days a week with additional walking on the days off
2. Intensity: 2 to 3 METs
   a) HR: 20 to 30 bpm above resting value
   b) RPE: 11 to 14
3. Time: Begin with 3- to 5-minute intervals. Allow for adequate rest and recovery between intervals. Aim for an overall exercise duration of 30 to 45 minutes.
4. Type: Low-intensity modes of exercise
   a) Treadmill (0% grade, low speed)
   b) Cycle ergometer
   c) Arm ergometer
   d) Elliptical
5. Progression: 5 to 2 METs as tolerated by the client
6. Monitoring: ECG, BP, RPE, and signs or symptoms of ischemia

References

1. Visich PS. The value of graded exercise testing in today's world. *Am J Lifestyle Med*. 2009;10:57–62.
2. McConnell TR. Exercise prescription when the guidelines do not work. *J Cardiopulm Rehabil*. 1996;16:34–7.
3. McConnell TR, Klinger, TA, Gardner JK, Laubach CA, Herman CE, Hauck CA. *J Cardiopulm Rehabil*. 1998;18:458–63.
4. American College of Sports Medicine. *ACSM's Guidelines for Exercise Testing and Prescription*.8th ed. Philadelphia (PA): Lippincott Williams & Wilkins; 2008.

Suggested Readings

ACSM's Exercise Management for Persons with Chronic Diseases and Disabilities —Provides a detailed overview on the approach on the proper development of an exercise prescription for persons in a diseased state.

Pollack's Textbook of Cardiovascular Disease and Rehabilitation — Provides comprehensive and detailed descriptions of the pathologic effects of CAD and effects on the exercise response.

TABLE 7.3 CLINICAL INDICATIONS AND CONTRAINDICATIONS FOR INPATIENT AND OUTPATIENT CARDIAC REHABILITATION

Indications	Contraindications
• Medically stable after MI • Stable angina • Coronary artery bypass graft surgery • Percutaneous transluminal coronary angioplasty or other transcatheter procedure • Compensated CHF • Cardiomyopathy • Heart or other organ transplantation • Other cardiac surgery, including valvular and pacemaker insertion (including implantable cardioverter defibrillator) • Peripheral arterial disease • High-risk CVD ineligible for surgical intervention • Sudden cardiac death syndrome • End-stage renal disease • At risk for CAD with diagnoses of diabetes mellitus, dyslipidemia, HTN, obesity, or other diseases and conditions • Other patients who may benefit from structured exercise and/or patient education based on physician referral and consensus of the rehabilitation team	• Unstable angina • Resting SBP >200 mm Hg or resting DBP >110 mm Hg that should be evaluated on a case-by-case basis • Orthostatic BP drop of >20 mm Hg with symptoms • Critical aortic stenosis (i.e., peak SBP gradient of >50 mm Hg with an aortic valve orifice area of <0.75 cm^2 in an average-size adult) • Acute systemic illness or fever • Uncontrolled atrial or ventricular dysrhythmias • Uncontrolled sinus tachycardia (>120 beats·min^{-1}) • Uncompensated CHF • Third-degree atrioventricular block without pacemaker • Active pericarditis or myocarditis • Recent embolism • Thrombophlebitis • Resting ST-segment depression or elevation (>2 mm) • Uncontrolled diabetes mellitus • Severe orthopedic conditions that would prohibit exercise • Other metabolic conditions, such as acute thyroiditis, hypokalemia, hyperkalemia, or hypovolemia

minute below the ischemic threshold (61). Although this exercise intensity is less than the exercise intensities usually set for maximizing cardiorespiratory fitness improvement and is the recognized intensity necessary for optimizing health-fitness benefits, this lower exercise intensity level will still increase functional capacity and reduce CVD risk (45).

- As fitness levels and exercise tolerance increase, the ischemic threshold is also increased and exercise intensity can be increased as warranted to ensure proper exercise progression while safety is maintained.
- Because HTN is a primary factor for CVD and other diseases, the likelihood for other medical emergencies is increased when blood pressure is elevated, and because a single dynamic exercise period will cause blood pressure to increase, the HFS must understand the hypertensive client's special considerations.
- The hypertensive client can exercise, once HTN is controlled (82). In the presence of severe HTN (>180/110 mm Hg), exercise is only engaged after initiating drug therapy (86). If resting SBP greater than 200 mm Hg or resting DBP greater than 115 mm Hg, even if blood pressure medications are being taken, exercise is contraindicated and is not engaged until blood pressure is under control (82).
- During exercise if SBP becomes greater than 220 mm Hg or DBP greater than 105 mm Hg, exercise is stopped, and blood pressure is allowed to return toward resting values (106). The next exercise period is completed at lower exercise intensity to ensure blood pressure stays less than 220/105 mm Hg (106).
- Also, many HTN medications present unique challenges for the HFS in prescribing proper exercise. For example β-blockers, a common medical treatment that can attenuate HR response by as much as 30 beats per minute (106). This attenuated HR response must be considered when prescribing exercise intensity. Clients taking these medications are advised to have longer cool-down periods, where blood pressure is monitored after exercise to ensure that blood pressure does not fall to unsafe levels (82).

Metabolic

Under normal conditions, blood glucose homeostasis is maintained by a precise coordination of hormones and metabolic events. Diabetes interrupts this delicate balance, and individuals with this condition do not respond normally to exercise. Nonetheless, diabetic patients are able to exercise but with precaution. Because diabetes involves multiple body systems resulting in a multitude of complications, the HFS must give careful consideration to the presence and severity of diabetes and its complications, medication regimens, and the schedule for these medications to ensure client safety.

- Diabetic patients need constant blood glucose monitoring, and the ability to measure is of upmost importance before, during, and after exercise (38).
- A readily available source of carbohydrate, such as fruit juice or hard candy, should be available if needed to increase blood glucose levels (95).
- If preexercise or during exercise blood glucose measurements are less than 70 or mg·dL^{-1}, a carbohydrate snack (~15 g) is administered, and a blood glucose reading of greater than 100 mg·dL^{-1} is obtained before starting or continuing exercise (95).
- When preexercise blood glucose values are greater than 250 mg·dL^{-1} with the presence of blood ketones or are greater than 300 mg·dL^{-1} with either presence or absence of ketones, blood glucose is lowered before initiating exercise (59). However, provided the patient feels well and is adequately hydrated and ketones are not present, postponing exercise is not compulsory based solely on hyperglycemia (99).
- When an active retinal hemorrhage is present or recent laser corrective surgery for retinopathy is completed, exercise is avoided (38). Postponing exercise will limit the risk of triggering vitreous hemorrhage and retinal detachment (95).
- Because diabetic patients experience greater time for proper healing process, exercising diabetic patients should practice good foot care by inspection of feet before and after exercise and by wearing proper shoes and cotton socks to avoid foot sores and blisters.
- Exercising with a partner or under the supervision of an HFS to reduce the risk of problems associated with hypoglycemic events (38).
- Consideration is always given to exercise timing and taking insulin or hypoglycemic agents. Exercise is not recommended during peak insulin action because hypoglycemia may result. Because delayed postexercise hypoglycemia is a known risk, late evening exercising is not recommended.
- Always carry medical identification.

Dyslipidemia present few, if any, exercise limitations, and individuals with elevated blood lipid levels are encouraged to engage in regular physical activity and exercise. To optimize blood lipid concentrations, dyslipidemic clients are encouraged to engage in longer exercise durations (43). Presently, clients with dyslipidemia are recommended to set a short-term goal of 150 minutes a week and a long-term goal of greater than 300 minutes a week and to expend more than 2,000 kcal of expenditure a week (49, 50). Both short-term and long-term goals are best achieved by exercising 5 or more days a week and, in some cases, by incorporating physical activity and exercise in multiple daily episodes. In general, most lipid-lowering drugs have no impact on exercise responses.

Obesity continues as a growing global health concern (11, 103). Both reducing energy intake by dietary restriction and increasing energy expenditure by exercise are targeted interventions for treating obesity (103).

- Obese individuals are often at risk for other chronic diseases and can need additional medical screening and appropriate supervision for exercise testing and programming.
- Obese individuals are recommended to engage in moderate physical activity at least 5, if not all, days of the week and progress to accumulate more than 2,000 kcal a week of energy expenditure (11).
- Because obese clients are at an increased risk for orthopedic injury and are usually in a deconditioned state, the exercise prescription should emphasize the use of low-impact or non–weight-bearing exercises such as the water-based, elliptical, and/or recumbent cycling. These types of exercises are recommended because of the reduced joint stress and the potential for less musculoskeletal injury.

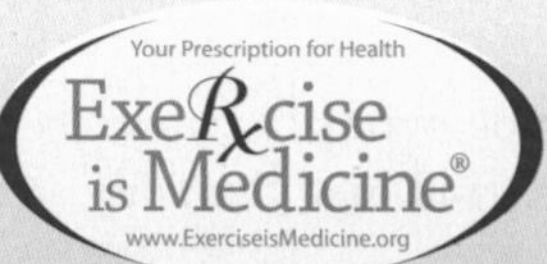

EXERCISE IS MEDICINE CONNECTION

Diabetes Prevention Program. National Institute of Health, National Institute of Diabetes and Digestive and Kidney diseases. Available from http://diabetes.niddk.nih.gov/dm/pubs/preventionprogram/

The U.S. Diabetes Prevention Program (DPP) was a multicenter trial that compared lifestyle modification with medication in the reduction in incidence of Type 2 diabetes mellitus. All of the participants (n = 3,234) were overweight and had either impaired glucose tolerance (IGT) or impaired fasting glucose (IFG) at the start of the study, and the main outcome measure was the development of Type 2 diabetes. Participants were randomly assigned to one of three groups: control, medication (metformin), or lifestyle modification. The lifestyle group included intensive dietary and physical activity modifications with a weight loss goal (5%–7% of current body weight) and 150 minutes of weekly aerobic activity. The lifestyle modification group reduced Type 2 diabetes incidence by 58%, and this was true across all participating ethnic groups and for both men and women. The metformin group realized a 31% reduction in diabetes incidence and was effective for both men and women, but it was least effective in people aged 45 and older.

The DPP's results indicate that weight loss and PA lower the risk of Type 2 diabetes by improving the body's ability to use insulin and process glucose.

- Because of likely low fitness level, an exercise prescription that has a slower intensity and duration progression will likely have fewer injuries.
- Obese clients may have a propensity for low motivation and drive for making lifestyle change, and thus, additional motivational strategies are often required to help make these changes (103). Incorporating lifestyle strategies such as realistic goal setting and balance sheets is an effective way to provide positive reinforcement and helps develop motivation to start and adhere to lifestyle change.
- Additional considerations for obese clients include adequate flexibility, warm-up and cool-down sessions, cool temperatures with low humidity, adequate hydration, and loose fitting clothing to allow for heat dissipation.

Pulmonary

The primary goal when developing an exercise prescription for COPD clients is to reduce barriers for activities of daily living and to help increase quality of life (88).

- Present scientific information is mixed as to whether exercise training has an impact on lessening the COPD disease state (34), but because exercise training improves muscle functionality, overall exercise tolerance is improved (88).
- Another exercise training goal for the COPD client is dyspnea desensitization — a condition characterized by shortness of breath that often limits exercise. The HFS must educate the COPD client to push past this feeling. Once learned, exercise can continue even when dyspnea is increasing, and thus greater exercise intensities and durations can be completed resulting in greater heath-fitness benefits (59, 88).
- Early in the exercise program, the COPD client will need constant monitoring until they are able to learn pulmonary triggering symptoms (34).
- To ensure safety, many COPD clients will need constant oxyhemoglobin saturation monitoring to maintain blood oxygen saturation greater than 90% (88). However, those patients needing this type of monitoring should exercise with closer medical supervision, which the HFS is not trained to provide.
- Fast-acting inhalers are kept close to hand at all times especially while exercising (34).

- A client with CRPD is treated in a similar fashion as a COPD client because they have similar exercise limitations and considerations (59).
- Additional considerations for patients with COPD include optimal exercise training time being mid- to late morning and avoiding extreme temperatures and high humidity as they can trigger symptoms and potentiate a medical incident (88).

EFFECT OF COMMON MEDICATIONS ON EXERCISE WITH CARDIOVASCULAR, METABOLIC, AND PULMONARY DISEASES

The vast majority of individuals with any form of CVD, metabolic, or pulmonary disease are likely to take one or more medications. Whether medications are over-the-counter (OTC) or prescription, many nonetheless may have an impact on exercise capacity. The expectation of the HFS is to have at least a cursory knowledge of the most common medications while keeping an updated drug reference guide handy. This preparation will allow the HFS to make appropriate and necessary adjustments in the exercise prescription while avoiding ischemic and/or other dangerous thresholds, and provide a safe and effective exercise experience.

OTC Drugs

OTC drug use is limited in treating individuals with a chronic condition. Aspirin, most commonly used for CVD individuals (57), does not pose any concerns when prescribing exercise (89). The same is true with most herbs, natural remedies, and minerals prescribed for CVD, metabolic, or pulmonary conditions. Nonetheless, these are not regulated by the FDA and should be used with extreme caution. The greater risk of OTC medications is drug interaction and the interactive effect that these drugs can have on many chronic conditions. OTC cold and flu medications often contain some form of ephedrine that has been shown to increase systemic blood pressure. These medications should be avoided or used cautiously in clients with CVD or HTN. When taken, consider postponing exercise for the day or adjusting exercise intensity and duration accordingly to avoid excessive blood pressure increases.

The diabetic patient should avoid any OTCs that contain alcohol or sugar, as they are likely to affect blood glucose levels. In addition, two common nonsteroidal anti-inflammatory drugs (NSAIDs) — ibuprofen and naproxen — are used cautiously in diabetic patients because both may increase the risk of hypoglycemia (90). Conflicting evidence exists regarding the effect of NSAIDs on blood pressure; therefore, HTN clients taking a NSAIDs are monitored closely (77, 83, 94). OTC cough suppressants can impede "productive cough" and are used cautiously in certain pulmonary patients, although the effect on exercise is negligible (52).

Prescription Drugs

An abundance of prescription drugs is available to treat CVD, metabolic, and pulmonary disorders/diseases, and many of these drugs impact exercise capacity. The most common class of CVD drugs includes β-blockers, CCBs, ACE inhibitors, digitalis, diuretics, and cholesterol-lowering medications. These drug classes are especially common in treating persons with a history of MI, ischemia, and HTN (69, 90).

β-Blockers are well known for decreasing mortality (47, 71, 92) and risk of a second MI (41, 44, 63), but also have a profound effect on exercise response. Although β-blockers lower HR and myocardial contractility, they also increase exercise capacity by decreasing coronary ischemia (47). This effect makes initial exercise intensity determination difficult, may limit functional capacity, inhibits using HR as an exercise intensity target, and requires more rigorous patient self-monitoring. β-Blockers may also block symptoms of hypoglycemia and increase the risk of undetected hypoglycemia during and after exercise (96).

CCBs (used for treating HTN and angina) and ACE inhibitors (used for treating HTN) both increase arterial diameter, thereby lessening blood pressure and decreasing the work by the heart.

CCBs effect is central while ACE inhibitors actions are more peripheral. Although CCBs have some effect on HR and contractility, the extent of this effect is not as much as that of β-blockers. Therefore, CCBs and ACE inhibitors pose much less concern regarding exercise responses, but the HFS must be aware of unusual changes in blood pressure or HR both before and during exercise. ACE inhibitors do work in the lungs and can produce an irritating dry cough; if this occurs, the HFS should refer the client to his or her physician.

Nitrates and cholesterol-lowering drugs tend to have very little effect on HR and contractility and thus no direct impact on exercise capacity or the exercise prescription. Because the liver is the site of action of these drugs, liver function should be checked regularly. Statins alone or in combination with fibric acid are often associated with unusual muscle soreness (76). Muscle soreness is an indication that a condition referred to as rhabdomyolysis might be evolving. When symptoms of this condition appear, the client should be referred to his or her physician. Clients taking this drug regimen and showing signs of this condition may need increased recovery time or lower exercise intensities.

Digitalis, commonly used in CHF and for certain persistent arrhythmias, increases contractility, slows rate, and mediates arrhythmias (97). In the CHF patient, digitalis typically increases exercise capacity. On the other hand, digitalis can cause ST-segment depression at rest or during exercise, so its use should be noted at all times (43).

Diuretics are used to control HTN and edema by triggering the kidney to excrete water (78). This increased water excretion may result in an increased resting and submaximal HR. The increased resting rate could be due to decreased blood volume and decreased blood pressure, which could have a slight negative impact on exercise capacity (78) as well as thermoregulation. Individuals using diuretics to control edema should check their body weight regularly.

In pulmonary disease, β_2-agonists are commonly used as a bronchodilator for both short-term (8) and long-term (14) relief and management of asthmatic symptoms. Strong evidence exists for using inhaled corticosteroids for managing asthmatic exacerbations and for longer-term treatment. However, steroid-based drugs carry long-term complications and are used cautiously.

There are a variety of oral medications available to treat diabetes. Mechanisms of action include increasing hepatic insulin output, lowering insulin resistance, and decreasing absorption of carbohydrates. These drugs may affect exercise capacity as some claim slight improvements in VO_2 (86) while others report no changes (73). Regardless, the diabetic exerciser needs to monitor blood glucose closely before, during, and after each exercise session.

Prescribing exercise for clients with CVD, metabolic disease, or pulmonary disease requires some knowledge of common medications, particularly their effect on exercise response, exercise capacity, and hemodynamics. The HFS is expected to be familiar with the most commonly prescribed medications and understand how to modify an exercise prescription accordingly. It is outside the scope of practice of the HFS to suggest medication changes; rather, the HFS should refer patients back to their attending physician for medication concerns.

TEACHING AND DEMONSTRATING SAFE AND EFFECTIVE EXERCISES FOR INDIVIDUALS WITH CONTROLLED CARDIOVASCULAR, METABOLIC, AND PULMONARY DISEASES

When developing a physical activity and exercise prescription for a medically cleared client, the HFS must complete a thorough review of the client's medical record to gain a full understanding of specific health conditions and possible exercise limitations and to develop an exercise plan. An orientation session is then scheduled to review this plan, discuss the importance of plan adherence to gain optimal health benefits as well as maintain safety, and demonstrate proper execution of all exercises.

Those individuals having incurred a recent medical event are encouraged to seek involvement in an organized rehabilitation setting to start an exercise program (66). The HFS reviews the medical history, notes, medication history, and any client limitations. This review provides the HFS with the background information needed to better understand the special health problems and needs surrounding the client's disease, to determine exercise contraindications and limitations, and to develop areas of emphasis in the exercise plan that will help optimize health-fitness benefits and maintain safety.

After a complete review of the client's file, the HFS is ready to meet and discuss all plan aspects. Individuals recently diagnosed with a chronic health condition and just starting an exercise program are probably concerned with safety and are often overwhelmed with making numerous lifestyle modifications. The HFS is never to assume client's knowledge of any part of the plan, goals, and specific exercise executions. Assumptions concerning client's exercise knowledge often lead to calamitous consequences, and for this reason, every aspect of the plan is reviewed and all exercises carefully explained and demonstrated with active participation by the client. Because making lifestyle modifications is difficult, a thorough explanation of the plan is critical in helping to overcome potential barriers and increase their chance for success in making change (9). On the other hand, if clients do not understand the goals of the program or are confused by incomplete information regarding proper exercise techniques, their likelihood of exercising outside their physical limitations is greatly increased and could result in muscle skeletal injury and excessive fatigue and/or incur an undesirable medical event. Injuries and extreme fatigue can lead to frustration and possible program discontinuation. In addition, because many chronic diseases pose adverse health effects, these individuals have unique limitations putting them at higher risk for injury and unwanted medical events.

Aerobic conditioning is an important component of the exercise program and is relatively easy to describe. Educational sessions provide a vital means for developing patient understanding while enhancing the likelihood in optimizing the FITT principle application. Careful explanation of exercise frequency as to the number of days each week that exercise is performed and providing information describing various ways to meet exercise frequency goals are essential; for example, suggesting multiple short exercise episodes per day versus one longer continuous exercise session may be appropriate. Exercise intensity is a measure of exercise difficulty or how hard exercise is being performed. Although several ways to measure intensity exist, HR measurement is most commonly used, while less quantitative means of measuring exercise intensity include the RPE scale (18) or the "Talk Test" (81). Once the exercise type or mode is selected, the HFS gives detailed exercise instructions using demonstrations and provides safety information regarding all exercises and the use of all exercise equipment. For best results, the client performs the exercise while the HFS observes, and adjustments to the client's program are made. In the early phase of any exercise program, the client is closely monitored for correct exercise movement and appropriate exercise responses. Client records for exercise frequency, intensity, time, and type are developed and kept on file.

Resistance exercise training requires more demonstration than aerobic conditioning because of different exercises used for the various muscle groups and types of resistance equipment. Clients with a chronic disease can have numerous exercise resistance contraindications, and the HFS must have a strong understanding of all various diseases and exercise contraindications to ensure client safety while optimizing health-fitness benefits (5). As in aerobic conditioning, the FITT principle is also used for developing the resistance exercise prescription (65). A detailed description of how 1 RM is used for determining the exercise intensity for resistance exercise may be provided. The RPE scale is also an effective indicator of resistance exercise intensity (65). The number of exercise repetitions and sets completed is a measure of the exercise time or duration. Unlike aerobic conditioning, a set of resistance conditioning exercises is developed for each major muscle group. Each exercise is described and completely demonstrated to show the appropriate range of motion with proper technique, number of repetitions performed, number of sets completed, and proper description of the concentric and eccentric portions of the motion (42). In conjunction with each exercise being demonstrated, an explanation regarding why each muscle group is exercised, how a particular exercise movement is beneficial, and what if any potential risks or dangers exist when improper technique is used or the client exercises outside the prescribed recommendations is warranted. In addition to the above-mentioned exercises, all clients should also be engaged in regular flexibility training, which is covered in greater detail in Chapter 5.

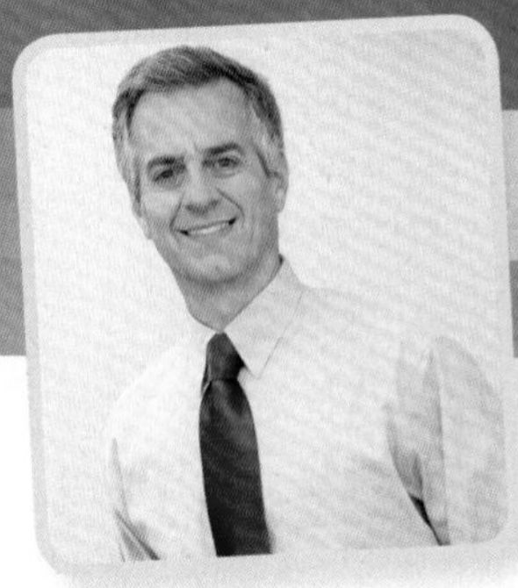

The Case of Frank

Submitted by **Benjamin Gordon, M.S., ACSM-CES, Larry Durstine, PhD, FACSM, Department of Exercise Science, University of South Carolina, Columbia, SC**

Frank is an unmotivated, physically inactive, middle-aged accountant. He has several risk factors for CVD, but has not been clinically diagnosed with a particular disease.

Narrative

From all outward appearances Frank seems to be an average middle-aged man. He has been an executive accountant for the past 28 years, and since starting this position as an accountant, Frank has consistently been physically inactive. Often he will enthusiastically start an exercise program, but is very unpredictable and inconsistent with exercising regularly and quits soon after starting. His eating choices and habits are poor and not consistent for good health. He consumes almost no vegetables, but lots of saturated fat while consuming several beers with most meals. His most recent endeavor into exercising was spurred on by his daughter, who recommended that he needed to see someone qualified to help him start a program and stay faithful to that exercise program. On this recommendation, Frank went to his college's wellness center to see one of the HFSs on staff. During the initial meeting, a comprehensive assessment was carried out to determine Frank's initial fitness level and his readiness to participate in a program.

Physical Information

Age: 49 years old
Height: 5′10″
Weight: 203 lb
BMI: 29.19 kg·m^{-2}
Body fat percentage (DEXA-scan): 29.22
Resting blood pressure:138/92 mm Hg
Resting HR: 64 bpm

ACSM Guidelines Risk Factors

Age: He is a man, 45 years or older.
Family history: His father had a heart attack at the age of 47.
Cigarette smoking: Does not smoke
Sedentary:
Obesity: None (but is considered overweight borderline obese by both his body fat and BMI)
Hypertension: DBP is within hypertensive levels, 138/92 mm Hg.
Dyslipidemia: Total cholesterol: 238 mg·dL^{-1}; LDL-C: 161 mg·dL^{-1}; HDL-C: 39 mg·dL^{-1}.
Prediabetes: None (resting blood glucose, 88 mg·dL^{-1})

The following results were from exercise testing:

Aerobic fitness ($\dot{V}O_{2max}$) (Balke protocol): Approximately 19.8 mL·kg^{-1}·min^{-1}
Bench press weight ratio for 1 RM: 0.77
Leg press weight ratio for 1 RM: 1.55
YMCA bench press test (total lifts): 15
Partial curl up test (total repetitions): 12
Forward flexion using a sit-and-reach box: 29 cm

The Case of Frank cont.

Frank's lifestyle is riddled with long periods of inactivity and no sustained exercise. His low fitness level is impacting his quality of life. He loses his breath and is easily fatigued from medial physical tasks. Unfortunately, Frank isn't really too worried about his health, but his daughter is. He only wants to exercise enough to stop his daughter from nagging him.

Questions

- What is the biggest problem concerning Frank's health right now?
- What sort of disease is Frank setting himself up for, and does he already have symptoms of the disease?
- Do you think that Frank's workouts should be supervised?
- Should Frank have his aerobic exercise broken up into intermittent exercise sessions or one longer continuous exercise session?

References

1. American College of Sports Medicine. *ACSM's Guidelines for Exercise Testing and Prescription*. 8th ed. Philadelphia (PA): Lippincott Williams & Wilkins; 2010.
2. American College of Sports Medicine. *ACSM's Resources for Clinical Exercise Physiology*. 2nd ed. Philadelphia (PA): Lippincott Williams & Wilkins; 2010.
3. American College of Sports Medicine. *ACSM's Resource Manual for Guidelines for Exercise Testing and Prescription*. 6th ed. Philadelphia (PA): Lippincott Williams & Wilkins; 2010.
4. Durstine JL, Moore GE, Painter PL, Roberts SO. *ACSM's Exercise Management for Persons With Chronic Diseases and Disabilities*. 3rd ed. Champaign (IL): Human Kinetics; 2009.

SUMMARY

Regular physical activity and exercise participation can provide primary and secondary prevention health-fitness benefits. Medications, specialized diets, and surgeries are generally viewed as first options before exercise is considered as an intervention. Nonetheless, daily physical activity and exercise training are effective tools in developing health-fitness benefits for persons with chronic diseases. Although exercise is beneficial, the challenges and limitations presented by diseases must be addressed to properly design the most effective and safest physical activity and exercise program. By adapting the ACSM (49) and U.S. Physical Activity Recommendations (21) for prescribing physical activity and exercise programs, the HFS is better able to meet the needs of the cardiovascular, metabolic, and pulmonary clients while ensuring program safety. The HFS must know the limitations and challenges these diseases present for the exercising client and how to adapt the physical activity and exercise programs accordingly.

STUDY QUESTIONS

1. Explain the pathophysiology of atherosclerosis, including the role of the major risk factors.
2. Explain why the asthmatic patient may have difficulty breathing, particularly during exercise.
3. Explain the major pathologic differences between Type 1 and Type 2 diabetes, within the context of exercise.
4. Briefly describe the effect of OTC medications on exercise in CAD and pulmonary disease.
5. Describe key differences in prescribing exercise for specific clinical populations.

REFERENCES

1. American College of Sports Medicine. *ACSM's Guidelines for Exercise Testing and Prescription*. 8th ed. Philadelphia (PA): Lippincott Williams & Wilkins; 2008. p. 260–2.
2. American College of Sports Medicine. *ACSM's Guidelines for Exercise Testing and Prescription*. 8th ed. Philadelphia (PA): Lippincott Williams & Wilkins; 2008. p. 160–4.
3. American College of Sports Medicine. *ACSM's Metabolic Calculations Handbook*. 1st ed. Baltimore, MD: Lippincott Williams and Wilkins; 2007.
4. American College of Sports Medicine. Position stand on exercise for patients with coronary artery disease. *Med Sci Sports Exerc*. 1994;26(3):i–v.
5. American College of Sports Medicine. Position stand on the recommended quantity and quality of exercise for developing and maintaining cardiorespiratory and muscular fitness, and flexibility in healthy adults. *Med Sci Sports Exerc*. 1998;30(6):975–91.
6. American Diabetes Association. Implications of the diabetes control and complications trial. *Diabetes Care*. 2003;26(1):S25–7.
7. American Diabetes Association. Diagnosis and classification of diabetes mellitus. *Diabetes Care*. 2007;30(1):S42–7.
8. American Pharmaceutical Association. A sample protocol for chronic management of asthma from the American Pharmaceutical Association Respiratory Disease Panelists and Reviewers. *Am Pharm*. 1995;NS35(11):30–5.
9. Ajzen I. *Attitudes, Personality and Behavior*. Chicago (IL): Dorsey Press; 1988. 116–27 p.
10. Balady GJ, Williams MA, Ades PA, et al. Core components of cardiac rehabilitation/secondary prevention programs: 2007 update: A scientific statement from the American Heart Association Exercise, Cardiac Rehabilitation, and Prevention Committee, the Council on Clinical Cardiology; the Councils on Cardiovascular Nursing, Epidemiology and Prevention, and Nutrition, Physical Activity, and Metabolism; and the American Association of Cardiovascular and Pulmonary Rehabilitation. *Circulation*. 2007;115(20):2675–82.
11. Barlow CE, Kohl HW III, Gibbons LW, Blair SN. Physical fitness, mortality and obesity. *Int J Obes Relat Metab Disord*. 1995;19(suppl 4):S41–4.
12. Barnard RJ, Gardner GW, Diaco NV, MacAlpin RN, Kattus AA. Cardiovascular responses to sudden strenuous exercise — heart rate, blood pressure, and ECG. *J Appl Physiol*. 1973;34(6):833–7.
13. Barnes P. Asthma management: Can we further improve compliance and outcomes. *Respir Med*. 2008;98:S8–9.
14. Barnes PJ. Immunology of asthma and chronic obstructive pulmonary disease. *Nat Rev. Immunol*. 2008;8(3):183–92.
15. Beevers G, Lip GY, O'Brien E. ABC of hypertension: The pathophysiology of hypertension *BMJ*. 2001;(332):912–6.
16. Belardinelli R, Georgiou D, Cianci G, Purcaro A. Randomized, controlled trial of long-term moderate exercise training in chronic heart failure: Effects on functional capacity, quality of life, and clinical outcome. *Circulation*. 1999;99(9):1173–82.
17. Blair SN, Kohl HW III, Barlow CE, Paffenbarger RS Jr, Gibbons LW, Macera CA. Changes in physical fitness and all-cause mortality. A prospective study of healthy and unhealthy men. *JAMA*. 1995;273(14):1093–8.
18. Borg GA. Perceived exertion. *Exerc Sport Sci Rev*. 1974;2:131–53.
19. Bouldin MJ, Ross LA, Sumrall CD, Loustalot FV, Low AK, Land KK. The effect of obesity surgery on obesity comorbidity. *Am J Med Sci*. 2006;331(4):183–93.
20. Boule NG, Haddad E, Kenny GP, Wells GA, Sigal RJ. Effects of exercise on glycemic control and body mass in type 2 diabetes mellitus: A meta-analysis of controlled clinical trials. *JAMA*. 2001;286(10):1218–27.
21. Buchner D. Physical activity guidelines for America. *2008 Physical Activity Guidelines for Americans*. Washington (DC): U.S. Department of Health and Human Services; 2008. p. 1–76.
22. Centers for Disease Control and Prevention Web Site [Internet]. Available from http://www.cdc.gov/heartdisease/facts.htm. Accessed on October 3, 2011.
23. Centers for Disease Control and Prevention Web Site [Internet]. Available from http://www.cdc.gov/nchs/data/series/sr_10/sr10_210.pdf. Accessed on October 3, 2011.
24. Centers for Disease Control and Prevention Web Site [Internet]. Available from http://www.cdc.gov/nchs/data/series/sr_10/sr10_215.pdf. Accessed on October 3, 2011.
25. Centers for Disease Control and Prevention Web Site [Internet]. Available from http://www.cdc.gov/nchs/data/series/sr_10/sr10_218.pdf. Accessed on October 3, 2011.
26. Centers for Disease Control and Prevention Web Site [Internet]. Available from http://www.cdc.gov/nchs/data/series/sr_10/sr10_222.pdf. Accessed on October 3, 2011.
27. Centers for Disease Control and Prevention Web Site [Internet]. Available from http://www.cdc.gov/nchs/data/series/sr_10/sr10_228.pdf. Accessed on October 3, 2011.
28. Centers for Disease Control and Prevention Web Site [Internet]. Available from http://www.cdc.gov/nchs/data/series/sr_10/sr10_232.pdf. Accessed on October 3, 2011.
29. Centers for Disease Control and Prevention Web Site [Internet]. Available from http://www.cdc.gov/nchs/data/series/sr_10/sr10_235.pdf. Accessed on October 3, 2011.
30. Centers for Disease Control and Prevention Web Site [Internet]. Available from http://www.cdc.gov/nchs/data/series/sr_10/sr10_240.pdf. Accessed on October 3, 2011.
31. Centers for Disease Control and Prevention Web Site [Internet]. Available from http://www.cdc.gov/nchs/data/series/sr_10/sr10_242.pdf. Accessed on October 3, 2011.
32. Centers for Disease Control and Prevention Web Site [Internet]. Available from http://www.cdc.gov/obesity/defining.html. Accessed on October 3, 2011.
33. Cnop M WN, Jonas JC, et al. Mechanisms of pancreatic beta-cell death in Type 1 and Type 2 diabetes: Many differences, few similarities. *Am Diabetes Assoc*. 2005;(54):S97–107.
34. Cooper CB. Exercise in chronic pulmonary disease: Aerobic exercise prescription. *Med Sci Sports Exerc*. 2001;33(7 suppl):S671–9.
35. Courser JI GR, Hamadeh MA, Kane CS. Pulmonary rehabilitation improves exercise capacity in older elderly patients with COPD. *Hypertension*. 2005;(45):667–75.
36. DeBusk RF, Haskell W. Symptom-limited vs heart-rate-limited exercise testing soon after myocardial infarction. *Circulation*. 1980;61(4):738–43.
37. Durstine JL, Moore GE, Polk, D. *ACSM's Exercise Management for Persons with Chronic Diseases and Disabilities*. Champaign (IL): Human Kinetics; 2009. p. 186–9.
38. Durstine JL, Moore GE, Polk D. *ACSM's Exercise Management for Persons with Chronic Diseases and Disabilities*. Champaign (IL): Human Kinetics; 2009. p. 192–4.
39. Durstine JL, Moore GE, Polk D. *ACSM's Exercise Management for Persons with Chronic Diseases and Disabilities*. Champaign (IL): Human Kinetics; 2009. p. 206–12.
40. Edmunds J, Ntoumanis N, Duda JL. Adherence and well-being in overweight and obese patients referred to

an exercise on prescription program. *Psychol Sport Exerc.* 2007;5(1):722–40.

41. Everly MJ, Heaton PC, Cluxton RJ Jr. Beta-blocker underuse in secondary prevention of myocardial infarction. *Ann Pharmacother.* 2004;38(2):286–93.
42. Fleck SJ, Kraemer WJ. *Designing Resistance Training Programs.* Champaign (IL): Human Kinetics Publishers Inc.; 2004.
43. Fletcher GF, Balady GJ, Amsterdam EA, et al. Exercise standards for testing and training: A statement for healthcare professionals from the American Heart Association. *Circulation.* 2001;104(14):1694–740.
44. Fonarow GC. Beta-blockers for the post-myocardial infarction patient: Current clinical evidence and practical considerations. *Rev Cardiovasc Med.* 2006;7(1):1–9.
45. Franklin BA. Myocardial infarction. In: Durstine LJ, Moore GE, Painter PL, Roberts SO, editors. *ACSM's Exercise Management for Person with Chronic Diseases and Disabilities.* Champaign (IL): Human Kinetics; 2009. p. 49–57.
46. Freese EC, Levine AS, Chapman DP, Hausman DB, Cureton KJ. Effects of acute sprint interval cycling and energy replacement on postprandial lipemia. *J Appl Physiol.* 2011;111(6):1584–9.
47. Friedman D, Roberts SO, Angina and silent ischemia In: Durstine LJ, Moore GE, Painter PL, Roberts SO, editors. ACSM's Exercise Management for Person with Chronic Diseases and Disabilities. Champaign (IL): *Human Kinetics*; 2009. p. 66–72.
48. Gaesser GA, Angadi SS, Sawyer BJ. Exercise and diet, independent of weight loss, improve cardiometabolic risk profile in overweight and obese individuals. *Phys Sportsmed.* 2011;39(2):87–97.
49. Garber CE, Blissmer B, Deschenes MR, et al. American College of Sports Medicine position stand. Quantity and quality of exercise for developing and maintaining cardiorespiratory, musculoskeletal, and neuromotor fitness in apparently healthy adults: Guidance for prescribing exercise. *Med Sci Sports Exerc.* 2011;43(7):1334–59.
50. Genest J, McPherson R, Frohlich J, et al. 2009 Canadian Cardiovascular Society/Canadian guidelines for the diagnosis and treatment of dyslipidemia and prevention of cardiovascular disease in the adult — 2009 recommendations. *Can J Cardiol.* 2009;25(10):567–79.
51. Giannuzzi P, Saner H, Bjornstad H, et al. Secondary prevention through cardiac rehabilitation: Position paper of the Working Group on Cardiac Rehabilitation and Exercise Physiology of the European Society of Cardiology. *Eur Heart J.* 2003;24(13):1273–8.
52. Giron AE, Stansbury DW, Fischer CE, Light RW. Lack of effect of dextromethorphan on breathlessness and exercise performance in patients with chronic obstructive pulmonary disease (COPD). *Eur Respir J.* 1991;4(5):532–5.
53. Goodman FK. *Pathology: Implications for the Physical Therapist.* China: Saunders Elsevier; 2009.
54. Gordon NF, Scott CB, Wilkinson WJ, Duncan JJ, Blair SN. Exercise and mild essential hypertension. Recommendations for adults. *Sports Med.* 1990;10(6):390–404.
55. Hansen D, Eijnde BO, Roelants M, et al. Clinical benefits of the addition of lower extremity low-intensity resistance muscle training to early aerobic endurance training intervention in patients with coronary artery disease: A randomized controlled trial. *J Rehabil Med.*2011;43(9):800–7.
56. Haskell WL, Lee IM, Pate RR, et al. Physical activity and public health: Updated recommendation for adults from the American College of Sports Medicine and the American Heart Association. *Med Sci Sports Exerc.* 2007;39(8):1423–34.
57. Hennekens CH, Dyken ML, Fuster V. Aspirin as a therapeutic agent in cardiovascular disease: A statement for healthcare professionals from the American Heart Association. *Circulation.* 1997;96(8):2751–3.
58. Horowitz MB, Littenberg B, Mahler DA. Dyspnea ratings for prescribing exercise intensity in patients with COPD. *Chest.* 1996;109(5):1169–75.
59. Hsia C. Chronic restrictive pulmonary disease. In: Durstine JL, Moore GE, Painter PL, et al, editors. *ACSM's Exercise Management for Persons with Chronic Diseases and Disabilities.* Champaign (IL): Human Kinetics; 2009. p. 167–74.
60. Hunt SA. ACC/AHA 2005 guideline update for the diagnosis and management of chronic heart failure in the adult: A report of the American College of Cardiology/American Heart Association Task Force on Practice Guidelines (Writing Committee to Update the 2001 Guidelines for the Evaluation and Management of Heart Failure). *J Am Coll Cardiol.* 2005;46(6):e1–82.
61. Juneau M, Roy N, Nigam A, Tardif JC, Larivee L. Exercise above the ischemic threshold and serum markers of myocardial injury. *Can J Cardiol.* 2009;25(10):e338–41.
62. Keteyian SJ. Exercise rehabilitation in chronic heart failure. *Coron Artery Dis.* 2006;17(3):233–7.
63. Kleiner SA, Vogt WB, Gladowski P, DeVries A, Levin G, Antonucci C, Fong J. Beta-blocker compliance, mortality, and reinfarction:Validation of clinical trial association using insurer claims data. *Am J Med Qual.* 2009;24(6):512–9.
64. Kohut ML, McCann DA, Russell DW, et al. Aerobic exercise, but not flexibility/resistance exercise, reduces serum IL-18, CRP, and IL-6 independent of beta-blockers, BMI, and psychosocial factors in older adults. *Brain Behav Immun.* 2006;20(3):201–9.
65. Kraemer WJ, Ratamess NA. Fundamentals of resistance training: Progression and exercise prescription. *Med Sci Sports Exerc.* 2004;36(4):674–88.
66. Kraus WE. *Physical Activity Status and Chronic Diseases.* 6th ed. Philadelphia (PA): Lippincott Williams & Wilkins; 2009. p. 166–80.
67. Leach RJ. Chronic obstructive airways disease. *Respir Dis Manag.* 2009;10:29–40.
68. Leon AS. Exercise following myocardial infarction. Current recommendations. *Sports Med.* 2000;29(5):301–11.
69. Li J , Zhang N, Ye B, et al. Non-steroidal anti-inflammatory drugs increase insulin release from beta cells by inhibiting ATP-sensitive potassium channels. *Br J Pharmacol.* 2007;151(4):483–93.
70. Libby P, Ridker PM. Inflammation and atherothrombosis: From population biology and bench research to clinical practice. *J Am Coll Cardiol.* 2006;48(9):A33–46.
71. Lindenauer PK, Pekow P, Wang K, Mamidi DK, Gutierrez B, Benjamin EM. Perioperative beta-blocker therapy and mortality after major noncardiac surgery. *N Engl J Med.* 2005;353(4):349–61.
72. Mallika V, Goswami B, Rajappa M. Atherosclerosis pathophysiology and the role of novel risk factors: A clinicobiochemical perspective. *Angiology.* 2007;58(5):513–22.
73. McGuire DK, Abdullah SM, See R, et al. Randomized comparison of the effects of rosiglitazone vs. placebo on peak integrated cardiovascular performance, cardiac structure, and function. *Eur Heart J.* 2010;31(18):2262–70.
74. Mittleman MA, Maclure M, Tofler GH, Sherwood JB, Goldberg RJ, Muller JE. Triggering of acute myocardial infarction by heavy physical exertion. Protection against triggering by regular exertion. Determinants of myocardial infarction onset study investigators. *N Engl J Med.* 1993;329(23):1677–83.
75. Naughton J, Raider R. Methods of exercise testing. In: Naughton JP, Hellerstein HK, Mohler IC, editors. *Exercise Testing and Exercise Training in Coronary Heart Disease.* New York (NY): Academic Press; 1973. p. 79–89.

76. Omar MA, Wilson JP, Cox TS. Rhabdomyolysis and HMG-CoA reductase inhibitors. *Ann Pharmacother.* 2001;35(9):1096–107.
77. Palmer R, Weiss R, Zusman RM, Haig A, Flavin S, MacDonald B. Effects of nabumetone, celecoxib, and ibuprofen on blood pressure control in hypertensive patients on angiotensin converting enzyme inhibitors. *Am J Hypertens.* 2003;16(2):135–9.
78. Parker JD, Parker AB, Farrell B, Parker JO. Effects of diuretic therapy on the development of tolerance to nitroglycerin and exercise capacity in patients with chronic stable angina. *Circulation.* 1996;93(4):691–6.
79. Patsch JR, Sailer S, Kostner G, Sandhofer F, Holasek A, Braunsteiner H. Separation of the main lipoprotein density classes from human plasma by rate-zonal ultracentrifugation. *J Lipid Res.* 1974;15(4):356–66.
80. Pauwels RA, Buist AS, Calverley PM, Jenkins CR, Hurd SS. Global strategy for the diagnosis, management, and prevention of chronic obstructive pulmonary disease. NHLBI/WHO Global Initiative for Chronic Obstructive Lung Disease (GOLD) Workshop summary. *Am J Respir Crit Care Med.* 2001;163(5):1256–76.
81. Persinger R, Foster C, Gibson M, Fater DC, Porcari JP. Consistency of the talk test for exercise prescription. *Med Sci Sports Exerc.* 2004;36(9):1632–6.
82. Pescatello LS, Franklin BA, Fagard R, Farquhar WB, Kelley GA, Ray CA. American College of Sports Medicine position stand. Exercise and hypertension. *Med Sci Sports Exerc.* 2004;36(3):533–53.
83. Pope JE, Anderson JJ, Felson DT. A meta-analysis of the effects of nonsteroidal anti-inflammatory drugs on blood pressure. *Arch Intern Med.* 1993;153(4):477–84.
84. Rabe KF, Beghe B, Luppi F, Fabbri LM. Update in chronic obstructive pulmonary disease 2006. *Am J Respir Crit Care Med.* 2007;175(12):1222–32.
85. Rabe KF, Hurd S, Anzueto A, et al. Global strategy for the diagnosis, management, and prevention of chronic obstructive pulmonary disease: GOLD executive summary. *Am J Respir Crit Care Med.* 2007;176(6):532–55.
86. Regensteiner JG, Bauer TA, Reusch JE. Rosiglitazone improves exercise capacity in individuals with type 2 diabetes. *Diabetes Care.* 2005;28(12):2877–83.
87. Rehman J, Li J, Parvathaneni L, et al. Exercise acutely increases circulating endothelial progenitor cells and monocyte-/macrophage-derived angiogenic cells. *J Am Coll Cardiol.* 2004;43(12):2314–8.
88. Ries AL, Bauldoff GS, Carlin BW, et al. Pulmonary rehabilitation: Joint ACCP/AACVPR evidence-based clinical practice guidelines. *Chest.* 2007;131(5 suppl):4S–42S.
89. Romer L. Pathophysiology and treatment of pulmonary disease. In: Ehrman JK, editor. *ACSM's Resource Manual for Guidelines for Exercise Testing and Prescription.* Philadelphia (PA): Lippincott Williams & Wilkins; 2010. p. 20–32.
90. Rosendorff C. Hypertension and coronary artery disease: A summary of the American Heart Association scientific statement. *J Clin Hypertens (Greenwich).* 2007;9(10):790–5.
91. Shah K, Villareal DT. Combination treatment to CONQUER obesity? *Lancet.* 2011;377(9774):1295–7.
92. Shekelle PG, Rich MW, Morton SC, et al. Efficacy of angiotensin-converting enzyme inhibitors and beta-blockers in the management of left ventricular systolic dysfunction according to race, gender, and diabetic status: A meta-analysis of major clinical trials. *J Am Coll Cardiol.* 2003;41(9):1529–38.
93. Shephard RJ, Balady GJ. Exercise as cardiovascular therapy. *Circulation.* 1999;99(7):963–72.
94. Sheridan R, Montgomery AA, Fahey T. NSAID use and BP in treated hypertensives: A retrospective controlled observational study. *J Hum Hypertens.* 2005;19(6):445–50.
95. Sigal RJ, Kenny GP, Wasserman DH, Castaneda-Sceppa C. Physical activity/exercise and type 2 diabetes. *Diabetes Care.* 2004;27(10):2518–39.
96. Sigal RJ, Purdon C, Bilinski D, Vranic M, Halter JB, Marliss EB. Glucoregulation during and after intense exercise: Effects of beta-blockade. *J Clin Endocrinol Metab.* 1994;78(2):359–66.
97. Sullivan M, Atwood JE, Myers J, et al. Increased exercise capacity after digoxin administration in patients with heart failure. *J Am Coll Cardiol.* 1989;13(5):1138–43.
98. Susic D. Hypertension, aging, and atherosclerosis. The endothelial interface. *Med Clin N Am.* 1997;81(5):1231–40.
99. Thompson PD. Exercise and physical activity in the prevention and treatment of atherosclerotic cardiovascular disease. *Arterioscler Thromb Vasc Biol.* 2003;23(8):1319–21.
100 .Thompson PD, Crouse SF, Goodpaster B, Kelley D, Moyna N, Pescatello L. The acute versus the chronic response to exercise. *Med Sci Sports Exerc.* 2001;33(6 suppl):S438–45; discussion S52–3.
101 .Verity L. Exercise prescription in patients with diabetes. In: Ehrman J, editor. *ACSM's Resource Manual for Guidelines for Exercise Testing and Prescription.* Philadelphia (PA): Lippincott Williams & Wilkins; 2010. p. 600–17.
102 .Villareal DT, Chode S, Parimi N, et al. Weight loss, exercise, or both and physical function in obese older adults. *N Engl J Med.* 2011;364(13):1218–29.
103 .Wallace JP, Shala R. Obesity. In: Durstine JL, Moore GE, Painter PL, et al, editors. *ACSM's Exercise Management for Persons with Chronic Diseases and Disabilities.* Champaign (IL): Human Kinetics; 2009. p. 192–9.
104 .Wang JS, Jen CJ, Chen HI. Effects of exercise training and deconditioning on platelet function in men. *Arterioscler Thromb Vasc Biol.* 1995;15(10):1668–74.
105 .Whelton SP, Chin A, Xin X, He J. Effects of aerobic exercise on blood pressure: A meta-analysis of randomized, controlled trials. *Ann Intern Med.* 2002;136(7):493–503.
106 .Williams B, Poulter NR, Brown MJ, et al. British Hypertension Society guidelines for hypertension management 2004 (BHS-IV): Summary. *BMJ.* 2004;328(7440):634–40.
107 .Willich SN, Lewis M, Lowel H, Arntz HR, Schubert F, Schroder R. Physical exertion as a trigger of acute myocardial infarction. Triggers and Mechanisms of Myocardial Infarction Study Group. *N Engl J Med.* 1993;329(23):1684–90.
108 .Xu JQ, Kochanek KD, Murphy SL, Tejada-Vera B. Deaths: Final data for 2007. *Natl Vital Stat Rep.* 58(19). Retrieved from Centers for Disease Control and Prevention. [Internet]. Hyattsville (MD): National Center for Health Statistics; [cited 2010 Sep 16]. Available from http://www.cdc.gov/nchs/

CHAPTER

8 Exercise Programming for Individuals with Musculoskeletal Limitations

John Sigg • Betsy Keller

CHAPTER OBJECTIVES

- To understand the causes of, effects of exercise on, and reduction of risks for traumatic injuries, overuse injuries, and selected musculoskeletal diseases.
- To apply appropriate exercise guidelines for traumatic injuries, overuse injuries, and selected musculoskeletal diseases.
- To modify exercise prescription appropriately for traumatic injuries, overuse injuries, and selected musculoskeletal diseases.

In previous chapters, you read about exercise prescription for individuals without limitations. In this chapter, we will review selected musculoskeletal injuries and pathologies and discuss causes of, effects of exercise on, and strategies to reduce risks associated with these conditions. The chapter is divided into three sections: traumatic injuries, overuse injuries, and chronic conditions. As you read through these sections, be reminded that safety is first and foremost for your clients. Therefore, it is important to work closely with qualified health care professionals as you develop and implement exercise programs for clients with musculoskeletal limitations.

TRAUMATIC MOVEMENT-RELATED INJURIES

Injury to a muscle or tendon is called a *strain,* whereas injury to a ligament, or tissue that connects bones, is called a *sprain.* Both strains and sprains occur in response to unaccustomed stress on the tissue, or in response to repeated lower level stress over time because of repetitive motion. In either case, an acute strain or sprain occurs most often when there is an eccentrically applied contractile force to tissue in an excessively stretched state (26).

Strains

The muscle-tendon unit (MTU) serves to generate force either by concentric contraction to create movement or by eccentric contraction to resist a load (26). Injury to the MTU can occur at any point along the MTU continuum, and the location of injury usually depends on the nature of the rate and magnitude of the applied force and type (intrinsic or extrinsic) of stress. Acute pain generally accompanies a muscle strain; however, muscle pain and dysfunction usually becomes more apparent 1 to 2 days after the injury because of delayed onset muscle soreness (DOMS). DOMS-related pain may be due to muscle fiber damage and inflammation that accompanies unaccustomed high-intensity eccentric contractions. In sport, the most common injury is to the muscle via direct impact that often causes a *contusion.* A contusion is a soft-tissue hemorrhage and/or hematoma that occurs after disruption of the muscle fibers, with subsequent inflammation and edema. Although muscle strains can occur in any MTU, they are most common in muscles of the calf (gastrocnemius, soleus) and thigh (quadriceps femoris, biceps femoris, semimembranosus, semitendinosus) (26).

The degree of MTU strain is graded from I to III and described in Table 8.1 with more severe strains generally rated as class III. Assessment of strain severity should be done by a trained health care professional to ascertain the degree of strain and appropriate treatment. In the case of a severe strain, imaging technology (MRI or X-ray) may be required to determine the degree of MTU damage and for follow-up assessment of tissue repair and joint function.

Sprains

Ligaments are collagenous fibrous structures that connect bone to bone and provide passive soft-tissue restraint of bone-to-bone contact. Like muscle strains, ligament sprains are graded according to severity as shown in Table 8.2. The most common site of a sprain is the ankle, and the most common mechanism for causing a sprain is inversion (foot falls inward) versus eversion. An inversion sprain typically occurs, for example, when a basketball player lands from a jump on another player's foot, causing the lateral ankle to roll outward while the foot falls inward. Diagnosis of a suspected moderate

TABLE 8.1 GRADING AND CHARACTERISTICS OF MTU STRAINS

Grade	Symptoms	Imaging Evidence	Treatment
I mild	Inflammation, edema, and/or hemorrhage usually near muscle-tendon unit (MTU), painful but strong muscle activity	MRI of muscle damage, although not required for diagnosis	RICE (rest, ice, compression, elevation) followed by therapeutic exercise for strength/flexibility
II moderate	Muscle pain and loss of strength, edema, and/or hemorrhage	MRI of partial tear of MTU; may not be required for diagnosis	RICE and possibly immobilization followed by therapeutic exercise for strength/flexibility
III severe	Painless, joint instability; complete tear of MTU	X-ray image of malalignment	RICE, immobilization, and/or surgical repair-referral

Adapted from Herzog R. Radiologic imaging in rehabilitation. In: Kibler W, Herring S, Press J, editors. *Functional Rehabilitation of Sports and Musculoskeletal Injuries.* 1st ed. Gaithersburg (MD): Aspen Publisher; 1998. p. 20–70; Booher J, Thibodeau G. Athletic injuries and related skin conditions. In: Booher J, Thibodeau G, editors. *Athletic Injury Assessment.* 4th ed. Boston (MA): McGraw-Hill; 2000. p. 77–106.

TABLE 8.2 GRADING AND CHARACTERISTICS OF LIGAMENT SPRAINS

Grade	Symptoms	Imaging Evidence	Treatment
I mild	Discomfort, no instability, little functional loss	MRI of microscopic fiber disruption, although not required for diagnosis	RICE, followed by therapeutic exercise for strength/flexibility
II moderate	Pain, inflammation, mild-to-moderate instability	MRI of partial macroscopic tear of ligament; may not be required for diagnosis	RICE and immobilization to ensure correct healing of torn fibers, followed by therapeutic exercise for strength/flexibility
III severe	Joint instability; complete tear of ligament	MRI/X-ray image of malalignment and detect possible avulsion of bone	RICE, immobilization, and/or surgical repair-referral

Adapted from Herzog R. Radiologic imaging in rehabilitation. In: Kibler W, Herring S, Press J, editors. *Functional Rehabilitation of Sports and Musculoskeletal Injuries.* 1st ed. Gaithersburg (MD): Aspen Publisher; 1998. p. 20–70; Booher J, Thibodeau G. Athletic injuries and related skin conditions. In: Booher J, Thibodeau G, editors. *Athletic Injury Assessment.* 4th ed. Boston (MA): McGraw-Hill; 2000. p. 77–106.

to serious ligament injury should be left to a trained health care professional who will obtain a detailed history, complete a physical examination, and perform special tests to assess joint stability.

If a client experiences a suspected strain or sprain, provide immediate care by having the injured person rest or restrict activity, apply ice with compression, and elevate the injured joint (RICE) (3). Support and maintain the joint in a position that presents no or minimum discomfort, thus protecting from further injury. Although this seems an obvious course of action, adding "protection" to the acronym RICE, or PRICE, may serve to remind of all steps for immediate care. Assist the client, as needed, in seeking medical attention.

Understanding the process of tissue healing is essential to providing safe and effective exercise guidance to an injured client. Although all types of tissue progress through the same phases of healing, the rate and length of each phase varies depending on the type of tissue and degree of tissue damage following injury/surgery. The initial *inflammatory* phase is about 2 to 3 days or longer. Inflammation occurs in response to acute tissue damage and is mediated chemically (*e.g.*, histamine and bradykinin) to increase blood flow and capillary permeability, causing edema. *Edema* is an accumulation of fluid in surrounding tissues that act as a brace or immobilizer and protects the damaged tissue. It does so by inhibiting contractile tissue activity and stimulating sensory nerves that cause pain to further inhibit activity. The inflammatory phase is important to prepare for the subsequent phase of tissue repair, and therefore this phase should be accompanied by relative rest and passive modalities or RICE. Exercise during this phase could interfere with and prolong tissue repair and therefore is not recommended at this time.

The *repair* phase begins within 3 to 5 days after injury and varies in length depending on the type of tissue and extent of damage, but could last up to 2 months. During this phase, damaged tissue is replaced with scar tissue. The quality of scar tissue development relies on proper management of the injury during this phase. As the scar tissue develops, exercise should be designed to prevent muscle atrophy and maintain joint integrity at the site of injury, and promote synthesis and optimum organization of new collagen fibers. Exercise should include gradual progression of low-load stress with no or minimal range of motion (ROM), such as isometric contractions. Exercise should be administered under the direction of a rehabilitative health care professional (*e.g.*, physical therapist, certified/licensed athletic trainer, or physician).

The final *remodeling* phase is characterized by weakened, repaired tissue. Exercise during this phase is to promote hypertrophy and strength of the newly formed scar tissue. Tissue remodeling can take up to 2 to 4 months, and exercise should be progressive and gradually work toward activity-specific exercises. Early stage progressive loading of tissue is important for collagen fiber alignment and muscle fiber hypertrophy, whereas later stage exercise should transition to activity-specific to prepare for return to activity (69). The three phases of tissue healing are summarized in Table 8.3.

TABLE 8.3 PHASES AND GOALS OF TISSUE REPAIR

Phase	Duration	Characteristics	Exercise Goals
Inflammation	2–3+ d	Pain, edema, redness, ↑ inflammatory cell activity	RICE for 20 min, 3–4 times a day
Repair	Up to 2 mo	Collagen fiber production, ↓ collagen fiber organization, ↓ inflammatory cell number	Progressive low-load stress isometric to ↓ muscle atrophy, ↑ joint integrity Low level stretching to recover ROM and heat to ↑ blood flow to damaged tissue
Remodeling	2–4 mo	Optimum collagen fiber alignment, ↑ tissue strength	Initial progressive loading exercises followed by transition to activity-specific exercises for return to activity

Adapted with permission from Potach D, Ellenbecker T. Clients with orthopedic, injury, and rehabilitation concerns. In: Earle R, Baechle T, editors. *NSCA's Essentials of Personal Training.* Champaign (IL): Human Kinetics; 2004. p. 533–56.

Medications for Strains and Sprains

The goal of medical therapy is to reduce pain during the acute phase of recovery. Medications commonly used to manage pain and inflammation after acute injury are listed in Table 8.4. Be advised that all medications are accompanied by a risk of toxicity and side effects, and knowledge of such risks should be fully understood prior to use. Recommendation of over-the-counter medications is best made by qualified health care providers, including medical doctors, physical therapists, nurse practitioners, physician assistants, and the like.

Exercise to Reduce Risk of Strains and Sprains

Appropriate exercises can mitigate the risks of strains and sprains. With regard to connective tissue, physiologic adaptations to resistance training increase ligament and tendon strength, and collagen content, to enhance the overall integrity of connective tissue (41). Similarly, muscle fiber size, fast twitch fibers, and rate of force production increase with resistance training as well, for an overall increase in muscle and connective tissue durability. To reduce the risk of muscle strain, encourage the client to practice the following preventative strategies:

1. Warm up 5 to 7 minutes prior to vigorous exercise using large muscle group activities such as walking, jogging, cycling, or rowing ergometry.

TABLE 8.4 COMMON MEDICATIONS FOR TREATMENT OF MUSCULOSKELETAL INJURIES

Class	Generic Name	Brand Name	Effect
NSAIDs	Ibuprofen	Motrin, Ibuprin	Analgesic, anti-inflammatory, antipyretic
	Naproxen	Naprosyn, Anaprox, Naprelan	
Analgesic	Acetaminophen	Tylenol, Feverall, Tempra	Pain control with sedating properties
	Hydrocodone + acetaminophen	Vicodin, Lorcet-HD, Lortab	
	Acetaminophen + codeine	Tylenol with Codeine	

Adapted with permission from Potach D, Ellenbecker T. Clients with orthopedic, injury, and rehabilitation concerns. In: Earle R, Baechle T, editors. *NSCA's Essentials of Strength Training and Conditioning.* Champaign (IL): Human Kinetics; 2004. p. 533–56.

2. Stretch tight muscles after the general warm-up, holding each stretch for 15 to 30 seconds.
3. Balance regular physical activities/sports with resistance exercises.
4. If possible, avoid exercise/sport when fatigued. Fatigue can increase the risk of injury (22). Balance this with the reality that at certain phases in an athlete's training program, fatigue is a desired outcome to induce specific adaptations.

OVERUSE INJURIES

Injuries are generally categorized as acute or overuse. Acute injuries typically occur with a single traumatic event such as joint sprains and muscle strains, joint dislocation, or fracture. Joint sprains and strains were discussed previously. This section will focus on overuse injuries that result from repetitive microtrauma and occur over time. Examples of overuse injury include tendinopathies, plantar fasciitis (PF), and low back pain (LBP).

Tendinopathy

Tendinopathy is a pathological change in the tendon because of repeated stress or microtraumas. The most common tendinopathies include tendinitis and tendinosis. *Tendinitis* is an acute inflammatory tendinopathy (83). *Tendinosis* describes a tendon with significant degenerative changes in the absence of an inflammatory response. Tendinosis is more common of the two as most individuals seek treatment only after the acute inflammatory process has resolved (66, 83). Common sites for tendinopathies include rotator cuff, common wrist flexor and extensor tendons, patellar tendon, and Achilles tendon (66).

Clinical Presentation/Assessment

Tendinopathies often result from overload injuries that disrupt the MTU. This overload usually occurs with an acute increase in activity or load. For example, increased mileage in the case of runners or increased repetitive motions in the case of those engaged in racquet sports (23, 40). These specific examples of overload are some of the most common mechanisms for tendinopathies. Other causes include premature return to occupational and/or sport and leisure activities after an injury. Individuals with tendinopathies often present with swelling (if acute) and pain, particularly with contraction or stretch of the involved muscle (23, 25). Assessment of tendinopathy includes evaluating strength and extensibility of the muscle and palpation of the involved tendon to determine tenderness (85).

Safe and Effective Exercise

For exercises that do not involve the affected joint/extremity, refer to Chapter 4 for exercise guidelines. For the affected area, the following considerations are important. Until pain has subsided, individuals should reduce activity of the affected muscle to decrease repetitive loading of the damaged tendon. Most individuals improve with conservative treatment that includes rest, stretching, ice, and/or use of analgesics (83). It should be noted that it might take up to 6 months for symptoms to subside. Once symptoms have decreased, strengthening of the affected area is appropriate. There is considerable evidence that supports the use of appropriately graded eccentric exercise as a safe and effective means for strengthening the MTU across the affected joint (44, 66, 83). Examples of exercises for tendinopathies can be found later in this section.

Exercise Considerations for Tendinopathies

The frequency, intensity, time, and type of eccentric exercise (FITT) is somewhat variable in the literature. However, a review of multiple studies reported a decrease in pain and return to activity with eccentric exercise (81). Refer to Table 8.5 for specific guidelines.

TABLE 8.5 EXERCISE GUIDELINES FOR TENDINOPATHIES AND PF

Condition	Type	
	Resistance	**Flexibility/Stretching**
Tendinosis		
Type	Eccentric until pain free; then add concentric and plyometrics as tolerated	Passive elongation of the muscle/tendon
Frequency	3–4 sessions·wk^{-1}	Daily
Intensity	6–15 reps 3–4 sets – use body weight with progressive loading as tolerated	3 reps • Gradual force to provide gentle stretch
Time	Completion of reps/sets or until pain level reaches threshold to stop exercise	Hold each rep 30 s
Special considerations	Concentric exercise should be avoided early in the healing process until nonsport activities are pain free (44)	
PF		
Type		• Gentle stretch of the fascia to the point of tension • Stretching: great toe flexors and gastroc soleus
Frequency		3 times a day
Intensity		10 reps (hold 10 s)
Time		To completion of reps
Special considerations	Pain determines exercise intensity and duration	

Plantar Fasciitis

Plantar fasciitis occurs most commonly with repeated trauma to the origin of the plantar fascia on the medial calcaneal tubercle. This is a common injury in athletes where running is involved. The pathology results from repeated stretching of the fascia during weight-bearing exercise (82)

Clinical Presentation/Assessment

Classic symptoms for PF include pain with first weight-bearing steps in the morning or during the first few minutes of running. Pain usually subsides with activity and increases after prolonged rest. Barefoot walking may exacerbate pain as well (6). Tight plantarflexor muscles along with either pes planus (flat foot) or pes cavus (high arch) may predispose an individual to PF (6, 23, 82).

Assessment of PF includes palpation along the plantar fascia, evaluating extensibility of the gastrocnemius, and a thorough client history. At the acute stage, PF is best managed with control of pain and minimal exercise. Pain management is often accomplished with nonsteroidal anti-inflammatory drugs (NSAIDs), ice massage, and minimizing excess stress on the fascia (*i.e.*, avoiding barefoot walking) (82).

Safe and Effective Exercise

As the acute phase subsides, it is important to introduce stretching of the plantar fascia as well as the plantarflexors (11, 51). Functional weight-bearing exercises may relieve stress on the plantar fascia by supporting the medial longitudinal arch. This is accomplished by strengthening the extrinsic (anterior and posterior tibialis and the peroneus longus) and the intrinsic (abductor hallucis, flexor hallucis brevis, flexor digitorum brevis, abductor digiti minimi, and dorsal interossei) musculature (19, 24). Examples of appropriate functional weight-bearing exercises include toe and heel raises (extrinsics) and short foot exercises (intrinsics) (35, 36). Qualified professionals may provide orthotic intervention, or taping may be beneficial in supporting the involved structures during weight-bearing exercises (51).

Examples of Safe and Effective Exercises for Overuse Injuries

As previously noted, exercises to address tendinopathies should focus initially on eccentric loading and stretching. Examples of these exercises are shown for calf, wrist, and foot in Figures 8.1 through 8.4.

Table 8.5 includes exercise guidelines for tendinopathies and PF. As indicated at the bottom of the table, pain should be the limiting factor in the intensity and duration of exercise, and the degree of stretch.

Low Back Pain

Low back pain (LBP) could be considered traumatic, acute, or chronic. It is estimated that LBP affects 60% to 80% of the adult population at some point in their lives, with an 80% recovery rate within 4 to 6 weeks, regardless of treatment (50). Unfortunately, unless the underlying cause of the pain is treated, the recurrence of LBP is quite high. There are many causes of LBP, including disc compression, degenerative changes in the lumbar spine, various joint and bone pathologies, and muscle imbalances (39). This discussion will center on general LBP resulting from issues of muscle imbalance.

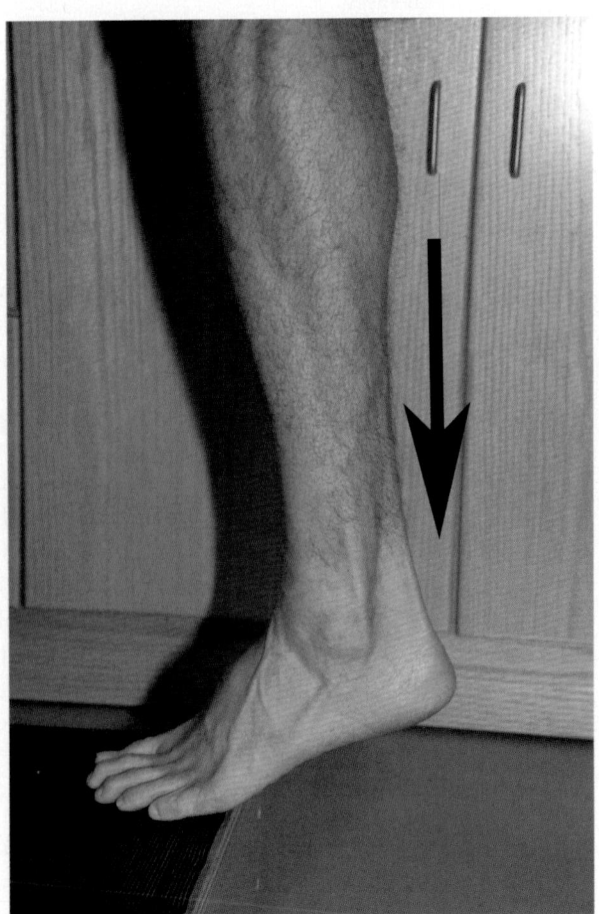

FIGURE 8.1. Eccentric loading of the gastrocnemius. Stand on the edge of a step. Using the uninvolved leg, raise up on toes (plantarflexed position), shift weight to involved leg, and slowly lower to start position. To avoid concentric contractions during the painful stage of healing, ensure that uninvolved limb is used to lift body weight.

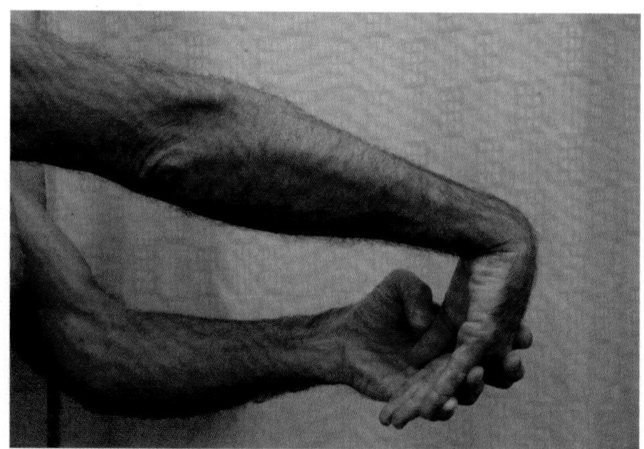

FIGURE 8.2. Stretching exercise for lateral epicondylitis. While sitting or standing, flex the wrist with opposite hand while elbow is extended. Apply pressure until a gentle stretch is felt at the elbow or forearm (wrist extensor) muscles.

Muscles important to the function of the spine are commonly referred to as the core, consisting of multiple layers of muscles that act to stabilize the spine, pelvis, and kinetic chain during functional movements (15). Core muscles are thought to provide a stable base of support to allow for optimal performance of the spine and extremities and help prevent injury. Also, endurance of core musculature is more critical to overall low back health than strength (Table 8.6) (49).

Clinical Presentation/Assessment

Research indicates that core muscle activity is different in clients with LBP. The inability of core muscles to adequately stabilize the spine can lead to pain, usually intensified with movement especially toward end of the range and with prolonged postures. Pain questionnaires and other outcome measures are often used to subjectively quantify pain and functional impairment. Examples are the *Oswestry Low Back Pain Scale* (14) and the *McGill Pain Scale* (53).

Safe and Effective Exercise

Core stabilization exercises do not fit the normal FITT template, but should be incorporated into daily activities and any general exercise program (74). Core stabilization programs progress through various stages of increasing difficulty or intensity. Stage I, which McGill (48) refers to as abdominal bracing, involves learning to engage the small, deep stabilizing muscles that include the transverse abdominis and multifidi muscles, primarily in a supine position. In stage II, cocontraction of these deep muscles of the core is required while in more challenging positions (*i.e.*, quadruped). Movement

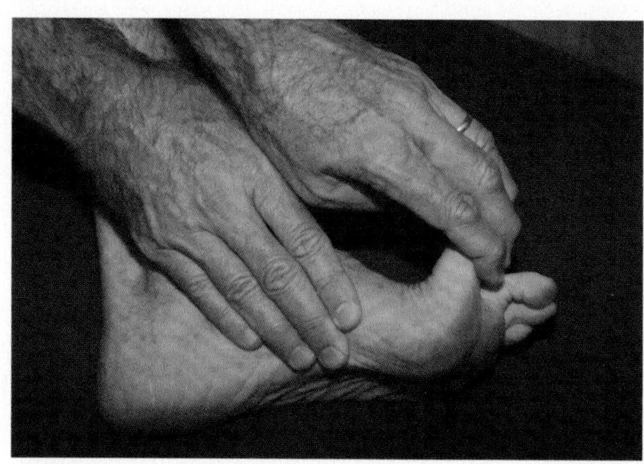

FIGURE 8.3. Stretching exercise for PF. Sitting with involved foot resting on opposite knee, apply stretch by extending great toe. Fingers of opposite hand can be used to massage tight fascia of arch.

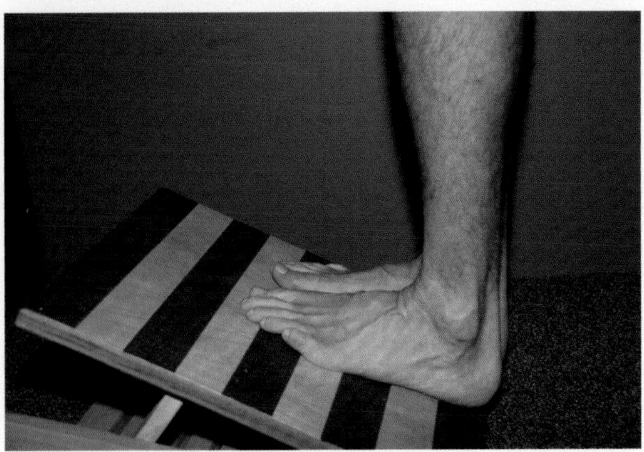

FIGURE 8.4. Stretching exercise for gastroc soleus. Stand on slanted surface, lean body forward keeping heels in contact with surface until a gentle stretch is felt in the posterior calf.

of the extremities is also added in this stage. Stage III focuses on maintaining cocontraction of the deep stabilizing muscles while performing exercises designed to recruit larger stabilizers in more functional positions. Regardless of the stage, it is critical for the client to maintain cocontraction of the deep stabilizers. When stabilization can no longer be maintained, the exercise should be stopped. Kolber and Beekhuizen (39) discuss safe and effective lumbar stabilization exercises for LBP, (see Table 8.6) and progressions of core exercises are illustrated elsewhere (15). Examples of selected core exercises are shown in Figures 8.5 through 8.7.

In stage I (Fig. 8.5), it is important to develop the abdominal drawing-in maneuver (39). This is referred to as "connecting your abdominals" and is a critical component of all core stabilization exercises.

Position: Lie on back with knees bent and arms relaxed.

Action: Tighten pelvic floor muscles (as if you were stopping the flow of urine); then draw in lower abdomen as if pulling belly button away from waistband. Think about pulling "up and in" like a zipper zipping up from your pelvis to your ribs (rather than down toward the mat).

TABLE 8.6 CORE MUSCULATURE

Classification	Muscle	Action
Global stabilizers	Erector spinae	Extension of vertebral column
	External obliques	Flexion of vertebral column with bilateral contraction and rotation of vertebral column with unilateral contraction
	Quadratus lumborum	Assists with extension, lateral flexion of lumbar vertebral column
	Rectus abdominis	Flexes vertebral column
Local stabilizers	Internal obliques	Flexion of vertebral column with bilateral contraction and rotation of vertebral column with unilateral contraction
	Multifidus	Extension of vertebral column with bilateral contraction and rotation of vertebral column with unilateral contraction
	Transversus abdominis	Draw abdominal wall toward spine. Helps maintain abdominal pressure

Adapted with permission from Kolber M, Beekhuizen K. Lumbar stabilization: An evidence-based approach for the athlete with low back pain. *Strength Cond J.* 2007;29(2):26–37.

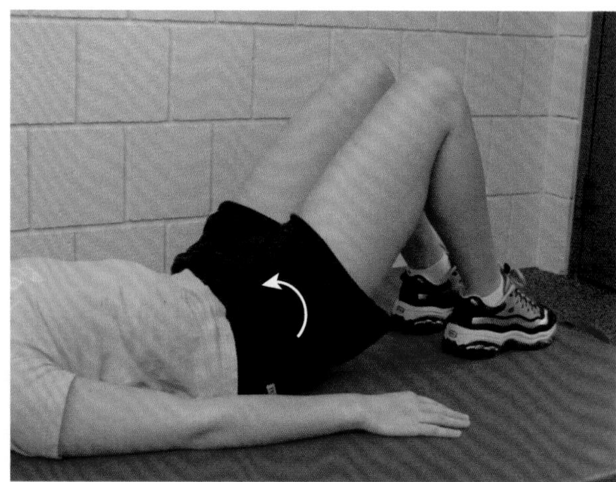

FIGURE 8.5. Example of stage I core stabilization exercise: isolating the transverse abdominis (TA).

Hold for a count of six; repeat four times. Avoid holding breath and flattening back (posterior pelvic tilt).

A stage II exercise shown in Figure 8.6 requires first a contraction of the transverse abdominis followed by simultaneously raising the diagonal arm and leg. Raise the arm to vertical and raise the leg to 45°. Return to starting position and repeat with the other diagonal pair, alternating in a rhythmic fashion. Maintain contact between the lumbar spine and the floor while moving arms and legs. The stage III exercise shown in Figure 8.7 requires connection of the abdominals followed by a lunge forward while maintaining pelvis and spine in a neutral (vertical) position. Return to starting position and repeat with other leg. Strive to maintain a vertical torso without side-to-side movement during the lunge.

Table 8.7 includes exercise guidelines for clients who suffer from LBP. Often, but not always, LBP may be alleviated through systematically strengthening the core muscles and posture training.

Medication for Overuse Injuries

Analgesics may be used to decrease pain and inflammation associated with tendinopathy. Although most over-the-counter analgesics are safe to use, it is important to know what type of analgesic is taken and its effect on pain, as it may mask or dampen pain that is a marker of exercise tolerance. Also, some analgesics such as NSAIDs may cause gastrointestinal (GI) bleeding with chronic use. Although there is limited evidence that steroid injections may have some positive short-term effects, multiple studies document the adverse effects of fascial or tendon degeneration and/or rupture resulting from injections (51).

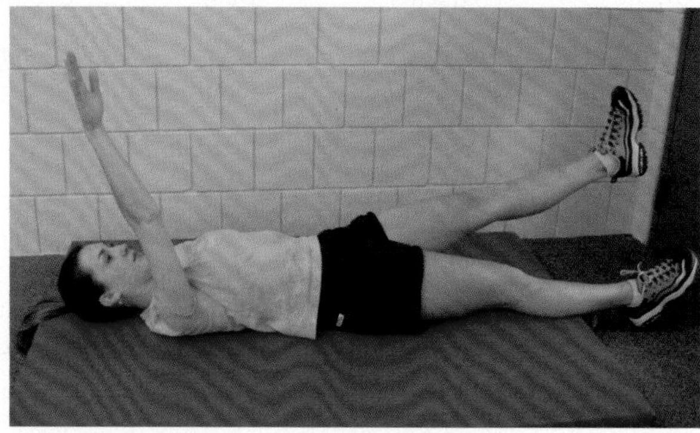

FIGURE 8.6. Example of stage II core stabilization exercise: opposing arm and leg.

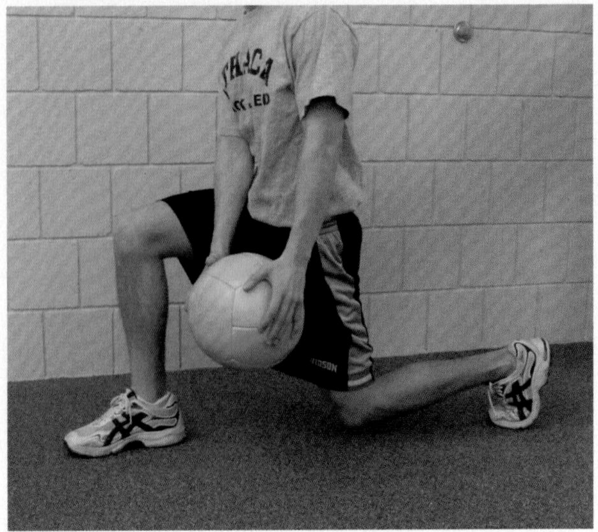

FIGURE 8.7. Example of stage III core stabilization exercise: lunge with medicine ball.

CHRONIC CONDITIONS

Chronic conditions are prolonged in duration and do not resolve spontaneously and are rarely cured completely. It is estimated that more than 75% of health care costs are due to treating chronic conditions (70). In this section, we will discuss two chronic conditions: arthritis and osteoporosis.

Arthritis

Arthritis is an inflammation of a joint. The two most common types of arthritis are rheumatoid arthritis and osteoarthritis (38).

TABLE 8.7 EXERCISE GUIDELINES FOR LBP

	Type		
	Weight-Bearing Aerobic	**Resistance**	**Flexibility/Stretching**
	Fast walking	Curl ups, bridging, bird dog	Limit exercises to unloaded flexion/extension
Frequency	Daily	2–3 times a week	
Intensity	% of maximum	High reps and low loads	
Time	Build up to 30 min·d^{-1}		
Special considerations	Exercise during the 1st or 2nd hour after rising from bed should be avoided because of disc hydration and subsequent loading. Any exercise that increases the intensity or frequency of pain should be discontinued, and the client should be referred for further evaluation. Exercises resulting in high-impact loading should be avoided		

Adapted with permission from McGill S. *Ultimate Back Fitness and Performance*. 3rd ed. Waterloo (ON): Backfitpro Inc.; 2006.

Rheumatoid Arthritis

Rheumatoid arthritis (RA) is an autoimmune, chronic inflammatory disease affecting the synovial lining of joints and other connective tissue. RA is a slowly progressing disease that, in the United States, affects 1 in 12 adult women and 1 in 20 adult men with symptoms that cycle through periods of exacerbation and remission (7).

Clinical Presentation/Assessment

Individuals with RA typically present with severe joint pain and inflammation, reduced muscle mass, decreased muscular strength and endurance, and decreased mobility and impaired physical activity. Loss of muscle strength is due to rheumatic cachexia, which creates a cytokine-driven hypermetabolism and protein degradation. RA is also associated with the increased risk of cardiovascular disease that appears to be independent of normal cardiovascular risk factors (5, 68).

Assessment of RA includes a thorough client history, ROM and strength tests, and appropriate outcome measures to determine the stage of the disease and the client's functional status. These assessments should be performed by a qualified health care professional.

Safe and Effective Exercise

Regular dynamic and isometric exercises are effective for improving muscular strength, cardiorespiratory function, and cardiovascular health in individuals with RA (57). Exercise can also reduce pain, morning joint stiffness, and fatigue. Individuals with RA can perform moderate-intensity exercises with little or no joint damage (80). Individuals with RA should be encouraged to pursue activities of daily living that require movement, as the benefits of an exercise program are lost when no longer continued (5, 68). Refer to Table 8.8 for specific exercise guidelines.

Osteoarthritis

Osteoarthritis (OA) is a relatively common chronic degenerative joint disease that is more prevalent with age (34). In the affected joint(s), OA first presents as deficits in articular cartilage of synovial

TABLE 8.8 EXERCISE GUIDELINES FOR RA AND OA

	Type		
	Weight-Bearing Aerobic	**Resistance**	**Flexibility/Stretching**
Type	Walking, cycling, rowing, swimming	Weight machines, isometric exercise, elastic bands	
Frequency	3–5 d·wk^{-1}	2–3 d·wk^{-1}	Daily
Intensity	60%–80% of maximum, RPE = 11–16	Use pain tolerance to set %MVC	
Time	Start with 5 min and build to 30 min per session	2–3 reps × 1 set building to 10–12 reps × 3 sets	
Special considerations for RA	With acute exacerbation, avoid high-intensity resistance exercises to minimize joint damage. Those with significant damage of large joints (assessed radiographically) should avoid moderate- to high-intensity weight-bearing exercise to avoid further damage (10)		
Special considerations for OA	Avoid overstretching unstable joints. Avoid high-resistance and high-impact exercise. Pain should be minimal. No strenuous exercise during acute flare-ups of OA and during periods of inflammation		

Adapted with permission from Minor M. Exercise in the treatment of osteoarthritis. *Rheum Dis Clin North Am.* 1999;25(2):397–415.

joints (58). As OA evolves, bone remodeling and overgrowth at the joint margins also occurs. OA is thought to be the result of mechanical injury due to excessive loading or repeated low-force stressors (38). The most common anatomical locations for OA are the large weight-bearing joints, including the hips and knees, the cervical and lumbar spine, the distal interphalangeal joints of the fingers, and carpometacarpal joint of the thumb (38).

Clinical Presentation/Assessment

Individuals with OA often present with pain, joint stiffness, decreased strength, and decreased cardiovascular fitness. Assessments for OA include a thorough client history, ROM and strength testing, and evaluation of cardiovascular fitness. As part of the client history, pain can be evaluated using a variety of pain questionnaires.

Safe and Effective Exercise

Evidence supports initiation or continuation of exercise for individuals with OA (13, 28, 57, 58). Exercise improves overall function and prevents disability. Improved flexibility, muscular strength, cardiovascular fitness, and quality of life, along with decreased pain, are reported with exercise. Exercise may include land-based or aquatic-based programs. Aquatic programs provide an alternative environment that may benefit clients who do not tolerate land-based exercise because of pain or obesity (27). Individuals should exercise at times when pain from OA is minimal or when pain medication is at peak effectiveness. Individuals with OA may experience discomfort during or immediately after exercise. However, if joint pain persists or increases beyond preexercise level, then duration and/or intensity should be reduced (79).

Medication Effects for RA and OA

Individuals should be aware that prolonged and/or excessive use of NSAIDs can cause GI bleeding (58). Also, RA-remitting drugs may cause secondary organ disease, including myopathy. Steroids may predispose individuals to stress fractures. Finally, oral corticosteroids may cause skeletal myopathy, truncal obesity, osteoporosis, and GI bleeding (57).

Exercise Guidelines for OA and RA

Examples of safe and effective aerobic and resistance exercises for RA and OA are shown in Figure 8.8 below. Additional details regarding exercise guidelines are supplied in Table 8.8. As indicated in the table, exercise should be avoided during periods of symptom flare-ups. However, regular, systematic exercise can be effective for preserving physical function and independence in those with RA and OA (20).

Osteoporosis

Osteoporosis, or the "silent disease," is characterized by low bone density or bone mass and deterioration of the bone microarchitecture and/or geometry that increases skeletal fragility and risk of fracture (8, 29, 31). It often goes undetected because early stages lack clear or overt symptoms. Diagnosis of osteoporosis is based on bone densitometry measured by dual-energy X-ray absorptiometry (DEXA or DXA) scan. Scan results are compared with those of an ethnicity- and gender-matched, 30-year-old reference. Bone density within +1.0 and -1.0 standard deviation (SD) unit (or T score) of the reference density is considered normal. A density score of -2.5 SD units or lower is deemed osteoporosis. *Osteopenia* is between normal and osteoporosis and describes those at risk for osteoporosis, with a density SD of -1.0 to -2.5 (12, 60).

It should be noted that DEXA does not evaluate trabecular bone architecture, an indicator of overall bone strength. However, imaging technology to measure bone architecture (quantitative computed tomography or QCT; peripheral QCT or pQCT; magnetic resonance imaging or MRI) is not used universally at this time, and thus the definitions for bone density status currently rely on the more commonly used DEXA measure of bone density (65).

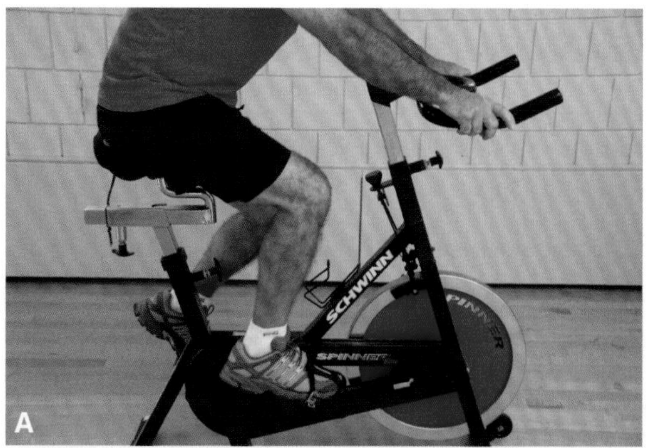

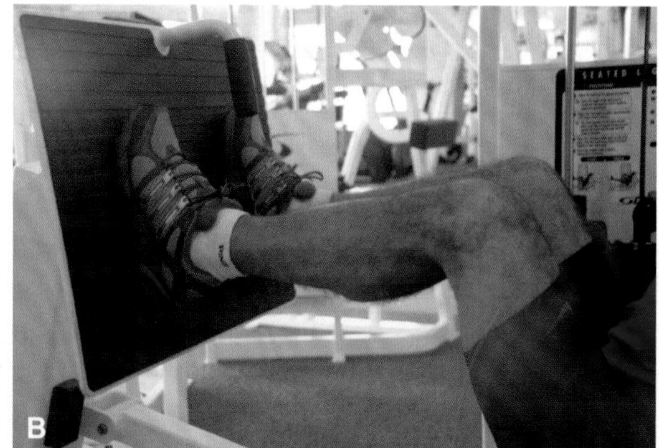

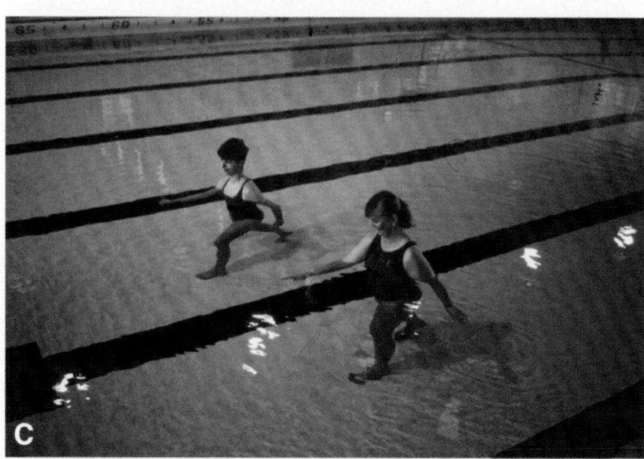

FIGURE 8.8. Types of aerobic and resistance exercises for persons with RA and OA.

Prevalence

Osteoporosis is largely preventable, yet is a serious public health concern that afflicts one in two women and one in five men older than 50 years (72). Women are three times more likely to suffer from osteoporosis (72). In the United States, there are approximately 10 million women and men who have osteoporosis, 34 million who are at risk for developing osteoporosis, and more than 1.5 million osteoporotic fractures per year (52). Because osteoporosis often leads to fracture, it may result in loss of workdays or employment and increased hospitalizations. The economic burden of osteoporotic fractures, including loss of work, loss of independence, and cost of treatment, is substantial and has been estimated to be $20 billion in the United States and $30 billion in the European Union (8). More significantly, the loss of function in older adults due to osteoporotic fractures or related pain is a risk factor for loss of independence. The most prevalent types of osteoporotic fracture in later life are of the hip, spine, and forearm (31). Treatment and rehabilitation can translate into a long hospital visit and subsequent physical therapy before one can manage on their own. However, disuse atrophy after surgical repair compounds a potentially long, arduous recovery, and the osteoporotic fracture can easily develop into a life-threatening event for an older adult (60). More than 70% of osteoporotic fractures occur in those older than 70 years and present a direct threat to aging independently — a goal of most older adults. In fact, up to 20% of older adults hospitalized with an acute fracture die within 6 months (73).

Risk Factors for Osteoporosis

In addition to those who have osteoporosis, many others have low bone density or osteopenia, which predisposes one to osteoporosis. There is much still to be learned about the cause(s) of osteoporosis and osteopenia; however, research indicates a number of risk factors for developing low

TABLE 8.9 RISK FACTORS FOR BONE LOSS, OSTEOPOROSIS, AND FRACTURE

Nonmodifiable Risk Factors	Modifiable Risk Factors	Disorders Associated with Osteoporosis
Female	Physical inactivity	Previous low body weight
Aging	Low calcium intake (<500–850 mg·d^{-1})	RA
Family history of osteoporosis or hip fracture	Vitamin D deficiency Smoker (current)	Malabsorption syndromes (including chronic liver disease, inflammatory bowel disease)
White or Asian ethnicity	Excessive alcohol consumption Excessive caffeine intake	Primary hyperparathyroidism
Loss of height and thoracic kyphosis	Excessive soda consumption	Long-term immobilization
Small body frame	Low strength/physical capability	
Natural or surgical menopause before age 45	Low body weight (BMI <19) Amenorrhea, including female athlete triad	
Previous fracture after low-energy trauma	Low testosterone in males Impaired vision Impaired hearing Postural hypotension Unstable/risky environment (low light, uneven floor, unsecured carpets) Poor fitting footwear, need for assistive devices Multiple medications	

Adapted from Finigan J, Greenfield DM, Blumsohn A, et al. Risk factors for vertebral and nonvertebral fracture over 10 years: A population-based study in women. *J Bone Miner Res.* 2008;23(1):75–85 (Ref. 16); Iacono MV. Osteoporosis: A national public health priority. *J Perianesth.* 2007;22(3):175–80; Keen R. Osteoporosis: Strategies for prevention and management. Best practice & research. *Clin Rheumatol.* 2007;21(1):109–22; Skinner JS, editor. *Exercise Testing and Exercise Prescription for Special Cases.* 3rd ed. Philadelphia (PA): Lippincott Williams & Wilkins; 2005. 173 p. (Ref. 75).

bone density. Table 8.9 includes both modifiable and nonmodifiable risk factors that increase the chances of developing osteoporosis. Modifiable risk factors can be influenced by lifestyle choices and indicate that we do have some control and influence over bone health.

Growth, Maturation, and Bone Density

Osteoporosis is classified as *primary* or *secondary*. Primary osteoporosis is age related, and secondary osteoporosis is due to other factors such as drug regimens for treating other diseases that can decrease bone at any time during the lifespan (47). The *female athlete triad* is an example of secondary osteoporosis and begins with disordered eating followed by amenorrhea and can result in early-onset osteoporosis (76).

Peak bone density, or highest lifetime bone density, is achieved in the 20s, and loss of bone density begins around the age of 25 to 30 (18). Recent longitudinal data indicate that bone loss begins earlier in men (25–39 yr) than women (40–44 yr) (2). Men and women lose bone at about the same rate until women begin to approach menopause, which occurs around the age of 52. Bone loss accelerates in women in late perimenopause (40–50 yr) and continues at an increased rate through early postmenopausal years (17, 55, 59, 62, 76). Although the rate of loss varies, within the early postmenopausal decade, bone loss is more evident in cortical bone and often signaled by a low-energy trauma fracture of the wrist/forearm (17, 45, 71, 78). A low-energy trauma occurs from forces due to a fall from standing height or lower (65). On the other hand, late postmenopause

(>10 yr after menopause) is marked by increased loss of trabecular bone, which comprises much of the hip and spine and contributes to the increased incidence of hip and vertebral crush fractures in older adults (17, 59). Following a 5- to 10-year period of rapid postmenopausal bone loss, rate of loss returns to premenopausal values or slows down again (46). The increased rate of loss after menopause and overall lower peak bone mass in women likely contribute to the higher incidence of osteoporosis and fragility fractures in women (64). However, men are also at risk for developing osteoporosis (59). Owing to a higher lifetime peak bone density in men, increased risk of osteoporotic fracture occurs about 10 years later than in women. That is, for men, fracture risk increases after age 65 (2).

Over the past two decades, studies of children indicate that most bone growth occurs by the end of the second decade of life, or the late teens to early 20s, with the achievement of peak bone mass and density in the 20s. The implication of this is critically important for our understanding of developing and maintaining healthy bone throughout the lifespan. Because all individuals will lose bone density and mass after the peak bone years, the goal for healthy aging of bone is to maximize the development of peak bone (achieve a high lifetime peak bone level) and minimize the rate of bone loss throughout the lifespan. In doing so, the lowest lifetime bone density, which usually occurs in later life, will still be high enough to protect from osteoporotic fracture. It appears that the age range around puberty (13–15 yr) is the time of peak bone velocity when bone growth occurs at the fastest lifetime rate. Bone growth that occurs during this critical period is highly associated with the amount of bone lost during the last four decades of life (30, 43). Although genetics plays an important role in overall bone mass, nutrition and physical activity are equally important influences on the development of bone. Therefore, particular attention should be paid to these lifestyle behaviors during the critical prepubertal years (10–12 yr) when bone is most responsive to the exercise stimulus. Maximizing bone growth during puberty will confer important benefits to bone health in later life (4, 43).

Inactivity and Bone Health

Cessation of bone-stimulating exercise may result in some loss of bone; however, the rate of loss and resultant bone density remains higher in young male athletes 5 years after retiring from competition, compared with their sedentary counterparts (63). The rate of loss and absolute amount of bone loss will likely vary, depending on other factors during one's lifetime (*e.g.*, bed rest, nutrition, medications, and alcohol use). Likewise, research indicates that exercise-induced bone gains in males and females, particularly during childhood and adolescence, confers benefits later in life and reduces the risk of developing osteoporosis and fragility fractures (63). In contrast, detraining studies indicate that low-exercise (low exercise intensity and volume) induced bone density in older adults is transient and may not persist after cessation of exercise (9, 33, 77, 84). Thus, for older adults who seek to maintain bone or minimize bone loss with age, it is important to continue to exercise.

Dietary Support for Bone Health

Nutritional support for bone growth and maintenance requires adequate amounts of calcium and vitamin D. The Institute of Medicine 2010 recommendations for calcium and vitamin D intake are shown in Table 8.10 (32). However, evidence indicates that overconsumption of these nutrients may be harmful, so knowledge of these nutrient sources is important.

Medications for Bone Health

There are several pharmacological agents to increase or preserve bone, or reduce bone loss. The common categories of agents to combat osteoporosis are shown in Table 8.11. Most are used in older adults, particularly postmenopausal women, and knowledge of risks associated with each drug should be considered before choosing to use a drug.

TABLE 8.10 DIETARY REFERENCE INTAKES FOR CALCIUM AND VITAMIN D

Age Group	Calcium			Vitamin D		
	Estimated Average Requirement (mg·d^{-1})	Recommended Dietary Allowance (mg·d^{-1})	Upper Level Intake (mg·d^{-1})	Estimated Average Requirement (mg·d^{-1})	Recommended Dietary Allowance (mg·d^{-1})	Upper Level Intake (mg·d^{-1})
0–6 mo	200	200	1,000	400	400	1,000
6–12 mo	260	260	1,500	400	400	1,500
1–3 yr	500	700	2,500	400	600	2,500
4–8 yr	800	1,000	2,500	400	600	3,000
9–13 yr	1,100	1,300	3,000	400	600	4,000
14–18 yr	1,300	1,300	3,000	400	600	4,000
19–30 yr	800	1,000	2,500	400	600	4,000
31–50 yr	800	1,000	2,500	400	600	4,000
51–70 yr males	800	1,000	2,000	400	600	4,000
51–70 yr females	1,000	1,200	2,000	400	600	4,000
>70 yr	1,000	1,200	2,000	400	600	4,000
14–18 yr pregnant/lactating	1,300	1,300	3,000	400	600	4,000
19–50 yr pregnant/lactating	800	1,000	2,500	400	600	4,000

Adapted from Institute of Medicine. DRIs for Calcium and Vitamin D Report [Internet]. Institute-of-Medicine; [cited 2011 Jul 12]. Available from: http://www.iom.edu/Reports/2010/Dietary-Reference-Intakes-for-Calcium-and-Vitamin-D.aspx

Exercise for Bone Health

Physical activity prevents osteoporosis by increasing bone-forming osteoblast cell activity and reducing the bone-resorbing osteoclast activity for an overall osteogenic effect of bone growth or slowing of bone loss. Bone adapts positively to sufficient and appropriate levels of stress. Strain magnitude (the quantity of load) and frequency of load (how rapidly load is imposed) on bone are imperative for bone growth and to minimize bone loss (42). Bone adaptation to stressors is site- and load-specific, meaning that only bone that is stressed appropriately will adapt favorably (9). This explains why activities such as jogging confer little benefit to appendicular bones of the upper body. Therefore, development of an appropriate and effective exercise program should consider the following: current state of bone health; site of adaption; appropriate degree of strain via force, torque, or compression; safety of exercise for the individual; and likelihood of compliance.

Bone-growing exercise is important at all ages; therefore, it is warranted to consider the age and other needs of the client when choosing appropriate and desirable exercises. However, appropriate forms of resistance-type exercise are necessary to stimulate bone at any age (29). For example, exercises for an adolescent or young adult may include agility or plyometrics and would likely differ from those for a postmenopausal woman who is largely sedentary. Also consider other needs of the client with respect to physical function and select exercises that may satisfy more than one objective such as exercises to improve balance and coordination and to reduce the risk of falls in older adults. Falls often result in fracture in older adults, so an exercise strategy to reduce fall risk and improve posture could indirectly benefit bone health

TABLE 8.11 PHARMACOLOGICAL AGENTS FOR TREATMENT OF OSTEOPOROSIS

Agent	Effect	Potential Side Effects	Comments
Calcium and vitamin D	Development and maintenance of bone	Calcium-gas, constipation. Vitamin D – generally none unless taking too much	Efficacy is questionable in those with already normal calcium and vitamin D levels
Selective estrogen receptor modulators (SERM)	Prevention and treatment. Estrogen agonist in bone and fat; antagonist in breast and endometrium	Hot flashes, leg cramps, and blood clots	May not be effective for nonvertebral fractures; decreased risk for breast cancer
Hormone replacement therapy (HRT)	Prevention only. Decreased risk for vertebral and nonvertebral fracture	Cancer, myocardial infarction, stroke, blood clot	Usually considered for short-term use for menopausal symptoms
Bisphosphonate	Prevention and treatment. Decreased bone resorption by osteoclast inhibition	GI disturbance (can use IV alternative); heartburn, esophageal irritation, headache, constipation, gas, diarrhea	Generally effective at all clinical bone sites. Long-term use may increase the risk of femur fracture (21, 61)
Strontium ranelate	Treatment only. Decreased bone resorption	GI disturbance, blood clot	Approved in EU, not in United States
Parathyroid hormone (PTH)	Treatment only. Increased bone deposition	Bone cancer in rat studies	Injection only. Continuous exposure to PTH causes (bone resorption
Calcitonin	Treatment only. Modest reduction in the risk of vertebral fractures	Stomach upset and flushing	May relieve pain associated with bone fractures

Adapted from Deal CL. Osteoporosis: Prevention, diagnosis, and management. *Am J Med.* 1997;102(1A):35S–9S and Keen R. Osteoporosis: Strategies for prevention and management. Best practice and research. *Clin Rheum.* 2007;21(1):109–22.

as well as overall physical function and independence. Likewise, back strengthening exercises for older adults to reduce thoracic hyperkyphosis (Dowager's hump) can reduce back pain and risk of falls (67).

Exercises that enhance bone growth and/or reduce loss of bone should be site-specific, be moderate-high compressive, and/or provide resistance, and must be pain free. Although there is no specific exercise prescription for those with or at risk for osteoporosis, it is recommended to alternate upper and lower body exercises to minimize risk of undue stress on tendons (65). Table 8.12 includes guidelines that incorporate characteristics of exercise important for improving or maintaining overall bone health. There is a wide variance in bone status among those with osteopenia and osteoporosis, and for that reason, prescribing exercise with particular attention to exercise intensity must be individualized and appropriate for each client.

Research in animals and humans indicates that whole body vibration (WBV; standing on a special, gently oscillating mechanical plate) for 10 to 20 minutes a day can reduce bone loss in the hip, although this is less clear for the spine (1). In addition, WBV can also increase lower limb muscle function to reduce fall risk (1). There is much still to learn about short- and long-term retention of WBV effects on bone and the dose-response relationship. Likewise, WBV is a higher risk type of exercise that must be administered under supervision and may not be appropriate for all older adults (1, 42, 54, 56).

Summary of Exercise Considerations for Osteoporosis

Intervention or prevention of osteoporosis is dependent on appropriate nutritional support and regular weight-bearing physical activity. To reduce the risk of fracture in later life, strategies to enhance bone health should begin early in life and seek to do the following (37):

- Maximize bone mass
- Maximize peak bone mass

TABLE 8.12 **EXERCISE GUIDELINES FOR PREVENTION AND TREATMENT OF OSTEOPOROSIS**

Condition	Type		
	Weight-Bearing Aerobic	**Resistance**	**Balance/ Posture/ Fall Prevention**
Healthy skeletal status			
Frequency	3–5 d·wk^{-1}	2–3 d·wk^{-1}	Daily
Intensity	Moderate to high	Moderate to high 60%–80% estimated 1 RM, 8–12 reps, progress to 80%–90% estimated 1 RM, 5–6 reps Impact jumps from floor, height of 1–2 in	
Time	30–60 min·d^{-1} — total exercise time (aerobic + resistance)		
At risk for osteoporosis			
Frequency	3–5 d·wk^{-1}	2–3 d·wk^{-1}	Daily
Intensity	Moderate to high	Moderate to high 60%–80% 1 RM, 8–12 reps progress slower to 80%–90% 1 RM, 5–6 reps Impact jumps from floor, height of 1–2 in	
Time	30–60 min·d^{-1} — total exercise time (aerobic + resistance)		
Osteoporosis			
Frequency	3–5 d·wk^{-1}	2–3 d·wk^{-1}	Daily
Intensity	40% to <60% Heart rate reserve or $\dot{V}O_{2max}$	Moderate Same as above, but consider individual circumstances	
Time	30–60 min·d^{-1} — total exercise time (aerobic + resistance + balance)		

Special Considerations

Avoid explosive, high-impact exercises, dynamic abdominal exercises (*e.g.*, sit-ups) exercises that involve twisting (*e.g.*, golf swing), bending, compression, or excessive flexion of spine. Provide posture education, fall prevention education, and movement education for lifting, bending, and carrying tasks to reduce fracture risk when doing activities of daily living.

Adapted from Petit F, Hughes C, Warpeha J. Exercise prescription for people with osteoporosis. In: Ehrman J, editor. *ACSM's Resource Manual for Guidelines for Exercise Testing and Prescription.* 6th ed. Philadelphia (PA): Wolters Kluwer/Lippincott Williams & Wilkins; 2010. p. 635–50; Pfeifer M, Sinaki M, Geusens P, Boonen S, Preisinger E, Minne HW. Musculoskeletal rehabilitation in osteoporosis: A review. *J Bone Miner Res.* 2004;19(8):1208–14; Skinner JS, editor. *Exercise Testing and Exercise Prescription for Special Cases.* 3rd ed. Philadelphia (PA): Lippincott Williams & Wilkins; 2005.

- Reduce age-related bone loss
- Prevent falls
- Avoid other risk factors for osteoporosis and fracture
- Reduce pain
- Reduce disability

Working with clients who are at risk for osteoporosis should include education about risk factors for osteoporosis and nutritional support, and an individualized exercise program, including weight-bearing aerobic, resistance, and core control exercises for balance, posture, and fall prevention. Exercise should be pain free, and the intensity should be guided by the strength and bone health status of the client. Physician clearance to exercise is warranted for a client diagnosed with osteoporosis. Further, clients with osteopenia or osteoporosis who have joint replacement should be cleared by a physician to exercise, and the Health Fitness Specialist should be aware of any and all physical activity limitations for these clients.

The rapidly increasing population of older adults means that osteoporosis will likely become even more prevalent in the near future (60). Knowledge of the disease process, risk factors, and exercise intervention strategies is essential to develop a safe and effective physical activity program for an osteoporotic client.

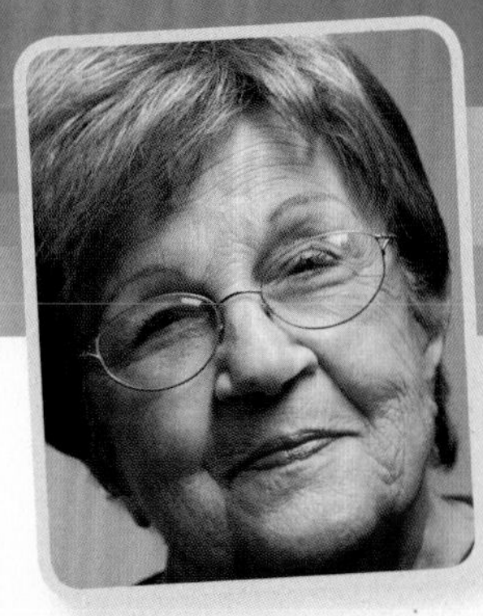

The Case of Mrs. Williams

Submitted by **Travis Michael Combest, RCEP, Walter Reed National Military Medical Center at Bethesda, Bethesda, MD**

A 75-year-old woman was recommended for exercise programming by her primary care physician to improve mobility and function and to decrease pain of OA symptoms. Mrs. Williams' exercise program for the past year was aquatic classes 45 minutes, 2 days a week. She came to her first appointment with symptom-limited ambulation and a walker, but a willingness to further her exercise program.

Narrative

A 75-year-old woman was recommended for exercise programming by her primary care physician to improve mobility and function and to decrease pain of OA symptoms. Mrs. Williams reports that her knee pain is "aching" and is 2–3/10 at rest. Notes from primary care physician indicates that Mrs. Williams has moderately severe OA in bilateral knees. She is symptom limited in walking more than 50 yards with pain of 5–6/10 and needing assistance with walking. Mrs. Williams reports for hospital visits, holding on to side rails of the walls and stopping every 50 yards. Mrs. Williams current exercise program for the past year are aquatic classes 45 minutes, 2 days a week. She came to her first appointment at the Fitness Center with symptom-limited ambulation and a walker, but a willingness to further her exercise program.

Physical Information

Height: 64 in
Weight: 171.7 lb
Body mass index (BMI): 29.5 kg·m^{-2}
Body fat percentage (measured by direct segmental bioelectrical impedance Inbody 520 by Biospace, Inc.): 51.4

The Case of Mrs. Williams cont.

Medical History from Primary Care Physician

Osteoarthritis
Type 2 diabetes
Hypertension
High cholesterol

Physical Assessments

Strength: dynamometer
Hip flexion: right, 20 lb; left, 18 lb
Leg extension: right, 15 lb; left, 10 lb
Physical activity limited by knee pain, lower body weakness

Activity Plan

Add progressive muscular and functional conditioning plan 2 days a week with aquatic aerobics.

Goals

1. Increase strength in lower extremities.
2. Increase mobility and function for quality of life.
3. Decrease pain at rest and during activity.

Exercise Program

Aerobic

Frequency: 4 days a week
Intensity: 65% to 75% target heart rate (THR)
Time: 10 to 45 minutes
Types: Aquatic aerobics, 45 minutes, 2 days a week
Stationary recumbent bike: Level 1, speed 60 to 80 rpm, start with 2 minute increments work/rest ratio to 10 minutes before muscular conditioning exercises
Progression: Increase to 30 minutes continuous exercise in 3 to 6 months

Muscular Conditioning

Two days a week, supervised
Exercise leg band light to start two to three sets low repetitions to start
Short-term progress to medium leg band and 10 to 12 repetitions in 2 to 3 months
In 3 to 6 months, progress to exercise circuit machines
Incorporate upper body bands medium to start for overall conditioning two to three sets of 12 to 15 reps
Types: Exercise leg band (cuffs) intensity light, two to three sets of five to eight repetitions exercises:
Lower body exercises: leg extension, hip flexion, partial squat, hip abduction and adduction, hamstring curl, isometric hold for 20 seconds × 3 sets
Upper body exercises: medium band: lateral raise, chest fly, row, bicep curl, and triceps extension.

Progression Updates

At 4 weeks

Mrs. Williams progressed to lower body light bands: three sets of 10 repetitions, and reported able to ambulate better, pain reported with walking 5/10 and rest 2–3/10. Upper body exercises: three sets of 12 to 15 reps medium remained the same.

The Case of Mrs. Williams cont.

At 8 weeks

Mrs. Williams progressed to medium lower body cuffs: three sets of 8 to 10 repetitions; patient reported able to walk with rest periods of approximately 100 yards and intermittently having to hold on to the handrails for support in Fitness Center to exercise appointments. She reported pain with walking 4–5/10 and rest 2/10. Upper body exercises: three sets of 15 reps, medium intensity remained for lateral raise, chest fly, hard intensity was increased for row, bicep curl, and tricep extension for three sets of 8 to 10 repetitions.

At 3 months

Mrs. Williams progressed to circuit training machines: two to three sets of 8 to 10 repetitions. Lower body: hamstring curl: 10 lb, leg press: 65 lb, hip abduction: 60 lb, hip adduction: 50 lb, assisted (holding on to upper bar) reebok step up two sets of eight repetitions. Upper body: lat pulldown: 35 lb, chest press: 20 lb, incline chest press: 10 lb, lateral raise: 15 lb, bicep curl: 10 lb, tricep extension: 25 lb. She reported able to walk approximately 200 1/3 of way to Fitness Center to exercise appointment and still intermittently holding to handrails for support. The patient reported pain with activity 4/10 and rest 2/10.

At 6 months

Mrs. Williams progressed to circuit training machines: three sets of 10 repetitions (upper 3 sets of 12 repetitions). Lower body: hamstring curl: 20 lb, leg press: 80 lb, hip abduction: 75 lb, hip adduction: 60 lb, assisted (holding on to upper bar) reebok step up three sets of 10 repetitions. Upper body: lat pulldown: 45 lb, chest press: 27.5 lb, incline chest press: 20 lb, bicep curl: 15 lb, lateral raise 22.5 lb, tricep extension: 32.5 lb. Aerobic: Mrs. Williams maintained aquatic aerobics 2 days a week, 45 minutes, stationary bike increased to level 2, and she was able to perform 10 minutes without stopping, and the following 10 minutes were work/rest ratios of 2 minutes. Mrs. Williams reported able to walk approximately 600 yards to Fitness Center to exercise appointment and rarely need handrails for support. The patient reported pain with activity 3–4/10 and rest 1–2/10.

At 1 year

Lower body: hamstring curl: 35 lb, leg press: 100 lb, hip abduction: 100 lb, hip adduction: 90 lb, no assistance needed reebok step up three sets of 10 repetitions. Upper body: lat pulldown: 55 lb, chest press: 40 lb, incline chest press: 37.5 lb, bicep curl: 30 lb, lateral raise 35 lb, tricep extension: 40 lb. Aerobic: She maintained aquatic aerobics 2 days a week, 45 minutes, stationary bike increased to level 3 speed 60 to 80 rpm, and she was able to perform 20 minutes without stopping, and the following 10 minutes were work/rest ratios of 2 minutes. Mrs. Williams reported ability to walk approximately 600 yards to Fitness Center to exercise appointment and did not need handrails for support. She reports pain with activity 2–3/10 and rest 0/10. She was able to participate in community outings walking in mall with friends, walked with friends to visit museums in Washington, DC, and was able to stand entire choir practice for 1 hour.

3-Year Assessment

Physical Data:

Height: 64 in, Weight: 160 lb, BMI: 27.5.
Body composition: Body fat percentage: 48.1 kg·m^{-2}, Inbody 520 DSM-BIA.

Fitness Data:

Muscular strength: Strength: dynamometer; hip flexion: R: 35 lb, L: 35 lb; leg extension: R: 30 lb, L: 30 lb
Lower body: Three sets of 10 reps: hamstring curl: 50 lb, leg press: 135 lb, hip abduction: 115 lb, hip adduction: 110 lb, no assistance needed reebok step up with 5 lb medicine ball, three sets of 10 repetitions, ball squat against the wall with 5 lb dumbbells.
Upper body: Three sets of 15 reps: lat pulldown: 60 lb, chest press: 50 lb, incline chest press: 40 lb, bicep curl: 35 lb, lateral raise 42.5 lb, tricep extension: 60 lb.
Aerobic: Mrs. Williams maintained aquatic aerobics 2 days a week for 45 minutes, stationary bike increased to level 3 speed 60 to 80 rpm and was able to perform 30 minutes without stopping.

***The Case of Mrs. Williams* cont.**

Mrs. Williams reports ability to perform exercise 3 days a week, recumbent bike, and muscular conditioning by herself. Instructed on proper progression from American College of Sports Medicine® and National Strength and Conditioning guidelines for muscular conditioning exercises and gave patient handout. Mrs. Williams reported pain in knees with walking after 2 miles 2/10, 0/10 at rest.

Conclusion

Mrs. Williams was able to progress to increase quality of life with managing OA by incorporating muscular and aerobic conditioning to routine. She was able to maintain 5 days a week for 45 to 60 minutes for more than 2 years, and pain was managed well. This client was motivated to increase ambulation and quality of life and was consistent with exercise programming over time. This may not be reflective of all clients, but gives an example for exercise programming if a client is consistent that this will help long-term exercise prescription goals.

Questions

- What would be a good starting muscular conditioning program for a client who has OA, in terms of days per week, number of sets, and repetitions?
- How often should you increase muscular conditioning exercises for an OA client?

References

1. American College of Sports Medicine. *ACSM's Guidelines for Exercise Testing and Prescription*. 9th ed. Baltimore (MD): Lippincott Williams & Wilkins; 2013.
2. Baechle T, Earle R, editors. *National Strength and Conditioning Association: Essentials of Strength Training and Conditioning*. 2nd ed. Champaign (IL): Human Kinetics; 2000.
3. Wallace JP. Obesity. In: Durstine J, Moore G, editors. *ACSM's Exercise Management for Persons with Chronic Diseases and Disabilities*. 2nd ed. Champaign (IL): American College of Sports Medicine, Human Kinetics; 2003.

SUMMARY

This chapter examines and provides guidelines for the exercise professional to effectively address common traumatic and overuse musculoskeletal injuries, and selected chronic musculoskeletal conditions related to physical activity or inactivity. Common causes of, role of exercise on, and strategies for reducing the risk of traumatic and overuse injuries and selected chronic conditions are covered. When applicable and within the scope of practice of the exercise professional, appropriate and current exercise guidelines are discussed with particular focus on modifying the exercise prescription to address special circumstances for these conditions.

Upon completion of this chapter, the reader should understand the etiology and mechanisms of common traumatic musculoskeletal injuries (strains and sprains), overuse injuries (tendinopathy, PF, and LBP), and chronic conditions (forms of arthritis and osteoporosis). Likewise, the reader will have knowledge of risk factors, commonly used medications, and exercise limitations and strategies to mitigate the effects of these conditions.

STUDY QUESTIONS

1. What recommendations would you make for maximizing bone health and reducing risk of osteoporosis to a client who is 55 years old? 25 years old? 12 years old?
2. Explain resistance exercise recommendations for a client diagnosed with osteoporosis of the spine who has physician clearance to exercise with appropriate limitations. What types of resistance exercises are appropriate and safe? How frequently should these exercises be performed and at what intensity?
3. A young client who is an athlete sprained her ankle (inversion) during soccer practice a day earlier, but did not want to miss a personal training session with you. She can walk, but the ankle is swollen and sore. What recommendations would you give this client regarding the injury and exercise?
4. Using the general guidelines presented, explain the progression of exercises for tendinopathies, including examples of types of exercise, frequency, and intensity.
5. Explain the difference between rheumatoid and OA, and taking into account special considerations for both, provide exercise recommendations.

REFERENCES

1. Beck BR, Norling TL. The effect of 8 mos of twice-weekly low- or higher intensity whole body vibration on risk factors for postmenopausal hip fracture. *Am J Phys Med Rehabil*. 2010;89(12):997–1009.
2. Berger C, Langsetmo L, Joseph L, et al. Change in bone mineral density as a function of age in women and men and association with the use of antiresorptive agents. *CMAJ*. 2008;178(13):1660–8.
3. Booher J, Thibodeau G. Athletic injuries and related skin conditions. In: Booher J, Thibodeau G, editors. *Athletic Injury Assessment*. 4th ed. Boston (MA): McGraw-Hill; 2000. p. 77–106.
4. Bradney M, Pearce G, Naughton G, et al. Moderate exercise during growth in prepubertal boys: Changes in bone mass, size, volumetric density, and bone strength: A controlled prospective study. *J Bone Miner Res*. 1998;13(12):1814–21.
5. Cooney JK, Law RJ, Matschke V, et al. Benefits of exercise in rheumatoid arthritis. *J Aging Res*. 2011;2011:681640.
6. Cosca D, Navazio F. Common problems in endurance athletes. *Am Fam Physician*. 2007;76(2):237–44.
7. Crowson C, Matteson E, Myasoedova E, et al. The lifetime risk of adult-onset rheumatoid arthritis and other inflammatory autoimmune rheumatic diseases. *Arthritis Rheum*. 2011;63(3):633–9.
8. Cummings SR, Melton LJ. Epidemiology and outcomes of osteoporotic fractures. *Lancet*. 2002;359(9319):1761–7.
9. Dalsky GP, Stocke KS, Ehsani AA, Slatopolsky E, Lee WC, Birge SJ Jr. Weight-bearing exercise training and lumbar bone mineral content in postmenopausal women. *Ann Intern Med*. 1988;108(6):824–8.
10. de Jong Z, Vliet Vlieland T. Safety of exercise in patients with rheumatoid arthritis. *Curr Opin Rheumatol*. 2005;17:177–82.
11. DiGiovanni BF, Nawoczenski DA, Lintal ME, et al. Tissue-specific plantar fascia-stretching exercise enhances outcomes in patients with chronic heel pain. A prospective, randomized study. *J Bone Joint Surg Am*. 2003;85-A(7):1270–7.
12. Epstein S. Update of current therapeutic options for the treatment of postmenopausal osteoporosis. *Clin Ther*. 2006;28(2):151–73.
13. Ettinger WH Jr, Burns R, Messier SP, et al. A randomized trial comparing aerobic exercise and resistance exercise with a health education program in older adults with knee osteoarthritis. The Fitness Arthritis and Seniors Trial (FAST). *JAMA*. 1997;277(1):25–31.
14. Fairbank J, Pynsent P. The Oswestry disability index. *Spine*. 2000;25(22):2940–53.
15. Faries M, Greenwood M. Core training: Stabilizing the confusion. *Strength Cond J*. 2007;29(2):10–25.
16. Finigan J, Greenfield DM, Blumsohn A, et al. Risk factors for vertebral and nonvertebral fracture over 10 years: A population-based study in women. *J Bone Miner Res*. 2008;23(1):75–85.
17. Finkelstein JS, Brockwell SE, Mehta V, et al. Bone mineral density changes during the menopause transition in a multiethnic cohort of women. *J Clin Endocrinol Metab*. 2008;93(3):861–8.
18. Firooznia H, Golimbu C, Rafii M, Schwartz MS, Alterman ER. Quantitative computed tomography assessment of spinal trabecular bone. I. Age-related regression in normal men and women. *J Comput Tomogr*. 1984;8(2):91–7.
19. Flokowski P, Brunt D, Bishop M, Woo R, Horodyski M. Intrinsic pedal musculature support of the medial longitudinal arch: An electromyography study. *J Foot Ankle Surg*. 2003;42(6):327–33.
20. Goksel Karatepe A, Gunaydin R, Turkmen G, Kaya T. Effects of home-based exercise program on the functional status and the quality of life in patients with rheumatoid arthritis: 1-year follow-up study. *Rheumatol Int*. 2011;31(2):171–6.

21. Gudena R, Werle J, Johnston K. Bilateral femoral insufficiency fractures likely related to long-term alendronate therapy. *J Osteoporos.* 2011;2011:810697.
22. Hall C, Thein-Brody L. Functional approach to therapeutic exercise for physiologic impairments. In: Hall C, Thein-Brody L, editors. *Therapeutic Exercise.* Philadelphia (PA): Lippincott Williams & Wilkins; 1999. p. 43–69.
23. Hart L. Exercise and soft tissue injury. *Bailliere's Clin Rheumatol.* 1994;8(1):137–48.
24. Headlee D, Leonard J, Hart J, Ingersoll C, Hertel J. Fatigue of the plantar intrinsic foot muscles increases navicular drop. *J Electromyogr Kinesiol.* 2007;18(3):420–5.
25. Herring S, Nilson KL. Introduction to overuse injuries. *Clin Sports Med.* 1987;6:225–39.
26. Herzog R. Radiologic imaging in rehabilitation. In: Kibler W, Herring S, Press J, editors. *Functional Rehabilitation of Sports and Musculoskeletal Injuries.* 1st ed. Gaithersburg (MD): Aspen Publisher; 1998. p. 20–70.
27. Hinman R, Heywood S, Day A. Aquatic physical therapy for hip and knee osteoarthritis: Results of a single-blind randomized controlled trial. *Phys Ther.* 2007;87:32–43.
28. Hopman-Rock M, Westhoff M. The effects of a health educational and exercise program for older adults with osteoarthritis for the hip or knee. *J Rheumatol.* 2000;27(8):1947–54.
29. Howe TE, Shea B, Dawson LJ, et al. Exercise for preventing and treating osteoporosis in postmenopausal women. *Cochrane Database Syst Rev.* 2011;(7):CD000333.
30. Hui SL, Slemenda CW, Johnston CC Jr. The contribution of bone loss to postmenopausal osteoporosis. *Osteoporos Int.* 1990;1(1):30–4.
31. Iacono MV. Osteoporosis: A national public health priority. *J Perianesth Nurs.* 2007;22(3):175–80.
32. Institute of Medicine. DRIs for Calcium and Vitamin D Report [Internet]. Institute-of-Medicine; [cited 2011 Jul 12]. Available from: http://www.iom.edu/Reports/2010/Dietary-Reference-Intakes-for-Calcium-and-Vitamin-D.aspx
33. Iwamoto J, Takeda T, Ichimura S. Effect of exercise training and detraining on bone mineral density in postmenopausal women with osteoporosis. *J Orthop Sci.* 2001;6(2):128–32.
34. Jan M-H, Lin J-J, Liau J-J, Lin Y-F, Lin D-H. Investigation of clinical effects of high and low-resistance training for patients with knee osteoarthritis: A randomized controlled trial. *Phys Ther.* 2008;88(4):427–36.
35. Janda V. *Muscle Function Testing.* London (UK): Butterworths; 1983.
36. Jung D-Y, Kim M-H, Koh E-K, Kwon O-Y. A comparison in the muscle activity of the abductor hallucis and the medial longitudinal arch angle during toe curl and short foot exercises. *Phys Ther Sport.* 2011;12(1):30–5.
37. Keen R. Osteoporosis: Strategies for prevention and management. Best practice & research. *Clin Rheumatol.* 2007;21(1):109–22.
38. Kisner C, Colby L. *Therapeutic Exercise Foundations and Techniques.* 5th ed. Philadelphia (PA): F.A. Davis Company; 2007. 309 p.
39. Kolber M, Beekhuizen K. Lumbar stabilization: An evidence-based approach for the athlete with low back pain. *Strength Cond J.* 2007;29(2):26–37.
40. Koplan JP, Powell KE, Sikes RK, Shirley RW, Campbell CC. An epidemiologic study of the benefits and risks of running. *JAMA.* 1982;248:3118–21.
41. Kubo K, Ikebukuor T, Yata H, Tsundoa N, Kanehisa H. Time course of changes in muscle and tendon properties during strength training and detraining. *J Strength Cond Res.* 2010;24(2):322–31.
42. Liu PY, Brummel-Smith K, Ilich JZ. Aerobic exercise and whole-body vibration in offsetting bone loss in older adults. *J Aging Res.* 2011;2011:379674.
43. Lloyd T, Petit MA, Lin HM, Beck TJ. Lifestyle factors and the development of bone mass and bone strength in young women. *J Pediatr.* 2004;144(6):776–82.
44. Lorenz D, Reiman M. The role and implementation of eccentric training in athletic rehabilitation: Tendinopathy, hamstring strains, and ACL reconstruction. *Int J Sports Phys Ther.* 2011;6(1):27–44.
45. Maggio D, Pacifici R, Cherubini A, et al. Age-related cortical bone loss at the metacarpal. *Calcif Tissue Int.* 1997;60(1):94–7.
46. Mazess RB. Bone mineral content in early-postmenopausal and postmenopausal osteoporotic women. *Radiology.* 1987;165(1):289–91.
47. Mazziotti G, Canalis E, Giustina A. Drug-induced osteoporosis: Mechanisms and clinical implications. *Am J Med.* 2010;123(10):877–84.
48. McGill S. *Low Back Disorders.* 1st ed. Champaign (IL): Human Kinetics; 2002. 210 p.
49. McGill S. *Ultimate Back Fitness and Performance.* 3rd ed. Waterloo (ON): Backfitpro Inc.; 2006. 221 p.
50. McKenzie RA, May S. *The Lumbar Spine: Mechanical Diagnosis and Therapy.* 2nd ed. Waikanae (New Zealand): Spinal Publications, New Zealand Ltd.; 2003.
51. McPoil T, Martin R, Cornwall M, Wukichj D, Irrgang J, Godges J. Heel pain: Plantar Fasciitis. *J Orthop Sports Phys Ther.* 2008;38(4):A1–18.
52. Melton L. Adverse outcomes of osteoporotic fractures in the general population. *J Bone Miner Res.* 2003;18(6):1139–41.
53. Melzack R. The McGill pain questionnaire: Major properties and scoring methods. *Pain.* 1975;1(3):277–99.
54. Merriman H, Jackson K. The effects of whole-body vibration training in aging adults: A systematic review. *J Geriatr Phys Ther.* 2009;32(3):134–45.
55. Meunier P, Courpron P, Edouard C, Bernard J, Bringuier J, Vignon G. Physiological senile involution and pathological rarefaction of bone. Quantitative and comparative histological data. *Clin Endocrinol Metab.* 1973;2(2):239–56.
56. Mikhael M, Orr R, Fiatarone Singh MA. The effect of whole body vibration exposure on muscle or bone morphology and function in older adults: A systematic review of the literature. *Maturitas.* 2010;66(2):150–7.
57. Minor M. Exercise in the treatment of osteoarthritis. *Rheum Dis Clin N Am.* 1999;25(2):397–415.
58. Minor M, Kay D. Arthritis. In: Durstine J, Moore G, editors. *ACSM's Exercise Management for Persons with Chronic Diseases and Disabilities.* 2nd ed. Champaign (IL): Human Kinetics; 2003. 374 p.
59. Mosekilde L. Sex differences in age-related loss of vertebral trabecular bone mass and structure — biomechanical consequences. *Bone.* 1989;10(6):425–32.
60. Mosely K, Jan de Beur S. Osteoporosis in men and women. In: Legato M, editor. *Principles of Gender-Specific Medicine.* 2nd ed. Cambridge (MA): Elsevier Inc.; 2010. p. 716–36.
61. Neviaser AS, Lane JM, Lenart BA, Edobor-Osula F, Lorich DG. Low-energy femoral shaft fractures associated with alendronate use. *J Orthop Trauma.* 2008;22(5):346–50.
62. Nilas L, Christiansen C. Rates of bone loss in normal women: Evidence of accelerated trabecular bone loss after the menopause. *Eur J Clin Invest.* 1988;18(5):529–34.
63. Nordström A, Karlsson C, Nyquist F, Olsson T, Nordström P, Karlsson M. Bone loss and fracture risk after reduced physical activity. *J Bone Miner Res.* 2005;20(2):202–7.
64. O'Flaherty EJ. Modeling normal aging bone loss, with consideration of bone loss in osteoporosis. *Toxicol Sci.* 2000;55(1):171–88.

65. Petit F, Hughes C, Warpeha J. Exercise prescription for people with osteoporosis. In: Ehrman J, editor. *ACSM's Resource Manual for Guidelines for Exercise Testing and Prescription.* 6th ed. Philadelphia (PA): Wolters Kluwer/Lippincott Williams & Wilkins; 2010. p. 635–50.
66. Pfefer M, Cooper S, Uhl N. Chiropractic management of tendinopathy: A literature synthesis. *J Manipulative Physiol Ther.* 2009;32(1):41–52.
67. Pfeifer M, Sinaki M, Geusens P, Boonen S, Preisinger E, Minne HW. Musculoskeletal rehabilitation in osteoporosis: A review. *J Bone Miner Res.* 2004;19(8):1208–14.
68. Plasqui G. The role of physical activity in rheumatoid arthritis. *Physiol Behav.* 2007;94:270–5.
69. Potach D, Ellenbecker T. Clients with orthopedic, injury, and rehabilitation concerns. In: Earle R, Baechle T, editors. *NSCA's Essentials of Personal Training.* Champaign (IL): Human Kinetics; 2004. p. 533–56.
70. Prevention CfDCa. Chronic Diseases The Power to Prevent, The Call to Control: At a Glance 2009 [Internet]. Available from: http://www.cdc.gov/chronicdisease/resources/publications/aag/chronic.htm
71. Rannevik G, Jeppsson S, Johnell O, Bjerre B, Laurell-Borulf Y, Svanberg L. A longitudinal study of the perimenopausal transition: Altered profiles of steroid and pituitary hormones, SHBG and bone mineral density. *Maturitas.* 1995;21(2):103–13.
72. Sambrook P, Cooper C. Osteoporosis. *Lancet.* 2006;367(9527):2010–8.
73. Sexson SB, Lehner JT. Factors affecting hip fracture mortality. *J Orthop Trauma.* 1987;1(4):298–305.
74. Simmonds M, Dreisinger T. *Lower Back Pain Syndrome.* 2nd ed. Champaign (IL): Human Kinetics; 2003. 218 p.
75. Skinner JS, editor. *Exercise Testing and Exercise Prescription for Special Cases.* 3rd ed. Philadelphia (PA): Lippincott Williams & Wilkins; 2005.
76. Smith R, Cullen D. Osteoporosis. In: LeMura L, von Duvillard S, editors. *Clinical Exercise Physiology.* Philadelphia (PA): Lippincott Williams & Wilkins; 2004. p. 485–502.
77. Snow CM, Shaw JM, Winters KM, Witzke KA. Long-term exercise using weighted vests prevents hip bone loss in postmenopausal women. *J Gerontol A Biol Sci Med Sci.* 2000;55(9):M489–91.
78. Sornay-Rendu E, Munoz F, Duboeuf F, Delmas PD. Rate of forearm bone loss is associated with an increased risk of fracture independently of bone mass in postmenopausal women: The OFELY study. *J Bone Miner Res.* 2005;20(11):1929–35.
79. Thompson W, Gordon N, Pescatello L, editors. *Exercise Prescriptions for other Clinical Populations.* 8th ed. Philadelphia (PA): Lippincott Williams & Wilkins; 2009.
80. van den Ende CH, Breedveld FC, le Cessie S, Dijkmans BA, de Mug AW, Hazes JM. Effect of intensive exercise on patients with active rheumatoid arthritis: A randomised clinical trial. *Ann Rheum Dis.* 2000;59:615–21.
81. Wasielewski NJ, Kotsko KM. Does eccentric exercise reduce pain and improve strength in physically active adults with symptomatic lower extremity tendinosis? A systematic review. *J Athletic Training.* 2007;42(3):409–21.
82. Williams III D. *Foot and Ankle.* 1st ed. London (UK): Churchill Livingstone; 2003. 451 p.
83. Wilson J, Best T. Common overuse tendon problems: A review and recommendations for treatment. *Am Fam Physician.* 2005;72(5):811–8.
84. Winters KM, Snow CM. Detraining reverses positive effects of exercise on the musculoskeletal system in premenopausal women. *J Bone Miner Res.* 2000;15(12):2495–503.
85. Zulia P, Prentice W. *Rehabilitation of the Elbow.* 1st ed. New York (NY): McGraw-Hill; 2001. 466 p.

CHAPTER

9 Exercise Programming Across the Lifespan: Children and Adolescents, Pregnant Women, and Older Adults

Laurie Milliken • Riggs Klika

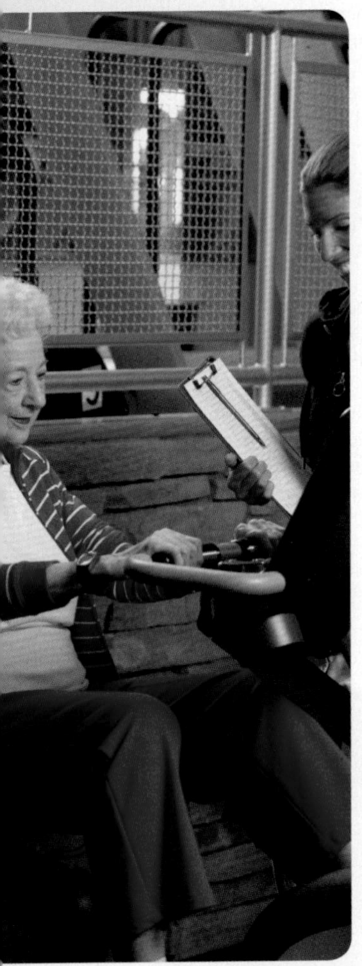

CHAPTER OBJECTIVES

- To understand the physical and selected physiological changes during the aging process (childhood to older adult).
- To understand the adaptations to training for children, adolescents, older adults, and pregnant women.
- To understand the differences in exercise prescriptions between children, adolescents, older adults, and pregnant women.
- To apply the ACSM's, AHA, and CDC guidelines to exercise prescriptions for children, adolescents, older adults, and pregnant women.

Individuals at any phase of the lifespan can respond positively to exercise training assuming the stimulus is appropriate and there is adequate time for recovery between stressors. However, placing an inappropriately low or high load on an immature, frail, or compromised system is ineffective or even contraindicated. Therefore, the goal of this chapter is to describe the impact of age and pregnancy on selected physiological systems and the benefits and limitations of training on those systems and to discuss practical applications of exercising programming across the lifespan.

This chapter will focus on three separate populations: children and adolescents, pregnant women, and older adults. Each population will be addressed in terms of physical and physiological changes, the impact of chronic exercise, and relevant exercise programming (*e.g.*, including specific exercise considerations and meeting activity recommendations). In accordance with the American College of Sports Medicine® (ACSM) Guidelines for Exercise Testing and Prescription (29), "children" are those who are younger than 13 years, "adolescents" are 13 through 18 years, and "older adults" are those 65 years and older or those 50 to 64 years who have significant physical or physiological limitations that affect physical movement or capacity.

This discussion of physical and physiological changes across the lifespan is important to understand exercise prescription and the unique exercise considerations for children, adolescents, pregnant women, and older adults. However, it is not the purpose of this chapter to provide a comprehensive discussion of growth, development, and aging. For a complete description, see Malina (14) for youth, Skinner (24) for aging, and Wolfe (35) for pregnancy. Instead, this chapter will focus on those areas that are pertinent to the safe and effective prescription of exercise by the Health Fitness Specialist (HFS) for children, adolescents, older adults, and pregnant women. Those pertinent areas include musculoskeletal system status and function, alterations in body composition, the function of the cardiorespiratory system during rest and exercise, endocrine system alterations, thermoregulation, and motor performance.

CHILDREN AND ADOLESCENTS

Children and adolescents in many ways are not simply miniature adults. In fact, most physiological systems are very different from an adult, and this directly impacts the way exercise is prescribed. In addition, many of the exercise measurement methods that were originally designed for adults are not scalable to children solely on the basis of body size. While not the main focus of this chapter, it should be noted that behavioral and psychological issues must also be considered when prescribing exercise for children and adolescents to ensure maximal participation.

PHYSICAL AND PHYSIOLOGICAL CHANGES

Body Size and Composition

The obvious physical change observed during childhood and adolescence is the increase in body size. Both weight and height increase with age, with rapid growth in infancy, steady increases in early childhood, an accelerated period of growth at puberty (about 12 years for girls and 14 years for boys), and slow gains until adult height and weight are attained (although weight tends to continue increasing into adulthood) (15). In general, girls stop growing in stature by 15 years of age, and boys reach their adult height by about 17 years of age (15). The longer period of growth in boys results in an adult gender difference in height, which is about 10 to 12 cm, or 4 to 5 in (15). The increase in height during childhood is achieved by long bone growth, where a layer of cartilage called the growth plate undergoes proliferation and subsequent ossification, resulting in longitudinal progression of the bone. This process eventually ceases once adult height is achieved (17).

There are also noticeable and important changes in the tissues that constitute body weight, which are bone mass, fat mass, and fat-free mass (17). Total body bone mass increases in a similar manner as height, but the increase continues to 20 years of age in males (17). Lower and upper extremity bone mass increases in childhood with accelerated growth in adolescence, whereas head and trunk bone mass remain fairly constant during these same periods (17). Fat-free mass, primarily skeletal muscle, increases in a manner similar to height in both boys and girls, resulting in adult females having about 30% less skeletal muscle mass than males. Fat mass increases for both boys and girls, whereas percentage body fat increases in girls, but decreases in boys because of the previously described increases in fat-free mass for boys (16).

Cardiorespiratory Function

As children grow, their cardiorespiratory system also develops. At birth, children have a high heart rate and respiration rates, both of which decline with age. Young children's heart rates in the seated position at rest are between 100 and 110 beats per minute, and their maximal heart rate is higher than adults. Respiratory frequency is also higher in children and continues to decrease throughout childhood and adolescence until adult values are achieved (19). Lung function measures increase as a function of height throughout youth (19). On the other hand, children seem to recover faster from a bout of exercise compared with adults, as heart rate, oxygen consumption, and minute ventilation return to resting values more quickly (12).

Although heart rate is higher in children, stroke volume is lower, resulting in cardiac output values that are lower than in adults (12). Systolic blood pressure, and to a lesser extent diastolic blood pressure, is lower in children than in adults both at rest and during exercise, yet resting blood pressure, especially systolic, increases with age (19). Hemoglobin concentration and red blood cell count increase during childhood, with an accelerated increase at puberty, with boys' values exceeding girls'. However, children have greater blood flow and oxygen extraction at the periphery during exercise (12). Despite this, children and adolescents have a greater oxygen cost during exercise than adults even after accounting for size differences. The relative inefficiency may be due to immature motor patterns, which improve with age. Peak $\dot{V}O_2$ measured in children is lower than in adults, but increases with age once size, adiposity, and gender are accounted for (12). A gender difference exists, however, with girls showing declines in peak $\dot{V}O_2$, which reflects not only the aforementioned gender differences in body composition and blood hemoglobin, but also the adoption of more sedentary behaviors in girls that occurs around puberty (12).

Muscular Strength, Flexibility, and Motor Performance

In both boys and girls, muscular strength increases with age and is related to the increases in body weight, height, fat-free mass, and muscle mass (18). The increases accelerate in boys during puberty and tend to plateau in girls in proportion to the slower increases in fat-free mass and muscle mass (16). Motor performance measures tend to follow the same pattern of improving with physical maturation (20). The smaller increases in girls, especially for weight-dependent performance measures such as vertical jump and long jump, may be due to the increase in fat mass at puberty. The decrease in exercise among girls at puberty probably also contributes to this trend. However, girls tend to outperform boys in flexibility measures and some measures of balance (20).

Perceived Exertion

Children and adolescents are able to distinguish between different levels of effort just as can adults. However, children tend to rate exertion lower than both adolescents and adults; adolescents also rate exertion lower than adults (12). Children may not be as able to reproduce an exercise intensity that corresponds to a particular exertion rating as are adults, although some studies have shown that they can do so during cycling exercise using the child-friendly OMNI scale (12). This scale is a 0 to 10 rating scale with pictures corresponding to different levels of effort both for walking/jogging and for cycling. A scale also exists for the perceived exertion of resistance exercise (7). A 6 to 20 scale or a 0 to 10 scale, however, without illustrations, has been less useful for children.

Thermoregulation

During exercise in hot environments, the evaporation of sweat is the main avenue for heat dissipation in humans. However, in children, the ability to produce sweat is lower than adults (12). Although children have more sweat glands, the output of each gland is lower than adults and the temperature where sweating starts is higher than in adults (12). The result is that children cannot sustain exercise for as long as adults when temperatures exceed 40°C, or approximately 100°F. This becomes exacerbated when the child is not well hydrated, which further limits the ability of a child to produce sweat, which in turn limits its thermoregulatory ability (12). Children or adolescents who are at special risk are those for whom proper hydration is not well maintained because of cognitive or physiological conditions. Staying well hydrated, particularly in warm conditions, should always be emphasized, encouraged, and even insisted by the HFS.

Obese children tend to acclimatize to heat stress more slowly and have a lower threshold for core temperature regulation. Although lean and obese children do not show a difference in heat tolerance, obese children exercising in the heat have increased core temperatures and higher heart rates at submaximal workloads (4). Mechanisms for lower-heat tolerance in obese children have not fully been examined, but adiposity has been shown to decrease abdominal heat transfer in adults and therefore may contribute to increase core temperature in children as well.

THE IMPACT OF CHRONIC EXERCISE

Exercise has been shown to be beneficial for the large majority of people, including children and adolescents (23, 30). Specifically, physically active youth will reap benefits such as improved cardiorespiratory and muscular fitness, metabolic health, cardiometabolic profiles, body composition, and for some, mental health (23, 30). Children performing exercise and training for certain sports can improve motor performance and efficiency and increase muscular strength and endurance, and those who include more intense aerobic activity can improve cardiorespiratory fitness and aerobic performance (5, 23, 30). As with adults, there is a dose-response effect in the benefits of exercise. Increases in the quantity and quality of exercise will result in more health-related improvements (5, 23, 30).

There is no evidence that exercise, including resistance training, weightlifting, and plyometric training, has any adverse effects on children and adolescents when exercises are performed properly and are supervised by qualified adults (5, 8, 13, 23, 30). In fact, resistance training and sports conditioning have been shown to reduce the rate of sports-related injuries (5). There is always the chance, as with any activity, that an injury that would damage the epiphyseal or growth plate and negatively impact growth can occur. There are also some children with undetected medical conditions that could result in sudden death, but the preponderance of evidence suggests that exercise is safe and that the benefits far outweigh the risks. Reasonable precautions should be taken, especially for children who have cardiometabolic risk factors, those who cannot adequately follow directions, or youth exercising in hot environments, to reduce the chance of injury or sudden death.

EXERCISE PROGRAMMING AND SPECIFIC EXERCISE CONSIDERATIONS

The recommended amount of activity for children and adolescents to reap the aforementioned benefits is described in detail by the Physical Activity Guidelines Advisory Committee (23). The Advisory Committee reports that children and adolescents should obtain at least 60 minutes of moderate or vigorous activity daily, with vigorous activity included on at least 3 days a week. Muscle and bone strengthening activities should be included within the 60 minutes on at least 3 days per week. Examples of moderate aerobic activity are brisk walking, hiking, casual biking, or activities that result in an effort of 5 to 6 on a scale of 0 to 10. Vigorous aerobic activities are those that are a 7 to 8 such as running, skipping, and jumping; chasing games such as tag and jump rope; or playing sports such as soccer or field hockey. Active video games may provide another avenue for obtaining the recommended amount of exercise. A recent review shows that most active video games provide light or moderate activity; however, there is not yet enough evidence to draw conclusions about the long-term role of these games for increasing exercise (3). For youth who do not meet the guidelines for activity, both the intensity and duration of activities should be progressed gradually until the minimum levels are achieved (23, 30, 33).

Muscle strengthening exercises are those that require moving against resistance, and can include resistance from body weight (push-ups, pull-ups, squats), free weights (dumbbells and barbells), or weight machines. Other examples of resistance training are playing on jungle gyms, using climbing walls, tree climbing, and playing tug of war. Bone strengthening exercises are those that result in a physical impact on the skeletal system, such as jumping, running, hopping, jumping rope, or gymnastics. Guidelines and recommendations exist for resistance training and plyometric training for youth (5, 13, 23, 30). In general, a muscle strengthening program should target large muscles of the whole body and should include a 5- to 10-minute warm-up and end with a cool-down. These exercises can be body weight exercises or machine-based exercises, depending on the child's ability to safely perform the exercises with proper form. For each exercise, 6 to 15 repetitions to fatigue can be performed in one to three sets on nonconsecutive days. One to three sets of power exercises can be performed for 3 to 6 repetitions. The HFS should monitor proper form, start with light weights, and progress the intensity gradually by 5% to 10%. One repetition maximum (1 RM) testing can also be performed under direct supervision of an HFS, ensuring to follow all of the recommended procedures (6). For all exercises, proper form with light weight should be emphasized first, followed by progression to heavier weights as tolerated by the child or adolescent. If a child consistently fails to perform resistance exercises safely, the child may not be emotionally mature enough to safely engage in resistance training, and consideration should be given to delay the onset of resistance training for that child.

Children

Parents and HFSs should encourage physical activities that are age-appropriate and enjoyable for children. Families should be encouraged to engage in active and fun activities together to establish positive lifelong PA habits. To this end, the HFS should realize that activity for children must be fun and intermittent for a child to perform it and enjoy it. The emphasis in programming should be on games or other fun activities and to provide opportunities for unstructured play. Rather than using an adult prescription paradigm, children should be allowed to self-regulate both the intensity and the duration of their activity (33). This means providing games or activities where intermittent rest opportunities are given and not penalized as part of the game. It is also recommended that games are chosen where children are not eliminated from play based on poor performance. A high-intensity game can be alternated with a low-intensity game, or safe zones can be included where children can have time to recover but are still included in the game. This is especially important for obese children whose cost of locomotion is higher than a smaller child. It is also important to focus on limiting sedentary behavior among children.

Adolescents

As children become adolescents, the activity paradigm can become more structured, but should still emphasize enjoyment (33). More complex games and activities requiring more maturity can be included. Where more play-based strengthening activities can be used for very young children, a more structured resistance training program can be well received by older children and adolescents. The use of child-sized resistance equipment and dumbbells can be incorporated on the basis of how well children follow directions. Children as young as 8 years can be successful in a structured resistance training program. Medicine balls and resistance bands can be incorporated as long as the child can respect the rules given by the teacher. This will vary depending on the child's ability to follow directions; most adolescents are mature enough to undertake a resistance training program that includes free weights, medicine balls, resistance bands, and weightlifting moves. Given adolescents at the same chronological age can have differing biological ages, it is important to consider the biological age when determining appropriate exercises for this population.

PREGNANT WOMEN

PHYSICAL AND PHYSIOLOGICAL CHANGES

Many changes occur to a woman's body with pregnancy, the most visible of which is an increase in body weight. Overall, about 12 kg or about 26 lb of weight are typically gained during the course of a pregnancy (35). However, the change in the distribution of weight, as the abdomen increasingly protrudes, causes a change in a women's center of gravity. As a result of this altered body carriage, half of pregnant women report lower back pain as pregnancy progresses (35). Significant hormonal changes also take place, including increases in estrogen and aldosterone, which contribute to water retention and increased blood volume. Relaxin, which is also released, is a hormone that limits uterine contractions, softens the cervix, and increases joint laxity in preparation for childbirth. Because of this, caution should be used during flexibility exercises so as not to overstretch the joints. Fatigue and nausea can also occur, especially during the first trimester, resulting from the hormonal changes that accompany pregnancy. Once the body adapts to these changes, these symptoms are reduced, usually after the first trimester (32). However, during times of nausea, a women's interest in being physically active may be understandably diminished.

Cardiovascular changes during pregnancy occur as a result of the increased blood volume. At rest, cardiac output, stroke volume, and heart rate increase, while vascular resistance decreases. Also, the heart may increase slightly in size because of the higher heart rate and stroke volume (32). However, during the third trimester, the expanded uterus may mechanically compress the inferior vena cava, causing a reduced venous return or less blood back to the heart (35). This is an important consideration for the HFS working with pregnant women, as supine exercise during the third trimester may exacerbate this situation and should be avoided whenever possible. The HFS must also be aware that blood pressure may fluctuate with changes on body position (33), and resting oxygen uptake increases by 20% to 30% because of fetal growth (35).

During exercise, heart rate for a pregnant woman is higher at lower intensities than a nonpregnant woman, yet lower at higher intensities with a lower overall maximum value. Therefore, the heart rate reserve, or the range of a women's heart rate, is smaller during pregnancy (35). Oxygen consumption during submaximal exercise is higher when pregnant, more so than would be expected by just from the increase in body weight. This is largely due to the increased oxygen cost of stabilization of the body from the displaced center of gravity plus the increased oxygen cost of respiration from the use of accessory muscles (35). The caloric need of pregnant women increases by about 150 calories a day in the first and second trimesters and by 300 calories a day in the third trimester (31).

THE IMPACT OF CHRONIC EXERCISE

Exercise training in women who are pregnant is beneficial for those who exercised prior to pregnancy and for those who start after becoming pregnant (32). Chronic exercise confers the same benefits to pregnant woman as it does for all, although there are benefits specific to pregnancy. Exercise improves circulation and tends to decrease the pregnancy-related edema that often occurs in the extremities (32). Exercise also improves mood and helps alleviate some of the general discomfort associated with pregnancy (31). Exercise training can reduce the chances for preeclampsia (high blood pressure and protein in the urine) and gestational diabetes (32). Chronic exercisers also tend to have smaller babies, though still in the normal range, and have a healthier weight gain during pregnancy, which can reduce complications (32).

The general consensus based on the most recent research is that there is no increased maternal or fetal risk caused by exercise training (1). Any woman with a normal pregnancy can start exercising or continue exercising without fear of harm to herself or her fetus (1). In fact, exercise is encouraged during pregnancy because of the benefits that can be reaped by adopting exercise, as is the case for all people.

EXERCISE PROGRAMMING AND SPECIFIC EXERCISE CONSIDERATIONS

The American College of Obstetricians and Gynecologists (ACOG) recommends that pregnant women accumulate 30 minutes of moderate-intensity exercise on all or most days of the week. This recommendation applies to all healthy pregnant women who have no absolute or relative contraindications for exercise (1). These contraindications are listed in Table 9.1. Those women who have or develop a medical condition while pregnant should consult with their physician before engaging in physical activities. The PARmed-X for Pregnancy health screening tool, developed by the Canadian Society for Exercise Physiology (available from www.csep.ca), should be used to screen all pregnant women seeking to start or continue exercising during pregnancy.

Although any activity is encouraged, the intensity recommended to reap health benefits is moderate, or 40% to 60% of heart rate reserve (29). Since pregnancy alters heart rate and $\dot{V}O_2$, intensity can be monitored by using perceived exertion. On a 6 to 20 scale, moderate intensity is 12 to 14 or an intensity where a woman can still maintain a conversation. Exercise heart rates for pregnancy have also been determined as follows: under 20 years, 140 to 155 beats per minute (bpm); 20 to 29 years, 135 to 150 bpm; 30 to 39 years, 130 to 145 bpm; and ≥40 years, 125 to 140 bpm (29).

Activities should be dynamic and involve the large muscles of the whole body, such as walking and cycling (dangers of outdoor cycling are high) (29). Pregnant women can safely participate in recreational sports, but should guard against trauma to the abdomen with the ACOG recommending against sports with a higher likelihood of abdominal trauma (ice hockey, soccer, and basketball) or with a high risk of falling (horseback riding, downhill skiing, gymnastics, or vigorous racquet sports) (1, 25). Also, scuba diving or exercise at altitudes more than 6,000 ft should be avoided so that fetal oxygen supply is not compromised, unless a woman already lives at high altitude (1). Exercising in the heat may also be safe, as no reports of fetal damage due to hyperthermia have

TABLE 9.1 CONTRAINDICATIONS FOR EXERCISE DURING PREGNANCY

Relative Contraindications	Absolute Contraindications
Severe anemia	Hemodynamically significant heart disease
Unevaluated maternal cardiac dysrhythmia	Restrictive lung disease
Chronic bronchitis	Incompetent cervix/cerclage
Poorly controlled Type 1 diabetes mellitus	Multiple gestation at risk for premature labor
Extreme morbid obesity	Persistent second- or third-trimester bleeding
Extreme underweight	Placenta previa after 26 wk of gestation
History of extremely sedentary lifestyle	Premature labor during the current pregnancy
Intrauterine growth restriction in current pregnancy	Ruptured membranes Preeclampsia/pregnancy-induced hypertension
Poorly controlled hypertension	
Orthopedic limitations	
Poorly controlled seizure disorder	
Poorly controlled hyperthyroidism	
Heavy smoker	

Reprinted with permission from American College of Obstetricians and Gynecologists. Exercise during pregnancy and the postpartum period. ACOG Committee Opinion No. 267. *Obstet Gynecol*. 2002;99:171–3.

been reported (1), yet it is important to modify intensity and duration and try to avoid the hottest parts of the day for exercise. Regardless, women should ensure that they are properly hydrated by ingesting a pint (~16 oz or 500 mL) of water prior to exercise and a cup every 20 minutes during exercise with the goal of replacing any fluid lost during exercise (25, 31). This will help ensure maximal thermoregulatory ability.

Women who undertake an exercise routine while pregnant should be aware of the warning signs or other conditions that could indicate increased risk. Women who develop a contraindication for exercise should consult with their physician who can help determine whether the risk of exercise outweighs the benefits. Also, exercise should be terminated and a physician consulted if any of the following occur (1): vaginal bleeding, shortness of breath prior to exertion, dizziness, headache, chest pain, muscle weakness, calf pain or swelling, preterm labor, decreased fetal movement, or a leaking of amniotic fluid. Women should also recognize that pregnancy increases caloric need and exercise results in an additional caloric cost. Caloric intake should therefore be adjusted so that the normal weight gain during pregnancy is achieved (26).

Finally, those women who begin exercising while pregnant should gradually increase the intensity and duration of exercise or activity until they meet the recommendations. All pregnant women should avoid extended periods of motionless standing and any activity that is conducted in a supine position, especially after the first trimester when venous return can become compromised (1). Resistance training, provided that all of the above recommendations are met, is also acceptable, although exercises should be modified to avoid the supine position and the Valsalva maneuver. If resistance training is conducted, exercises should be dynamic in nature and focus on the large muscles of the whole body. A resistance that produces a moderate level of muscular fatigue within 12 to 15 repetitions is recommended (29).

OLDER ADULTS

Older adults and those who are younger but severely deconditioned present the fitness professionals with unique challenges. The process of aging affects every system to some extent and these changes are inevitable. Of course, a healthy lifestyle in most people alters the rate of these changes resulting in increased longevity and better physical functioning. However, the older adult populations tend to have more disease conditions and also tend to be further progressed in those conditions. Several disease states are discussed in Chapters 7 and 8 in this book. The discussion here focuses on the relatively healthy older adult who is free from the advanced stages of disease but may be sedentary and generally deconditioned.

PHYSICAL AND PHYSIOLOGICAL CHANGES

Body Composition and Musculoskeletal Function

During adulthood, individuals tend to gain body weight and fat mass and tend to lose fat-free mass, height, and bone. However, the increases in percentage fat and body weight in older adults may be largely lifestyle related rather than a natural consequence of aging (24). Mirroring the loss of fat-free mass is a loss of muscular strength and the associated decreases in physical function (2). The loss of strength, muscle mass, and bone density are larger in women than in men (2). In the very old adult, there is also a loss of body weight and body cell mass (10), and this loss of weight is associated with a higher mortality rate (22). As the total body water content decreases with age, so does the elasticity and pliability of tissues such as cartilage and connective tissues that are found within joints among other places. Range of motion becomes reduced, the effects of which are compounded by the low levels of activity in many older adults (24, 34). Neuromotor function also deteriorates with age because of a reduction in the number of neurons resulting in reduced coordination, reaction time, balance, and agility (24, 34).

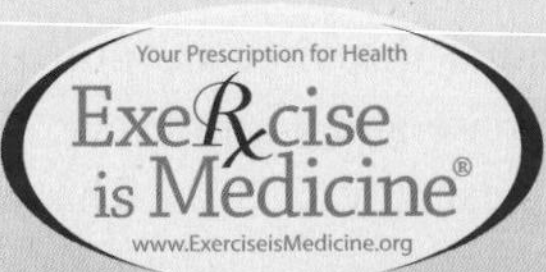

EXERCISE IS MEDICINE CONNECTION

Figueroa A, Park SY, Seo DY, Sanchez-Gonzalez MA, Baek YH. Combined resistance and endurance exercise training improves arterial stiffness, blood pressure, and muscle strength in postmenopausal women. Menopause.2011;18(9):980–4.

Figueroa and colleagues (2011) conducted a study in which postmenopausal women engaged in resistance and endurance exercise over 12 weeks. Arterial stiffness (at the ankle), blood pressure, and muscle strength were evaluated. This randomized controlled trial compared the control group with the treatment group who completed a circuit resistance training program followed by endurance (aerobic) training at 60% of age-predicted HR_{max} 3 day·week^{-1}. Participants included 24 postmenopausal women who were between 47 and 68 years of age. Results indicated that postmenopausal women in the treatment group had significantly better ankle blood flow, lower mean systolic and diastolic blood pressure, and greater dynamic leg strength and isometric handgrip strength than those in the control group. The authors of this study reported that combined resistance and aerobic training had favorable outcomes on risk factors associated with hypertension and frailty in postmenopausal women.

Cardiorespiratory Function and Thermoregulation

The cardiorespiratory system is affected by aging and by a sedentary lifestyle. Vessels become stiffer, and elasticity is lost in cardiac tissue, including the heart values. This results in higher blood pressure and higher resistance to flow, which creates more work for the heart (24). During submaximal exercise, aging tends to result in higher ventilation, blood pressure and oxygen extraction, lower cardiac output and stroke volume, and little change in heart rate and oxygen uptake (24). At maximal levels of exercise, oxygen uptake, ventilation, cardiac output, heart rate, stroke volume, oxygen extraction, and lactic acid concentrations are higher while total peripheral resistance and blood pressure is higher than in a younger person (24). Because collagen fibers in the lungs also lose elasticity and bronchioles lose their tone, less air can be moved per minute in an older adult (34). The result of these processes, and what is important for the HFS to recognize, is that older individuals have a lower overall exercise capacity and that any given submaximal exercise intensity represents a higher percentage of their maximum.

Thermoregulatory ability also declines with aging. The number and activity of sweat glands decreases with age and the capillary density also decreases. This results in a lower ability of the body to benefit from evaporative or radiant cooling. Older adults, as well as younger groups, also cannot withstand the cold because of a reduced ability to divert blood flow toward deeper tissues. In the very old, this is exacerbated by the loss of subcutaneous body fat (34).

THE IMPACT OF CHRONIC EXERCISE

It is not the purpose of this discussion to provide a comprehensive literature review on the benefits of chronic exercise since this has been well documented elsewhere (9, 11, 21, 23, 30). However, there is strong evidence that an adequate amount and type of exercise lowers the risks of several cancers, cardiovascular disease, some metabolic diseases, and premature death in older adults (9, 11, 21, 23, 30). Exercise results in a more favorable cardiovascular risk profile, increases physical function, prevents falls, improves some mental health outcomes, improves fitness, and helps with achieving a healthy weight (9, 11, 21, 23, 30). In fact, many of the age-related declines in fat-free mass, strength, and motor performance are at least partially reversible with the onset of a regular exercise program (21, 24). There is evidence that these benefits can be reaped even in sedentary older adults who initiate an exercise program late in life (9, 21, 23).

Nelson (21) outlines in detail the benefits of regular exercise in older adults. Specifically, in addition to the benefits that are reaped for all adults, regular exercise in older adults reduces the risk of falls, injuries from falls, and functional limitations and improves the management of many conditions, including dementia, anxiety, and back pain. There is some evidence that exercise improves sleep in old adults and can prevent or delay the negative cognitive changes that often occur with aging (21).

EXERCISE PROGRAMMING AND SPECIFIC EXERCISE CONSIDERATIONS

As is the case for all adults, the HFS should perform proper baseline assessments, health screenings, and risk factor stratification for an older adult to determine whether contraindications for exercise exist as well as to determine the type, intensity, and quantity of exercise that can be safely performed. Individualized approaches to promoting exercise can be designed on the basis of this risk. This process is discussed in Chapter 3 and is described in ACSM's Guidelines for Exercise Testing and Prescription book (27). ACSM's Resource Manual for Guidelines of Exercise Testing and Prescription presents an evaluation tool to help an exercise professional determine the appropriateness of exercise prescription in older adults (2). The following general guidelines are recommended for older adults who are healthy but may be deconditioned.

Aerobic Activity

Older adults should strive for the same amount of aerobic activity that is recommended for all adults: at least 30 minutes of moderate-intensity activity for 5 or more days a week, or at least 20 minutes of vigorous activity for 3 days a week, or a combination of vigorous and moderate for 3 to 5 days a week — see Chapter 3 and Garber (9). Greater levels of activity should be encouraged in those who are able to do so safely, as exceeding these minimal recommendations will result in further health benefits and will improve an older adult's ability to manage existing conditions and further reduce disease risk (21). However, any person who is at moderate or high risk should be medically cleared before engaging in vigorous activity (28).

Because of the heterogeneity of aerobic capacities in the older adult population, a different definition of moderate versus vigorous intensity is required (21). Since the subjective rating of an activity may be vastly different for an unconditioned person compared with a well-conditioned person, an exercise that is easy for one person may be very difficult for another. For adults, intensity is defined in absolute terms, but for older adults, a subjective rating system is used to determine the intensity of exercise, which accounts for differences in the level of conditioning. Moderate intensity is a 5 or 6 on a 0 to 10 scale (where 0 is sitting and 10 is a maximal effort) and is that which produces a noticeable change in breathing and heart rate. A vigorous effort would be a 7 or 8 on the same scale and would produce large increases in heart rate and breathing. It should also be noted that any activity is beneficial, so the HFS should also emphasize reducing sedentary behaviors as well as a gradual approach to adopting exercise. Very deconditioned adults may initially aim for light-intensity activity (<5 subjective rating of effort) and perform exercise in shorter bouts until more continuous exercise can be sustained (21).

Muscle-Strengthening Activity

All adults are recommended to perform muscle-strengthening activities for 2 to 3 nonconsecutive days a week, targeting the major muscle groups (see Chapter 4 and Garber [9]). Older adults should choose a weight or resistance that can be performed 10 to 15 times, which produces a level of effort that is moderate to high. A perception rating of 5 to 6 is moderate and a 7 to 8 is considered high on a 10-point scale (where 0 is no movement and 10 is a maximal muscular effort) (21). As with all individuals, a lighter initial weight with a focus on proper form followed by progressively increasing loads based on each person's ability is recommended. Achieving more than the minimum recommendations for muscle strengthening activity will confer proportionally greater health benefits and should be encouraged, if possible, on the basis of how well exercise is tolerated (21).

Flexibility Activity and Neuromotor Exercises

Exercises that target joint mobility are recommended for all adults. Stretching exercises that are held for 10 to 30 seconds to a point of tightness or mild discomfort for the major muscle groups (after a warm-up) and performed 2 to 3 days a week are recommended (see Chapter 5 and Garber [9]). For older adults, stretches may produce greater benefits when they are held for 30 to 60 seconds. The total time for flexibility training should reach about 10 minutes per session and should occur on at least 2 days a week. Neuromotor exercises that help improve balance, coordination, agility, gait and proprioception are recommended for older adults to reduce the number and severity of falls, aid in functional tasks, and improve the quality of life (9, 21). Tai chi, qigong, and yoga have been studied for this, but there is not enough evidence to recommend a frequency, duration, or intensity for these activities (9).

Thermoregulation

As with children and other vulnerable populations, the HFS should protect against a heat injury in the older adult by conducting exercise in a thermoneutral environment and encouraging clients to avoid exercise in the hottest times of day. It is also important to ensure adequate hydration so that evaporative cooling is maximized. For exercise in the cold, older adults should dress in layers for increased warmth and for the ability to add or remove layers as needed.

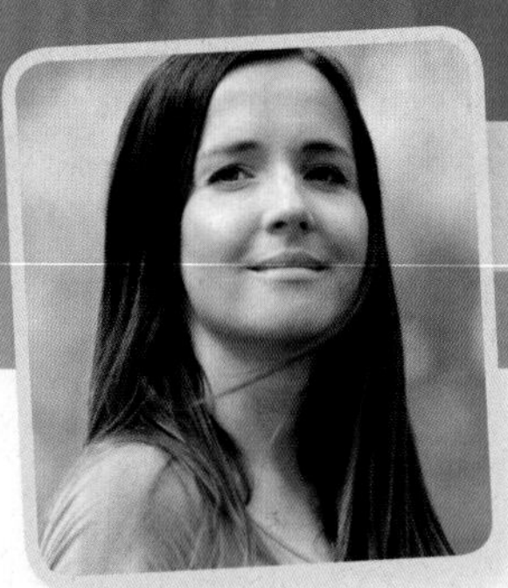

The Case of Katie

Submitted by **Kim DeLaFuente, MA, ACSM PD, Spectrum Health Healthier Communities Department, Grand Rapids, MI**

Katie is a 26-year-old pregnant mother of one with a history of gestational diabetes. She is interested in exercising safely during her pregnancy while maintaining her endurance and strength levels.

Narrative

Katie is a 26-year-old woman who is 15 weeks pregnant with her second child. She is a part-time nurse who works 24 hours a week on an ICU floor. Her work is stressful and demands a lot of time on her feet with limited rest periods. In addition, she has a young child at home that requires much of her attention.

Health Appraisal

Age: 26 years old
Family history: none
Cigarette smoking: none
Sedentary lifestyle: regularly participated in an exercise program, up until becoming pregnant. She suffered from morning sickness during the first trimester of her pregnancy and did little physical activity during this time.

The Case of Katie cont.

Obesity: none; body mass index (BMI) was 26.7 (overweight) before becoming pregnant
Hypertension: none
Dyslipidemia: none
Diabetes: history of gestational diabetes with first pregnancy and family history of diabetes
Risk classification: low risk, after consultation with physician to determine blood glucose level

Physical Data

Height: 5′ 4″
Weight: 155 lb (before pregnancy); 162 lb (current weight)
% Body fat: NA
BMI: 26.6 kg·m^{-2} before pregnancy (overweight)
Blood pressure: 120/74 mm Hg
Resting heart rate: 86 bpm
Fasting blood sugar: 96
No exercise test was done.

To date, Katie's pregnancy is uncomplicated. During her first pregnancy, Katie gained 50 lb and she was not physically active outside of work and activities of daily living. She has a family history of Type II diabetes and a diagnosis of gestational diabetes in her first pregnancy. She became motivated to exercise regularly and has maintained an exercise program that consists of jogging for 30 minutes, 4 days a week, at a rating of perceived exertion (RPE) of 15 and resistance training 2 days a week. Nausea and vomiting during the first trimester has reduced her exercise to walking a few times a week. Now that she is feeling better, Katie is interested in increasing her exercise again. Since she did not exercise during her first pregnancy, she is unsure how much or what type of exercise she should be doing.

Goals

Her goals include healthy weight gain, maintaining endurance and strength levels and safe exercise.
Goal 1: In addition to walking, start a prenatal water aerobics class, 2 days a week (RPE 11).
Goal 2: Restart a muscular strength program, 2 days a week, using resistance bands and a stability ball.
Goal 3: Learn and apply exercise guidelines related to pregnancy. What other considerations need to be made with physical activity during pregnancy?

Questions

- Identify exercise precautions that should be taken during pregnancy.
- Identify four conditions that would require exercise be terminated if a woman is pregnant.
- Identify four appropriate modes of exercise during pregnancy.

References

1. American College of Sports Medicine. *ACSM's Guidelines for Exercise Testing and Prescription*. 8th ed. Philadelphia (PA): Lippincott Williams & Wilkins; 2010.
2. American Congress of Obstetrics and Gynecology. *Exercise During Pregnancy* [Internet]. 2003 [cited 2010 Oct 8]. Available from: http://www.acog.org/publications/patient_education/bp119.cfm.
3. Colberg SR, Albright AL, Blissmer BJ, et al. Exercise and type II diabetes: American College of Sports Medicine and the American Diabetes Association: Joint position statement. *Med Sci Sports Exerc*. 2010;42(12):2282–303.

SUMMARY

Exercise is beneficial for all individuals regardless of age or activity status; however, the HFS must be aware of the unique concerns of older individuals, the young, and pregnant women. Benefits can be achieved for each of these populations once exercise type, quantity, and intensity have been adjusted on the basis of unique individual needs.

STUDY QUESTIONS

1. Which modes of exercise should be avoided by children for safety reasons?
2. Describe how exercise should be modified for pregnant women.
3. Under what conditions should a pregnant woman stop exercising?
4. What are different ways exercise intensity should be gauged for older adults and why?
5. What are some exercise precautions that should be taken when children, pregnant women, or older adults are exercising in the heat?

REFERENCES

1. American College of Obstetricians and Gynecologists. Exercise during pregnancy and the postpartum period. *Obstet Gynecol.* 2002;99:171–3.
2. Coe DP, Fiatarone-Singh MA. Exercise prescription for special populations: Women, pregnancy, children and the elderly. In: Ehrman JK, editor. *ACSM's Resource Manual for Guidelines for Exercise Testing and Prescription.* Baltimore (MD): Lippincott Williams & Wilkins; 2010. p. 665–95.
3. Biddiss E, Irwin J. Active video games to promote physical activity in children and youth: A systematic review. *Arch Pediatr Adoles Med.* 2010;164(7):664–72.
4. Dougherty KA, Chow M, Kenney WL. Critical environmental limits for exercising heat-acclimated lean and obese boys. *Eur J Appl. Physiol.* 2010;108(4):779–89.
5. Faigenbaum AD, Kraemer WJ, Blimkie CJR. Youth resistance training: Updated position statement paper from the National Strength and Conditioning Association. *J Strength Cond Res.* 2009;23(5):S60–79.
6. Faigenbaum AD, Milliken LA, Westcott W. Maximal strength testing in children. *J Strength Cond Res.* 2003;17:162–6.
7. Faigenbaum AD, Milliken LA, Cloutier G, Westcott WL. Perceived exertion during resistance exercise in children. *Percept Mot Skills.* 2004;98:627–37.
8. Faigenbaum AD, McFarland J. Relative safety of weightlifting movements for youth. *Strength Cond J.* 2008;30(6):23–5.
9. Garber CE, Blissmer B, Deschenes MR, et al. Quantity and quality of exercise for developing and maintaining cardiorespiratory, musculoskeletal, and neuromotor fitness in apparently healthy adults: Guidance for prescribing exercise. *Med Sci Sports Exerc.* 2011;43(7):1334–59.
10. Going S, Williams DP, Lohman TG. Aging and body composition: Biological changes and methodological issues. *Exerc Sport Sci Rev.* 1995;23:411–58.
11. Haskell WL, Lee IM, Pate RR, et al. Physical activity and public health: Updated recommendation for adults from the American College of Sports Medicine and the American Heart Association. *Med Sci Sports Exerc.* 2007;39(8):1423–34.
12. Hebestreit HU, Bar-Or O. Differences between children and adults for exercise testing and prescription. In: Skinner JS, editor. *Exercise Testing and Exercise Prescription for Special Cases.* 3rd ed. Baltimore (MD): Lippincott Williams & Wilkins; 2005. p. 68–84.
13. Johnson BA, Salzberg CL, Stevenson DA. A systematic review: Plyometric training programs for young children. *J Strength Cond Res.* 2011;25(9):2623.
14. Malina RM, Bouchard C, Bar-Or O. *Growth, Maturation, and Physical Activity.* 2nd ed. Champaign (IL): Human Kinetics; 2004.
15. Malina RM, Bouchard C, Bar-Or O. Somatic growth. In: *Growth, Maturation, and Physical Activity.* 2nd ed. Champaign (IL): Human Kinetics; 2004. p. 41–81.
16. Malina RM, Bouchard C, Bar-Or O. Body composition. In: *Growth, Maturation, and Physical Activity.* 2nd ed. Champaign (IL): Human Kinetics; 2004. p. 101–19.

17. Malina RM, Bouchard C, Bar-Or O. Bone tissue in skeletal growth and body composition. In: *Growth, Maturation, and Physical Activity.* 2nd ed. Champaign (IL): Human Kinetics; 2004. p. 121–35.
18. Malina RM, Bouchard C, Bar-Or O. Skeletal muscle tissue. In: *Growth, Maturation, and Physical Activity.* 2nd ed. Champaign (IL): Human Kinetics; 2004. p. 137–57.
19. Malina RM, Bouchard C, Bar-Or O. Heart, blood and lungs. In: *Growth, Maturation, and Physical Activity.* 2nd ed. Champaign (IL): Human Kinetics; 2004. p. 181–93.
20. Malina RM, Bouchard C, Bar-Or O. Strength and motor performance. In: *Growth, Maturation, and Physical Activity.* 2nd ed. Champaign (IL): Human Kinetics; 2004. p. 215–33.
21. Nelson ME, Rejeski WJ, Blair SN, et al. Physical activity and public health in older adults: Recommendation from the ACSM and the AHA. *Circulation.* 2007;116:1094–104.
22. Newman AB, Yanez D, Harris T, et al. Weight change in old age and its association with mortality. *J Am Geriatr Soc.* 2001;49:1309–18.
23. Physical Activity Guidelines Advisory Committee. *Physical Activity Guidelines Advisory Committee Report, 2008.* Washington (DC): U.S. Department of Health and Human Services; 2008.
24. Skinner JS. Aging for exercise testing and exercise prescription. In: Skinner JS, editor. *Exercise Testing and Exercise Prescription for Special Cases.* 3rd ed. Baltimore (MD): Lippincott Williams & Wilkins; 2005. p. 85–99.
25. Stevenson L. Exercise in pregnancy. Part 1: Update on pathophysiology. *Can Fam Physician.* 1997;43:97–104.
26. Stevenson L. Exercise in pregnancy. Part 2 Recommendations for individuals. *Can Fam Physician.* 1997;43:107–11.
27. Thompson WR, editor. *ACSM's Guidelines for Exercise Testing and Prescription.* 8th ed. Philadelphia (PA); Lippincott Williams & Wilkins; 2010.
28. Thompson WR, editor. Preparticipation health screening and risk stratification. In: *ACSM's Guidelines for Exercise Testing and Prescription.* 8th ed. Baltimore (MD); Lippincott Williams & Wilkins; 2010. p. 18–39.
29. Thompson WR, editor. Exercise prescription for health populations and special considerations. In: *ACSM's Guidelines for Exercise Testing and Prescription.* 8th ed. Baltimore (MD); Lippincott Williams & Wilkins; 2010. p. 183–206.
30. U.S. Department of Health and Human Services Web site [Internet]. *2008 Physical Activity Guidelines for Americans.* Atlanta (GA): USDHHS; [cited 2010 Jan 1]. Available from: www.health.gov/paguidelines
31. Wang TW, Apgar BS. Exercise during pregnancy. *Am Fam Physician.* 1998;57(8):1846–52.
32. Williamson P. Exercise during Pregnancy. In: *Exercise for Special Populations.* Baltimore (MD): Lippincott Williams & Wilkins; 2011. p. 46–81.
33. Williamson P. Exercise for youth. In: *Exercise for Special Populations.* Baltimore (MD): Lippincott Williams & Wilkins; 2011. p. 82–120.
34. Williamson P. Exercise for senior adults. In: *Exercise for Special Populations.* Baltimore (MD): Lippincott Williams & Wilkins; 2011. p. 121–78.
35. Wolfe LA. Pregnancy. In: Skinner JS, editor. *Exercise Testing and Exercise Prescription for Special Cases.* 3rd ed. Baltimore (MD): Lippincott Williams & Wilkins; 2005. p. 377–91.

Additional Resources

Ehrman JK, editor. *ACSM's Resource Manual for Guidelines for Exercise Testing and Prescription.* 6th ed. Baltimore (MD): Lippincott Williams & Wilkins; 2010.

PART

IV

Behavior Change

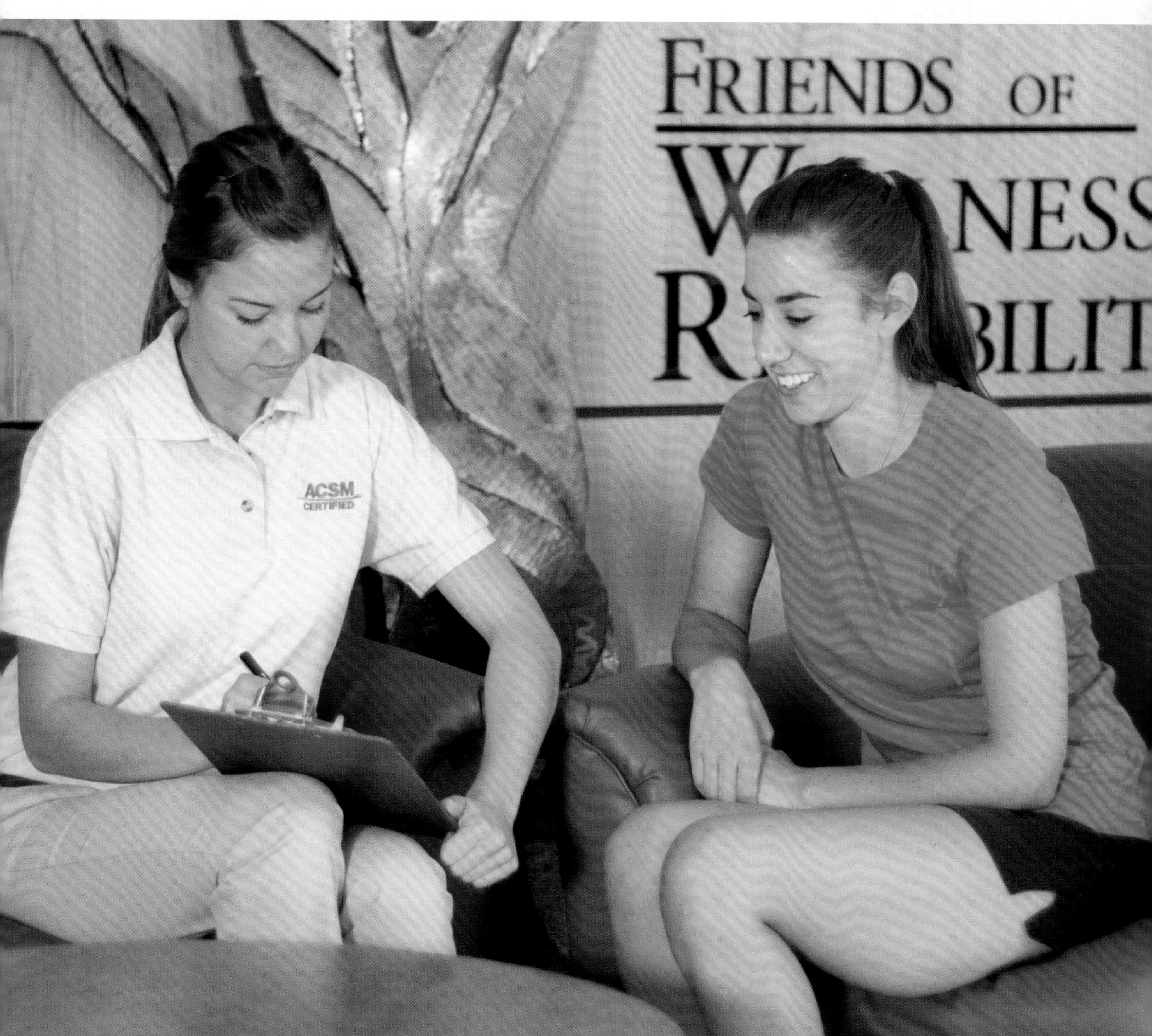

CHAPTER

10 Theories of Behavior Change

Beth Lewis • Katie Schuver

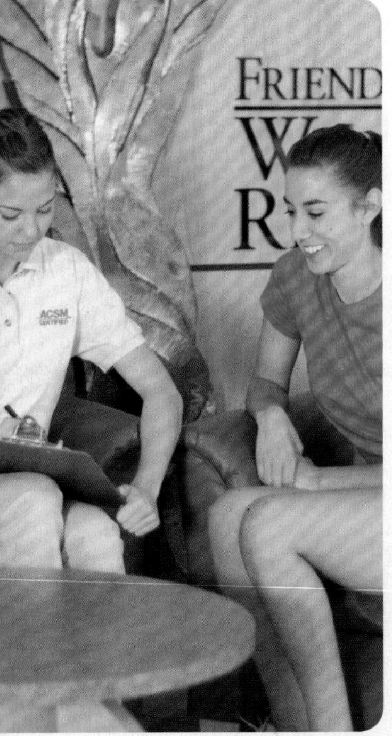

CHAPTER OBJECTIVES

- To identify and describe the theories and models used to explain physical activity behaviors.
- To understand key terminology as it relates to behavior change.
- To summarize the empirical support for the theories and models.
- To understand the practical application of the concepts presented in the chapter.

This chapter summarizes theories and models believed to be important for physical activity behavior change, including the transtheoretical model (TTM), social cognitive theory (SCT), social ecological model, health belief model, theory of planned behavior (TPB), and self-determination theory. The evidence supporting each of the theories will also be briefly outlined. In addition, the practical application of the theories will be briefly described. Chapter 11 will expand on this chapter by summarizing how the various theories and models are applied to interventions designed to motivate individuals to adopt physical activity. Before the specific models and theories are reviewed, the difference between and importance of models and theories will be explored.

WHAT IS THE DIFFERENCE BETWEEN A THEORY AND A MODEL?

A theory refers to a systematic view of a behavior by specifying relationships between variables and predicting specific behaviors and situations (23). Nutbeam and Harris (44) stated that there are three essential elements of a theory, including (a) variables that influence the particular behavior, (b) the relationship between the variables, and (c) understanding the conditions in which the relationships occur or do not occur. Specifically related to physical activity, a theory would explain the variables that influence physical activity, how these variables interact with one another to influence physical activity, and the conditions under which physical activity occurs. Theories can also help in designing interventions for physical activity promotion. A model, on the other hand, is defined as a hypothetical depiction of a behavior or situation (24). Models do not attempt to understand the variables underlying a particular behavior, but rather to represent what is happening with a particular behavior. It is important to note that these definitions are general guidelines, and researchers will occasionally use the terms *theory* and *model* interchangeably.

IMPORTANCE OF THEORIES AND MODELS

There are a number of reasons why it is important to utilize theories and models for physical activity. First, theories and models provide a framework for better understanding physical activity adoption. For example, practitioners may identify that their clients have low self-efficacy toward physical activity, which refers to one's confidence in his or her ability to engage in physical activity. Self-efficacy is derived from social cognitive theory, which will be discussed later in this chapter. The practitioner may be more successful at increasing physical activity in the client after discussing with him or her different strategies to increase self-efficacy. Second, theories and models can help practitioners understand why a client has stopped his or her physical activity participation. For example, the barrier of time is a frequently reported variable for stopping physical activity and thus could be addressed with the client. Third, theories and models allow the practitioner to identify which types of clients respond to which types of physical activity promotion strategies. For example, it may be especially important for adults with children to have spousal support for engaging in physical activity, yet this may not be necessary for people without children living at home. In summary, models and theories provide the foundation for better understanding physical activity adoption and maintenance and can provide helpful tools for practitioners attempting to increase physical activity among their clients.

TRANSTHEORETICAL MODEL

When discussing theories or models, it is important to understand that both cognitive theories and behavioral strategies exist. Cognitive processes are used to change the way we think about activity, whereas behavioral processes are used to change/initiate the actual behavior itself.

The transtheoretical model (TTM) has also been used to understand physical activity behavior and to create physical activity interventions (35). Research indicates that physical activity interventions based on the TTM are efficacious for increasing physical activity among sedentary adults (37, 38, 43, 46, 50) and other groups. The TTM proposes that individuals move through a series of stages ("stages of change") during physical activity adoption (13, 48): (a) precontemplation, (b) contemplation, (c) preparation, (d) adoption, and (e) maintenance (35). These specific stages are outlined in Table 10.1.

Specific behavioral and cognitive processes occur as individuals move through the various stages of change. The various processes are thought to receive differential emphasis during particular stages of change (13, 14, 48). Cognitive processes of change include increasing knowledge, being aware of risks, caring about consequences to others, comprehending benefits, and increasing healthy opportunities. Behavioral processes of change include substituting alternatives, enlisting social support, rewarding yourself, committing yourself, and reminding yourself (34). These processes

TABLE 10.1 **THE TTM: STAGES OF CHANGE**

Stage of Change	Progression Through the Five Stages	Application to Physical Activity
Precontemplation	Individuals in this stage are not intending to take action within the next 6 mo. There may be a variety of reasons why an individual would be in the precontemplation stage – uninformed about the health effects of a sedentary lifestyle, uninformed about the consequences, not motivated to make changes, or have made several failed attempts at physical activity adoption and is now discouraged or debilitated	Stage 1: Inactive and not thinking about becoming more active These individuals do not currently engage in physical activity and do not plan on doing so in the near future
Contemplation	Individuals in this stage are intending to alter their behavior within the next 6 mo. They may be becoming more aware of the pros of engaging in physical activity; however, the costs associated with physical activity may still outweigh the benefits	Stage 2: Inactive and thinking about becoming more active These individuals are thinking about adopting physical activity and are planning to become more physically active within a reasonable time frame
Preparation	Individuals in this stage are intending to increase their physical activity in the immediate future. These individuals may have a specific plan to change behavior and may be seeking out resources for assistance	Stage 3: Doing some physical activity These individuals are currently doing physical activity, but are not meeting the standards and guidelines identified by the American College of Sports Medicine
Action	Individuals in this stage have made specific, measureable changes in their physical activity in the past 6 mo	Stage 4: Doing enough physical activity These individuals are currently engaging in physical activity 5 $d \cdot wk^{-1}$ for at least 30 min each session. These individuals have participated in regular physical activity for <6 mo
Maintenance	Individuals in this stage are maintaining their physical activity and are working to prevent relapse to old habits	Stage 5: Making physical activity a habit These individuals have been participating in regular physical activity at the recommended levels for at least 6 mo

represent principles of change in behavior and are considered responsible for movement through the various stages of the TTM.

Sufficient evidence exists to support the use of the TTM in facilitating physical activity behavior change regardless of the medium of physical activity intervention (36). Both print- and phone-based exercise interventions have been coupled with the TTM, and each shows individuals increasing levels of moderate-intensity physical activity for at least 6 months, especially compared with controls. Further, receiving a physical activity intervention through the TTM appears to allow individuals to increase their behavioral strategies, cognitive processes, decisional balance (*i.e.*, weighing the pros and cons of becoming physically active when moving through the stages), and self-efficacy.

SOCIAL COGNITIVE THEORY

Social cognitive theory (SCT) (4, 6, 7), first known as social learning theory, is one of the most popular theoretical frameworks for understanding physical activity adoption (39, 60). SCT emphasizes reciprocal determinism, which is the interaction between individuals and their environments

(Fig. 10.1). SCT identifies three main factors that influence behavior and behavioral choices: (a) the environment (*e.g.*, neighborhood and proximity to gym), (b) individual personality characteristics and/or experience (including cognitions), and (c) behavioral factors. Behavior is the product of the interplay between these three factors. In other words, the environment can influence individuals and groups, but individuals and groups can also influence their environments, and in turn, govern their own behaviors.

A key concept identified in SCT is self-efficacy (4–6). Self-efficacy is the confidence in one's ability to successfully engage in and perform a specific behavior. This would differ from self-confidence, which indicates a belief in being able to sustain the exercise regardless of challenges faced. Self-efficacy, as part of the SCT, postulates that the more confident one feels in their capabilities and skills to succeed, the more likely they will engage in that behavior (6). Capabilities and skills refer to the organization and execution of the necessary course of action required to produce the desired results. Intervention studies indicate that self-efficacy is likely an important component of physical activity behavior change for apparently healthy adults (34), children and older adults (15, 61, 63), and those with controlled disease (25, 39, 40, 57).

According to Bandura (6), self-efficacy is a product of (and therefore can be influenced by) four sources of information: (a) enactive mastery experience, (b) vicarious experience, (c) verbal persuasion, and (d) physiological or affective states. First, enactive mastery experience is the successful performance of the target behavior (in this case, physical activity), which should enhance perception of efficacy, while failure to perform the behavior sabotages it. For example, an individual who is able to successfully maintain a regular physical activity program for 6 weeks would demonstrate higher levels of perceived self-efficacy. Second, vicarious experience refers to seeing a similar individual successfully perform a behavior and comparing one's own performance with the performance of the

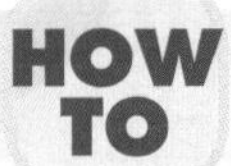

Determine an Individual's Stage or Change for Physical Activity

According to the TTM, interventions should be tailored to the individual depending on his or her stage of change. Specific to physical activity, it may be helpful to ask the following questions to determine an individual's stage of change:

1. Are you currently accumulating at least 150 minutes of moderate-intensity physical activity each week? (If yes, in action or maintenance stage and go to question 2. If no, go to question 3).
2. Have you been regularly physically active over the past 6 months? (If yes, in maintenance stage and stop questions. If no, in action stage and stop questions).
3. Are you doing any physical activity? (If yes, in the preparation change and stop questions. If no, ask question 4).
4. Have you made any actions and/or concrete plans in increasing your physical activity (*i.e.*, gym membership, purchasing exercise equipment, and hiring a trainer)? (If yes, in preparation stage and stop questions. If no, ask question 5).
5. Do you plan on becoming more physically active over the next 6 months? (If yes, in contemplation. If no, in precontemplation).

Once you have answers to the above questions, you can better develop a plan of action specific to each client and tailored to their current stage or readiness. For those clients in the maintenance stage, the plan might just involve introducing new exercises or goals. For those in the contemplation or preparation stages, the plan will need to be more detailed and include guidance on how to handle setbacks.

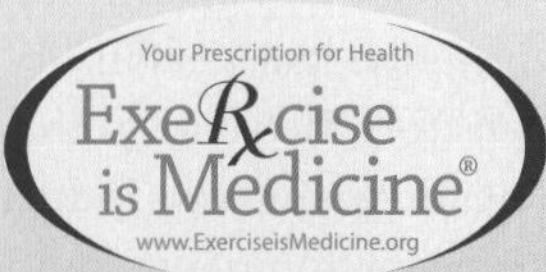

EXERCISE IS MEDICINE CONNECTION

Wilcox S, Dowda M, Leviton LC, et al. Active for life: Final results from the translation of two physical activity programs. *Am J Prev Med.* 2008;35:340–51.

Wilcox and colleagues (2008) conducted a study in which two theory-based physical activity interventions shown to be efficacious were translated into real-world setting. The interventions were "Active Choices" and "Active Living Everyday." Both interventions were based on SCT and the TTM. Active Choices lasted 6 months and included a face-to-face contact and up to eight telephone contacts. Participants were given a physical activity log, a pedometer, and a resource guide at the face-to-face visit. Participants set physical activity goals and were given strategies on the basis of SCT and TTM (*e.g.*, overcoming barriers and self-monitoring). Active Living Everyday was originally a 20-week program, but was based on feedback from the disseminating organizations, and was modified to a 12-week program. This physical activity program was delivered in small groups. There were nine organizations that disseminated the programs. Examples included Blue Shield of California, the Council on Aging of Southwestern Ohio, and the Berkeley Public Health Department. Participants included individuals who were at least 50 years of age and who were sedentary or underactive. Results indicated that the number of individuals meeting or exceeding the ACSM/CDC physical activity guidelines increased from pre- to posttest. The authors of this study reported that the interventions were adapted to meet the needs of the organization while maintaining high treatment fidelity. This study indicated that theory-based efficacious physical activity interventions can be successfully disseminated into real world settings.

other individual. Third, verbal persuasion occurs when others express faith in the individual's capabilities. Finally, correcting misinterpretations of physiological messages, reducing negative emotional states, and increasing positive emotional states have a positive influence on self-efficacy.

Substantial evidence supports the SCT as an effective means of influencing human behavior. Results compiled from multiple studies indicate that the most successful behavioral interventions for enhancing self-efficacy were found when vicarious experiences and feedback techniques (*e.g.*, providing feedback by comparing participants' performance with the performance of others, providing feedback on the participants' past performances) were used in an intervention (3). In addition, monitoring an individual's behavior and performance based on task mastery and skill development may also have a positive influence on self-efficacy. Setting a specific detailed plan and encouraging individuals to set a specific intention of how to adopt physical activity are common among successful intervention programs (64).

Interestingly, there is emerging literature indicating that focusing on relapse prevention techniques and identifying physical activity barriers may actually have a negative impact on physical activity and therefore are not recommended to enhance physical activity self-efficacy. Instead, the focus of interventions should be on what the individual can do to achieve the desired behavior

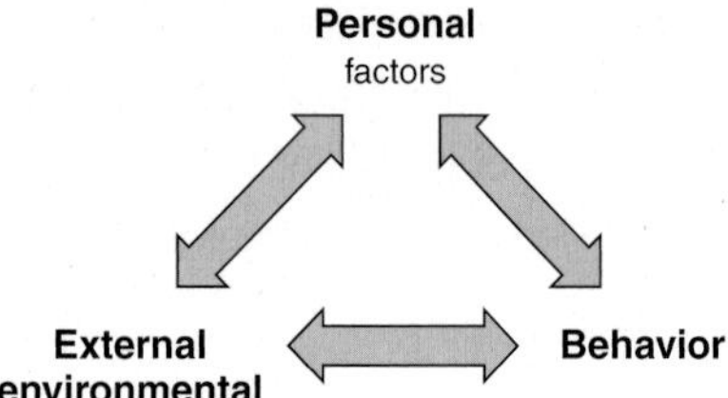

FIGURE 10.1. Reciprocal determinism: Based on Bandura's social cognitive theory. (Reproduced with permission from Bandura A. *Social Foundations of Thought and Action: A Social Cognitive Theory.* Englewood Cliffs (NJ): Prentice-Hall Inc.; 1986.)

change rather than emphasizing on what they cannot do. This is believed to be the most effective means of improving self-efficacy toward physical activity (3, 64).

Although there are numerous correlates of physical activity, including attitudes, perceived barriers, enjoyment, expected benefits, and so on, the prevailing evidence supports self-efficacy as possibly the most important component of physical activity behavior change (60). However, despite this strong evidence, results of various self-efficacy–based interventions have been inconsistent. In general, there are consistent increases in physical activity (64), but inconsistent improvements in self-efficacy (27, 28, 34).

On the basis of SCT, there is still sufficient evidence to support the Health Fitness Specialist (HFS) focusing on increasing client's physical activity self-efficacy. Some techniques that could be used in building physical activity self-efficacy include the following:

- Verbal persuasion to reinforce task mastery.
- Provide exposure to positive vicarious experiences.
- Explain and reinforce the positive physiological states achieved from exercise.
- Encourage various forms of physical activity, noting what is most enjoyed.
- Encourage client recall of previous successful behavior change.
- Maintain a physical activity log to help track successes and progressions.
- Encourage reasonable, specific physical activity goals that can be achieved in a short time.
- Encourage perseverance and praise efforts to achieve goals, not just the attainment of goals.

SOCIAL ECOLOGICAL MODEL

The social ecological model is a comprehensive approach integrating multiple variables or layers that influence behavior. These layers include intra- and interpersonal factors, community and organizational factors, institutional factors, environmental factors, and public policies (Fig. 10.2). Within this model, each layer has a resulting impact on the next layer. For example, an individual's social environment of family, friends, and workplace are embedded within the physical environment of geography and community facilities. This is then embedded within and influenced by the policy environment of government or other official bodies. All levels of the social ecological model influence the behavior of the individual (10).

There are many versions of the social ecological model for physical activity, including systems theory, ecological model of health behavior, and social ecology model for health promotion. Each of these applications uses slightly different classifications of environmental influences. Systems theory uses "microsystem" (personal interactions between family members, work groups, etc.), "mesosystem" (physical settings for family, school, and work), and "exosystem" (the larger social influences of economics, policies, culture, and politics) (10). The social ecological model is specific to an individual's health behaviors and includes factors such as intrapersonal, interpersonal processes, institutional influences, community factors, and public policies (41). The social ecology model is specific to the promotion of health behaviors and focuses on assumptions related to influences of the physical and social environments; multidimensional environments; interactions between individuals, families, communities, and so on; and how individuals influence their surroundings (58, 59).

Many of the traditional ecological models were meant to apply broadly across a variety of behaviors, yet more recent models have been developed to apply specifically to health behaviors (41, 58, 59). Researchers and practitioners have begun to acknowledge the significant role that the environment plays on health behaviors. Many health behaviors, including physical activity, are too complex to be adequately evaluated and understood by simply addressing the individual. Research suggests that coordinating and planning efforts among the agencies responsible for transportation, urban planning, school zoning, access to facilities and programs, and supporting social environments that encourage activity (*e.g.*, walking and biking trails, sidewalks, and reduction of crime) may influence physical activity behavior (12, 20, 30, 55).

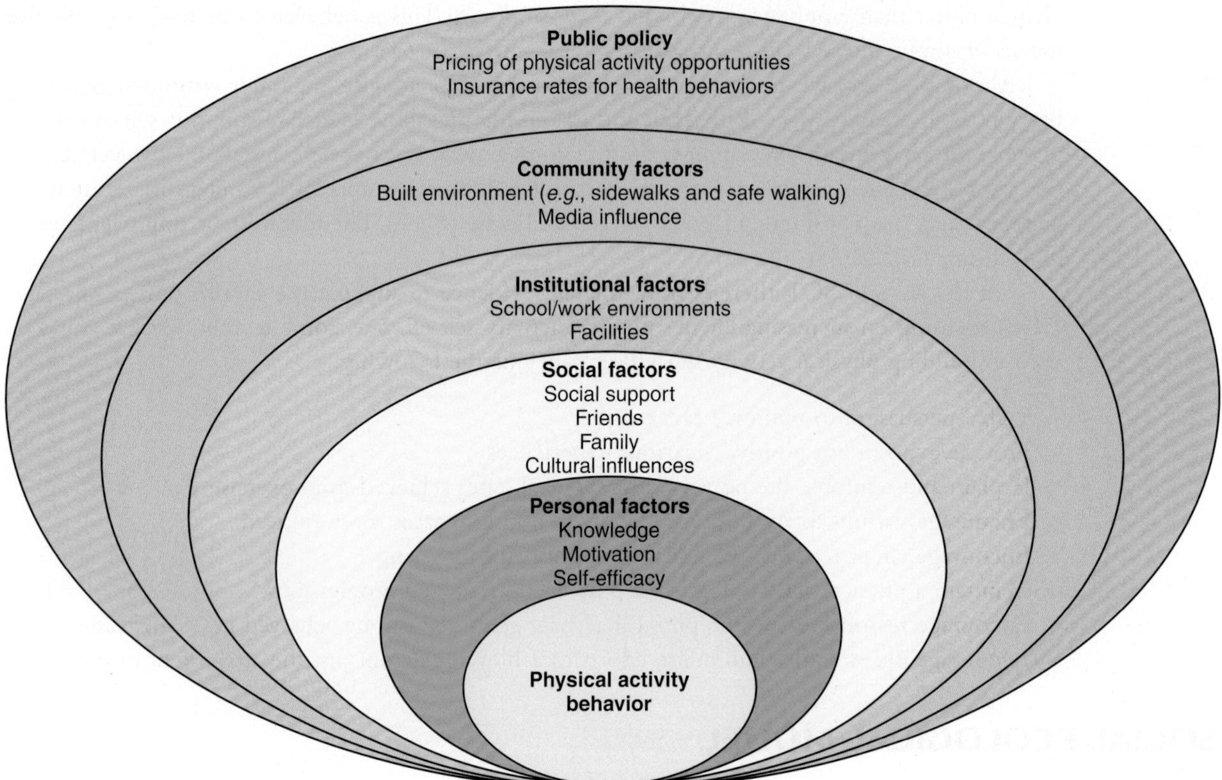

FIGURE 10.2. Social ecological model of physical activity behavior: Based on Bronfenbrenner's social ecological model. (Reproduced with permission from Bronfenbrenner U. *The Ecology of Human Development: Experiments by Nature and Design*. Cambridge (MA): Harvard University Press; 1979.)

Uncovering the motivational factors that underlie the successful adoption and maintenance of physical activity programs requires a multidimensional approach that considers not only behavioral change and intrapersonal factors, but also social and environmental factors. The socioeconomic approach incorporates these considerations; however, the application of socioeconomic models can be difficult, as they need to be tailored and refined to meet the needs of specific behaviors and populations. A number of multidimensional models, specific to the physical activity domain, have been proposed and empirically supported (9, 18, 54). Elder and colleagues (18) described a framework that was created to promote physical activity

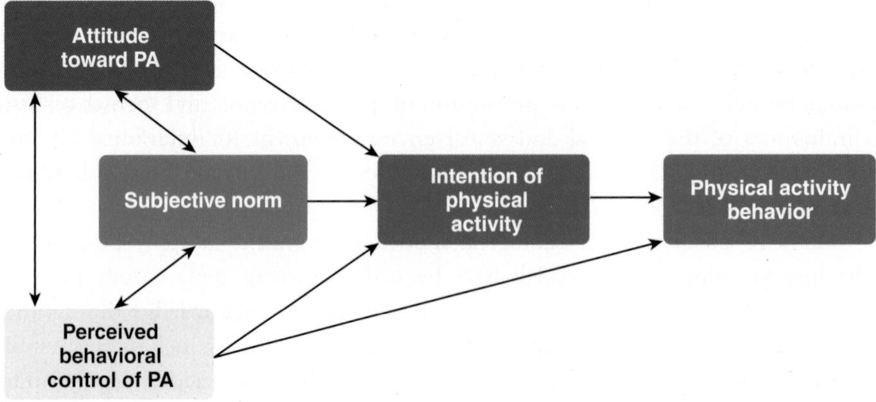

FIGURE 10.3. Theory of planned behavior: Based on Ajzen's theory of planned behavior. (Adapted from Ajzen I. The theory of planned behavior. *Organ Behav Hum Decis Process.* 1991;50(2):179–211 and Marcus BH, Forsyth LH. *Motivating People to be Physically Active.* 2nd ed. Champaign (IL): Human Kinetics; 2009.)

behavior among adolescent girls. This framework, which guided the intervention known as TAAG (trial of activity for adolescent girls), adopted principles from behavioral modification, social cognitive, and organizational change theories to influence physical activity behavior in adolescent girls' intrapersonal, school, and community environments. The TAAG approach has been used to promote positive physical activity behaviors in middle school girls, and when incorporated in a school and community-based environment, girls in the intervention schools demonstrated a trend of increased physical activity in comparison with those in the schools that did not receive the TAAG program (19, 62).

The social ecological model provides a useful framework for better understanding the multiple factors and barriers that influence physical activity behavior. Empirical evidence suggests that the social, physical, and policy environments influence physical activity participation. Behavior can be difficult to change, especially in an environment that does not support change. To increase physical activity, efforts may need to focus on both the behavior choices of each individual and factors that influence those choices. The social ecological model helps identify opportunities to promote participation in physical activity by recognizing the multiple variables that may influence an individual's choices.

As advocates of regular physical activity, the HFS may find that they are more successful at influencing an individual's physical activity when multiple levels of influence are addressed at the same time. According to this model, in order for physical activity interventions to be effective, the HFS must go beyond simple exercise prescriptions. Other factors that influence physical activity behavior choices must also be addressed. For example, the HFS may help the client choose new exercise equipment for the home, employ family members to join the physical activity program, decrease overall sedentary behavior, and assist in identifying possible environmental barriers to exercise. This holistic approach in providing physical activity guidance may help the HFS develop more appropriate, sensitive, and effective motivational and intervention strategies.

Additional strategies the HFS can use to create an environment that promotes physical activity include the following:

- Assist clients in identifying the wide variety of physical activity options that exist within proximity to their home. This may include parks, gyms, community centers, clubs, hiking trails, and the like.
- Discuss with your client the existing potential environmental barriers that deter him or her from regular physical activity.
- Encourage your client to join a walking or jogging club or training group.

HEALTH BELIEF MODEL

The health belief model is a conceptual framework that outlines an individual's health behavior based on his or her health beliefs (52). The model ascertains that as individuals take greater investment in their personal health, they are more likely to make relevant and meaningful behavior changes. The model identifies four main components that may influence an individual's health behavior choices as follows:

1. Perception of susceptibility or risk of the identified health threat.
2. Perception of the severity of the identified health threat, including clinical and/or medical and social consequences.
   a. Combined, these two factors create a "perceived threat" to each individual that will largely determine his or her level of interest in initiating change.
3. Perception of the benefits from taking action to reduce the identified health threat.
4. Perception of barriers and/or costs of taking action to reduce the identified health threat.
   a. Combined, these two factors create a potential action plan for any given individual, assuming the perceived threat is great enough to create the need for action.

According to the health belief model, an individual examines the negative aspects of a particular health action and/or behavior and weighs those "costs" with the benefits of the health action. If benefits outweigh the costs, then the individual is more likely to participate in the health action. For example, an individual may weigh the barriers of physical activity (*e.g.*, time-consuming, inconvenience, cost, and unpleasant) against the perceived benefits of physical activity (*e.g.*, reduction in risk of disease, weight management, and social connection). If the individual decides that the reduction in disease risk and weight loss (benefits) outweighs the cost of the inconvenience of physical activity, then they may experience higher levels of motivation to begin and/or maintain a regular exercise program. This can also be considered an equation in which (a) (susceptibility + seriousness) = perceived threat, (b) (benefits + barriers) = outcome expectation, and (c) (threat + expectations) = likelihood of action.

A comprehensive review of literature notes that the most powerful determinants of health behaviors were the perception of barriers and/or the costs of taking action (31). Perceived severity was the least powerful predictor of health behaviors, yet the health belief model has been shown to have support when examining health behaviors and compliance with medical recommendation, particularly in older persons (8, 29). However, the support for the health belief model applied to physical activity has been mixed (42, 45).

Koch (32) examined the health belief model in women with Type 2 diabetes mellitus and found that women who exercised regularly reported fewer barriers to exercise and perceived greater benefits from adhering to a regular exercise regimen than women who reported lower levels of physical activity. In addition, women indicated that the belief in the perceived benefits of exercise (health belief) was most strongly linked to desired behaviors (regular physical activity).

Although empirical evidence is inconclusive regarding the importance of the health belief model for physical activity adoption, practitioners can benefit from using this model. On the basis of the health belief model's hypothesis of predicting health-related behaviors, the HFS can do the following to assist his or her clients in adopting and maintaining a regular fitness regime:

1. Assist clients in identifying their personal susceptibility and potential severity of disease if regular physical activity does not become a lifestyle behavior.
2. Educate clients regarding the risk of a sedentary lifestyle on the basis of empirically supported research.
3. Assist clients in identifying the potential benefits of a regular physical activity program on the basis of their personal goals and motivation.
4. Prepare clients for the potential barriers of maintaining a regular physical activity program (*e.g.*, time, cost, sickness, family-related obligations, and work) and develop a plan for maintaining physical activity even when potential barriers appear to outweigh the benefits.

THEORY OF PLANNED BEHAVIOR

The theory of planned behavior (TPB) is an intention-based model used to explain physical activity behavior across many populations (1, 26). The TPB is an extension of the theory of reasoned action (21) and identifies intention as the primary influence in determining behavior (see Figure 10.3). Intention directly reflects the individual's level of motivation (*i.e.*, willingness and amount of effort exerted) to perform the desired behavior. According to the TPB, one's attitude, subjective norms, and perceived behavioral control influence intention, which then influences actual behavior. Specifically related to physical activity, attitude is defined as a positive or negative evaluation of physical activity. Subjective norm is the individual's perception of social pressure to participate, or not, in physical activity. Perceived behavioral control is the individual's perception of the ease or difficulty for engaging in physical activity. This can be perceived as similar to self-efficacy because it involves an individual's perception that he or she has the ability to execute the desired behavior.

The research literature is mixed in terms of support for intention predicting physical activity behavior (2, 16, 33). Intention generally appears to be the most influential factor in predicting behavior, yet perceived behavioral control significantly adds to the prediction of actual behavior

(22). In addition, it is suggested that perceived behavioral control may also directly impact behavior itself (16). Therefore, each can stand on its own to predict behavior; however, combined, they have a much stronger effect.

In using the TPB in practice, the HFS may assist the client in identifying and developing their intentions. These intentions will then be influenced by the individual's attitude, perceived level of behavioral control, and subjective norm. An HFS can encourage physical activity behavior by assisting the development of self-efficacy, helping the client create an environment of support by recruiting coworkers and friends to be reminder cues for physical activity (subjective norm), and finally making physical activity easily accessible (perceived behavioral control). With these changes, the client's intention for physical activity behavior will be increased, causing an improvement in actual behavior.

SELF-DETERMINATION THEORY

Self-determination theory states that individuals have three basic psychological needs that must be met in order to be motivated to engage in a behavior: (a) competence, (b) relatedness, and (c) autonomy (53). Competence is the sense of being capable of completing an activity or mastering a task and the perception of being effective in that task. Relatedness is the need to be connected and involved with the social world. Autonomy is characterized by maintaining a perceived internal locus of control and a sense that behaviors are freely chosen. When a behavior is self-determined, then an individual perceives that the locus of control is internal to himself or herself. However, when an individual feels that a behavior is controlled, then they perceive the locus of control to be external to himself or herself. The more the individual feels he or she is engaging in self-directed behavior with a perceived internal locus of control, the more likely that individual will continue the desired behavior. For example, when individuals have an opportunity to freely choose which physical activities they engage in (perceived internal locus of control) versus being told specifically which mode of physical activity to engage in (perceived external locus of control), according to self-determination theory, those individuals will be more likely to adhere with the desired physical activity behavior.

Self-determination theory proposes that the extent to which the needs (*i.e.*, competence, relatedness, and autonomy) are met describes how motivated an individual is to complete a task. In other words, when an individual is in a social context in which he or she feels competent, related, and autonomous, he or she will be motivated to participate in an activity and the motivation will be based on self-determination rather than an external factor.

Motivation is described as a continuum and ranges from amotivation, or a complete lack of motivation, to intrinsic motivation, or the inherent willingness to engage. According to self-determination theory, an individual who is closer to the intrinsically motivated end of the continuum will be more motivated to participate in an activity than an individual who falls closer to the amotivation end of the continuum, which is often related to those with extrinsic motivation. An individual who is intrinsically motivated to participate in physical activity would be motivated by the genuine love of physical activity. An extrinsically motivated individual would engage in physical activity for reasons such as weight control, weight loss, and stress reduction. An amotivated person wouldn't engage in physical activity regardless.

Also within the motivation continuum exists a threshold of autonomy, as not all extrinsic motives are the same and there may be a nonlinear prediction along the continuum. In addition, it is important to note that truly intrinsic motivation toward physical activity, or many other behaviors, is actually quite rare and shouldn't be considered a key construct for successful change. In fact, a person can exercise to avoid disease or exercise because being healthy is important; these may seem similar on the surface, but they are very different from a theoretical perspective.

Self-determination theory is a holistic, inclusive approach that can help gain a stronger understanding of exercise behavior and a better understanding of the intrapersonal (*e.g.*, psychological needs) and interpersonal (*e.g.*, influence of exercise environment) factors that influence physical activity. Self-determination theory considers the social contact in which the individual operates. According to self-determination theory, individuals who are in an autonomy supportive climate (a climate in which the client plays an active role in choosing how and/or what he or she learns) are more likely to feel like their needs of autonomy, relatedness, and competence are being met (53), which promotes greater intrinsic motivation. In addition, events that are interpreted by the individual to be informational, rather than controlling or amotivating, will result in the endorsement of intrinsic motivating behaviors. According to this theory, sociocontextual variables can be manipulated to create an environment conducive to exercise. Therefore, this theory can provide insight into why individuals intend to adopt and maintain physical activity, as preliminary research supports self-determination theory as a predictor motivating individuals to engage in physical activity (17, 65).

Self-determination theory offers promise in explaining the behaviors that influence an individual's motivation. On the basis of the foundational principles of self-determination theory, the HFS may see improved levels of motivation for physical activity if the three innate psychological needs of autonomy, competence, and relatedness are met. Autonomy can be encouraged by allowing the client to have input on the physical activity plan, including choice of activity mode and intensity. Competence can be encouraged by making sure the client is entering a physical activity environment in which he or she will feel challenged, yet successful. For example, if working with a client who is just returning to running, encourage him or her to join a beginner group that would likely lead to success. Finally, the HFS should encourage clients to exercise with others to meet the relatedness need of self-determination theory.

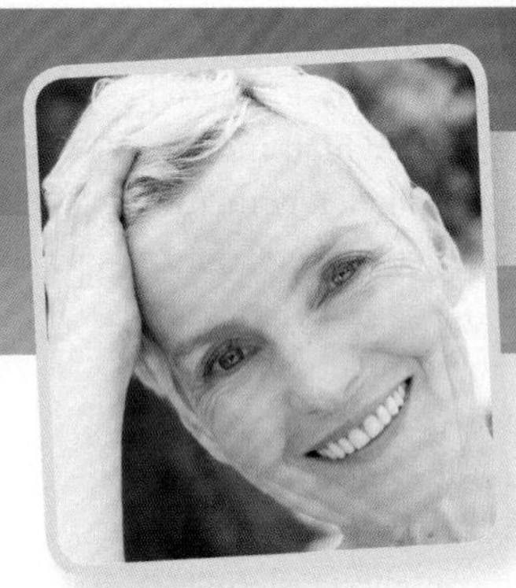

The Case of Anna

Submitted by **Steve McClaran, PhD, ACSM-HFS, Associate Professor, Colorado State University-Pueblo, Pueblo, CO**

Anna was an almost 60-year-old woman who could barely walk four blocks before beginning an exercise program. Anna had a history of attempting an exercise programs in the past, but had low adherence to these programs.

Narrative

When I first met Anna, we decided to go for a walk — she barely made it four blocks. Five years later after exercising regularly, she had lost more than 150 lb and walked a half marathon in 4 hours! She was almost 60 when we started our project, and we concentrated on the process of behavior change. What were the best practices to stay motivated for exercise? We started with three questions:

1. Where are you now? To help with this question, we did a fitness assessment. As a note, we redid the fitness assessment after the first 3 months, again after 6 months, after a year, and then yearly for the next 5 years.
2. Where do you want to go? To help with this, we felt that first we wanted to personalize the goal. Anna had tried many times to be successful and had failed a lot! We started off slowly and used short-term goals every month. Of course, we had long-term goals, but we concentrated on the short-term goals to keep building her confidence in the long-term success. We continuously asked what the potential positive outcome was and then molded the goal to optimize the long-term outcome. Lastly (and maybe most importantly), we concentrated on making our goals measurable behavior goals versus outcome. There was a strong sense that in Anna's past attempts, she concentrated on the outcomes as opposed to the behaviors that would lead to these positive outcomes. I feel that the behavior goals are the important and sustainable pieces of long-term behavior change.
3. How are you going to get there? We found that attention to behavior change skills was extremely helpful.

The Case of Anna cont.

I know this has been discussed a lot, but we concentrated on discussion of benefits of physical activity, barriers or obstacles to long-term success, goal setting, social support, and monitoring her activities. It started with a commitment: we devised together a behavior change contract, and our responsibilities to the cause were delineated and signed. As far as benefits, not only is it the knowledge of what the benefits are but there was also a discussion of what she was feeling toward our original list of benefits every time during our weekly exercise walks. We felt that realizing the benefits during the behavior change process was critical for continued motivation. Social support strategies include practical support (logistics will be discussed below in the barriers section), technical support (I found a lot of shared experiences on the Internet and would find something each month to discuss during our weekly walks), group support (she joined a gym and did aerobics classes at the Senior Center), and emotional motivational support (she shared the experience with her sister, daughter, son, and her colleagues at work).

Barriers or obstacles were our next order of business to solve. We started with a list of five obstacles and then came up with creative and workable solutions to each of the issues. We looked on each of the obstacles as a challenge, and we revisited the five at the end of every 3 months to determine our progress. We also felt that logistics were the practical steps she needed to be successful with behavior change. As obvious and simple as logistics are, any failure to pay attention to logistical details is often a cause of relapse. If plan A didn't work for some reason, having plans B and C ready helped our chances of success. Planning for weather changes was essential for exercise; walking in cold weather means you need either different gear or an inside track. We found that scheduling exercise before work was logistically more effective than planning to do it later, when complications may interfere. Logistical problems were never completely solved, so you want to help your client adopt the mindset of finding a solution to any problem that arises. We felt that environment control was an important consideration. First, we discussed removing herself from the presence of temptation. Anna owned her own business with four other women. Prior to her starting her journey toward the half-marathon, there was always some form of fattening pastries at the office, so she asked her partners if it was all right to bring in fruit and vegetable platters to replace the pastries and they all agreed. Maybe more importantly was putting her in the presence of the desired behavior: She joined a gym and signed up for aerobics classes at the senior center. Concentrating on emotional control reduced both the risk of returning to the old behavior and increased the opportunity to engage in the new behavior. Anna also sets up a stationary bike and a Bowflex in the basement, which helped with those times that weather was an issue. As a further note, Anna found music when exercising in her basement! She would often share with me those songs that were the most inspirational. By the end of the third year, she had a library of more than 500 songs she could use and rock out to in her basement.

Reward systems worked for us. It seems that some people simply make a decision to do something, and do it, with no other need for rewards. Most of us need a system of reward that includes external incentives followed by internal ones. Some of us use disincentives, or punishments. A further variation is a balance system of earning rewards, such as working out to use the number of calories in the dessert we plan to have after dinner. Anna liked to put stickers on her calendar when she completed a desired behavior, and then she gave herself a reward when she earned a certain number of stickers. Eventually, her continued success brought its own reward, and we felt that external rewards became more unnecessary. Another idea she came up with was to give her clothes away to charity as she lost weight and waist size. Anna felt that giving the clothes away would close that part of her life and make it more difficult to go back to the fit of those clothes.

Maybe one of the biggest reasons for Anna's success was the continued monitoring and reporting she did. Once she had completed her exercise for the week, she e-mailed me every Sunday evening. She is a pretty competitive person that in the first year and a half, she would sometimes exercise later in the week just so she wouldn't have to send in a low-volume exercise report. This I believe worked to help the new behavior become a habit. One interesting part about our monitoring and reporting plan was the first and second yearly summaries. After the first year, I used a computer graphing package to make a picture of how much she exercised every week – I made an average weekly amount of exercise line that went through each of the 52 bars that represented the amount of exercise for that week. As all of the weekly volume bars

***The Case of Anna* cont.**

were on one page, both of us could see when the good and less good periods were. We then made some goals that would improve the amount of exercise time for those periods for the next year. This helped a lot with motivation. Eventually, we went with pedometers, which we believed significantly help by reminding and challenging her to achieve success. I crossed that finish line at the end of the half-marathon with Anna and her daughter.

It is difficult to describe how great it was to see how happy she was at accomplishing those many goals along her journey. Her daughter had cameras and video evidence, and many family members were there to help her celebrate. I have since moved half way across the country, but we still keep in touch. She sends me postcards from Africa, South America, and Europe as she and her sister do many hiking adventures that were essentially unavailable to her before she went on her successful exercise journey.

Question

- How important are benefits?
- What is the process of successful behavior change?
- What were the most important aspects of the process you emphasized?

SUMMARY

The TTM, SCT, social ecological model, health belief model, TPB, and self-determination theory have been used to better understand physical activity behavior. The TTM has been researched most frequently followed by SCT and the TBP (51). The self-determination theory is newer, yet has also been receiving greater interest more recently (11, 56). Even though there is less support for the social ecological model, health belief model, and the TBP, HFSs can use tools from these models to motivate individuals to adopt physical activity. For any HFS, there is a need to fully understand the psychological processes that influence the adoption and maintenance of physical activity across all populations. Otherwise, simply prescribing an exercise prescription without thought to the behavioral aspect of why someone may or may not fully engage in physical activity is likely to lead to low retention rates.

The purpose of this chapter was to outline the basic tenets of various theories and models that have been applied to physical activity behavior. Chapter 11 will explore in more detail how these theories have been specifically applied to interventions and how the HFS can provide these theory-based interventions to their clients.

STUDY QUESTIONS

1. What is the difference between a theory and a model?
2. What are the five stages of change, as identified by the TTM? How would an HFS use the five stages of change to assess his or her client's readiness to participate in physical activity?
3. What are the four sources of self-efficacy? What techniques would an HFS use to improve self-efficacy?
4. Briefly describe other models of change (SCT, health belief model, self-determination theory) and how the HFS could use them to increase physical activity participation.

REFERENCES

1. Ajzen I. The theory of planned behavior. *Organ Behav Hum Decis Process*. 1991;50(2):179–211.
2. Armitage C. Can the theory of planned behavior predict the maintenance of physical activity? *Health Psychol.* 2005;24(3):235–45.
3. Ashford S, Edmunds J, French DP. What is the best way to change self-efficacy to promote lifestyle and recreational physical activity? A systematic review with meta-analysis. *Br J Health Psychol.* 2010;15(2):265–88.
4. Bandura A. *Self Efficacy: The Exercise of Control.* New York (NY): W.H. Freeman and Company; 1997.
5. Bandura A. Self-efficacy mechanism in psychobiologic functioning. In: Schwarzer R, editor. *Self-efficacy: Thought Control of Action.* Washington (DC): Hemisphere Publishing Corp.; 1992. p. 355–94.
6. Bandura A. Self-efficacy: Toward a unifying theory of behavioral change. *Psychol. Rev.* 1977;84(2):191–215.
7. Bandura A. *Social Foundations of Thought and Action: A Social Cognitive Theory.* Englewood Cliffs (NJ): Prentice-Hall Inc.; 1986.
8. Becker MH, Maiman LA, Kirscht JP, Don PH, Drachman RH. The health belief model and prediction of dietary compliance: A field experiment. *J Health Soc Behav.* 1977;18(4):348–66.
9. Booth SL, Sallis JF, Ritenbaugh C, et al. Environmental and societal factors affect food choice and physical activity: Rationale, influences, and leverage points. *Nut Rev.* 2001;59(3):S21–36.
10. Bronfenbrenner U. *The Ecology of Human Development: Experiments by Nature and Design.* Cambridge (MA): Harvard University Press; 1979.
11. Chatzisarantis NL, Hagger MS. Effects of an intervention based on self-determination theory on self-reported leisure-time physical activity participation. *Psychol Health.* 2009;24:29–48.
12. Davison K, Lawson C. Do attributes in the physical environment influence children's physical activity? A review of the literature. *Int J Behav Nut Phys Act.* 2006;3(1):19.
13. DiClemente CC, Prochaska JO, Fairhurst SK, Velicer WF, Velasquez MM, Rossi JS. The process of smoking cessation: An analysis of precontemplation, contemplation, and preparation stages of change. *J Consult Clin Psychol.* 1991;59(2):295–304.
14. DiClemente CC, Prochaska JO. Self-change and therapy change of smoking behavior: A comparison of processes of change in cessation and maintenance. *Addict Behav.* 1982;7(2):133–42.
15. Dishman RK, Motl RW, Saunders R, et al. Self-efficacy partially mediates the effect of a school-based physical-activity intervention among adolescent girls. *Prev Med.* 2004;38:628–36.
16. Duncan MJ, Rivis A, Jordan C. Understanding intention to be physically active and physical activity behaviour in adolescents from a low socio-economic status background: An application of the theory of planned behaviour. *J Adolesc.* 2011;35:761–4.
17. Edmunds J, Ntoumanis N, Duda JL. Testing a self-determination theory-based teaching style intervention in the exercise domain. *Eur J Soc Psychol.* 2008;38(2):375–88.
18. Elder JP, Lytle L, Sallis JF, et al. A description of the social-ecological framework used in the trial of activity for adolescent girls (TAAG). *Health Educ Res.* 2007;22(2):155–65.
19. Elder JP, Lytle L, Sallis JF, et al. A description of the social-ecological framework used in the trial of activity for adolescent girls (TAAG). *Health Educ Res.* 2007;22(2):155–65.
20. Ewing R, Schmid T, Killingsworth R, Zlot A, Raudenbush S. Relationship between urban sprawl and physical activity, obesity, and morbidity. *Am J Health Promot.* 2003;18(1):47–57.
21. Fishbein M, Ajzen I. *Belief, Attitude, Intention, and Behavior: An Introduction to Theory and Research.* Reading (MA): Addison-Wesley Pub. Co.; 1975.
22. Godin G, Kok G. The theory of planned behavior: A review of its applications to health-related behaviors. *Am J Health Promot.* 1996;11(2):87–98.
23. Glanz K, Lewis FM, Rimer BK. Theory, research, and practice in health behavior and health education. In: Glanz K, Rimer BK, Lewis FM, editors. *Health Behavior and Health Education: Theory, Research, and Practice.* 3rd ed. San Francisco (CA): Joseey-Bass; 2002.
24. Glanz K, Rimer BK. *Theory at a Glance: A Guide for Health Promotion Practice* [NIH Pub. No. 95-3896]. Washington (DC): National Cancer Institute; 1995.
25. Haas BK. Fatigue, self-efficacy, physical activity, and quality of life in women with breast cancer. *Cancer Nurs.* 2011;34(4):322–34. doi:10.1097/NCC.0b013e3181f9a300.
26. Hagger MS, Chatzisarantis NLD, Biddle SJH. A meta-analytic review of the theories of reasoned action and planned behavior in physical activity: Predictive validity and the contribution of additional variables. *J Sport Exerc Psychol.* 2002;24(1):3–32.
27. Hallam J, Petosa R. A worksite intervention to enhance social cognitive theory constructs to promote exercise adherence. *Am J Health Promot.* 1998;13(1):4–7.
28. Hallam JS, Petosa R. The long-term impact of a four-session work-site intervention on selected social cognitive theory variables linked to adult exercise adherence. *Health Educ Behav.* 2004;31(1):88–100.
29. Harrison JA, Mullen PD, Green LW. A meta-analysis of studies of the Health Belief Model with adults. *Health Educ Res.* 1992;7(1):107–16.
30. Heath GW, Brownson RC, Kruger J, et al. The effectiveness of urban design and land use and transport policies and practices to increase physical activity: A systematic review. *J Phys Act Health.* 2006;3(suppl 1):S55–76.
31. Janz NK, Becker MH. The health belief model: A decade later. *Health Educ Behav.* 1984;11(1):1–47.
32. Koch J. The role of exercise in the African-American woman with type 2 diabetes mellitus: Application of the health belief model. *J Am Acad Nurse Pract.* 2002;14(3):126–30.
33. Kwan MYW, Bray SR, Ginis KAM. Predicting physical activity of first-year university students: An application of the theory of planned behavior. *J Am Coll Health.* 2009;58(1):45–52.
34. Lewis BA, Marcus BH, Pate RR, Dunn AL. Psychosocial mediators of physical activity behavior among adults and children. *Am J Prev Med.* 2002;23(2 suppl 1):26–35.
35. Marcus BH, Forsyth LH. *Motivating People to be Physically Active.* 2nd ed. Champaign (IL): Human Kinetics; 2009.
36. Marcus BH, Napolitano MA, King AC, et al. Telephone versus print delivery of an individualized motivationally tailored physical activity intervention: Project STRIDE. *Health Psychol.* 2007;26(4):401–9.
37. Marcus BH, Rossi JS, Selby VC, Niaura RS, Abrams DB. The stages and processes of exercise adoption

and maintenance in a worksite sample. *Health Psychol.* 1992;11(6):386–95.
38. Marshall S, Biddle S. The transtheoretical model of behavior change: A meta-analysis of applications to physical activity and exercise. *Ann Behav Med.* 2001;23(4):229–46.
39. McAuley E, Blissmer B. Self-efficacy determinants and consequences of physical activity. *Exerc Sport Sci Rev.* 2000;28(2):85–8.
40. McAuley E, White SM, Rogers LQ, Motl RW, Courneya KS. Physical activity and fatigue in breast cancer and multiple sclerosis: Psychosocial mechanisms. *Psychosom Med.* 2010;72(1):88–96.
41. McLeroy KR, Bibeau D, Steckler A, Glanz K. An ecological perspective on health promotion programs. *Health Educ Behav.* 1988;15(4):351–77.
42. Mirotznik J, Feldman L, Stein R. The health belief model and adherence with a community center-based, supervised coronary heart disease exercise program. *J Community Health.* 1995;20(3):233–47.
43. Nigg CR, Courneya KS. Transtheoretical model: Examining adolescent exercise behavior. *J Adolesc Health.* 1998;22(3):214–24.
44. Nutbeam D, Harris E. *Theory in a Nutshell: A Guide to Health Promotion Theory.* Sydney (Australia): The McGraw-Hill Companies Inc.; 1999.
45. O'Connell JK, Price JH, Roberts SM, Jurs SG, McKinley R. Utilizing the health belief model to predict dieting and exercising behavior of obese and nonobese adolescents. *Health Educ Behav.* 1985;12(4):343–51.
46. Plotnikoff RC, Lubans DR, Costigan SA, et al. A Test of the theory of planned behavior to explain physical activity in a large population sample of adolescents from Alberta, Canada. *J Adolesc Health.* 2011;49(5):547–9.
47. Prochaska JO, DiClemente CC, Norcross JC. In search of how people change: Applications to addictive behaviors. *Am Psychol.* 1992;47(9):1102–14.
48. Prochaska JO, DiClemente CC. Stages and processes of self-change of smoking: Toward an integrative model of change. *J Consult Clin Psychol.* 1983;51(3):390–5.
49. Prochaska JO, Velicer WF, DiClemente CC, Fava J. Measuring processes of change: Applications to the cessation of smoking. *J Consult Clin Psychol.* 1988;56(4):520–8.
50. Prochaska JO, Velicer WF, Rossi JS, et al. Stages of change and decisional balance for 12 problem behaviors. *Health Psychol.* 1994;13(1):39–46.
51. Rhodes RE, Pfaeffli LA. Mediators of physical activity behavior change among adult non-clinical populations: A review update. *Int J Behav Nut Phys Act.* 2010;7:37.
52. Rosenstock I. Historical origins of the health belief model. *Health Educ Monogr.* 1974;2:328–35.
53. Ryan RM, Deci EL. Self-determination theory and the facilitation of intrinsic motivation, social development, and well-being. *Am Psychol.* 2000;55(1):68–78.
54. Saelens B, Sallis J, Frank L. Environmental correlates of walking and cycling: Findings from the transportation, urban design, and planning literatures. *Ann Behav Med.* 2003;25(2):80–91.
55. Sallis JF, Bauman A, Pratt M. Environmental and policy interventions to promote physical activity. *Am J Prev Med.* 1998;15(4):379–97.
56. Silva MN, Vieira PN, Coutinho SR, et al. Using self-determination theory to promote physical activity and weight control: A randomized controlled trial in women. *J Behav Med.* 2009;33:110–22.
57. Snook EM, Motl RW. Physical activity behaviors in individuals with multiple sclerosis: Roles of overall and specific symptoms, and self-efficacy. *J Pain Symptom Manage.* 2008;36(1):46–53.
58. Stokols D, Grzywacz JG, McMahan S, Phillips K. Increasing the health promotive capacity of human environments. *Am J Health Promot.* 2003;18(1):4–13.
59. Stokols D. Establishing and maintaining healthy environments: Toward a social ecology of health promotion. *Am Psychol.* 1992;47(1):6–22.
60. Trost SG, Owen N, Bauman AE, Sallis JF, Brown W. Correlates of adults' participation in physical activity: Review and update. *Med Sci Sports Exerc.* 2002;34(12):1996–2001.
61. Valois RF, Umstattd MR, Zullig KJ, Paxton RJ. Physical activity behaviors and emotional self-efficacy: Is there a relationship for adolescents? *J Sch Health.* 2008;78(6):321–7.
62. Webber LS, Catellier DJ, Lytle LA, et al. Promoting physical activity in middle school girls: Trial of activity for adolescent girls. *Am J Prev Med.* 2008;34(3):173–84.
63. White SM, Wójcicki TR, McAuley E. Social cognitive influences on physical activity behavior in middle-aged and older adults. *J Gerontol B Psychol Sci Soc Sci.* 2011;67(1):18–26.
64. Williams SL, French DP. What are the most effective intervention techniques for changing physical activity self-efficacy and physical activity behaviour — and are they the same? *Health Educ Res.* 2011;26(2):308–22.
65. Wilson PM, Rodgers WM. The relationship between perceived autonomy support, exercise regulations and behavioral intentions in women. *Psychol Sport Exerc.* 2004;5(3):229–42.

CHAPTER

11 Facilitating Health Behavior Change

Ernestine Jennings • Sarah Linke • Bess Marcus

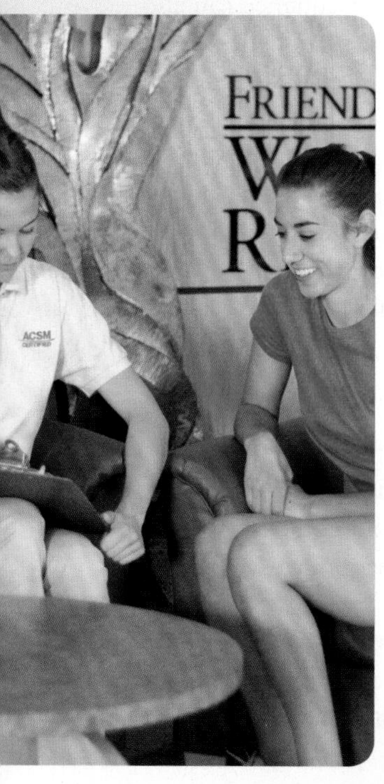

CHAPTER OBJECTIVES

- To describe the interventions strategies related to learning theory, including identifying antecedents and consequences, rewards, self-monitoring, and goal setting.
- To understand the various barriers to exercise adherence and describe strategies to overcome these barriers.
- To summarize several intervention strategies, including increasing social support, improving enjoyment of exercise, engaging in motivational interviewing with the client, visual imagery, and relapse prevention.
- To describe effective communication strategies when interacting with the client.

Theory-based behavioral interventions are an effective means for increasing physical activity among sedentary adults (*e.g.*, Marcus et al. [23]). These interventions can provide the Health Fitness Specialist (HFS) with a framework for helping clients adopt a new exercise program or adhere to an existing exercise program. More specifically, theory-based interventions that are tailored to each individual's specific interests, preferences, and readiness for change can teach behavioral skills that help individuals incorporate exercise into their daily routines (16, 30).

The purpose of this chapter is to expand on Chapter 10, which discussed various theories related to exercise promotion, by applying these various theories to practice. The following chapter outlines specific strategies for promoting the adoption and maintenance of exercise. Specifically, this chapter will summarize several intervention strategies, including using rewards, engaging in self-regulation strategies, overcoming barriers to exercise, increasing social support, improving enjoyment of physical activity, identifying outcome expectancies, and engaging in motivational interviewing, visual imagery, relapse prevention, and communication.

INTERVENTION STRATEGIES BASED ON LEARNING THEORY

Intervention strategies based on learning theory (42) can assist the HFS in facilitating the initiation and maintenance of a physical activity program. Learning theory describes how individuals acquire, enhance, or make changes in one's knowledge, skills, and values (42); reflects the process through which a physical activity behavior change occurs; and provides strategies for facilitating this behavior change (13).

According to learning theory, there are antecedents and consequences to behavior. An antecedent is a preceding event or circumstance that prompts a behavior, such as exercise. A consequence is the result of the antecedent behavior, which, in this case, would be performing the exercise and reaping the immediate benefits (consequence). Of course, the antecedent and consequence can also produce decreases in physical activity or other negative health outcomes.

Relating to exercise, the HFS can identify what factors (*i.e.*, stimuli) increase the likelihood of adhering to an exercise program. Simply put, stimulus control describes when a behavior is triggered by the presence or absence of some stimulus. Therefore, recognizing these factors, or stimuli, can help a client increase the stimuli for exercise and/or decrease the stimuli that prompt sedentary behavior. In general, people who receive learning theory–based strategies increase their exercise adherence considerably more than participants who attempt to start exercise programs with no theory-based strategies (23).

Identifying Rewards

Derived from learning theory, *rewards* help maintain motivation throughout the behavior change process. Without effective rewards in place, progress tends to wane. Rewards can be earned by achieving short-term goals en route to overall long-term goals. Rewards can also be used to help individuals increase their likelihood of engaging in one or more specific behaviors that have a low probability of occurring.

Like motivation, rewards can be classified as intrinsic or extrinsic (9). The term *intrinsic reward* describes anything that is fulfilling because of the internal pleasure derived from achieving or completing a task or goal. For example, the feeling of pride that often follows a job well done is intrinsically rewarding. Common intrinsic rewards include feeling proud of completing a specific workout or exercise plan for a period and feeling healthy and vibrant after a workout. *Extrinsic rewards,* which are external, typically include tangible things earned in response to completing a task or accomplishing a goal. Extrinsic rewards can also increase morale and motivation to adhere to an exercise routine or complete a specific exercise session. Well-known extrinsic rewards related to exercise include treats (*e.g.*, movie and a night out), awards in competitive sports (*e.g.*, medals, trophies, and prize money), and body/appearance changes (*e.g.*, weight loss, increased muscle tone, and smaller clothing size).

Intrinsic rewards tend to be more sustainable over time because, unlike extrinsic rewards, they do not rely on an outside source. However, intrinsic rewards are not always reliable, particularly in response to exercise. For example, individuals who usually experience positive feelings after completing an exercise session may not experience these feelings after every workout. In fact, individuals may occasionally feel worse while exercising, which may decrease the likelihood that they participate in their next exercise session. Therefore, using extrinsic rewards may help individuals adhere to their exercise plan when intrinsic rewards are not present. It is important to note that the novelty of extrinsic rewards decreases over time and that extrinsic rewards can reduce the value of intrinsic rewards (8). Thus, extrinsic rewards should be incorporated with caution when intrinsic rewards are in place.

It is important for the HFS to consider whether his or her client is motivated intrinsically, extrinsically, or a combination of both when using strategies to increase exercise adherence. For example, a client may dislike exercise and report that he or she perceives no joy or benefit from physical activity. The client only maintains exercise to please a physician. In this case, the client is extrinsically motivated. The HFS should identify extrinsic rewards that can keep the client motivated over time.

Another example is a client who loses a considerable amount of weight. Previously, during the weight loss period, the client had a significant amount of extrinsic reinforcement (*e.g.*, individuals congratulating them on their weight loss). However, this extrinsic reward may lose its potency over time, and the HFS needs to work with the client to identify other extrinsic rewards and attempt to make exercise more intrinsically rewarding (*e.g.*, identifying how exercise makes the person feel immediately after and throughout the day).

Research examining the functions of intrinsic versus extrinsic rewards in the context of exercise behavior has suggested that the two types of rewards may be especially useful at different points during the behavior change process. Specifically, extrinsic rewards seem to help increase adherence to exercise during the adoption phase of behavior change (*i.e.*, beginning an exercise program), whereas intrinsic rewards appear to help maintain exercise adherence in the long term (15). Intrinsic versus extrinsic rewards have been considered in the context of the transtheoretical model (TTM) (3, 7), with indications that extrinsic rewards help increase motivation in the initial stages of change (precontemplation, contemplation, preparation) and intrinsic rewards help sustain motivation during the latter stages of change (action, maintenance; see Chapter 10 for more information on the TTM).

Self-Regulation Strategies

Behavioral exercise interventions that include self-monitoring and goal setting are also intervention strategies derived from learning theory. These strategies have had a positive effect on the adoption of health-related behaviors (5, 20, 42, 46). These strategies can also increase self-efficacy by helping individuals identify ways to initiate and maintain exercise and build their confidence about their ability to succeed. Self-monitoring is a process whereby an individual observes and manually monitors his or her own behavior. The individual then evaluates the outcomes through comparisons with performance standards or goals. One example of self-monitoring is having the individual document the type, intensity, and duration of exercise on a log resembling a calendar. Self-monitoring can help the individual self-reinforce and set realistic goals for the future. Daily self-monitoring in the early days of exercise adoption is especially important for establishing the individual's baseline level of exercise. Ideally, regular self-monitoring should continue during the entire adoption phase of exercise, which could last for up to 6 months. Once exercise becomes routine, the need for daily self-monitoring isn't as critical; however, it should still occur periodically.

The HFS should work with the client to determine which type of self-monitoring works best. For example, some clients may prefer to simply document their exercise on a calendar or notebook. Others may prefer to track their success online or through their mobile phones. There are publically available Web sites where clients can track their progress for free (*e.g.*, www.startwalkingnow.org/). One particular method is not necessarily better than another. Instead, the focus should be on identifying which particular method fits with the client's lifestyle such that it will be sustained and helpful. The HFS should discuss with the client potential barriers toward implementing self-monitoring (*e.g.*, forgetting to document exercise and losing the calendar) and work to develop a plan for increasing adherence such as taping the calendar to the wall to remind the client to document his or her activity. The client may want to start with just documenting yes/no on his or her calendar and then work toward providing greater detail (*e.g.*, duration and intensity) as familiarity increases with the monitoring and recording of exercise. The HFS should consider establishing an exercise contract with his or her clients as part of the goal setting process. Adherence to this contract could be monitored through the use of an exercise log as described above. The exercise contract should help motivate the individual to exercise regularly by creating intrinsic motivation, consistency of goals, and teaching independence and self-control. This contract should be specific and individualized with measureable and observable objectives. Moreover, using self-monitoring strategies to track progress allows individuals to see their progress and adjust their goals appropriately.

Goal setting has long been established as an effective strategy for exercise adherence (41). Therefore, goal setting is an important component of the exercise contract. Goals refer to inherently valued, futuristic outcomes that are derived from a level of dissatisfaction with the present condition or circumstance. Goals should direct effort and attention toward activities that are goal-relevant and away from those that are irrelevant (19). Goals also increase persistence, knowledge, and skill attainment. The strategies and tools used to set health behavior–related goals vary; however, the majority of goals should address the following key components to ensure that goals are SMART:

Specific: exactly what are you going to do, or how are you going to do it;
Measureable: can you track your daily exercise and the progress, or lack thereof;
Attainable: losing 10 lb is attainable for most, fitting into your high school clothes is not usually;
Realistic: starting a jogging program is realistic, finishing a marathon may not be; and
Time-bound: short-term goals tend to be more successful than long-term goals (29).

Explicit goals ("I will go to the store to buy new exercise pants tomorrow after work") reduce the ambiguity of the task, which makes the achievement of the goal more likely. However, setting goals that are too vague ("will start running every day"), complex, or difficult can lead to little chance of success and therefore negatively impact one's confidence to exercise (44). Setting specific short-term goals in the context of a long-term goal is a more successful approach to enhancing performance than setting a long-term goal in isolation (18). Effective goal setting also requires people to monitor progress and assess capabilities, adjust the strategy and goal as needed, and set a new goal when the present one is attained. It is important for the HFS to provide regular feedback and encouragement regarding the individual's progress toward his or her goals and work with the individual to create new goals when the previous goals are attained (19).

ASSESSING BARRIERS TO PHYSICAL ACTIVITY

Understanding common barriers to exercise and creating strategies to address these issues are important steps to help people make exercise a part of their daily lives (30). Common exercise barriers include lack of time, environmental challenges, fear of injury, and lack of enjoyable activities. When working with people to increase their activity, anticipating and problem solving for these specific situations are important. For example, when addressing time as a barrier, one might begin with selecting short exercise durations, working with the client to find the most convenient time of the day to exercise, and using time management strategies to schedule activities. Also, completing a 24-hour time diary will allow a client to see how he or she currently utilizes time and where adjustments can be made to accommodate exercise.

The environment is another potential barrier to exercise. Environmental barriers include bad weather, lack of exercise facilities, cost, and safety issues. When addressing environmental challenges, exercise may need to be tailored to accommodate these environmental constraints. It is important for the HFS to help the client find alternatives when impacted by these factors. Where there is a lack of exercise facilities, walking may be the best option. Where the weather is a challenge (too hot or too cold), finding indoor alternatives is essential. Also, terrain can be an issue if someone lives in a particularly hilly area, and therefore exercise plans may need to be adjusted accordingly.

Fear of injury or negative past experiences with exercise are both potential barriers. If someone has never enjoyed exercise, or worse, been hurt from exercise, he or she will be more hesitant to start. In these cases, it is critical to have the client identify an activity of interest instead of the HFS choosing an activity. If past injury is an issue, discuss the benefits of exercise while also taking extra care to ease into anything new.

Most but not all barriers to exercise are perceived and therefore can be modified to make exercise more realistic. For example, the client may report lack of time as a perceived barrier; however, after further discussion, he or she may realize it is more a lack of prioritization. By identifying what is truly driving the barrier, the HFS can work with the client more effectively to meet his or her exercise goals. In addition, addressing the barriers, along with setting small, realistic, and achievable goals, is critical to the success of the new exercise adopter.

Social Support

Social support is associated with various health behavior theories and models, including social cognitive theory (SCT) (see Chapter 10). Research indicates that social support from family and friends is an important component for exercise adherence (1, 2, 11, 43). Social support refers to anything a friend or family member does to help increase the individual's exercise level. Examples of social support strategies include encouraging the individual to exercise, exercising with the individual, watching the individual's children so that he or she can exercise, providing monetary support for attending exercise facilities, and obtaining support from a professional health educator support (*e.g.*, telephone counseling and mail follow-up). Specific social support can take on a variety of forms, including but not limited to regular check-ins (*i.e.*, inquiring about progress toward the goal) and reward provision (*i.e.*, withholding and releasing rewards according to a preset arrangement). In the exercise setting, social support is often achieved via active participation, which enables two individuals to strive for the common goal of increasing their exercise levels — a win-win situation.

A common theme that binds all types of social support is that the individual must share his or her goal with family and friends to allow them to provide support to the individual. The very act of sharing a goal with significant others increases the odds of success by creating a greater sense of obligation and ownership of the goal. Individuals tend to feel more compelled to follow through with a goal by sharing it with others for a number of reasons, including the fear of embarrassment, shame, and/or disappointment if the goal is not attained. However, the number of people with whom a goal is shared for maximal effectiveness varies from person to person. For example, one person may experience an extreme amount of distress by sharing his or her goals with too many people and may therefore be better off sharing the goal with only a few close family members or friends. Another person may experience an abundance of motivation by publicly sharing his or her goal with a large network of people. Thus, the amount and type of social support that is most helpful may vary widely from one individual to another.

Enjoyment

It is important to encourage individuals to engage in exercise that they find enjoyable (54). Enjoyment of exercise is easy to overlook, but is a critically important concept for facilitating exercise adherence. Taking time to explore enjoyable activities may increase the likelihood that he or she will exercise regularly and become more physically active. Inactive individuals who are beginning an exercise program may ask what the "best" type of exercise is to obtain their desired results (*e.g.*, improved overall health, weight loss, and toning). The best answer to this question is "Whichever type of exercise you enjoy the most" because enjoyment increases the odds of exercise adoption and maintenance (47). And if the client is new to exercise, there may need to be a trial period in which he or she tries many different modes of exercise before determining which is most liked. Regardless of the most efficient/effective exercise for reaching a given goal, no form of activity will lead to the desired results if it is not done regularly (39). In this scenario, enjoyment is a mediator of exercise and expected results (10).

Enjoyment may also be the desired outcome of engaging in exercise. Indeed, many individuals engage in exercise primarily for participatory enjoyment, and it is one of the best predictors of long-term exercise adherence. Although sports are often played for enjoyment, interestingly, many people lose that sense of enjoyment when they engage in exercise for reasons such as health benefits and weight loss. Helping clients to select activities that are enjoyable and understanding the benefits of participation will undoubtedly increase their activity levels more than requiring them to engage in preselected activities that they may or may not enjoy at all (47).

OUTCOME EXPECTANCIES

The concept of *outcome expectancy* refers to what individuals generally expect to attain as a result of exercise and how much they value that outcome. For instance, individuals may expect that exercise will lead to a better mood. The successful adoption of exercise will depend on how likely individuals believe that exercise will enhance their mood and how much they value experiencing an enhanced mood. In designing exercise interventions, outcome expectancies may be effectively targeted by helping individuals shape their environments in ways that lead them to expect real and immediate positive outcomes from exercise. For example, perhaps the individual will feel more of an energy boost throughout the day when he or she exercises in the morning rather than in the evening. The HFS should brainstorm with the individual to identify various positive outcomes related to exercise and how they can best be implemented. Outcome expectancy in the exercise setting is typically used in theories such as SCT. Also, positive outcome expectancy appears to be more predictive of physical activity in older adults than in young and middle-aged adults, and personal barriers appear to be the most predictive subtype of negative outcome expectancy (50). Indeed, the Outcome Expectations for Exercise Scale was developed to strategically evaluate the positive and negative outcomes that older adults associate with exercise engagement (32). This scale uses the phrase "exercise will . . . " and then asks individuals to rate their response (strongly agree to strongly disagree) to questions such as "exercise will improve my social standing," or "exercise will improve my mood." Using this type of scale will allow the HFS to gain a solid understanding of the client's outcome expectations and therefore help in developing an exercise initiation plan that addresses both positive and negative expectations. In addition, outcome expectancies are not the exclusive domain of older individuals, as they in fact have relevance for younger people considering exercise behavior as well (40, 35).

USING MOTIVATIONAL INTERVIEWING

Motivational interviewing (MI) is a person-centered technique used to elicit and strengthen motivation for change (26) and is based on the premise that individuals become more committed to what they say to themselves than what they hear from others (12). The strategy is especially helpful for clients to explore and resolve ambivalence. MI attempts to shift behavioral responsibility to the individual and away from any external source. Although there are many "treatment" options for increasing exercise, the MI approach is considered at least as effective as most others and is superior to placebo or no treatment at all (4). Although the use of MI for exercise has only recently begun and therefore the research results are limited, there appears to be a positive effect in this area (25, 38). MI strategies include eliciting the person's priorities, needs, and values; building rapport; supporting autonomy; resisting the temptation to prescribe prematurely; and tailoring counseling to address the two dimensions necessary for change (importance and confidence about successfully changing). See the "How to" box to understand how to incorporate MI.

When attempting to adopt a new behavior, individuals frequently experience feelings of ambivalence, not really sure if they want to commit or not. The purpose of a MI intervention is to help individuals explore and resolve their ambivalence about the possible change (37). Four general principles underlie this approach to resolving ambivalence (37):

1. Expressing empathy
   a. Know that acceptance facilitates change
   b. Use reflective listening
   c. Be empathetic to the ambivavlence
2. Developing discrepancy
   a. Change is motivated by a perceived discrepancy between present behavior and important personal goals or values
   b. The client, rather than the coach, should present the arguments for change
3. Rolling with resistance
   a. Avoid arguing for change
   b. Do not directly oppose resistance
   c. New perspectives are invited, but not imposed
   d. The client is a primary resource in finding answers and solutions
   e. Resistance is a signal to respond differently

HOW TO Perform a MI

First, perform the readiness assessment:

Readiness assessment

0 5 10

1. If "0" is not ready to make changes in physical activity and "10" is ready to make changes, what score would you give yourself?

   You gave yourself a score of X. Why do you think you are X, and not ___ (a lower number)?

   or

   You gave yourself a score of X. What would have to happen to move up to ___ (higher number)?

Then, determine decisional balance. Discuss what the client perceives to be the short-term and long-term benefits and drawbacks of making healthy changes. Encourage the person to generate personal costs and benefits, and then openly discuss these to identify barriers and goals.

	Short-Term Costs	Short-Term Benefits
1.		
2.		
3.		
4.		
5.		

	Long-Term Costs	Long-Term Benefits
1.		
2.		
3.		
4.		
5.		

Instructions and Tips

Complete these steps at each session to provide feedback. The Readiness-to-Change Ruler can be used as a quick assessment of a person's present motivational state relative to changing a specific behavior, and can serve as a way to elicit behavior change, a key indicator of commitment to change. In addition, you will be able to identify barriers that may be holding a client back from attempting to change his or her behavior.

4. Supporting self-efficacy (*i.e.*, confidence)
   a. A person's belief in the possibility of change is an important motivator
   b. The client, not the coach, is responsible for choosing and carrying out change
   c. The coach's belief in the client's ability to change becomes a self-fulfilling prophecy

As individuals discuss their ambivalence about behavior change, they typically produce two types of talk regarding their behavior. First, "sustain talk" refers to talking about the costs of changing and the benefits of not changing. Sustain talk is used as a way for the client to not feel obligated to adopt any change. Second is "change talk," which refers to talk about the benefits of changing a client's behavior and the costs of not changing. The goal of an MI intervention is to generate change talk, as this indicates the client having moved to a point of readiness to adopt change. This is accomplished by asking open-ended questions, making summaries, and skillfully using reflective listening to express empathy and direct the conversation toward more change talk.

More specifically, as the HFS talks with the client in an attempt to elicit more change talk, he or she must keep in mind some basic MI principles of conversation. First, it is important to make observations, not evaluations. It is quite important for the HFS to limit the tendency to judge, exaggerate, interpret, generalize, catastrophize, assume, or criticize. For example, stating "you failed to exercise last week," is an evaluation or judgment, while "you went to the gym one time last week," is an observation.

Next is the ability to express feelings, not thoughts. Although grammatically correct, none of the following sentences express feelings: "I feel like a failure," "I feel it is useless," "I feel that my boss is controlling," and "I feel inadequate." These are thoughts, masquerading as feelings, and are not useful in expressing empathy. Encouraging the client to express his or her true feelings about exercise is an important step toward change (*e.g.*, "I do not enjoy exercising" and "Exercising takes too much of my time"). The HFS can identify feelings by asking probing questions such as how the client feels before and after exercise (referring to both energy level and mood). Third is to identify needs, not strategies. This implies a distinction between universal human needs and specific strategies to meet those needs. "I need you to stop at the store," "I need to work out every day," and "I need to eat better." None of these actually represent the needs themselves, but instead these are strategies for meeting the need. Instead, the needs would be needing to eat and improving health. Finally, make requests, not demands. Once a client is clear about his or her feelings and underlying needs, it's time to either confirm a mutual understanding or agree on an action. "What agreements would you be willing to make with regard to exercise in the coming week?" is an example of both an understanding and potential action, and this also allows the HFS to respect both the autonomy of the person and the possibility of the moment.

VISUAL IMAGERY

Imagery is a term used to describe the process of visualizing oneself engaging in a specific behavior or set of behaviors en route to achieving a desired outcome. Imagery may increase self-efficacy, help individuals identify and address potential barriers to achieving specific goals or behaviors, and also increase the likelihood that they will successfully perform specific behaviors. Imagery is also used to improve muscle memory for specific physical tasks that involve intricate movements or fine motor skills, such as in sports (48) and surgical procedures (36). This process has also been used to enhance physical rehabilitation after injury or trauma, such as in stroke patients who must relearn how to use their limbs in the recovery process (52). Evidence suggests that this process, also called mental rehearsal or mental practice, may strengthen cortical connections in the brain that are involved in the actual physical performance of the target task (17). From this perspective, imagery's effectiveness should theoretically increase, as more senses are included because of the use of additional brain connections and regions (28). For example, a golfer might improve his or her swing to a greater extent using imagery if he or she imagines the smell of the golf course, the feel of the golf club, the sight of the ball on the green, the sound of the club cutting through the air, and the movement of his or her body going through the motions of the swing. However, scientific evidence supporting the importance of multiple sensory inputs is sparse (48).

Imagery usually entails visualizing in your "mind's eye" a scene associated with a goal or plan and can be completed from an *internal* or *external perspective.* When internal, individuals imagine a scene in which they are inside their own body and thus experience it as they would in real life. In other words, the person is going through the motions, seeing the environment from an internal perspective, and enacting or rehearsing the scene. Specifically, the HFS can encourage clients to imagine how it feels to be riding their bikes along a pleasant country road during the fall foliage, or how good the warm water feels while swimming in a pool. When completed from an external perspective, individuals imagine a scene in which they are outside of their own body and thus experience it as an observer or audience might; in other words, they are watching themselves in and out of body type experience. These two perspectives can be equally effective, so individuals can choose to use whichever type they prefer.

Although imagery is more often associated with sports or physical rehabilitation than general exercise, it can be quite helpful for individuals who would like to increase their exercise. Imagery could be helpful for overcoming barriers that deter regular exercise participation (6) since many individuals may have difficulty following through on an exercise plan. For example, they may repeatedly push the snooze button on their alarm clock, realize at the last minute that they do not have any clean workout clothes, or wake up to the sound of rain on a morning they had planned to go outside for a walk. Imagery can address these barriers by helping individuals anticipate and overcome these barriers by visualizing themselves overcoming the barriers prior to the barrier occurring, thus increasing their confidence that they can overcome the barrier if it should occur.

The Exercise Imagery Questionnaire (EIQ) was designed on the basis of the idea that exercise imagery may serve cognitive and motivational functions similar to those it serves in sport, plus the questionnaire has guided most of the research in exercise imagery to date (14). The EIQ yields three types/functions of exercise imagery, including energy, appearance, and technique. Energy imagery includes mental images related to becoming more energized or relieving stress. Appearance imagery involves images associated with a leaner, fitter, and healthier appearance. Technique imagery includes imagery related to the execution of proper body positioning and form while exercising.

Specific types of images may be more or less effective for different individuals, depending on what motivates them to exercise. For example, younger individuals who frequently exercise for appearance reasons may be especially motivated by images of themselves looking fit or lean (6). Appearance imagery is also the most frequently used type among older individuals who are often concerned about looking older than their age; however, younger adults report using appearance imagery more often than their older adult counterparts (27). Furthermore, older adults also report exercising to feel more energetic and "psyched up" and thus also frequently engage in so-called energy imagery (49). Although the EIQ and the three types of imagery it measures still dominate in the exercise imagery field, research suggests that additional types of exercise imagery (*e.g.*, health, self-efficacy, and routines) may also influence exercise behavior (45).

ADDRESSING RELAPSE

Although initial health behavior change is difficult to attain, maintaining behavior change over time may be even more difficult because it requires a lifelong commitment to change. In fact, individuals are notoriously poor at maintaining health behavior changes for an extended period. Although the timeline varies according to different theories and types of behavior, 6 months is often used as the barometer for the "maintenance phase" of behavior change, when the goal shifts from initiating to maintaining behavior change (31). *Relapse prevention* is an ongoing process in which efforts are made to prevent a return to former, undesirable behaviors after a period of abstinence (24). Relapse prevention has been particularly well described in the context of substance abuse, but has been applied to a variety of other health behaviors as well (14). In terms of exercise, the relapse prevention model's goal is to prevent an individual from returning to an inactive lifestyle after establishing a regular exercise routine.

Relapse prevention incorporates various techniques, many of which are also used during the initial behavior change process. For example, goal setting, self-monitoring, and rewards are often used in both the initiation of behavior change and relapse prevention processes. Once habits are established in the initial behavior change process, some of these techniques may be used less frequently or intensely because they are no longer required to maintain the desired behavior. However, eliminating them entirely may lead to a gradual (or steep) decline and return to previous, undesired behaviors. Regular check-ins with a practitioner, friend, group, or another trusted confidante are often incorporated into the relapse prevention process.

Despite their similarities, relapse prevention and the initial behavior change process differ in that relapse prevention focuses largely on self-regulation and anticipation (22). The initial behavior change process relies heavily on the relationship between the HFS and clients. However, long-term exercise maintenance may only involve "booster sessions" reviewing exercise adherence and may rely more on the client's own self-monitoring. Planning ahead is a simple but crucial component of the relapse prevention model. Anticipating events or circumstances that could ultimately lead to a relapse is an important component of relapse prevention. The individual should be prepared to follow a specific plan of how to deal with decreasing exercise levels if a relapse occurs. Although relapses are often spontaneous or unforeseeable, they typically result from a series of events that could have been prevented if more caution was used. Incorporating community resources to maintain exercise may be a helpful step in the relapse prevention stage (Table 11.1).

TABLE 11.1 PHYSICAL ACTIVITY COMMUNITY RESOURCES

YMCAs	• Nationwide locations • Membership fees often lower than those of other gyms, and financial assistance available for low-income individuals and families • Childcare, camps, and lessons/programs typically available for children • Group exercise classes and personal trainers usually available (some for additional costs) • Knowledgeable and well-trained/friendly staff members
Parks and recreation departments	• Local/community oriented • Range of program types offered (varies widely) • Usually free or low cost, often with financial assistance available • Programs offered for children and older adults • Transportation sometimes offered for older adults • Outdoor and indoor programs typically offered, depending on season and geographic location
Parks, trails, and outdoor spaces	• Free/open to public • Exercising in nature/natural environments is linked to higher enjoyment levels and enhanced mood • Opportunities to meet others • Physical fitness/obstacle equipment often located on grounds to incorporate strength training, balance, and/or stretching along with aerobic activity (*e.g.*, walking/running around park space or trail
Miscellaneous	• Indoor and outdoor shopping malls (place to walk, no charge if not purchasing anything) • Gyms (available year-round, multiple options and locations, group exercise classes, personal trainers) • Yoga and pilates (can be done at gyms, specialty centers, home with DVDs, or outdoors) • Swimming pools (good for those with joint problems and/or musculoskeletal injuries) • Walking or bicycling to run errands/active transportation (reduces or eliminates time sitting in traffic, promotes multitasking, reduces carbon emissions from automobiles) • Taking the stairs instead of the escalator/elevator (increases overall steps/activity) • Libraries can be a good place to check out exercise DVDs/videos or can order online (*e.g.*, http://www.nia.nih.gov/health/publication/go4life-dvd-everyday-exercises-national-institute-aging) • Local walking/running clubs (*e.g.*, some sports store serve as an organizing center for group runs/walks, grassroots walking group clubs) • Getting on local listservs that send e-mails about active events in the community, etc. • Universities/colleges may also have physical activity opportunities that might be open to the general public • Local departments of public health may have programs/opportunities • Check out various Internet Web sites (*e.g.*, http://www.heart.org)

COMMUNICATION

Effective communication is vital in the behavior change process. *Communication* involves at least two parties: sender and receiver. The sender conveys the message and the receiver interprets and responds to it (at which point the sender and receiver roles are reversed). Messages are sent both verbally and nonverbally. Verbal communication comprises words the speaker says aloud. Nonverbal communication includes messages that are conveyed in several ways, including hand gestures, eye contact, and posture. These nonverbal cues are often as or even more informative than the actual spoken words. Nonverbal cues convey emotions, level of engagement in the communication process, and an array of other internal processes. Listening is as important as speaking in the communication process. Active listening is a specific type of listening that demonstrates a more complete comprehension of the message by listening with undivided attention and repeating back to the speaker the message that was heard to ensure accuracy of interpretation. After the sender and receiver agree that the original message has been accurately conveyed and interpreted, feedback, which isa response to the received message, may be offered.

To facilitate behavior change, the HFS strives to convey messages in a manner that ideally inspires and motivates his or her clients. By first actively listening to the client, the HFS can tailor health behavior messages appropriately. For example, if the client reports low self-efficacy for exercise, the HFS could provide specific strategies for increasing self-efficacy. The HFS can generally begin by eliciting information about the client past and current patterns of exercise as well as his or her goals for the future, while then offering relevant feedback. It is critical that the messages received by the HFS match the messages sent by the client. Other important components of communication that facilitate exercise include conveying supportive messages to clients and demonstrating to

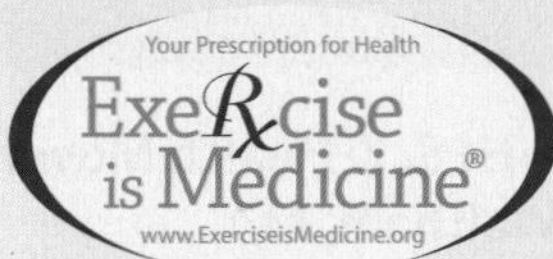

EXERCISE IS MEDICINE CONNECTION

Williams D, Papandonatos G, Jennings E, et al. Does tailoring on additional theoretical constructs enhance the efficacy of a print-based physical activity promotion intervention? *Health Psychol.* 2011;30(4):432–41.

Physical inactivity is an important public health area for intervention. A recent meta-analysis has shown greater health behavior intervention efficacy when tailoring includes a greater number of theoretical constructs. Thus, we sought to enhance a previously efficacious individually tailored physical activity (PA) intervention by adding theoretical constructs to the tailored feedback. We randomly assigned 248 healthy, underactive (moderate-vigorous physical activity [MVPA] $<$90 min·wk^{-1}) adults (mean age = 48.8; SD = 10.0) to receive either (a) a theoretically tailored (five constructs based on the TTM and SCT) print-based PA promotion intervention (Print) or (b) the same theoretically tailored print-based PA promotion intervention plus enhanced tailoring addressing five additional SCT constructs (Enhanced Print). The 7-day Physical Activity Recall was administered at baseline, month 6, and month 12, with outcomes operationalized as percentage achieving 150 minutes·week^{-1} of MVPA and continuous minutes per week of MVPA. When controlling for covariates, there was a nonsignificant trend in favor of Enhanced Print, reflecting 46% and 50% greater odds of achieving 150 minutes·week^{-1} of MVPA at the 6-month and 12-month follow-ups, respectively. Regarding continuous outcomes, a time-by-treatment interaction showed that mean minutes per week of MVPA among Enhanced Print participants remained stable between months 6 and 12 (132–137 min·wk^{-1} MVPA; P value n.s.), whereas Print arm participants experienced a decrease from month 6 to 12 (141 to 97 min·wk^{-1} MVPA; p = .012). The results suggest that enhanced tailoring based on additional theoretical constructs may result in marginal improvements in physical activity outcomes.

them that they will be accepted regardless of their success or failure in their attempt to increase their exercise. On the contrary, clients also need to feel adequately challenged so that their efforts seem worthwhile.

Clients vary in their relative responsiveness to feedback on the unconditional support versus challenge spectrum in the exercise change process. Therefore, assessing each person's preference for style of feedback, rather than making assumptions or using a one-style-fits-all approach, is critical and well described as the preferred method of communication toward behavior change (33). Print materials (*e.g.*, brochures, letters, and booklets) are the most extensively researched format for delivering tailored health communication to date; however, tailored health communication via the Internet is growing in popularity and will likely surpass print materials at some point in the near future. The solicitation of the background information required to provide tailored feedback may be done verbally, but it is commonly done via standardized assessments, which can be delivered in person to the client or through non–face-to-face strategies (*e.g.*, mail or Internet). Interactive health communication programs have become increasingly popular over the past two decades, increasing the accessibility of tailored health messages and enabling even individuals in remote areas to receive evidence-based, tailored feedback for a variety of conditions/problems (34).

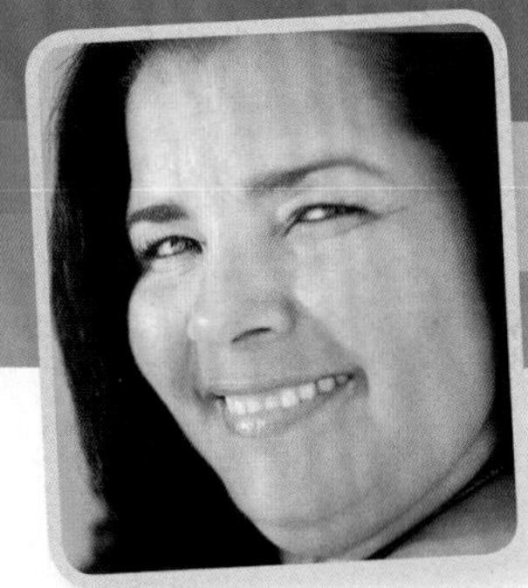

The Case of Brenda

Submitted by **Joyce Dendy, MS, RD, ACSM-HFS, Z-Health Movement Performance Specialist (R, I, S, T), Affirmative Fitness, Waltham, MA**

This case describes how MI is used to effect change over time with a 52-year-old client.

Narrative

Brenda is a 52-year-old married woman who has two children in college and is actively involved in the care of her aging parents. She left her job as an attorney more than 9 years ago. Brenda has gained 30 lb over the past 3 years because of an increase in sedentary behaviors and a lack of routine in her day. With her role as caretaker and a history of anxiety, she found it increasingly difficult to "find" the time to exercise and to consider her health needs. Brenda was active in high school, where she played basketball and softball. In college, she played varsity basketball and did some occasional running.

Brenda has been working with a Training and Performance Coach/Registered Dietitian/HFS for the past 6 years, meeting with her twice a month. During this period, Brenda has worked with her coach at clarifying her long-term goals, identifying barriers, and planning and completing her weekly exercise, specifically spinning and tai chi.

Weight History

Height: 5′9½″
Heaviest weight: 180 lb
Current weight: 165 lb
Goal weight: 155 lb
Lowest weight: 138 lb
Pregnancy weight: 195 lb

continues

The Case of Brenda cont.

Medical History

Postmenopausal, anxiety, tinnitus
No history of coronary artery disease, hypertension, diabetes mellitus, cancer, smoking
No surgeries
Bone density — NA
Labs: Complete blood count and lipid profile: normal; vitamin D <30 ng·mL^{-1}
Medications/supplements: Vitamin D

Eating Habits

Three meals per day plus snacks. Brenda eats mostly organic foods and avoids meat and chicken; protein sources include fish, dairy, eggs, cheese, Greek yogurt, nuts, and legumes; vegetables and greens are from a farmers market or home grown; she limits sugar and sweet intake; beverages include decaffeinated tea, water, about two glasses (6–8 oz) of wine in the evening.

Physical complaints: Neck and upper back pain due to tension and left knee pain with squatting and lunging
Sleep: Approximately 7 hours a night, reports sleeping well throughout the night
Respiration: Paradoxical breathing, upper chest breathing pattern, mouth breathing
Social support: Serves on multiple committees, organizes group gatherings with friends, belongs to a book club and a singing group, serves as a trainer/coach, and so on.

Objective

Utilizing MI strategies, the coach guides, listens, and elicits information from the client to encourage the process of change. (Please note that this was a conversation that took place as coach and client over the span of several months after we had spent a significant amount of time together.)

Conversation 1

Brenda: I really want to lose the weight I've gained, but don't think I'll ever be able to lose it.
Coach: What makes you say that?
Brenda: I've always heard that being postmenopausal makes it harder to lose the weight.
Coach: So, tell me about what your eating habits are like.
Brenda: [See diet history, eating habits.]
Coach: It sounds like you eat really healthy and have good knowledge about nutrition.
Brenda: I really think I do, but I just don't know what to do.
Coach: What have you tried in the past to help lose weight?
Brenda: I don't like diets. I just try to eat healthy, but it's not coming off. I eat healthy foods like salads, maybe my portion size is too big, I don't know.
Coach: What are your thoughts about keeping a food diary so that we could get a good sense of what's going on?
Brenda: I don't want to do food records! (Breathing rate and anxiety level go up.)
Coach: I hear what you're saying. They can be really time-consuming, especially when you've got a lot going on.
Brenda: I'd prefer to see if we could do this without food records.
Coach: OK. Sounds like food records are not the right plan for you now. Let's see if you can identify foods or beverages that are contributing extra calories. What foods or beverages, if any, would you say are contributing extra calories?
Brenda: Wine. I could easily cut back on this. I'm drinking two glasses per night with my husband.
Coach: Sounds like a great way to save some calories! I wouldn't want you to miss out on the social benefits of spending time with your husband. So what beverage(s) would be a good replacement?

The Case of Brenda cont.

Brenda: I think a cup of tea would be best (client solution).
Coach: How would that work for you?
Brenda: I think having tea instead of wine is fine.
Coach: Give it a whirl over the next week and let me know how it goes!

Conversation 2 (2 wk later)

Coach: How did your goal of cutting down on your wine consumption go?
Brenda: I cut back to having it only one or two nights a week. And I actually lost a few pounds.
Coach: Nice job! How did you feel about not having the wine at night?
Brenda: I found the nights that I didn't drink the wine I actually felt better in the morning.
Coach: Sounds like this is something you wouldn't have been aware of if you had continued to drink the wine at night.
Brenda: I didn't realize it, but it really makes a difference. But I really want to lose this weight!
Coach: You really are committed to making changes that make a difference you can see! [reinforcing change talk]
Coach: Let me summarize where we are at. Last time we met we talked about the challenges to monitoring your food intake. I know that keeping a food record is something you prefer not to do and eating healthier is not where you want to focus right now and because you are already eating healthy foods. Does this sound right?
Brenda: Yes, that's right.
Coach: The question then becomes "Where do we go from here?" Most people tend to focus on the food, but focusing on a few small behaviors can make a huge impact on weight loss. So, let's take a look at this "menu of behaviors" I brought for you.

Menu of behaviors

Become a conscious eater.
Do not eat in the car.
Do not eat in front of the TV.
Eat all meals and snacks sitting down.
Take smaller bites.
Put your fork down between bites.
Take several breaths before eating.

Brenda: WOW! I have a tendency to eat while I'm standing up, especially when I'm cooking; I eat off my plate as I'm walking to the table before I sit down; and I frequently grab a handful of almonds when I'm stressed and I eat them while I walk through the kitchen. And I definitely don't put my fork down between bites either!
Coach: Well, it sounds like you've hit on some things that are contributing to extra calories. Which one do you think would be the biggest priority for you?
Brenda: I really think I need to eat all my meals and snacks seated. That way I can stop myself if I'm not really hungry and I'm eating just because I'm stressed (commitment).
Coach: Great! We have a plan!

Follow-Up

A few months later, Brenda had lost a total of 13 lb without keeping a food dairy. She continues to work on the repetition of these habits. Over the past year, she has kept the weight off and has even been able to lose a few more pounds. Gaining confidence in her ability to create change has motivated her to work on other goals.

continues

The Case of Brenda cont.

A Message from the Coach

This was a real client with a common problem, the inability to make change happen to reach a goal. Reflecting back on my experience of working with clients over the past 20 years, I learned that to facilitate behavior change, my communication skills needed to change. I had plenty of education and knew all the reasons why people needed to change their behaviors. And most people know they would be healthier by exercising more, losing weight, getting more sleep, eating healthier foods, and so on. Accepting that the ideas and solutions for change need to come from the client is really important. But knowing how to recognize the clues to ambivalence and how to get the client to "argue for change" by guiding him or her through a conversation (DARN-C) about his or her Desires, Abilities, Reasons, and Needs for change, and ultimately getting someone to Commit, is just the beginning. Changing behavior takes time, patience, trial and error, and repetition on both the coach's and client's parts.

Questions

- Define MI and describe how the coach used this approach with his or her client.
- With guidance from the coach, the client was able to identify several antecedents that were preventing him or her from losing weight. Define antecedent and consequence, and identify them from this conversation.
- What is ambivalence? When someone is ambivalent, what "stage of change" is this person at? From the conversation above, what statement from the client provides a clue to the coach to know this?

References

1. Coyle D. *The Talent Code: Greatness isn't Born. It's Grown. Here's How.* New York (NY): Bantam Books; 2009.
2. Goulston M. *Just Listen: Discover the Secret to Getting Through to Absolutely Anyone.* New York (NY): AMACOM; 2010.
3. Patterson K, Grenny J, Maxfied D, McMillan R, Switzler A. *Change Anything: The New Science of Personal Success.* New York (NY): Business Plus; 2011.
4. Prochaska JO, Norcross J, Diclemente C. *Changing For Good: A Revolutionary Six-Stage Program for Overcoming Bad Habits and Moving Your Life Positively Forward.* New York (NY): Avon Books; 1994.
5. Rollnick S, Miller W, Butler C. *Motivational Interviewing in Health Care: Helping Patients Change Behavior (Applications of Motivational Interviewing).* New York (NY): Guilford Press; 2008.

SUMMARY

Theory-based behavioral interventions provide clients with the strategies necessary to incorporate exercise into their daily routines. When the HFS can tailor these programs to each individual's specific interests, preferences, and readiness for change, an increase in the likelihood of exercise adoption and maintenance can be expected. Simply providing knowledge about the importance of increasing an individuals' exercise is often not sufficient to evoke the desired behavior change; rather, assessing their readiness for change and providing a tailored intervention based on their receptivity are important, if not critical. Therefore, it is necessary for the HFS to incorporate specific skills and strategies to aid clients in moving through the change process (21). This chapter has offered and explained several strategies and skills that may be used when focusing on the behavioral aspects of adopting and maintaining a regular exercise program.

STUDY QUESTIONS

1. Describe the differences between intrinsic and extrinsic rewards, and provide an example of each type.
2. What does the acronym SMART stand for in the context of goal setting?
3. Name three examples of social support for exercise.
4. Describe MI and the related strategies used to elicit change.
5. What is imagery, and how can it be used in the context of increasing or maintaining exercise behavior?

REFERENCES

1. Anderson ES, Wojcik JR, Winett RA, Williams DM. Social-cognitive determinants of physical activity: The influence of social support, self-efficacy, outcome expectations, and self-regulation among participants in a church-based health promotion study. *Health Psychol.* 2006;25:510–20.
2. Anderson ES, Winett RA, Wojcik JR, Williams DM. Social cognitive mediators of change in a group randomized nutrition and physical activity intervention. *J Health Psychol.* 2010;15:21–32.
3. Buckworth J, Lee RE, Regan G, Schneider LK, DiClemente CC. Decomposing intrinsic and extrinsic motivation for exercise: Application to stages of motivational readiness. *Psychol Sport Exerc.* 2007;8(4):441–61.
4. Burke BL, Arkowitz H, Menchola M. The efficacy of motivational interviewing: A meta-analysis of controlled clinical trials. *J Consult Clin Psychol.* 2003;71(5):843–61.
5. Clark M, Hampson S E, Avery L, Simpson R. Effects of a tailored lifestyle self-management intervention in patients with type 2 diabetes. *Br J Health Psychol.* 2004;9:365–79.
6. Cumming J. Investigating the relationship between exercise imagery, leisure-time exercise behavior, and self-efficacy. *J Appl Sport Psychol.* 2008;20(2):184–98.
7. Dacey M, Baltzell A, Zaichkowsky L. Older adults' intrinsic and extrinsic motivation toward physical activity. *Am J Health Behav.* 2008;32(6):570–82.
8. Deci EL, Koestner R, Ryan RM. A meta-analytic review of experiments examining the effects of extrinsic rewards on intrinsic motivation. *Psychol Bull.* 1999;125:627–68.
9. Deci EL, Ryan RM. *Intrinsic Motivation and Self-determination in Human Behavior.* New York (NY): Plenum Press; 1985.
10. Dishman RK, Motl RW, Saunders R, et al. Enjoyment mediates effects of a school-based physical-activity intervention. *Med Sci Sports Exerc.* 2005;37:478–87.
11. Eyler AA, Brownson RC, Donatelle RJ, et al. Physical activity social support and middle- and older-aged minority women: Results from a US survey. *Soc Sci Med.* 1999;49:781–9.
12. Gaume J, Gmel G, Faouzi M, Daeppen JB. Counselor behaviors and patient language during brief motivational interventions: A sequential analysis of speech. *Addiction.* 2008;103:1793–800.
13. Glanz K, Rimer BK. *Theory at a Glance: Application to Health Promotion and Health Behavior.* 2nd ed. National Cancer Institute, NIH, Public Health Service, U.S. Government Printing Office; 2005. NIH Publication No. 05-3896.
14. Hausenblas HA, Hall CR, Rodgers WM, Munroe K J. Exercise imagery: Its nature and measurement. *J Appl Sport Psychol.* 1999;11:171–80.
15. Ingledew D K, Markland D, Medley AR. Exercise motives and stages of change. *J Health Psychol.* 1998;3:477–89.
16. Kahn EB, Ramsey LT, Brownson R, et al. The effectiveness of interventions to increase physical activity: A systematic review. *Am J Prev Med.* 2002;22(4S):73–107.
17. Kosslyn SM, Ganis G, Thompson WL. Neural foundations of imagery. *Nat Rev Neurosci.* 2001;2(9):635–42.
18. Kyllo LB, Landers DM. Goal setting in sport and exercise: A research synthesis to resolve the controversy. *J Sport Exerc Psychol.* 1995;17:117–37.
19. Locke EA, Latham GP. Building a practically useful theory of goal setting and task motivation: A 35-year odyssey. *Am Psychol.* 2002;57:705–17.
20. Lorig K, Ritter P, Stewart AL, et al. Chronic disease self-management program: 2 year health status and health care utilization outcomes. *Med Care.* 2001;39:1217–23.
21. Marcus BH, Ciccolo J, Whitehead D, King TK, Bock BC. Adherence to physical activity recommendations and interventions. In Shumaker SA, Ockene JK, Reikert K, editors. *The Handbook of Health Behavior Change.* 3rd ed. New York (NY): Springer; 2009. p. 23–51.
22. Marcus BH, Dubbert PM, Forsyth LH, et al. Physical activity behavior change: Issues in adoption and maintenance. *Health Psychol.* 2000;19(1 suppl):32–41.
23. Marcus BH, Williams DM, Dubbert PM, et al. What we know and what we need to know: A scientific statement from the American Heart Association Council on nutrition, physical activity, and metabolism (subcommittee on physical activity); Council on cardiovascular disease in the young; and the Interdisciplinary Working Group on quality of care and outcomes research. *Circulation.* 2006;114:2739–52.

24. Marlatt GA, George WH. Relapse prevention: Introduction and overview of the model. *Br J Addict.* 1984;79(3):261–73.
25. Martins RK, McNeil DW: Review of Motivational Interviewing in promoting health behaviors. *Clin Psychol Rev.* 2009;29:283–93.
26. Miller WR, Rollnick S. *Motivational Interviewing: Preparing People for Change.* New York (NY): Guilford Press; 2002.
27. Milne MI, Burke SM, Hall C, Nederhof E, Gammage KL. Comparing the imagery use of older and younger exercisers. *Imagin Cognit Pers.* 2005;25:59–67.
28. Moran A. Cognitive psychology in sport: Progress and prospects. *Psychol Sport Exerc.* 2009;10(4):420–6.
29. Pearson ES. Goal setting as a health behavior change strategy in overweight and obese adults: A systematic literature review examining intervention components. *Patient Educ Couns.* 2012;87:32–42. Epub 2011 Aug 17.
30. Physical Activity Guidelines Advisory Committee. *Physical Activity Guidelines Advisory Committee Report.* Washington (DC): U.S. Department of Health and Human Services; 2008.
31. Prochaska JO. *Systems of Psychotherapy: A Transtheoretical Analysis.* Homewood (IL): Dorsey Press; 1979.
32. Resnick B, Zimmerman SI, Orwig D, Furstenberg A-L, Magaziner J. Outcome expectations for exercise scale: Utility and psychometrics. *J Gerontol B Psychol Sci Soc Sci.* 2000;55:S352–6.
33. Rimer BK, Kreuter MW. Advancing tailored health communication: A persuasion and message effects perspective. *J Commun.* 2006;56:S184–201.
34. Robinson TN, Patrick K, Eng TR, Gustafson D, The Science Panel on Interactive Communication Health. An evidence-based approach to interactive health communication. *JAMA.* 1998;280(14):1264–9.
35. Rodgers WM, Brawley LR. The influence of outcome expectancy and self-efficacy on the behavioral intentions of novice exercisers. *J Appl Soc Psychol.* 1996;26:618–34.
36. Rogers RG. Mental practice and acquisition of motor skills: Examples from sports training and surgical education. *Obstet Gynecol Clin North Am.* 2006;33(2):297–304.
37. Rollnick S, Miller WR, Butler CC. *Motivational Interviewing in Health Care: Helping Patients Change Behavior (Applications of Motivational Interviewing).* New York (NY): The Guilford Press; 2008.
38. Rubak S, Sandbaek A, Lauritzen T, Christensen B. Motivational interviewing: A systematic review and meta-analysis. *Br J Gen Pract.* 2005;55(513):305–12.
39. Salmon J, Owen N, Crawford D, Bauman A, Sallis JF. Physical activity and sedentary behavior: A population-based study of barriers, enjoyment, and preference. *Health Psychol.* 2003;22:178–88.
40. Sears SR, Stanton AL. Expectancy-value constructs and expectancy violation as predictors of exercise adherence in previously sedentary women. *Health Psychol.* 2001;20:326–33.
41. Shiltz MK, Horowitz M, Townsend MS. Goal setting as a strategy for dietary and physical activity behavior change: A review of the literature. *Sci Health Promot.* 2004;19(2):81–93.
42. Skinner BF. *Science and Human Behavior.* New York (NY): Macmillan; 1953.
43. Spanier PA, Allison KR. General social support and physical activity: An analysis of the Ontario Health Survey. *Can J Public Health.* 2001;92(3):210–3.
44. Strecher VJ, Seijts GH, Kok GJ, Latham GP, Glasgow R, DeVellis B. Goal setting as a strategy for health behavior change. *Health Educ Q.* 1995;22(2):190–200.
45. Thøgersen-Ntoumani C, Cumming J, Ntoumanis N, Nikitaras N. Exercise imagery and its correlates in older adults. *Psychol Sport Exerc.* 2012;13(1):19–25.
46. Tsai AC, Morton SC, Mangione CM, Keeler EB. A meta-analysis of interventions to improve care for chronic illnesses. *Am J Manag Care.* 2005;11(8):478–88.
47. Wankel LM. The importance of enjoyment to adherence and psychological benefits from physical activity. *Int J Sport Psychol.* 1993;24:151–69.
48. Weinberg R. Does imagery work? Effects on performance and mental skills. *J Imagery Res Sport Phys Act.* 2008;3(1):1–21.
49. Wesch NN, Milne MI, Burke SM, Hall CR. Self-efficacy and imagery use in older adult exercisers. *Eur J Sport Sci.* 2006;6(4):197–203.
50. Williams DM, Anderson ES, Winett RA. A review of the outcome expectancy construct in physical activity research. *Ann Behav Med.* 2005;29:70–9.
51. Williams DM, Dunsiger S, Ciccolo JT, Lewis BA, Albrecht AE, Marcus BH. Acute affective response to a moderate-intensity exercise stimulus predicts physical activity participation 6 and 12 months later. *Psychol Sport Exerc.* 2008;9(3):231–45.
52. Zimmermann-Schlatter A, Schuster C, Puhan M, Siekierka E, Steurer J. Efficacy of motor imagery in post-stroke rehabilitation: A systematic review. *J Neuroeng Rehabil.* 2008;5(1):8.

CHAPTER

12 Healthy Stress Management

Rob Motl • Madeline Weikert

CHAPTER OBJECTIVES

- To provide a working definition of stress.
- To examine the effects of stress on health and well-being.
- To identify different techniques for managing and coping with stress.

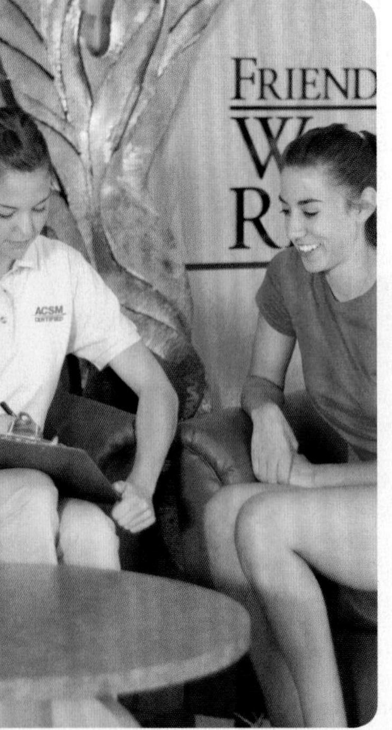

Stress occupies a central presence in medicine, health care, and the media. Stress has been linked with the common cold, the development of chronic conditions, including cardiovascular disease and stroke, the worsening of autonomic diseases such as multiple sclerosis (MS), and premature death (22). In addition, the fast-pace and demanding nature of our society and culture provide the optimal condition for the frequent occurrence of stress in the home, workplace, and community. Interestingly, although stress has become interweaved into the very fabric of our lives, we still do not have the clearest of definitions. In addition, we do not have an adequate understanding of what stress is or the breadth of how it affects the human body. Hans Selye (95), the father of modern stress research, wrote that "the term stress has been used so loosely, and so many confusing definitions have been formulated," and it is easier to list what stress is not than provide an operational definition (p. 61).

DEFINITION AND CHARACTERISTICS OF STRESS

Stress has become a popular term in today's modern vocabulary, and many different races and cultures have adopted this word into regular, everyday language (87). People often use the word stress to express uncomfortable situations in life, with phrases such as "I feel stressed out" or "my job is stressful," and the word is often used to refer to pressure or tension (87, p. 17). Stress, however, is defined as the *process* by which one responds to an environmental demand that is perceived as threatening (87). The scientific concept of stress is based on the interaction between the environment and the person — essentially stress occurs whenever an environmental demand taxes or exceeds one's resources and endangers one's well-being (51). This discrepancy between the demand and resources elicits a response pattern from the organism that compensates for the external disturbance and restores normal equilibrium (homeostasis). The response pattern may be physical, behavioral, psychological, or a combination (87). The inability of the body to cope properly and restore homeostasis after exposure to a stressor can yield to biological or psychological damage and possibly even death (74).

The demand or stimulus itself is otherwise known as a stressor, and stressors have a diverse set of characteristics and sources. Stressors can vary in frequency, from infrequently to very often, and intensity, from mild to severe. The duration of a stressor can be acute, as in "flight or fight" or major life event, or chronic, as in the steady accumulation of minor, everyday perturbations (67). Chronic stress could be described as "the long-term grinding kind" of stress, and some examples of this might be "living in poverty, living in a bad relationship, or remaining in a high-stress job," (102, p. 158). The stressors that are severe, occur often, and last longer are considered to be the most damaging.

The source of a stressor can stem from within the person, the family, the community, or the society. Person-bound stressors can include living with a physical ailment such as arthritis, fibromyalgia, or MS. Family-bound stressors could be a major life event such as divorce, loss of job, or death of loved one. Community-bound stressors can include a sudden increase in crime rates, traffic construction, or pollution. Lastly, stressors in society can be catastrophic events such as a hurricane, tsunami, or earthquake and can also include global issues (*e.g.*, civil unrest and war between nations). Even small incidents in everyday life (*i.e.*, daily hassles) such as giving a speech, encountering heavy traffic, or misplacing keys can be perceived as stressful and possibly have a cumulative effect.

There are different categories or types of stress, namely eustress and distress. Eustress or good stress is considered to be a "pleasant and stimulating experience" that promotes growth, development, and improvement in performance; an example of this type of stress might be a marriage, addition to the family, or a job promotion (87, p. 17). Conversely, distress or bad stress is negative and damaging. An example of this type of stress could include being diagnosed with an incurable illness or loss of employment. However, the decision or view that an event is stressful depends entirely on the individual, the appraisal process, and one's resources.

Appraisal of Stress

Stress is largely based on one's cognitive appraisal of two components, namely the event and available resources. There are two types of appraisals, including primary and secondary appraisals (23, 50, 51). Primary appraisal is when one evaluates the significance of an event and its associated threat or harm. Individuals gauge their perceptions for susceptibility to a threat and severity of the threat by asking questions such as "What does this mean to me?" and "Will I be in trouble?" During this appraisal, stressors are classified as either threatening with the expectation of future harm or challenging with the expectation of achieving growth, mastery, and profit (91). With secondary appraisal, one evaluates the controllability of the stressor and the person's coping resources to alter the situation or manage his or her emotional reaction. Individuals evaluate (a) resources available to cope with the stressor (perceived control over the threat), (b) emotional reaction (perceived control over feelings), and (c) finally, the ability to deal effectively with the resources concerning the burden of stress (coping self-efficacy [36]).

The transactional model of stress and coping suggests that these two types of appraisals influence and predict the coping processes during a stressful event (51). According to the original model, coping efforts were conceptualized in two-dimensions, problem management and emotional regulation. Problem management coping is focused on changing the stressful situation, where one takes an active role in problem solving and information seeking (36). Emotional regulation is a more passive coping effort, with one altering feelings or thoughts about the stressful situation or denying and avoiding the situation (36). One is likely to adopt a problem management coping strategy when the situation is appraised as changeable, thereby resulting in the perception of control and self-efficacy (36). By comparison, when a stressor is appraised as uncontrollable or highly threatening, individuals adopt disengaging or passive coping strategies (103). This escape-avoidance behavior (*e.g.*, hiding feelings, refusing to think about illness or situation) has been associated with higher levels of psychological distress and poorer quality of life (6, 106).

Response to Stress

When an event or stimulus is determined to be stressful, the body elicits an immediate response to counteract the disturbance and restore homeostasis or balance. The stress response has three main stages of variable and undefined duration; the response itself depends on the appraisal and reaction of the person. If stressors begin to accumulate and there is no period for restoration, then eventually the person will reach a limit called allostasis.

General Adaptation Syndrome

The physiologic stress response of the body was first theorized by Hans Selye (1956), who later became known as the father of stress research (94). Selye conducted experiments that exposed animals to various and diverse homeostatic challenges such as heat, cold, infection, and toxic substances and objectively measured physiological changes. The reaction to each stressor varied respectively according to its unique characteristics, but his primary finding was an underlying nonspecific response pattern that was consistent across the different stressors. This stereotypical response pattern of stress was coined the general adaptation syndrome (GAS).

The GAS consists of three broad stages, each with a wide variety of nonspecific and specific responses, all working together to restore homeostasis and ensure the survival of the organism (93, 57). The first stage is called the *alarm reaction,* where the stressor is first recognized by the system and a fight-or-flight response is initiated (94). The second stage is that of *resistance,* where a cascade of metabolic, hormonal, and immune changes is generated as a compensatory stress reaction until biochemical substrates have been depleted (94). During this stage, some compensatory reaction may include the release of glucocorticosteroids, the activation of the hypothalamic–pituitary–adrenal (HPA) axis, and change in autonomic neurotransmitters and inflammatory cytokines (69). The last stage is that of *exhaustion,* when the organism has depleted all resources and is no longer able to mount a defense to the stressor. This has the capacity to result in death. On the basis of GAS, the impact of repeated stress exposure can be problematic because individuals who remain in the resistance phase have difficulty withstanding additional challenges (94).

Allostatic Load Model

Allostasis is "the ability to achieve stability through change," and the allostatic load model refers to the rapid activation of bodily systems to cope with the stressor and restore homeostasis as effectively and efficiently as possible (67, p. 171). In regard to allostasis, all of the systems in the body are involved, including the autonomic nervous system and HPA axis along with the cardiovascular, immune, and metabolic systems (67). However, if the body does not compensate well and the wear and tear of repeated stressors on the body accumulates (*i.e.*, allostatic load), then there is an increased risk of the development of physical ailments (68). Overactivity of the allostatic systems, where there is limited to no time for rest and restitution, can increase the risk of atherosclerosis and, consequently, myocardial infarction (59). If the body is unable to stop or shut off the stress response after the stressor has been resolved, then the systems can be driven to exhaustion resulting in the breakdown of feedback mechanisms and overexposure to stress hormones such as cortisol (59). Stress, chronic and acute, minor and severe, can have an impact on the functioning of an individual, and any accumulation or combination of these stressors together can be damaging to one's health.

HOW DOES STRESS IMPACT HEALTH?

Stress has a combined and interrelated impact on the physiological and psychological aspects of a person, including bodily systems, mental processes, and behaviors. The physiological and psychological response of a person to a stressor is called strain, and that strain, if severe or prolonged, can negatively affect the functioning and health of a person, increase illness vulnerability, and worsen disease progression and activity.

Stress and Physical Illness

When an individual experiences stress, there are three primary systems of the body that are activated and affected: the cardiovascular, endocrine, and immune systems (91). If the stressor continues and activation of these systems is extended for a long period, the bodily systems can eventually break down and result in dysfunction of major organs (*e.g.*, heart or brain). These physical changes in response to chronic or intense stress can lead to, contribute to, or worsen life-threatening and altering conditions such as myocardial infarction, stroke, cancer, or autonomic diseases.

Cardiovascular and Metabolic Diseases

Unresolved, chronic stress profoundly affects the cardiovascular system, including the heart, blood vessels, and blood itself. High levels of job stress have been associated with abnormally enlarged hearts and hypertension (92). These changes in the heart and blood vessels can increase cardiovascular reactivity to a stressor, which is considered a risk factor for the development of coronary heart disease (65, 98). Persons under stress have higher concentrations of activated platelets (64, 79) and more triglycerides, free fatty acids, and lipoproteins in the blood (78, 109). These changes in blood composition likely promote quick blood clotting in case of physical trauma, but over time, the elevated blood lipid levels promote the development and growth of plaques in the arteries, or arthrosclerosis. These plaques harden and narrow the blood vessels, increasing blood pressure and the likelihood of myocardial infarction and stroke (91).

Corticosteroids, specifically cortisol, are released in response to a stressful event, but high concentrations of cortisol in the blood over time can increase the risks of cardiovascular disease and Type 2 diabetes and reduce immune function and cognitive performance (60). High levels of cortisol influence free fatty acid levels in the plasma and block blood glucose from being taken up by cells, which significantly affects cardiovascular and metabolic functioning (59). Cortisol contributes to the accumulation of fat in the abdominal region, and this visceral fat is readily released into the bloodstream. This increase of free fatty acids in the bloodstream is another risk factor for cardiovascular disease (60). By blocking the uptake of glucose from the cells, high levels of cortisol increase insulin resistance and can lead to the development of Type 2 diabetes (60). Overall, stress can have a major impact on the functioning of the cardiovascular and metabolic systems and can lead to the development and progression of cardiovascular pathologies.

Immune Suppression, Cancer, and MS

Persons exposed to chronic, severe stress have increased vulnerability to infections, meaning that the immune system can be suppressed during stress (21). Indeed, Selye observed that animals exposed to a stressor had a reduction in the size of immune system organs, such as the thymus gland (94, 58). The sympathetic nervous system activity and the release of cortisol after a stressful event suppress the immune system, which limits the number of lymphocytes that are activated in response to a viral challenge (58). For example, among mice exposed to repeated restraint stress, there was a decrease in the production of antibodies and activation of T cells in response to the influenza virus (97). Among humans who were exposed to the "common cold" virus, 47% of those who had high stress developed cold symptoms compared with only 27% of those who had low stress (25). Collectively, both animals and humans demonstrate immune suppression after repeated stress exposure, and this attenuation can leave a person more susceptible to contracting a virus or disease.

Similarly, psychological stress has been correlated with a reduction in natural killer (NK) cells and NK cell activity. This is a significant problem because NK cells combat cancerous tumor cells and monitor neoplastic (new and abnormal) growth (39, 37, 57). The NK cell activity is considered to be important to survival rates in certain types of cancers, specifically breast cancer (53). Although stress overall has not been linked with the onset of cancer, specific stressors such as loss of social support can influence the onset and course of cancer (102). Major social stressors, such as marital divorce, infidelity, quarreling, and financial problems have been associated with an increased risk or likelihood of being diagnosed with cervical cancer (27).

Chronic, autoimmune diseases such as AIDS and MS are impacted by psychological stress, and several studies provide evidence of a consistent relationship between stress and disease activity. Depression, stress, and trauma have all adversely affected disease progression in patients with HIV, and negative beliefs and expectations about the disease and one's future are associated with declines in helper T cells (CD4) and the onset of AIDS (93, 52). Regarding MS, one meta-analysis of 14 empirical studies reported a significant association between stressful life events (SLEs) and relapse incidence (75), indicating the significant impact of stress on disease activity. One longitudinal study of 23 women with MS reported an average annual relapse rate of 2.6 relapses a year, and 85% of those relapses were associated with one or more SLEs occurring in the 6 weeks prior (2). These findings support the existence of a relationship between stress and disease activity among patients with HIV and MS, and likely with other diseases and conditions. Overall, the functioning of the immune system in fighting off viruses, infections, cancer, and autonomic diseases can be severely compromised because of stress.

Stress and Mental Health

The impact of stress is not limited to the physical body. Stress can affect psychological well-being, cognition function, emotion, social involvement, and behavior. There are several psychological conditions that can be influenced by chronic stress such as anxiety, depression, fatigue, insomnia, and burnout, and these conditions can have a profound negative impact on quality of life.

Cognition

The HPA axis is activated in response to stress and glucocorticoids (GCs), and cortisol in humans and corticosterone in animals are released as end products. High levels of GCs have been related to cognitive impairment, specifically in hippocampal spatial memory tasks (60, 14, 88). This may be because the elevated levels of GCs are associated with degeneration of the hippocampus, including neuronal loss, dendritic atrophy, and reductions in the hippocampal volume (66). One hypothesis, called the "glucocorticoid cascade hypothesis" (89), more recently known as the "neurotoxicity hypothesis" (63), postulates that long periods of exposure to elevated levels of GCs can "exert a deleterious effect on HPA-axis regulation that cumulatively impacts hippocampal volume and memory performance" (66, p. 2). Although there is high variability among humans regarding their stress reactivity, GC secretion, and cognitive performance, there is evidence that the release of GCs, specifically cortisol in humans, is related to memory impairment and hippocampal atrophy (61, 62).

Psychological Distress, Depression, and Burnout

Chronic stress has been shown to promote psychological distress and the development of psychological disorders (47, 102). Research studies have shown that people who report exposure to chronic stress in their marriage, household functioning, parenting, or jobs have an increased likelihood of being psychologically distressed (80). Another study looked at only married men and women and found that chronic stress was a greater predictor of depressive symptoms than acute stress, and this was consistent between sexes (71). It has been suggested that chronic stress for only 2 years can lead to the development of depression and that chronic stress of any type can magnify the impact of life events on clinical depression (15). Personality can also accentuate the severity of distress and depression experienced in response to a stressor. For example, a person with high negativity affectivity (*i.e.*, neuroticism and negative mood) is more prone to heavy drinking, depression, and suicidal gestures after experiencing life stressors (102).

Persons who continually deal with exposure to high levels of occupational stress can develop a psychological response called burnout, which is characterized by physical, mental, and emotional exhaustion (87). Burnout was defined by Veniga and Spradley (87) as "a debilitating psychological condition brought about by unrelieved work stress, which results in: 1) depleted energy reserves, 2) lowered resistance to illness, 3) increased dissatisfactions and pessimism, and 4) increased absenteeism and inefficiency at work" (p. 79). Employees who experience burnout may develop a variety of symptoms, including overall job dissatisfaction, lack of energy and insomnia, and tension headaches and ulcers (87). Eventually, the individual can reach a stage of crisis and final breakdown if the stressor is not relieved (87). Burnout is a serious condition of chronic stress that has received only a limited amount of attention in the research field, but burnout symptoms have been associated with cognitive failures in everyday life, increased inhibition errors, and variability in performance on attention tasks (108).

Common Disorders and Symptoms of Excessive Stress

Ulcers, inflammatory bowel disease, and irritable bowel syndrome are all disorders in the digestive tract that are influenced by stress (91). Ulcers are due to an increase in gastric juices and erosion of the lining of the stomach, duodenum, or upper small intestine. Inflammatory bowel disease may involve inflammation of the colon and small intestine, whereas irritable bowel syndrome may involve diarrhea, constipation, and abdominal pain (91). Intense headaches can also be a physical disorder that results from exposure to chronic stress; the two most common recurrent headaches are migraines and tension-type headaches (4, 56, 83). Tension-type headaches are the result of the contraction and tightening of muscles in the neck and head, which is a common reaction of person's under stress (3, 91). The effect of chronic stress can be quite damaging and lead to the development of a variety of symptoms. The American Institute of Stress (29) has listed several common signs and symptoms of excessive stress (Table 12.1), and this list includes physical and emotional responses and conditions, some of which are more serious and severe than others. This list is certainly not exhaustive, but includes common physical and emotional responses reported by persons who have appraised and expressed feelings of stress. These symptoms range from blushing to headaches to social isolation and excessive drug use.

HEALTHY STRESS MANAGEMENT

Although stressful events are unavoidable in daily life, the majority of people would prefer to limit or manage the amount of exposure to stress. Currently, there is no drug that can be taken or ritual that can be performed to make people "immune" to stress and stressors, but there are several strategies for coping and managing stress. Both cognitive and behavioral approaches exist for decreasing the negative impact of stress. Certain strategies are more effective for some people than others, but all play a role in preventing or reducing stress and stress reactivity.

TABLE 12.1 SIGNS AND SYMPTOMS OF EXCESSIVE STRESS

1. Frequent headaches, jaw clenching, or pain	26. Insomnia, nightmares, disturbing dreams
2. Gritting, grinding teeth	27. Difficulty concentrating, racing thoughts
3. Stuttering or stammering	28. Trouble learning new information
4. Tremors, trembling of lips, hands	29. Forgetfulness, disorganization, confusion
5. Neck ache, back pain, muscle spasms	30. Difficulty in making decisions
6. Light-headedness, faintness, dizziness	31. Feeling overloaded or overwhelmed
7. Ringing, buzzing, or popping sounds	32. Frequent crying spells or suicidal thoughts
8. Frequent blushing, sweating	33. Feelings of loneliness or worthlessness
9. Cold or sweaty hands, feet	34. Little interest in appearance, punctuality
10. Dry mouth, problems swallowing	35. Nervous habits, fidgeting, feet tapping
11. Frequent colds, infections, herpes sores	36. Increased frustration, irritability, edginess
12. Rashes, itching, hives, "goose bumps"	37. Overreaction to petty annoyances
13. Unexplained or frequent "allergy" attacks	38. Increased number of minor accidents
14. Heartburn, stomach pain, nausea	39. Obsessive or compulsive behavior
15. Excess belching, flatulence	40. Reduced work efficiency or productivity
16. Constipation, diarrhea	41. Lies or excuses to cover up poor work
17. Difficulty breathing, sighing	42. Rapid or mumbled speech
18. Sudden attacks of panic	43. Excessive defensiveness or suspiciousness
19. Chest pain, palpitations	44. Problems in communication, sharing
20. Frequent urination	45. Social withdrawal and isolation
21. Poor sexual desire or performance	46. Constant tiredness, weakness, fatigue
22. Excess anxiety, worry, guilt, nervousness	47. Frequent use of over-the-counter drugs
23. Increased anger, frustration, hostility	48. Weight gain or loss without diet
24. Depression, frequent, or wild mood swings	49. Increased smoking, alcohol, or drug use
25. Increased or decreased appetite	50. Excessive gambling or impulse buying

Source: Adapted with permission from http://www.stress.org/topic-effects.htm

Coping

Coping has become the term for what people do to alleviate, eliminate, or manage stress, and this term has as many meanings as the term *stress.* Coping activities are "geared toward decreasing the person's appraisal of, or concern of the discrepancy" between the demands of the situation and the resources of the person (91, p. 134). Coping is an ongoing, dynamic process that involves "continuous appraisals and reappraisals of the shifting person–environment relationships" (51, p. 142). To neutralize or reduce stress, a person will attempt to change either the environment or its perception or meaning.

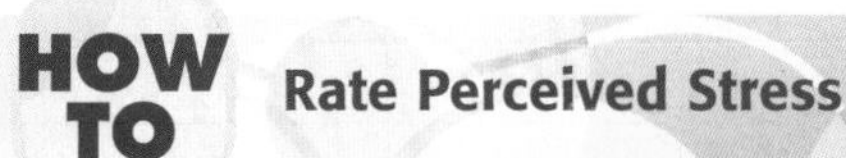

HOW TO Rate Perceived Stress

The most common instrument used to assess perception of stress is the ***Perceived Stress Scale*** (PSS). It is a 10-item questionnaire that measures a person's perception of stress over the previous month. The results of this questionnaire have been used to determine whether perceived stress is associated with susceptibility to disease, smoking behavior, and compromised health (1).

Instructions and Tips

1. Read each question.
2. After reading each question, consider and estimate how often you have felt or thought that way over the past month. Beside each item, mark the frequency as: N = never, AN = almost never, S = sometimes, FO = fairly often, and VO = very often.
3. The best approach is to answer fairly quickly. That is, don't try to count up the number of times you felt a particular way that month, but rather choose the option that seems like a reasonable estimate.
4. After answering each question, use the table called "Perceived Stress Scale Scoring" to determine your numerical grade for each response and write your scores in the box called "Score."
5. Add the numbers for each response in the "Score" column together for the total PSS score.

Question	Rating	Score
1. How often have you been upset because of something that happened unexpectedly?		
2. How often have you felt that you were unable to control the important things in your life?		
3. How often have you felt nervous and "stressed"?		
4. How often have you felt confident about your ability to handle your personal problems?		
5. How often have you felt that things were going your way?		
6. How often have you found that you could not cope with all the things that you had to do?		
7. How often have you been able to control irritations in your life?		
8. How often have you felt that you were on top of things?		
9. How often have you been angered because of things that happened that were outside of your control?		
10. How often have you felt difficulties were piling up so high that you could not overcome them?		

Perceived Stress Scale Scoring

Question	Never	Almost Never	Sometimes	Fairly Often	Very Often
1					
2					
3					

4					
5					
6					
7					
8					
9					
10					
Total score:					

Interpretation and Normative Values

The scores can range from 0 to 40, and higher scores reflect a higher level of perceived stress. High scores on the PSS-10 questionnaire have been associated with increased difficulty in making lifestyle changes such as quitting smoking and increased susceptibility to stress-induced illness (1). Normative values for the PSS-10 questionnaire were acquired through a large probability study (*N* = 2,387) that was conducted by Louis Harris and Associates, Inc., in 1983 (2). Although these values are not recent, they provide a baseline reference of mean PSS-10 scores for men and women of different ages, races, education levels, and household sizes in the United States. This table of values was modified from Cohen and Williamson, 1988 (2).

Category	Mean ± SD	Category	Mean ± SD
Sex		**Race**	
Male (*N* = 926)	12.1	White (*N* = 1,924)	12.8
Female (*N* = 1,344)	13.7	Hispanic (*N* = 98)	14.0
		Black (*N* = 176)	14.7
		Other minority (*N* = 50)	14.1
Education		**Number of People in Household**	
Less than H.S.	13.4	One	12.6
H.S. graduate	13.1	Two	12.3
Some college	13.1	Three	13.2
Four-year college	12.0	Four or five	13.7
Some grad school	12.2	Six or more	14.4
Advanced degree	11.4		

Note: SD, standard deviation; H.S., high school.

References

Cohen S, Karmarck T, Mermelstein R. A global measure of perceived stress. *J Health Soc Behav*. 1983:24;385–96.

Cohen S, Williamson GM. Perceived stress in a probability sample of the United States. In: Spacapan S, Oskamp S, editors. *The Social Psychology of Health*. Newbury Park (CA): Sage Publications; 1988. p. 31–68.

There are different methods of coping with stress, but those ways of coping can be separated into two broad categories: problem-focused or emotion-focused coping. Table 12.2 lists and describes several coping strategies with specific examples of cognitive and behavioral efforts that would typically fall under each category of coping. Depending on the situation, a person will be more inclined to engage in problem-focused or emotion-focused coping, but both are necessary because both are used and sometimes even in combination with each other.

Problem-Focused Coping

In problem-focused coping, the person attempts to reduce "the demands of the stressful situation or expand their resources to deal with it," (91, p. 135–136). This type of coping may include seeking out information, talking with a professional or friend to get advice on how to handle the problem, or drawing from previous experience and knowledge. Examples of problem-focused coping in everyday life would be negotiating an extension on an assignment, learning a new skill, or quitting a stressful job (91). This type of coping is most often used when people believe that either personal resources or the demands of the situation are changeable (51).

Emotion-Focused Coping

In emotion-focused coping, the person attempts to control or manage the emotional response to the stressful event. In this type of coping, people change the behavior such as "seeking emotional support from friends and family, drinking alcohol or using drugs, or engaging in activities like sports or watching TV to distract their attention from the problem" (91, p. 135). People tend to use this emotion-focused coping when they believe that the circumstances they are facing are fixed and they cannot change their stressful condition (51). Moreover, some persons use a combination of both problem-focused and emotion-focused coping to solve problems and manage their stress. Table 12.2 lists and describes different coping mechanisms that were proposed by Folkman and Lazarus in 1986 (35) and then again in 1988 (34).

Modifiers or Buffers of Stress

Enhancing Social Support

Social support is a common method of managing dire, stressful situations. People typically seek out and rely on help and comfort from friends, neighbors, classmates, coworkers, significant others, and health professionals. Four types or functions of social support exist, adapted from House (1981):

- *Emotional support* — the provision of empathy, love, trust, and caring (*e.g.*, significant other actively listening to concerns)
- *Instrumental support* — the provision of tangible aid and services that directly meet a need (*e.g.*, providing childcare to provide time to accomplish tasks)
- *Informational support* — the provision of advice and information concerning the problem (*e.g.*, understanding why an issue is causing significant stress)
- *Appraisal support* — the provision of information useful for self-evaluation purposes such as constructive feedback and affirmation (*e.g.*, friend helping individual brainstorm possible solutions to a problem)

TABLE 12.2 COPING METHODS: PROBLEM-FOCUSED COPING VERSUS EMOTION-FOCUSED COPING

Problem-Focused Coping	Emotion-Focused Coping
Planning and problem solving: This involves analyzing the situation and developing possible solutions to address and correct the problem	*Distancing:* This involves detaching oneself from the reality of the situation and attempting to develop a positive outlook
Confrontation: This involves taking assertive action, which may include feelings of anger or risk-taking behaviors	*Escape-avoidance:* This involves taking action to remove oneself from the situation and escaping or avoiding it all together
Seeking social support: This involves making new relationships to increase informational or emotional support	*Self-control:* This involves trying to modulate our feelings and actions about the situation to establish feelings or perceptions of control
	Accepting responsibility: This involves acknowledging the role they played in the situation and trying to make things right
	Positive reappraisal: This involves choosing to create a positive meaning from the situation, rather than a negative meaning

Adapted from Folkman S, Lazarus RS. Coping as a mediator of emotion. *J Pers Soc Psychol.* 1988;54:466–75; and Folkman S, Lazarus RS, Dunkel-Schetter C, DeLongis A, Gruen RJ. Dynamics of a stressful encounter: Cognitive appraisal, coping, and encounter outcomes. *J Pers Soc Psychol.* 1986;50:992–1003.

The matching hypothesis suggests that social support is most beneficial when it meets the needs caused by a stressful event (24, 26). For example, if the pet of a friend or roommate dies, the person needs emotional support such as active listening and empathy rather than information about where to bury the pet. Social support could potentially reduce uncertainty and unpredictability about a stressful situation, which would promote a greater sense of personal control and the use of problem-solving coping methods (38). The mechanism for how social support improves health and well-being is still unknown, but there is evidence indicating that social support has a buffering effect on the harmful physical and mental effects of stress exposure (104).

People can enhance perceptions of social support by strengthening existing relationships with friends or significant others or by developing new relationships that broaden a social network (38, 42). Social relationships that provide daily contact may be the most effective sources of social support (*e.g.*, spouse, partner, and close friend [99, 107]). Another way to increase social support is by getting involved in a community organization, such as a religious, special interest, or self-help group (91). These organizations bring together people of similar interests and problems, and this allows the opportunity for members to share and help each other through tough, stressful situations. Communities can "play a valuable role in enhancing people's resources for social support by creating programs to help individuals," and to increase their social network (101, 91, p. 141). Social support has been suggested to enhance well-being and health, regardless of stress levels (12), and may improve coping with increased access to networks and resources in the community (38).

Improving Personal Control and Self-Efficacy

Another psychosocial factor that modifies the evaluation of stress is personal control. When persons feel like they have a good sense of agency or control, they feel like they are able to effectively make decisions and execute a plan of action to produce the outcome desired and avoid the outcome undesired (85, 91). There are four types of control (5, 20, 72, 105), adapted from Sarafino (2002):

1. *Behavioral control* — when a person can take concrete action to reduce the impact of stress
2. *Cognitive control* — when a person can use thought processes and strategies to manipulate and modify the impact of the stressor

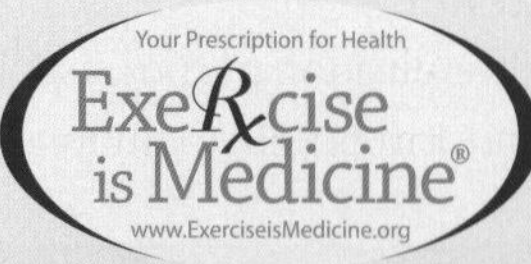

EXERCISE IS MEDICINE CONNECTION

Suh Y, Weikert M, Dlugonski D, Sandroff B, Motl RW. Physical activity, social support, and depression: Possible independent and indirect associations in persons with multiple sclerosis. *Psychol Health Med.* 2012;17:196–206. Epub 2011 Jul 25.

Social support and physical activity both independently influence perceived stress and indirectly effect mood and depressive symptoms. Special populations more prone to depressive symptoms, such as persons with MS, would strongly benefit from interventions that improve their physical activity and broaden their circles of social support. Lack of social support and low levels of physical activity have been associated with more severe and frequent depressive symptoms in persons with MS (99). In a large cross-sectional study of 218 persons with MS, physical activity and social support were both inversely related with depressive symptoms (r = 70.3 and r = 70.4, respectively). Further investigation using multiple linear regression and path analysis showed that the relationship between physical activity, social support, and depressive symptoms is mediated through perceived stress (99). Therefore, future direction in stress research may be to implement exercise interventions that specifically promote social support in diseased populations or in persons more prone to depressive symptomology.

3. *Decisional control* — when a person can choose between different courses of action
4. *Informational control* — when a person can glean knowledge about the stressful event and the potential consequences of the situation

There is evidence that people who have a strong sense of personal control experience less strain with stressors, compared with those who feel they have no control over their lives (70, 82, 86, 100).

Individuals who believe that they have control over their lives are considered to have an internal locus of control. On the other hand, individuals who believe that their lives are dictated by forces outside of themselves, such as destiny, fate, or faith, have an external locus of control (81, 85). These two types of locus of control have a major impact on health, and even management of chronic diseases, such as MS. For example, evidence shows that patients with relapsing-remitting MS who have an internal locus of control in regard to their health decisions and efforts show higher individual, social, and occupational functioning and a better prognosis than patients with external orientation (110). These same people have less disease activity with fewer clinical relapses (49, 73).

Another aspect of personal control is self-efficacy, which is defined as the belief or "conviction that one can successfully execute the behavior required to produce the outcomes" desired (7, p. 193). People evaluate their chances of success in handling an activity, such as quitting smoking or starting an exercise program, to determine whether they are efficacious to overcome in the situation. In the decision process, the person must determine his or her expectations about whether the behavior can be properly carried out and whether the change would lead to a favorable outcome. People who are highly efficacious show less psychological and physiological strain than those who are less efficacious, when facing a stressful activity (9, 10, 40).

Exercise

Physical exercise has been broadcasted from every popular media source, including television, radio, magazines, newspapers, and the Internet, as a possible method for buffering the impact of stress. Stress can be alleviated by engaging in some aerobic activity, such as walking, running, cycling, or swimming, because the repetitive movement of large muscle groups and the high rate of oxygen consumption promote stress-reducing benefits (55). In addition, the social aspects of exercise (*e.g.*, walking with a friend) or listening to music may be beneficial for stress reduction. The benefits of exercise can be physical including improvement in cardiovascular function, muscle tone, fluidity of joints, and sleep patterns (87). Acute bouts of exercise improve vigor, self-esteem, self-efficacy, and alertness, and those are all important psychological states that influence stress appraisal and reaction (91).

There is evidence that people who are more physically fit or who exercise more report less depression, anxiety, and tension in comparison with those who are less fit or do not exercise (1, 13, 28, 41). In a study with 135 college students, students dealing with high stress who engaged in low levels of leisure physical activity experienced approximately 37% more physical symptoms and 21% more anxiety compared with those engaging in high levels of physical activity (19). Aerobic training in a sample of highly stressed police officers has also shown physical and psychological improvements, including gains in cardiovascular fitness, reductions in perceived job stress, and enhancements in quality of life (77). These findings suggest that individuals who engage in higher levels of physical activity are less susceptible to the consequences of stress, such as anxiety and physical symptoms.

The psychological benefits that follow exercise are not necessarily related to improvements in physical fitness (32). For example, a meta-regression analysis conducted by Jackson and Dishman (43) reported that physical fitness does not mitigate the cardiovascular reaction to a psychological stressor, meaning that a strenuous exercise training program may reduce heart rate and blood pressure, but these changes are not responsible for the reduction in feelings and perceptions of stress reported after exercise. There are four prominent explanations that suggest how exercise leads to these benefits of stress reduction. The distraction hypothesis suggests that people who engage in exercise are distracted and that their thought processes about stress are momentarily reduced. The cognitive dissonance explanation suggests that people create and perceive benefits to exercise so as to justify the time and effort it takes for them to perform exercise (55). Another popular explanation that originated with the social cognitive theory with Bandura (8) is the self-efficacy explanation, stating that people who engage and maintain an active lifestyle may see themselves as more in control of their lives and more capable of handling a stressful life event. Lastly, the expectancy theory suggests that exercisers may hold "a set of positive expectancies regarding social norms endorsing exercise," (54, p. 72). All these explanations provide a possible mechanism for how exercise impacts stress and support the practice and maintenance of regular exercise habits (55).

Techniques for Reducing Stress

Progressive Muscle Relaxation and Yoga

The opposite of stress and arousal is relaxation; progressive muscle relaxation and yoga are techniques that individuals can learn and practice to help promote relaxation and decrease the feelings of stress. Progressive muscle relaxation is a technique where people learn to control and target their feelings of tension by focusing on certain muscle groups and alternatively tightening and contracting these muscles (90). This long-standing practice instructs persons to focus on the sensation of relaxation in certain muscle groups as they flex and then release the muscle (44). Researchers have postulated that muscle relaxation may promote feelings of pleasure and arouse pleasant thoughts in the individual, which counteract the negative thoughts of stress (81). The individual first identifies certain areas of the body that tighten and hold tension when they are under stress (*e.g.*, jaw clamps shut, shoulders tighten up, and fingers cramp). Whenever persons feel tension rising in these areas, they can stop what they are doing for 5 to 10 minutes, breathe deeply, tighten and relax the affected muscles, and then return to their work after their short break (102). Yoga has also been shown to promote health benefits, such as more positive emotions and lower inflammatory responses to stress (102). Research indicates that those who regularly practice yoga have 41% lower serum interleukin 6 levels compared with novice yoga attendees, meaning that yoga has the ability to minimize the inflammatory response to stressful encounters (48).

Relaxation Therapy

Massage is the external application of pressure to muscles and tendons that can range from smooth, light pressure to deep kneading motion depending on preference. Deep tissue massage has been an effective method for reducing stress, muscle tension, pain, and asthma symptoms, and has been shown to boost immune function (91, 30, 31). The deep tissue massage is the application of forceful, penetrating pressure that is applied to the muscles and joints by a trained masseuse. Breast cancer patients in the earlier stages of the disease have shown positive results after 3 weeks of massage therapy, such as a decrease in anxiety, depression, mood, and anger (39). These patients also showed a boost in their dopamine and serotonin levels and number of NK immune cells and lymphocytes, which could potentially promote a better and faster recovery (39).

Hypnosis is an enticing practice that influences states of consciousness so as to change perception, memory, and even behavior. The practice of hypnosis is one of the oldest techniques for managing pain, but can be used as a relaxing, therapeutic technique in stress management. Persons can undergo hypnosis with the assistance of a technician, who directs them to relax and to empty their mind and then makes statements to alter the way they think about stress or pain (102). The hypnotic trance can provide relief from stress using relaxation, reinterpretation, and distraction; the composite effects of these methods may actually be the cause for stress relief, or hypnosis itself may lead to an altered state of consciousness that completes the experience (102). In a small case study with 30 persons, hypnosis treatment (*i.e.*, hypnotic analgesia) was reported to be significantly beneficial by increasing perceived control over painful symptoms, reducing levels of perceived stress, and improving relaxation and well-being (45). Most research studies on hypnosis and stress management focus on more formalized and intense situations such as during and after medical operative procedures (33, 18) or in treatment of posttraumatic stress disorder and acute stress disorder (16). The major limitation of hypnosis is that the success of this therapeutic method is heavily dependent on the suggestibility of the patient. The use of hypnosis to help alleviate stress in everyday life is still not yet fully understood, but current research suggests that hypnosis may be a useful and helpful tool in stress management (45, 16, 91).

Meditation is the practice of "exercising the mind," in which the individual focuses on calming and quieting the body while keeping the mind alert (87). There are several forms of meditation: (a) Mantra meditation focuses on sounds and phrases, and the same word or verse is repeated over and over again to promote concentration, (b) Yantra meditation uses a visual image, and the person focuses on that image to eradicate distracting thoughts from the mind, and (c) Transcendental meditation incorporates breathing, visualization, relaxation, and repetition (87). The transcendental meditation has been shown to reduce stress and improve mental and physical health by decreasing blood pressure, heart rate, and respiratory response (11, 87).

Cognitive Manipulation: Systematic Desensitization and Biofeedback

A state of relaxation is not always easy to attain for certain individuals, and there are two cognitive manipulation techniques that can assist individuals in reducing fear and anxiety. The first method is systematic desensitization, which is a method based on classical conditioning, that attempts to transform a "feared" object or situation into a pleasant or neutral event. The process of desensitization can last for a couple of hours to several weekly appointments. The procedure includes counterconditioning, in which the individual is shown or comes in contact with the feared object and a "calming" response is trained to be associated with the item. Desensitization has been effective for both children and adults in reducing a variety of fears, such as fear of dentist, public speaking, and taking a test (54, 76, 90). The patient is slowly exposed to the feared object in a series of 10 to 15 steps, with each step involving a closer and more intimate exposure to the feared object. The patient is not supposed to move on to the next step until they reach a state of calmness and relaxation with each exposure. Completing the entire procedure may be relatively quick, with only several hours divided into multiple sessions; this is considered relatively quick for reversing a persons' cognitive appraisal of an item or situation as stressful.

Another cognitive manipulation method is biofeedback, a method of gaining control over bodily process such as heart rate and muscle tension in response to a stressor (102). The procedure involves attaching device monitors that provide immediate biophysiological feedback to the person on how his or her body is responding to the stressor. This information helps individuals attain voluntary control of their bodily response to a stressor. This process is called operant conditioning and shows patients when their body is overacting. Patients are encouraged to change their bodily response to the stressor, for instance, one may be asked to slow down a speeding heart rate by blocking out all sounds and breathing deeply until the heart rate reduces and returns to normal. Biofeedback has been useful in treating stress-related health problems such as chronic muscle tension headaches (17).

Medication

There are several medication brands that physicians can prescribe to help patients manage and reduce their stress levels, but they all primarily fall into one of two categories: benzodiazepines and β-blockers. The two types of drugs are usually prescribed by physicians because they decrease physiological arousal and feelings of anxiety (91, 84, 96). Benzodiazepines, such as chlordiazepoxide (Librium) and diazepam (Valium), have been on the pharmaceutical market for the past 50 years, and they appear to facilitate the binding of neurotransmitter γ-aminobutyric acid (46). Benzodiazepines decrease neural transmission in the central nervous system, by causing hyperpolarization of the postsynaptic neuron, and result in sedative, anxiolytic, muscle relaxant, and amnesic action (46). β-Blockers, on the other hand, influence the peripheral nervous system and block endogenous catecholamines (*i.e.*, epinephrine and norepinephrine) as well as stress hormones from stimulating and activating the sympathetic nervous system, which is responsible for the "fight or flight" response (91). Although these medications are usually only prescribed for temporary assistance in reducing and managing a stressful circumstance, such as a major life event, progressively more patients are requiring medications for long-term care and maintenance of chronic stress (91).

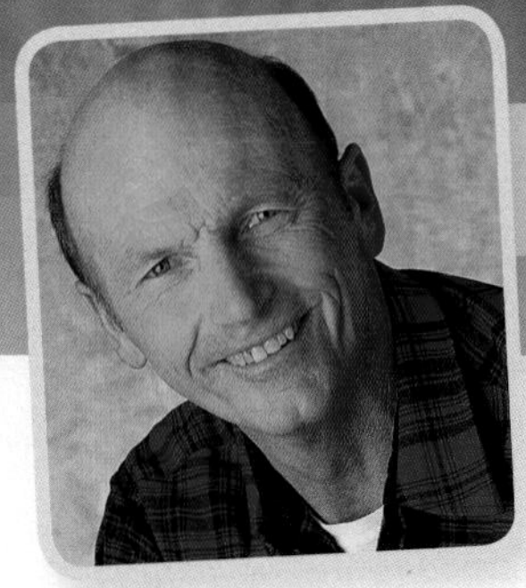

The Case of Paul

Submitted by **William Raymond VanWye, PT, DPT, ACSM-RCEP, CSCS, Active Physical Therapy, Hilliard, OH**

Paul is a 54-year-old man with low back pain (LBP) who was referred to an American College of Sports Medicine® (ACSM) credentialed professional to establish an exercise program. Paul had a history of diverticulitis as well as anxiety and depression.

Narrative

Paul is a 54-year-old man who was referred to an ACSM professional by an orthopedic physician to establish an exercise program that would address Paul's fitness and low mood. Paul reported diagnosis of nonspecific LBP, diverticulitis, and abdominal surgery as well as anxiety and depression. He recently completed cardiovascular screening as well as further follow-up testing related to his abdominal surgery. His surgeon and primary care physician deemed his medical condition to be well managed and appropriate for regular exercise as recommended by his orthopedic physician. Unfortunately, Paul had been experiencing a high level of stress as well as anxiety and depression since his abdominal surgery a year ago. He had returned to working full time, taking his mental health medications as prescribed, and felt ready to address his physical fitness to better manage his LBP. He reported no history of any medical or mental health conditions before his surgery and no family history of these issues as well. He worked full time as an owner of a large trucking company, which required long hours and high-stress decisions. He is married and reports having very good family support. He noted that before becoming ill and having surgery, he was extremely confident, outgoing, and able to provide for his family. His goal was to begin a regular exercise program under the supervision of an exercise professional at five times a week for 8 weeks. He would then progress to independent exercise at a fitness facility for life-long exercise and improved health. He hoped this would help manage his LBP and mental health for reducing anxiety and depression as well as improve his confidence.

Health Fitness Examination

Screening tools and Outcome Measures: SF 36: Paul reported negative health beliefs (scores $<$50 on scale of 0–100) for all dimensions.

Modified Oswestry Low Back Questionnaire: 13/50, where greater score = more disability related to LBP.

Functional Based Pain Scale: Present pain 2/10, at worst 4/10, where 0 is no pain and 10 is emergency room pain.

Risk Stratification: Moderate (man ≥45 years old).

Vitals

Age: 54 years
Resting HR: 65 bpm
Resting BP: 115/60 mm Hg
BMI: 25.1
Height: 6′5″
Weight: 211 lb

continues

***The Case of Paul* cont.**

Cardiorespiratory Fitness

Rockport One-Mile Fitness Walking Test Predicted $\dot{V}O_{2max}$ = 40 mL·kg^{-1}·min^{-1}, 65th percentile for age.

Muscular strength – 1 RM upper body bench press: 110 lb; 110/211 = 0.52 or 10th percentile. Lower body leg press: 390 lb; 390/211 = 1.85 or 90th percentile. Muscular endurance: push-up: 8 reps, fair for age.

Range of motion (ROM)/flexibility: ROM: Goniometric measures were within functional limits and equal bilateral upper and lower extremity, as well as for the neck and trunk. Mild pain (2/10) noted with trunk flexion.

Questions

- What testing and/or outcome measures should be used in this case besides health fitness testing?
- Are there indications for use of exercise in clients with LBP?
- Are there indications for use of exercise in clients with diverticulitis?

References

Bize R, Johnson JA, Plotnikoff RC. Physical activity level and health-related quality of life in the general adult population: A systematic review. *Prev Med.* 2007;45(6):401–15. Epub 2007 Jul 21.

Carek PJ, Laibstain SE, Carek SM. Exercise for the treatment of depression and anxiety. *Int J Psychiatry Med.* 2011;41(1):15–28.

Lavie CJ, Milani RV, O'Keefe JH, Lavie TJ. Impact of exercise training on psychological risk factors. *Prog Cardiovasc Dis.* 2011;53(6):464–70.

Strate LL, Liu YL, Aldoori WH, Giovannucci EL. Physical activity decreases diverticular complications. *Am J Gastroenterol.* 2009;104(5):1221–30. Epub 2009 Apr 14.

George SZ, Wittmer VT, Fillingim RB, Robinson ME. Comparison of graded exercise and graded exposure clinical outcomes for patients with chronic low back pain. *J Orthop Sports Phys Ther.* 2010;40(11):694–704.

American College of Sports Medicine. *ACSM's Guidelines for Exercise Testing and Prescription.* 8th ed. Philadelphia (PA): Lippincott Williams & Wilkins; 2009.

SUMMARY

Stress is a variable condition across individuals. The occurrence and perception of an event as stressful depends entirely on the person and his or her resources to deal with the stressors. Contrary to popular belief, stress is not always negative; stress can act as a positive challenge that encourages individuals to rise to the occasion and possibly even face their phobias or anxieties. How a stressful situation is perceived is completely unique to each individual. Situations that are perceived to be stressful can cause a variety of symptoms, including ulcers, migraines, and muscle spasms. Long-term chronic stressors can increase the risk of life-threatening conditions, including cardiovascular disease, stroke, and cancer. Stress cannot be cured, but there are many tactics and strategies for changing the psychological perception of a stressor and for decreasing the physiological response to a stressor. This chapter has offered and explained a wide variety of methods for buffering and decreasing the negative impact of stress on the individual. A person may prefer one method over another, but no matter what therapeutic method implemented, "stress" should be addressed by the health and clinical community with the same level of importance as any other life-threatening condition. Stress left untreated or unresolved can lead to serious psychological and physiological damage. Stress may or may not be "America's No. 1 Health Problem," as stated in *Time* magazine (1983), but it is certainly a pervasive health problem that needs to be recognized, diagnosed, and properly addressed by the clinical community.

STUDY QUESTIONS

1. Understanding stress: What is stress? How is stress different from stressors? Are all stressors bad? What are some examples of good stress (*i.e.*, eustress)?
2. Discuss the consequences of stress on the development and progression of disease.
3. What is the reasoning behind certain people not becoming stressed when they encounter a demanding situation? Explain the two coping mechanisms that can be implemented to minimize the impact of stress.
4. Before encountering a stressful event, how can a person can prepare himself or herself to ideally handle the event and avoid becoming stressed? Discuss some of the strategies for buffering the impact of stress such as social support and exercise.
5. What is healthy stress management? Discuss three techniques or approaches for handling and decreasing perceived stress, including the potential benefits and consequences of each method.

REFERENCES

1. Abele A, Brehm W. Mood effects of exercise versus sports games: Findings and implications for well-being and health. In: Maes S, Leventhal H, Johnston M, editors. *International Review of Health Psychology.* Vol 2. New York (NY): Wiley; 1993.
2. Ackerman KD, Heyman R, Rabin BS, et al. Stressful life events precede exacerbations of multiple sclerosis. *Psychosom Med.* 2002;64:916–20.
3. AMA (American Medical Association). *The American Medical Association Encyclopedia of Medicine.* New York (NY): Random House; 1989.
4. Andrasik F, Blake DD, McCarran MS. A biobehavioral analysis of pediatric headache. In: Krasnegor NA, Arasteh JD, Cataldo MF, editors. *Child Health Behavior: A Behavioral Pediatrics Perspective.* New York (NY): Wiley; 1986.
5. Averill JR. Personal control over aversive stimuli and its relationship to stress. *Psychol Bull.* 1973;80:286–303.
6. Baider L, Perry S, Sison A, Holland J, Uziely B, DeNour AK. The role of psychological variables in a group of melanoma patients: An Israeli sample. *Psychosomatics.* 1997;38:45–53.
7. Bandura A. Self-efficacy: Toward a unifying theory of behavioral change. *Psychol Rev.* 1977;84:191–215.
8. Bandura A. *Self-efficacy: The Exercise of Control.* New York (NY): W. H. Freeman; 1997.
9. Bandura A, Reese L, Adams NE. Microanalysis of action and fear arousal as a function of differential levels of perceived self-efficacy. *J Pers Soc Psychol.* 1982;43:5–21.
10. Bandura A, Taylor CB, Williams SL, Mefford IN, Barchas JD. Catecholamine secretion as a function of perceived coping self-efficacy. *J Consult Clin Psychol.* 1985;53:406–14.
11. Benson H. *Beyond the Relaxation Response.* New York (NY): Time Books; 1984.
12. Berkman LF, Glass T. Social integration, social networks, social support, and health. In: Berman LF, Kawachi I, editors. *Social Epidemiology.* New York (NY): Oxford University Press; 2000.
13. Blumenthal JA, McCubbin JA. Physical exercise as stress management. In: Baum A, Singer JE, editors. *Handbook of Psychology and Health.* Vol 5. Hillsdale (NJ): Erlbaum; 1987.
14. Borcel E, Perez-Alvarez L, Herrero AI, et al. Chronic stress in adulthood followed by intermittent stress impairs spatial memory and the survival of newborn hippocampal cells in aging animals: Prevention by FGL, a peptide mimetic of neural cell adhesion molecule. *Behav Pharmacol.* 2008;19:41–9.
15. Brown GW, Harris T. *Social Origins of Depression: A Study of Psychiatric Disorder in Women.* New York (NY): Free Press; 1978.
16. Bryant RA, Moulds ML, Guthrie RM, Nixon RD. The additive benefit of hypnosis and cognitive-behavioral therapy in treating acute stress disorder. *J Consult Clin Psychol.* 2005;73:334–40.
17. Budzynski TH, Stoyva JM, Adler CS, Mullaney DJ. EMG biofeedback and tension headache: A controlled outcome study. *Psychosom Med.* 1973;35:484–96.
18. Butler LD, Symons BK, Henderson SL, Shortliff LD, Spiegel D. Hypnosis reduces distress and duration of an invasive medical procedure for children. *Pediatrics.* 2005;115:E77–85.
19. Carmack CL, Boudreaux E, Amaral-Melendez M, Brantley PJ, de Moor C. Aerobic fitness and leisure physical activity as moderators of the stress-illness relation. *Ann Behav Med.* 1999;21:251–7.
20. Cohen S, Evans GW, Stokols D, Krantz DS. *Behavior, Health, and Environmental Stress.* New York (NY): Plenum; 1986.
21. Cohen S, Frank E, Doyle WJ, Skoner DP, Rabin BS, Gwaltney JM. Types of stressors that increase susceptibility to the common cold in healthy adults. *Health Psychol.* 1998;17:214–23.
22. Cohen S, Janicki-Deverts D, Miller GE. Psychological stress and disease. *JAMA.* 2007;298(14):1685–7.

23. Cohen F, Lazarus RS. Coping and adaptation in health and illness. In: Mechanic D, editor. *Handbook of Health, Health Care, and the Health Professions.* New York (NY): Free Press; 1983.
24. Cohen S, McKay G. Social support, stress, and the buffering hypothesis: A theoretical analysis. In: Baum A, Taylor SE, Singer JE, editors. *Handbook of Psychology and Health.* Hillsdale (NJ): Erlbaum; 1984.
25. Cohen S, Tyrrell DA, Smith AP. Psychological stress and susceptibility to the common cold. *N Engl J Med.* 1991;325:606–12.
26. Cohen S, Wills TA. Stress, social support, and the buffering hypothesis. *Psychol Bull.* 1985;98:310–57.
27. Coker AL, Bond S, Madeleine MM, Luchok K, Pirisi L. Psychological stress and cervical neoplasia risk. *Psychosom Med.* 2003;65:644–51.
28. Dishman RK. Mental health. In: Seefeldt V, editor. *Physical Activity and Well-being.* Reston (VA): American Alliance for Health, Physical Education, Recreation, and Dance; 1986.
29. Effects of Stress. Fort Worth (TX): American Institute of Stress; [cited 2011 Jul 27]. Available from: http://www.stress.org/topic-effects.htm
30. Field TM. Touch therapies across the life span. In: Kato PM, Mann T, editors. *Handbook of Diversity Issues in Health Psychology.* New York (NY): Plenum; 1996.
31. Field TM. Massage therapy effects. Am Psychol. 1998;53:1270–81.
32. Flood KR, Long BC. Understanding exercise as a method of stress management: A constructionist framework. In: Kerr J, Griffiths A, Cox T, editors. *Workplace Health, Employee Fitness and Exercise.* London (England): Taylor & Francis; 1996. p. 117–28.
33. Flory N, Salazar GM, Lang EV. Hypnosis for acute distress management during medical procedures. *Int J Clin Exp Hypn.* 2007;55:303–17.
34. Folkman S, Lazarus RS. Coping as a mediator of emotion. *J Pers Soc Psychol.* 1988;54:466–75.
35. Folkman S, Lazarus RS, Dunkel-Schetter C, DeLongis A, Gruen RJ. Dynamics of a stressful encounter: Cognitive appraisal, coping, and encounter outcomes. *J Pers Soc Psychol.* 1986;50:992–1003.
36. Glanz K, Schwartz MD. Stress, coping, and health behavior. In: Glanz K, Rimer BK, Viswanath K, editors. *Health Behavior and Health Education: Theory, Research, and Practice.* 4th ed. San Franscisco (CA): Jossey-Bass; 2008. p. 209–36.
37. Glaser R, Rice J, Speicher CE, Stout JC, Kiecolt-Glaser JK. Stress depresses interferon production by leukocytes concomitant with a decrease in natural killer cell activity. *Behav Neurosci.* 1986;100:675–8.
38. Heaney CA, Israel BA. Social networks and social support. In: Glanz K, Rimer BK, Viswanath K, editors. *Health Behavior and Health Education: Theory, Research, and Practice.* 4th ed. San Francisco (CA): Jossey-Bass; 2008. p. 189–210.
39. Hernandez-Reif M, Ironson G, Field T, et al. Breast cancer patients have improved immune and neuroendocrine functions following massage therapy. *J Psychosom Res.* 2004;57:45–52.
40. Holahan CK, Holahan CJ, Belk SS. Adjustment in aging: The roles of life stress, hassles, and self-efficacy. *Health Psychol.* 1984;3:315–28.
41. Holmes DS. Aerobic fitness and the response to psychological stress. In: Seraganian P, editor. *Exercise Psychology: The Influence of Physical Exercise on Psychological Processes.* New York (NY): Wiley; 1993.
42. House JS. *Work Stress and Social Support.* Reading (MA): Addison-Wesley; 1981.
43. Jackson EM, Dishman RK. Cardiorespiratory fitness and laboratory stress: A meta-regression analysis. *Psychophysiology.* 2006;43:57–72.
44. Jacobson EJ. *Progressive Relaxation.* Chicago (IL): University of Chicago Press; 1938.
45. Jensen MP, McArthur KD, Barber J, et al. Satisfaction with, and the beneficial side effects of, hypnotic analgesia. *Int J Clin Exp Hypn.* 2006;54:432–47.
46. Julien RM, Advokat CD, Comaty JE. *A primer of Drug Action: A Comprehensive Guide to the Actions, Uses, and Side Effects of Psychoactive Drugs.* 11th ed. New York (NY): Worth Publishers; 2008.
47. Kahn JR, Pearlin LI. Financial strain over the life course and health among older adults. *J Health Soc Behav.* 2006;47:17–31.
48. Kiecolt-Glaser JK, Christian L, Preston H, et al. Stress, inflammation, and yoga practice. *Psychosom Med.* 2010;72:113–21.
49. Lasar M, Kotterba S. Locus of control of patients with a phasic encephalomyelitis disseminate course. *Schweiz Arch Neurol Psychiatr.* 1993;144:147–62.
50. Lazarus RS. *Stress and Emotion: A New Synthesis.* New York (NY): Springer; 1999.
51. Lazarus RS, Folkman S. *Stress, Appraisal, and Coping.* New York (NY): Springer Publishing Company; 1984. 142 p.
52. Leserman J. Role of depression, stress, and trauma in HIV disease progression. *Psychosom Med.* 2008;70:539–45.
53. Levy S, Herberman R, Lippman M, D'Angelo T, Lee J. Immunological and psychosocial predictors of disease recurrence in patients with early-stage breast cancer. *Behav Med.* 1991;17:67–75.
54. Lichstein KL. *Clinical Relaxation Strategies.* New York (NY): Wiley; 1988.
55. Linden W. *Stress Management: From Basic Science to Better Practice.* Thousand Oaks (CA): Sage Publications; 2005.
56. Lipton RB, Silberstein SD, Stewart WF. An update on the epidemiology of migraine. *Headache.* 1994;34: 319–28.
57. Locke S, Kraus L, Leserman J, Hurst M, Heisel S, Williams M. Life change stress, psychiatric symptoms and natural killer cell activity. *Psychosom Med.* 1984;46:441–53.
58. Lovallo WR. *Stress & Health: Biological and Psychological Interactions.* 2nd ed. Thousand Oaks (CA): Sage Publications; 2005. p. 35–8.
59. Lundberg U. Coping with stress: Neuroendocrine reactions and implications for health. *Noise Health.* 1999;1:67–74.
60. Lundberg U. Stress hormones in health and illness: The roles of work and gender. *Psychoneuroendocrinology.* 2005;30:1017–21.
61. Lupien S, Lecours AR, Lussier I, Schwartz G, Nair NPV, Meaney MJ. Basal cortisol-levels and cognitive deficits in human aging. *J Neurosci.* 1994;14:2893–903.
62. Lupien SJ, de Leon M, de Santi S, et al. Cortisol levels during human aging predict hippocampal atrophy and memory deficits. *Nat Neurosci.* 1998;1:69–73.
63. Lupien SJ, Evans A, Lord C, et al. Hippocampal volume is as variable in young as in older adults: Implications for the notion of hippocampal atrophy in humans. *Neuroimage.* 2007;34:479–85.
64. Malkoff SB, Muldoon MF, Zeigler ZR, Manuck SB. Blood platelet responsivity to acute mental stress. *Psychosom Med.* 1993;55:477–82.
65. Manuck SB. Cardiovascular reactivity in cardiovascular disease: "Once more unto the breach." *Int J Behav Med.* 1994;1:4–31.
66. Marin M-F, Lord C, Andrews J, et al. Chronic stress, cognitive functioning, and mental health. *Neurobiol Learn Mem.* 2011;96:583–95. Epub 2011 Mar 2.
67. McEwen BS. Protective and damaging effects of stress mediators. *N Engl J Med.* 1998;338:171–9.

68. McEwen BS, Stellar E. Stress and the individual: Mechanisms leading to disease. *Arch Intern Med.* 1993;153:2093–101.
69. McEwen BS, Wingfield JC. The concept of allostasis in biology and biomedicine. *Horm Behav.* 2003;43:2–15.
70. McFarlane AH, Norman GR, Streiner DL, Roy RG. The process of social stress: Stable, reciprocal, and mediating relationships. *J Health Soc Behav.* 1983;24:160–73.
71. McGonagle KA, Kessler RC. Chronic stress, acute stress, and depressive symptoms. *Am J Community Psychol.* 1990;18:681–706.
72. Miller SM. Controllability and human stress: Method, evidence, and theory. *Behav Res Ther.* 1979;17:287–304.
73. Mitsonis CI, Potagas C, Zervas I, Sfagos K. The effects of stressful life events on the course of multiple sclerosis: A review. *Int J Neurosci.* 2009;119:315–35.
74. Mohr DC. Stress and multiple sclerosis. *J Neurol.* 2007;254:II/65–8.
75. Mohr DC, Hart SL, Julian L, Cox D, Pelletier D. Association between stressful life events and exacerbation in multiple sclerosis: A meta-analysis. *BMJ.* 2004;328:731–6.
76. Morris RJ, Kratochwill TR. *Treating Children's Fears and Phobias: A Behavioral Approach.* New York (NY): Pergamon; 1983.
77. Norris R, Carroll D, Cochrane R. The effects of aerobic and anaerobic training on fitness, blood pressure, and psychological stress and well-being. *J Psychosom Res.* 1990;34:367–75.
78. Patterson SM, Matthews KA, Allen MT, Owens JF. Stress-induced hemoconcentration of blood cells and lipids in healthy women during acute psychological stress. *Health Psychol.* 1995;14–24.
79. Patterson SM, Zakowski SG, Hall MH, Cohen L, Wollman K, Baum A. Psychological stress and platelet activation: Differences in platelet reactivity in healthy men during active and passive stressors. *Health Psychol.* 1994;13:34–8.
80. Pearlin LI, Schooler C. The structure of coping. *J Health Soc Behav.* 1978;19:2–21.
81. Peveler RC, Johnston DW. Subjective and cognitive effects of relaxation. *Behav Res Ther.* 1986;24:413–9.
82. Phares EJ. Locus of control. In: Corsini RJ, editor. *Concise Encyclopedia of Psychology.* New York (NY): Wiley; 1987.
83. Pothmann R, Frankenberg SV, Muller B, Sartory G, Hellmeier W. Epidemiology of headache in children and adolescents: Evidence of high prevalence of migraine among girls under 10. *Int J Behav Med.* 1994;1:76–89.
84. Priest RG. Benzodiazepines: The search for tranquility. In: Christie MJ, Mellett PG, editors. *The Psychosomatic Approach: Contemporary Practice of Whole-Person Care.* New York (NY): Wiley; 1986.
85. Rodin J. Health, control, and aging. In: Baltes MM, Baltes PB, editors. *The Psychology of Control and Aging.* Hillsdale (NJ): Erlbaum; 1986.
86. Rotter JB. Generalized expectancies for the internal versus external control of reinforcement. *Psychol Monogr.* 1966;90:1–28.
87. Rout UR, Rout JK. *Stress Management for Primary Health Care Professionals.* New York (NY): Kluwer Academic; 2002. 17, 78 p.
88. Sandi C, Davies HA, Cordero MI, Rodriguez JJ, Popov VI, Stewart MG. Rapid reversal of stress induced loss of synapses in CA3 of rat hippocampus following water maze training. *Eur J Neurosci.* 2003;17:2447–56.
89. Sapolsky RM, Krey LC, McEwen BS. The neuroendocrinology of stress and aging: The glucocorticoid cascade hypothesis. *Endocr Rev.* 1986;7:284–301.
90. Sarafino EP. *Behavior Modification: Principles of Behavior Change.* 2nd ed. Mountain View (CA): Mayfield; 2001.
91. Sarafino EP. *Health Psychology: Biopsychosocial Interactions.* 4th ed. New York (NY): John Wiley & Sons; 2002.
92. Schnall PL, Pieper C, Schwartz JE, et al. The relationship between "job strain," workplace diastolic blood pressure, and left ventricular mass index: Results of a case-control study. *JAMA.* 1990;263:1929–35.
93. Segerstrom SC, Taylor SE, Kemeny ME, Reed GM, Visscher BR. Causal attributions predict rate of immune decline in HIV-seropositive gay men. *Health Psychol.* 1996;15:485–93.
94. Selye H. *The Stress of Life.* New York (NY): McGraw-Hill; 1956.
95. Selye H. *The Stress of Life.* New York (NY): McGraw-Hill; 1976.
96. Shapipro AP, Krantz DS, Grim CE. Pharmacologic agents as modulators of stress. In: Matthews KA, Weiss SM, Detre T, et al., editors. *Handbook of Stress, Reactivity, and Cardiovascular Disease.* New York (NY): Wiley; 1986.
97. Sheridan JF, Dobbs CM. Stress, viral pathogenesis, and immunity. In: Glaser R, Kiecolt-Glaser J, editors. *Handbook of Human Stress and Immunity.* San Diego (CA): Academic Press; 1994. p. 101–23.
98. Sherwood A, Turner JR. Hemodynamic responses during psychological stress: Implications for studying disease processes. *Int J Behav Med.* 1995;2:193–218.
99. Stetler CA, Miller GE. Social integration of daily activities and cortisol secretion: A laboratory based manipulation. *J Behav Med.* 2008;31:249–57.
100. Suls J, Mullen B. Life change and psychological distress: The role of perceived control and desirability. *J Appl Soc Psychol.* 1981;11:379–89.
101. Taylor RL, Lam DJ, Roppel CE, Barter JT. Friends can be good medicine: Excursion into mental health promotion. *Community Ment Health J.* 1984;20:294–303.
102. Taylor SE. *Health Psychology.* 8th ed. New York (NY): McGraw-Hill; 2012. 158 p.
103. Taylor SE, Kemeny ME, Aspinwall LG, Schneider SG, Rodriguez R, Herbert M. Optimism, coping, psychological distress, and high-risk sexual behavior among men at risk for acquired immunodeficiency syndrome (AIDS). *J Pers Soc Psychol.* 1992;63:460–73.
104. Thoits PA. Mechanisms linking social ties and support to physical and mental health. *J Health Soc Behav.* 2011;52:145–61.
105. Thompson SC. Will it hurt less if I can control it? A complex answer to a simple question. *Psychol Bull.* 1981;90:89–101.
106. Trask PC, Paterson AG, Hayasaka S, Dunn RL, Riba M, Johnson T. Psychosocial characteristics of individuals with non-stage IV melanoma. *J Clin Oncol.* 2001;11:2844–50.
107. Umberson D. Family status and health behaviors: Social control as a dimension of social integration. *J Health Soc Behav.* 1987;28:306–19.
108. Van der Linden D, Keijsers GPJ, Eling P, Van Schaijk R. Work stress and attentional difficulties: An initial study on burnout and cognitive failure. *Work Stress.* 2005;19:23–36.
109. Vitaliano PP, Russo J, Niaura R. Plasma lipids and their relationships with psychosocial factors in older adults. *J Gerontol B Psychol Sci Soc Sci.* 1995;50:18–24.
110. Wassem R. A test of the relationship between health locus of control and the course of multiple sclerosis. *Rehabil Nurs.* 1991;16:189–93.

PART

V

Business

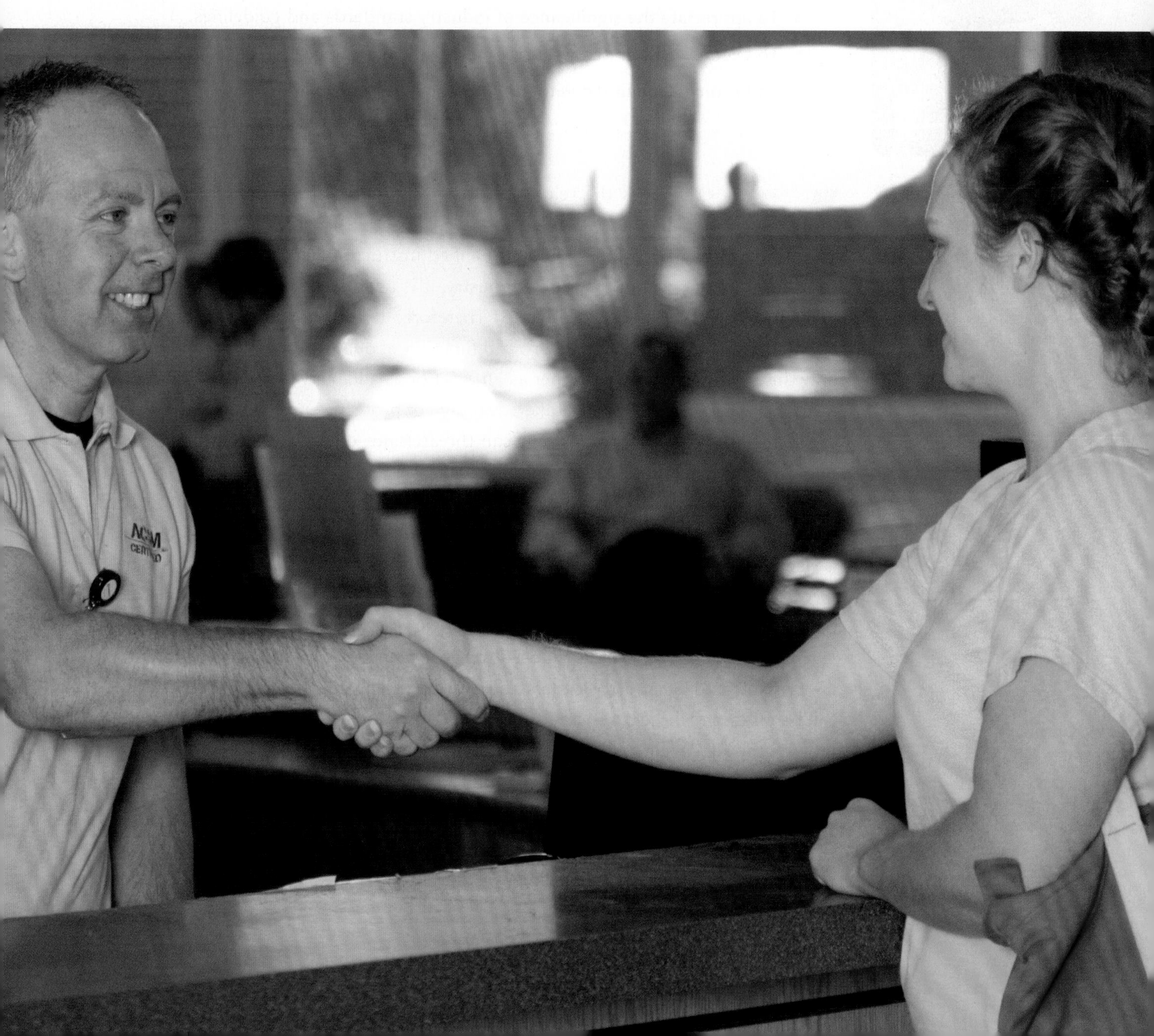

CHAPTER

13 Legal Structure and Terminology

Anthony A. Abbott

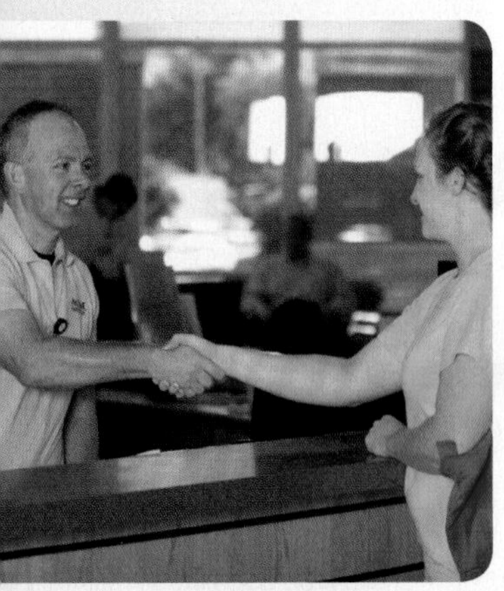

CHAPTER OBJECTIVES

- To understand basic concepts of the law and legal system.
- To understand the potential for legal liability and areas of primary concern.
- To appreciate the significance of industry standards and guidelines.
- To become acquainted with risk management strategies.
- To become acquainted with administrative responsibilities.

What is the relevance of understanding the law and legal system by the Health Fitness Specialist (HFS)? With the recognition that the HFS is a more qualified instructor than those typically found within the fitness industry, it is understandable that he or she will be held to a higher "standard of care." Therefore, it is incumbent on the HFS to be knowledgeable of the basic structure and function of our legal system. Being aware of how this system may be used either as an asset or as a liability to the client–instructor relationship enables the HFS to take advantage of protective mechanisms afforded by the system and to avoid pitfalls that can threaten not only the safety of their clients but also the livelihood of the HFS.

The HFS who trains within a fitness facility will most likely find that an injured party will pursue a claim against the facility rather than the HFS because the facility is viewed as having more extensive financial resources. Nevertheless, claims have been filed jointly against facilities and instructors wherein multiple judgments have been rendered.

In this chapter, the HFS is exposed to those tenets of the "standard of care" that are promulgated by industry leaders and available to protect the instructor. The focus will be on essential client services and, more importantly, protective actions that help insulate the HFS against litigation while simultaneously promoting professionalism.

THE LAW AND LEGAL SYSTEM

The HFS must be knowledgeable about the basic concepts of the law and the legal system. Along with this is the accompanying terminology that will provide the HFS with insight into issues affecting his or her business and potential exposure to liability. The HFS needs to understand the various divisions of the law, and especially the division of civil law, where tortuous and contract claims are areas within which the HFS is most likely to become legally embroiled. The anatomy of a lawsuit should be understood such that the HFS can navigate the sequence of legal proceedings and requirements to successfully support or defend a negligence claim or contract violation.

The HFS must understand that negligence is defined as one's failure to act, or as more likely will be the case, one's substandard performance. There are four elements of a negligence claim that must be documented to bring a successful suit against the HFS. If in fact these elements are substantiated, then the court can assess monetary damages against the HFS. Each element will be discussed in more detail later in this chapter.

The HFS needs to be aware of those varied situations wherein an instructor may create a risk of insult, injury, or possibly death, as these all present a potential case of negligence. There exist a myriad of settings to be considered when determining one's susceptibility to a negligence lawsuit, and these areas of vulnerability can primarily be found within the five stages of the instructor–client relationship. In short, if the HFS can remember the acronym STEPS (Fig. 13.1), this will be helpful in avoiding the distressing experience of litigation. By being attentive and applying the standard of care to the details of each one of the five steps, the HFS can successfully navigate through potentially litigious waters (2).

PRIMARY SOURCES OF LAW

The primary sources of law can be divided into four categories: (a) constitutional law, (b) statutory law, (c) case law, and (d) administrative law. The federal government and all states have constitutions that not only provide the authority for government, but also define how it will function and what its responsibilities are. Statutory laws or legislative laws are enacted by mandates from federal, state, and municipal governments, and this codification of law imposes duties or restrictions upon individuals. However, in the case of the Good Samaritan law, immunity is granted to those persons who in good faith try to protect, serve, and tend to others who are injured or ill. It should be noted, though, that the Good Samaritan law does not apply to HFS while on the job. Case law, sometimes referred to as common law, is based on decisions of courts and administrative tribunals. Common law is founded on unwritten law (not codified) and is based on customs and general usages, whereas case law is based on reported judicial decisions of selected lower and appellate courts. Administrative law

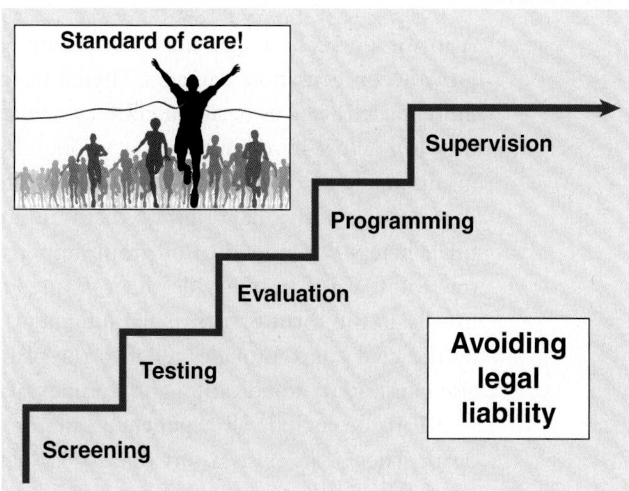

FIGURE 13.1. STEPS to success: avoiding legal liability.

is found within specialized bodies or agencies that have been granted law-making power to regulate specific activities. Federal agencies such as the Occupational Safety and Health Administration (OSHA), along with numerous state agencies, draft and enforce regulations that impact a wide range of individuals and entities, including fitness instructors and health facilities (3). Primary sources of law then are official bodies with the authority to make laws that can affect the legal rights of citizens.

In addition, our system of jurisprudence is subdivided into the two domains of criminal law and civil law, both of which dispose the citizenry to act in a way that benefits society. Whereas criminal law governs the conduct of both individuals and groups toward society as a whole, civil law pertains to personal responsibilities that an individual or a group must observe when dealing with other individuals or groups. This division of law addresses expressed grievances and judicial remedies between individuals, between an individual and a group, or between groups.

When individuals or groups violate criminal laws, they are subject to the penalties for misdemeanors and felonies, including fines, imprisonment, or both. Although the HFS is less likely to violate criminal law, there is the possibility that he or she could be charged with the unauthorized practice of medicine or unauthorized practice of an allied health field such as physical therapy or dietetics. For example, after screening a client for resting blood pressure, the HFS cannot diagnose him or her as hypertensive, as such a diagnosis remains only within the purview of a licensed physician. It could also be considering encroaching upon the realm of physical therapy by conducting postural analyses and providing corrective exercises, or encroaching upon the field of dietetics by providing clients with specific meal plans to correct nutritional deficiencies. The HFS could be found guilty of committing a first-degree misdemeanor that not only is punishable by a severe fine, but also could be punishable by imprisonment. Therefore, it is especially wise for the HFS, and any other unlicensed provider, to remain well within his or her scope of practice.

When individuals or groups violate civil law, they are subject to the jurisprudence of civil courts that adjudicate noncriminal cases. Civil lawsuits handle disputes between individuals, organizations, businesses, and governmental agencies wherein two parties, the plaintiff (*e.g.*, the injured party or representative of an injured or deceased individual) and the defendant (*e.g.*, the HFS and/or the facility that he or she represents) present their cases for litigation (3). Whereas criminal law requires that a prosecutor provide proof beyond a reasonable doubt to find the defendant guilty, civil law only requires that the plaintiff demonstrate that the preponderance of the evidence supports his or her claim to find the defendant liable. This again emphasizes that the HFS should stay within the stated scope or practice, as to avoid any potential issues of negligence that may lead to litigation.

When considering lawsuits against instructor personnel and fitness facilities, the plurality of such cases falls within the domain of civil law. The typical civil law violation falls under the categories of either tort law or contract law.

Tort Law

A tort is a breach of legal duty amounting to a civil wrong or injury for which a court of law will provide compensation/damages. Therefore, tort law governs the legal rights and obligations between individuals as well as between collective bodies in relationship to injuries, deaths, or civil wrongdoings (4). A tort by definition is a wrongful act, whether intentional or accidental, from which an insult, injury, or death occurs to another person or perhaps an organization that sustains pecuniary damage. The individual or group that is injured or sustains pecuniary damage is known as the plaintiff, whereas the individual or group responsible for the tortuous act is known as the defendant or tortfeasor. When an injury, death, or wrong is documented and attributed to the defendant, a remedy, usually in the form of a financial judgment, is then levied against the defendant. This levy, applied by the civil court, provides relief to the plaintiff. A tort does not include a breach of contract that also can lead to adjudication and compensation in the form of monetary damages.

Torts do include all negligence cases as well as intentional wrongdoings that result in injury or death. There also exists a tort due to "no fault" conduct. Therefore, tortuous acts are divided into the following three categories: (a) intentional misconduct, (b) negligent conduct, and (c) "no fault" conduct. "No fault" conduct falls under the category of Strict Liability and relates to ultrahazardous activities and product liability that will not be addressed in this chapter. An intentional tort is indicative of an act that willfully caused an injury, a death, a financial distress, or a damaged reputation. Since it is extremely difficult to document an intentional tort, courts typically give the benefit of doubt to the defendant and presume that the tort is one of negligence.

Negligence

When considering the lawsuits filed against fitness facilities and/or fitness instructors, the overwhelming majority are suits alleging negligence. The definitions of "negligence" and "standard of care" are similar in that they both are concerned with prudence and caution in dealing with clients. Standard of care refers to the application of a degree of prudence and caution required by an individual or organization that owes a duty of care. As it relates to the fitness industry, the standard of care is the degree of care that a reasonably prudent fitness instructor or reasonably prudent facility management would utilize under similar circumstances. A failure to exercise that degree of care utilized by prudent instructors or management represents negligence. The failure to do, or the failure to avoid, that which the prudent instructor would have done or not done may lead an individual to becoming liable for negligence. As a certified practitioner, the HFS will be held to a higher standard than most other instructors. Figure 13.2 provides an image of the components of negligence.

For the plaintiff to prosecute a successful tort claim, four basic elements of negligence must be well documented (5). First, a legal duty must be established from the relationship between the client and the HFS, a duty in which the HFS is required to provide safe and effective instruction without exposure to risks that could be the cause of injury and, perhaps, even death. Second, a breach of that legal duty, which is either substandard performance or a failure to act, is determined to have taken place. Third, the breach of duty owed was the factual or proximate cause of the injury or death. Fourth, the negligent act or failure to act resulted in well-documented damages or losses to the plaintiff, both economic damages (*e.g.*, medical costs and lost wages) and noneconomic damages (*e.g.*, pain and suffering).

HFSs can use three major risk management strategies to lessen the chances of becoming embroiled in legal liability with a negligence tort. First, the HFS must adhere to the standard of care in the screening process, fitness profiling, evaluation, programming, and supervision of clients. Second, the HFS must use waivers and assumption of risk forms in varied venues of the client–instructor relationship. Third, the HFS must ensure that he or she has purchased appropriate liability insurance for the activities in which his or her client is engaged.

Regarding adherence to the standard of care, the grasp of safe and effective fitness practices is dealt with in other chapters within this resource manual. However, the prudent and cautious HFS is unlikely to be faced with litigation because of his or her commitment to providing such safe and effective practices. This is the first line of defense in risk management. Waivers and assumption of risk forms provide a second line of defense and must be understood in light of their implementation and limitations.

Protective legal documents exist in different forms, of which the three most common are informed consent, agreement to participate, and prospective waivers or releases. However, before discussing the legal protection each of the above documents provide, it is necessary to review the three major causes of injury or death associated with physical activity:

- *Inherent:* injuries due to accidents that are not preventable and are no one's fault
- *Negligence:* injuries due to the fault of the defendant (sometimes the plaintiff)
- *Extreme forms of negligence:* injuries due to the gross negligence, willful and wanton, or reckless conduct of the defendant (6)

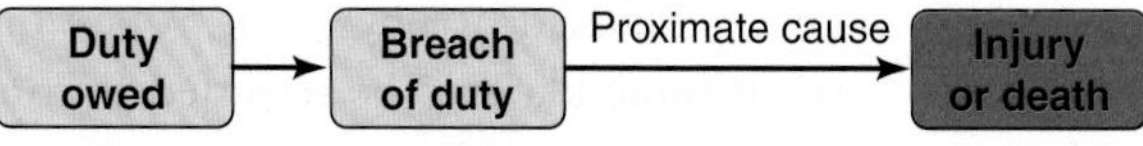

FIGURE 13.2. Minimizing negligence through risk management.

When lawsuits are filed due to an inherent injury such as a sprained ankle on a fitness facility's basketball court, an informed consent or agreement to participate provides the best legal protection by strengthening what is termed an assumption of risk defense. For this reason, informed consents are utilized prior to fitness testing or exercise programming and participation. Therefore, despite the fact that the client has been advised and warned of the risks, he or she declares that the risks are understood, appreciated, and voluntarily assumed. Although this defense is generally upheld in court for injuries due to inherent causes, it is sometimes used unsuccessfully be defendants for various reasons; for example, the injury was due to negligence of the defendant or the plaintiff did not fully understand and appreciate the inherent risks prior to participation. Chapter 2 of this text covers preparticipation screening in greater detail.

When lawsuits are filed due to negligence on the part of the instructor, a prospective waiver or release provides the best legal protection to thwart potential liability. Within the waiver, there exists an "exculpatory" clause explicitly stating that the instructor is released from liability due to any negligence. This clause is designed to document that the client has relinquished his or her right to pursue litigation. The validity of waivers to provide protection from negligent torts is determined by state law, which can vary greatly from state to state. In some states, waivers provide no protection from liability due to negligence, whereas in other states, lenient, moderate, or rigorous requirements (7) must be upheld to protect the instructor from negligence.

To ensure that waivers and releases are legally binding, HFSs should engage legal counsel to draft their exculpatory forms, recognizing that state laws not only vary but also change periodically. Therefore, if the HFS has been using waivers or releases for an extended period, it is wise to have legal counsel review the forms to ensure that they remain compliant with current law. Frequently, the HFS can obtain samples of waivers and releases from seminars or copies in texts such as American College of Sports Medicine® (ACSM) Health/Fitness Facility Standards and Guidelines (10). Although this may save the cost of hiring a lawyer, the HFS should be aware that these documents might not be applicable and legally enforceable in their state.

When lawsuits are filed due to extreme or gross negligence, there are generally no protective legal documents. A few states may permit the use of a waiver or release to provide such protection, but this is rarely the case (7). Extreme forms of negligence exist when the defendant is aware of the potential danger and risk of an activity or exercise but fails to warn the client and instead allows the performance of that activity or exercise. In such cases, punitive damages may be awarded, and normally liability insurance policies will not cover the instructor liable of extreme negligence.

As discussed, protective legal documents are an important line of defense for the HFS in that they can provide evidence in a court of law that the client was made aware of risks but decided to assume such risks as outlined. In addition, an exculpatory clause may provide a defense in case of an inadvertent lapse in the HFS's performance related to either an act of commission or an act of omission. Frequently, protective legal documents in the form of prospectively signed waivers or exculpatory agreements may prevent a claim from going forward, as a judge can dismiss a case through a pretrial motion termed a summary judgment.

Insurance Coverage

As previously stated, liability insurance is an important component of an HFS's risk management strategy. There are multiple types of insurance coverage available to the HFS; however, those of interest should be "general" and "professional" liability insurance that affords protection from negligence claims. The HFS can obtain a general liability insurance policy, which protects from "ordinary" negligence, from a commercial general liability firm, or CGL (1).

Professional liability insurance (PLI), also called professional indemnity insurance (PII) but more commonly known as errors and omissions (E&O), protects individuals who provide professional advice and service as part of their job responsibility. This insurance is similar to malpractice insurance purchased by physicians. When the HFS is employed in a health care provider setting, he or she is more likely to be regarded as conducting professional services and therefore should have PII.

However, because CGLs may attempt to avoid a payoff by claiming their policy excludes coverage for "professional services," the HFS should hold both general and PLI.

The last line of defense in risk management is the possession of both general and PLI. With this coverage, the HFS can be assured that an untoward event at work resulting in a negligence claim will not dampen his or her future but that he or she can continue to enjoy a personally rewarding and financially secure career as a fitness professional.

FEDERAL LAWS

Key laws that employers and HFSs should be well versed in include those pertaining to sexual harassment, workplace safety, and maintaining privacy of clients and employees. Each of these is critical to promoting a safe and inviting environment and conducting business in the most professional manner possible. Ideally, legal counseling will be retained to make sure the place of business is in compliance with the various aspects of each law.

Sexual Harassment

The definition of sexual harassment is any kind of intimidation, browbeating, bullying, or coercion of a sexual nature, or the inappropriate promise of promotions in exchange for sexual favors, or the threat of loss of job security for failure to provide such favors. Both sexes may be guilty of sexual harassment although more often complaints are lodged against men. The HFS could be the victim of sexual harassment by peers as well as superiors; of course, the HFS could also be accused of sexual harassment in relation to clients. Sexual harassment is a form of sex discrimination and as such can lead to litigation.

Title VII of the Civil Rights Act of 1964 prohibits sex discrimination in the workplace, and since that time, the courts have extended this prohibition to include sexual harassment. In 1980, the Equal Employment Opportunity Commission amended its "Guidelines on Discrimination Because of Sex" to include sexual harassment and helped solidify judicial acceptance of this cause of action (8).

Sexual harassment could include a range of behaviors from seemingly mild transgressions and annoyances to actual sexual abuse or sexual assault. In some circumstances, sexual harassment may be not only unethical but also illegal and, therefore, a violation of criminal law. In the workplace, sexual harassment is a form of illegal employment discrimination. For many fitness facilities, preventing sexual harassment among personnel and defending employees from sexual harassment charges have become key goals of managers.

The HFS must be aware that charges of sexual harassment by clients can be made against him or her, and therefore, the HFS needs to choose his or her words carefully, to be cautious with touching as in assisting and spotting clients, and to avoid any suggestion of impropriety. For example, when the male HFS is conducting body fat testing with skinfold calipers within the confines of a testing center, it would be wise to have a female employee assisting, thereby ensuring that no unjust accusations may be directed against the examiner.

OSHA Guidelines

Under the U.S. Department of Labor, the OSHA is the principal federal agency charged with the enforcement of safety and health legislation in the workplace. In an effort to improve worker safety, OSHA has established regulations that have some specific implications for the fitness industry. The health code relating to blood-borne pathogens presents a formidable challenge to facility managers and often their HFSs who, as a result of their higher level of certification, are assigned the task of implementing a safety policy to prevent the possibility of employees contracting HIV and hepatitis B and C viruses.

HFSs frequently become responsible for understanding, recognizing, and dealing with the blood-borne pathogen threat inherent within fitness center operations, especially during an emergency response. There are potential dangers for pathogen exposure to both staff and members, and therefore the HFS may have to educate employees how to protect not only themselves, but also their members through necessary preventive techniques.

HFSs should become familiar with OSHA's published guidelines that provide directives on the training and record-keeping procedures of how to avoid and handle blood-borne pathogens. To adequately protect both staff and members, the HFS may need to educate facility employees on the following:

- What is a blood-borne pathogen?
- What is meant by *occupational exposure* to blood-borne pathogens?
- What are potential infectious materials and how to prevent exposure to them?
- What are the possible methods of disease transmission and how can they be controlled?
- What protective equipment is required to safeguard the first responder in an emergency situation (9)?

An explanation of the above concerns along with additional information of interest is available from OSHA, with regional offices located throughout the country that can provide fitness facility personnel with written materials and advice on how to meet OSHA requirements and how to improve workplace safety. Furthermore, the International Health Racquet and Sportsclub Association (IHRSA), the professional trade association of the fitness industry, has published a briefing paper for its member facilities regarding the OSHA blood-borne pathogens requirements. Failure to meet OSHA's legally enforceable standards may result in facility citations and penalties.

Besides blood-borne pathogens, employees and perhaps even facility members may be exposed to potentially hazardous substances such as swimming pool chemicals and cleaning agents. Therefore, the HFS may be assigned the task of advising facility employees, including independent contractors, of potentially harmful materials other than blood-borne pathogens. This may be accomplished through the posting of placards, notices, and memoranda. To this end, the ACSM's *Health/Fitness Facility Standards and Guidelines* (10, 2) indicates "standard 5" as follows: "Facilities must have in place a written system for sharing information with users and employees or independent contractors regarding the handling of potentially hazardous materials, including the handling of bodily fluids by staff in accordance with OSHA standards."

HIPAA Guidelines and Recommendations

Under the Department of Health and Human Services, the Health Insurance Portability and Accountability Act (HIPAA) of 1996 was established to protect the privacy of health information. The Office for Civil Rights is provided the legal authority to enforce the HIPAA Privacy Rule, a rule that protects the privacy of an individual's identifiable health information. The HIPAA Security Rule sets national standards for the security of electronically protected health information and also for the confidentiality of such information (11).

HIPAA requires that all information gathered about a client's health status must be kept confidential in the fitness facility. The HFS will frequently oversee the health screening process and therefore needs to guarantee that all information from medical histories, physical exam reports, and lifestyle questionnaires is only available to the appropriate individuals and that this information will be properly maintained and secured.

The HIPAA Privacy Rule provides federal protections for personal health information held by covered entities such as health care providers, health plans, and health care clearinghouses. The rule gives patients an array of rights regarding the privacy of their information. Concurrently, the Privacy Rule is balanced by permitting the disclosure of personal health information that is required by legitimate health care professionals for patient care. Although fitness facilities are not technically listed as covered entities, because they have access to a member's health information, they have an obligation to guarantee the confidentiality, integrity, and security of that information, or they could be found in violation of the Privacy Rule.

CLIENT RIGHTS AND RESPONSIBILITIES

The HFS is expected to have a mature grasp of instructor–client relations and what it means to provide professional service to his or her clientele. The HFS should know what is included in the rights of the client, such as making informed choices and knowing how to voice grievances. Likewise, it is often the duty of the HFS to ensure that clients in turn know their responsibilities to the facility and instructor, which could mean being truthful about their health history and assisting in keeping the workout environment safe.

Client Rights

Clients have the right to receive quality service that is provided in a respectful manner without offensive or defamatory remarks or any form of discrimination. Clients should be provided with an overview of services provided and what would be typical health and fitness requirements to safely participate in these physical activities. This information allows clients to make informed choices about services and programs that would be suitable to their needs and capabilities.

Clients have the right to know the qualifications of staff members and the educational requirements met to achieve different certifications. Client should be well informed about any activities in which they will be exposed and any inherent risks as well as risks created through the inability to carry out activities as directed by instructors.

Clients not only have the right to an appropriate health screening, but also have the necessity to be screened prior to physical activity. In addition, they have the right for a thorough orientation to the facility, operation of equipment to be used, and physical activity programs available, while also being advised of how to respond to potential emergencies within the facility.

Clients have a right to timely responses to their requests and inquiries along with reasonable continuity and coordination of any services provided. Any charges for services should be openly disclosed and discussed, and if there are any complaints, clients have a right to know how to voice their grievances about services provided or omitted.

In line with the HIPAA Privacy Rule as well as described in ethical statements published by ACSM and other professional organizations, clients have the right to expect confidentiality regarding health information that is disclosed to facility staff. In addition, if there is other personal and financial information shared with a facility, it must be handled discreetly and securely.

Client Responsibilities

Clients have the responsibility to give accurate information about their physical and mental health, any substance abuse, or any other conditions or circumstances that could adversely impact their physical activity programming. If during activities clients experience pain or any injuries, it is their responsibility to report such concerns to instructor personnel in a timely and forthright manner.

Clients are to assist instructor personnel in maintaining a neat and safe environment, such as in putting weights back in their racks or not leaving clothing or bottles on the floor where they could become a hazard to others. This means respecting not only the workout areas, but also other areas such as lounges or locker rooms.

Personal training clients are responsible for notifying their trainers well in advance if they cannot make appointments or if appointments need to be rescheduled. Likewise, clients should also notify facilities well in advance if they have to suspend a membership. If clients' addresses or phone numbers have changed, facilities must be advised. Clients are responsible for working with their instructors or trainers in reviewing, planning, or changing programs to ensure that programs meet their needs, capabilities, and schedules. In this respect, clients should also be quick to inform instructors or trainers if they are having any concerns or problems with the service being provided.

Both IHRSA and the ACSM have addressed a facility's responsibilities to its membership and therefore the rights to be anticipated by clients (10, 12). Both IHRSA's "Standards Facilitation Guide" and ACSM's "Health/Fitness Facility Standards and Guidelines" publications outline important responsibilities addressing preactivity screening, orientations, education, and supervision of membership; risk management; and emergency policies. These responsibilities, and more, are owed to the client; in addition, there are responsibilities outlined that the member/client has to the facility and its staff.

Contract Law

The law of contracts governs agreements that are enforceable in court. Contracts are agreements pertaining to the legal rights and obligations between individuals as well as between collective bodies. The contract is a stipulation to which both parties consent and recognize as legally enforceable. This agreement or promise gives rise to a legal obligation that one will perform or not perform some activity or venture. An offer is proposed by one party and then accepted by the other. In effect, there exists a promised exchange between the parties, and this promised exchange may be written, oral, and even implied. This agreement or promised exchange within the health and fitness industry usually amounts to a service (availability of a facility and exercise instruction) for money (financial remuneration). Examples of contracts used in the health fitness field are (a) employment contracts for employees and independent contractors, (b) informed consents, (c) waivers, and (d) membership contracts.

Employer and Employee Rights and Responsibilities

When individuals are hired by a facility to work as an HFS, there is in effect a contract regarding the rights and responsibilities of the employee. The employee has agreed to perform certain services for which he or she will be remunerated. And the employee has the recognizable expectation that he or she will be treated with a degree of propriety and decorum while in the conduct of his or her service, whether it be from fellow workers, management, or even clientele.

Employers and employees have responsibilities to each other, and they should expect their rights to be upheld while their responsibilities are met. Regarding employee rights, one expects that he or she will be presented with a well-defined job description and that there will be periodic reviews of work performance with accompanying critiques and recommendations for improvement or, hopefully, recognition for exemplary performance.

Employees can expect that the provision of their terms and conditions of employment will be explicitly spelled out. They can expect that the terms and conditions will set forth what their primary and secondary duties are, to whom they are accountable, their rates of pay, and other entitlements such as vacation time, health benefits, sick leave, and the like.

Employees can expect that there will be no discrimination of any kind (to include sexual harassment) and that there will be equal opportunities for advancement with appropriate pay adjustments. Equal opportunity legislation mandates that all employees must receive the same pay and same work conditions for carrying out the same or similar work. There are also specific laws relating to gender, racial, and disability discrimination (13).

Employees are expected to conduct their services in a manner that has regard to the safety of others, both staff and clientele. In this vein, employees have a serious obligation to educate clients about the safe operation of exercise equipment, in addition to the safety practices involved with all physical activities that clients perform not only in the facility but also outside of the facility.

Regarding OSHA requirements, employees must be advised and have every right to expect that management will caution them about any potential hazards, whether of a physical or chemical nature. This caution may be delivered through verbal warnings or written and posted notices that are readily observable. As previously stated, there exist specific regulations about the manner in which potentially harmful substances should be used, stored, and recognized by both staff and clientele, and this information should be clearly posted for all to see.

In light of the above requirements, employers are expected to abide by numerous regulations such as providing safe equipment, carrying out regular maintenance and safety checks, ensuring the training of employees in health and safety issues, and carrying out a risk assessment to assess the dangers of the unique work environment within fitness facilities. In short, during their employment, workers can anticipate that management will place a priority on their health and safety.

Employers and employees are expected to meet minimum legal requirements in the area of health and safety at work, as well as minimum standards and conditions related to hours, pay scales, and the treatment of people in the workplace. Along with rights for employees, there are corresponding responsibilities such as the expectation that employees will work in a safe manner and will have regard for the safety of their colleagues and clientele. In addition, employees are responsible for conducting all their relations with management, fellow workers, and clientele with the respect and decorum, reflecting ethical and collegial behavior.

Federal Employment Laws

When in a position to hire personnel, the HFS must understand the myriad laws that govern hiring. These laws cover issues related to civil rights, disabilities, and more; such laws are continually changing. It is not legally defensible to simply claim that a hiring law changed and you were unaware. Instead, similar to what was mentioned regarding earlier federal laws, legal counsel should be retained to ensure complete compliance with all local, state, and federal hiring laws.

Hiring and Prehiring Statutes

There are federal employment regulations or statutes regarding the hiring and prehiring of individuals and related regulations that apply to the fitness industry and other industries. The two important federal laws that prohibit employment discrimination related to preemployment inquiries include the Civil Rights Act of 1964 and the Americans with Disabilities Act (ADA) of 1990.

The Civil Rights Act of 1964 prohibits discrimination on the basis of race, color, gender, religion, and national origin (14). Therefore, unfair inquiries related to the above characteristics or preferences within job application forms, preemployment interviews, or any type of inquiry made of job applicants are unlawful. Questions that appear to take a candidate's race, creed, color, national origin, age, gender, marital status, or any physical, mental, or sensory handicap into consideration for discriminatory purposes must be avoided. However, these rules do not prevent employers from asking questions to determine which candidates are most qualified to perform the specific functions or tasks of a given job. These rules were developed to prevent characteristics or conditions that have nothing to do with an individual's ability to perform the job from influencing the process of candidate selection. Understandably, certain physical and mental conditions in addition to personality traits would prevent some individuals from successfully performing various staff duties within a fitness facility, including exercise instruction.

The ADA prohibits employment discrimination on the basis of disabilities or perceived disabilities (15). The ADA addresses the "Dos and Don'ts" regarding preemployment inquiries, specifically those questions to be avoided at the preoffer stage. This means that employers cannot directly ask whether an applicant has a particular disability or ask questions that are closely related to disability issues at anytime during the hiring process. The reason for this prohibition is that this information has been used in the past to exclude applicants with disabilities prior to an evaluation of their ability to perform the job.

Both the Civil Rights Act and the American Disabilities Act make it clear that anyone involved in the interviewing process must avoid asking unfair preemployment questions. Interview questions are considered fair only when they specifically relate to an individual's ability to perform the actual duties of the job. Within the fitness industry, there are many staff positions that can be handled by disabled individuals. In addition, there are disabled individuals who can carry out many of the functions of an HFS and, in some cases, may be the ideal candidate to offer classes for disabled individuals.

In light of the ADA, it is unfortunate that many barriers still exist that prevent disabled individuals from participating in mainstream society. Sadly, too many fitness facilities cannot accommodate disabled individuals, even though federal requirements mandate such accommodation. In addition to limited accessibility to the fitness facility as a whole, which in itself is an impediment to hiring, it is not uncommon to find rooms within the facility so overcrowded with exercise equipment that individuals who use a wheelchair cannot maneuver between machines nor have proper access to them, which is a clear violation of the American Disabilities Act.

There are two other federal employment regulations related to hiring, which bear mentioning, background checks, and drug testing. A background investigation is normally the process of researching criminal records, commercial records, and in some cases financial records of an individual. Background checks are frequently requested by employers interviewing job applicants, especially applicants pursuing positions that require high security or substantial trust, such as in a schools, hospitals, financial institutions, airports, and government. As background checks are normally conducted by government agencies or private enterprises for a fee, most fitness facilities conduct their own checks and are principally interested in criminal history and past employment verification. Such checks allow management to also evaluate qualifications such as education and certifications, along with character.

However, although a fitness facility may want more information on an applicant than that stated above, management does not have unlimited rights to investigate an applicant's background and personal life. As employees have a right to privacy in certain areas of their life, they can take legal action if they feel these rights have been violated. Consequently, it is essential that management understand what is permitted when doing further investigation on a potential employee's background and work history.

Under the Federal Trade Commission's Fair Credit Reporting Act (FCRA), applicants must give written permission to prospective employers if employers wish to obtain applicants' credit reports (16). If an employer decides not to hire an applicant or to promote an existing employee based on his or her credit report, then that applicant or employee must be provided a copy of the report, so he or she may challenge the veracity of the report. Statutes regulating the use of investigations of credit reports vary from state to state, and some states have very serious restrictions on obtaining credit reports.

As stated above, although fitness facilities have a vested interest in an applicant's potential criminal past, the extent to which a facility's management may consider one's criminal history in making a hiring decision varies from state to state. Owing to this wide variation, management should consult a lawyer or do further legal research on state laws before probing into whether or not an applicant does in fact have a criminal past.

The Drug-Free Workplace Act of 1988 and the mandatory guidelines for federal drug testing programs were specifically designed for federal employees with certain sensitive occupations relating to safety and security (17). Although the Act only applied to federal employees, many state and local governments followed suit and adopted similar programs under state laws and drug-free workplace programs. However, challenges to drug testing arose based on contested violations of the fourth and fifth amendments to the constitution. Generally, applicants are deemed to have a lesser expectation of privacy than current employees, and therefore, employers do enjoy greater freedom to test applicants without the same concerns of constitutional violations being invoked.

Drug testing may be of interest to the fitness facility not only because non–drug users make better employees, but also because some facilities may insist that staff, particularly instructors, not engage in the use of steroids or other quasi-illegal performance enhancing drugs. Although employers rightfully argue that the safety of clientele and coworkers may depend on the alertness of fellow employees and that employers will be liable if an employee under the influence of narcotics or alcohol injures a staff member or client, there are understandable concerns about the invasion of one's privacy. This idea of invasion of one's privacy is not only of concern to the American Civil Liberties Union (ACLU), but also deeply upsetting to many Americans who value their rights and privacy of person and property.

Owing to the above concerns, there has been the tendency to limit the type and extent of drug testing in the workplace. Specifically, some states have found their courts more restrictive than the federal legislature in regard to preemployment drug testing as well as ongoing drug testing in the workplace. Consequently, it is essential that before designing a drug-free workplace with a testing program, management not only familiarize itself with both state and federal regulations, but also secure legal counsel specializing in labor relations and law.

An additional federal regulation and requirement related to prehiring and hiring is the Equal Pay Act of 1963, which prohibits different pay rates on the basis of gender (18). This act was necessitated because over the years, women have received lower wages for the exact same duties performed by men. Another employment regulation is the Age Discrimination in Employment Act (ADEA), which prohibits discrimination on the basis of age for people older than 40 years (19). Yet another necessary regulation is the Immigration Reform and Control Act of 1986 (IRCA), which requires all employers to complete an employment eligibility verification form on individuals hired after November 6, 1986 (20).

These are but a few of the important requirements that employers need to address when hiring staff for their fitness facilities. In order to be thoroughly versed with prehiring and hiring requirements, employers should visit the U.S. Department of Labor Web site and search under the "hiring" section for information related to these and numerous other concerns such as affirmative action, the hiring of veterans and foreign workers, and the employment of workers younger than 18 years (21).

Facility Policies and Procedures

A fitness facility's policies and procedures represent a type of contract with employees as the applicant is agreeing to abide by such policies and procedures as a term of his or her employment. The development and implementation of policies and procedures provides businesses, such as fitness facilities, with operational uniformity and consistency. The adherence to policies and procedures is recognized to be one of the most important keys to profitability within a business. Policies and procedures are guidelines as well as mandates to the daily operation of a facility, and observing these assists employees in becoming more proficient because of the implied consistency of practice. This consistency, and proficiency, is noted by members and engenders greater confidence in the staff as a whole.

There are numerous policies and procedures related to the efficient conduct of business and financial operations within a facility. Unfortunately, many facilities fail to develop a comprehensive policy and procedure manual, and instead it is the responsibility of the HFS to work with management to develop and implement such a manual. Once developed, the number one priority of any facility should be the health and safety of its membership. Within this context of health and safety, there are certain policies and procedures that should take precedence: membership screening, fitness testing, orientations, instructor qualifications, supervision, equipment maintenance, facility cleanliness, and emergency procedures.

Screening members through health risk appraisals is essential to determine whether they are ready for the stress of exercise or whether medical clearance is needed. The health risk appraisalis the procedure by which a facility can identify those members who are at an increased risk for experiencing exercise-related cardiovascular incidents as well as musculoskeletal problems and the consequent need for physician referral before exercise programming can commence. The current standard of care dictates that screening procedures be practiced without exception.

Although it is possible for facilities to require that all members undergo a fitness assessment in conjunction with their health appraisal, it is typical that most facilities only offer and, hopefully, encourage members to avail themselves of this valuable service. There are numerous advantages for the member to participate in such an assessment or profiling; however, minimizing the chances of injuries, and thereby lessening the potential for litigation, is a high priority for any facility.

Managers have a primary responsibility to ensure that facility members receive a formal and comprehensive orientation related to the effectiveness and safety in exercise programming. During the orientation, members should be apprised of the advantages of personal training, to include fitness profiling, which will enhance their chances of program success. Other program services and benefits can be outlined with appropriate cautionary notes regarding one's preparedness for some of the more demanding activities. A walk-through of the facility highlighting both aerobic and resistance equipment should be available, with an emphasis on equipment operation and safety concerns. There are numerous topics to be covered during the orientation, and these should be explicitly detailed in the procedure manual.

Of paramount importance are policies relating to instructor qualifications, particularly regarding education, certifications, and prior work experience. In addition to the required knowledge, skills, and ability, instructors must be evaluated and advised on their interpersonal relations with fellow workers and members. Hiring policies must be clear as to which qualifications are most desirable and which qualifications meet minimal requirements. Performance reviews, along with continuing education expectations, should also be clearly detailed in the policy and procedure manual.

Policies regarding supervisory responsibilities ensure that personnel are always available to assist members having difficulty with equipment operation or the technique of specific exercises. Floor supervisors must be aware of potentially unsafe activities and alert to their anticipated implementation. Safe floor monitoring also requires that equipment is arranged in a manner that allows for all areas to be readily visible by personnel on duty and that there are no blind spots in which a member could become endangered without being observed.

Policies regarding equipment maintenance should be in writing and regularly observed. There are general, everyday maintenance requirements and inspections that can be carried out by staff members such as checking cables, pull-pin security, loose belts, gated snap hooks, and so on, along with the routine cleaning and wiping down of equipment. Policies regarding equipment should also include timely and proper reporting of any defects to be listed in maintenance and repair logs. Posted warnings or out-of-order signage is to be visibly secured on inoperable equipment if the equipment cannot be removed from the floor. Besides in-house inspection and cleaning, management should have service contracts with outside vendors who are certified in the inspection and repair of equipment. In addition to regularly scheduled appointments for servicing aerobic and resistive equipment, vendors should also be available for short notice or emergency calls.

Policies regarding facility cleanliness not only lead to member satisfaction and retention, but also, more importantly, lead to hygienic safety that can lessen the potential for litigation. An undercover investigation of fitness facilities indicated that "gyms" are some of the most likely environments for the transmission of germs (1). Accordingly, management needs to establish policy and procedures for daily equipment cleaning and hiring a professional cleaning service for nightly or early morning operations. Increased awareness of germ transmission has led many fitness facilities to provide members with clean towels and, more recently, with antiseptic spray bottles, germicidal wipes, paper towel dispensers, and antibacterial hand gel throughout the exercise floor. However, this cannot take the place of policies requiring regular and thorough cleaning provided by staff and professional services.

Of all facility policies, the emergency policy, and particularly the emergency medical policy, is the most consequential. It is incumbent on management to develop a written, venue-specific emergency response plan to deal with any reasonably foreseeable untoward event within the facility. The emergency plan's primary purpose is to ensure that minor problems do not escalate into major incidents and that major incidents do not intensify to fatal events. Possible emergencies could be fires, floods, tornadoes, earthquakes, hurricanes, severe storms, bomb threats, and even terrorist activities.

However, the most likely emergency is a "Code Blue" or "member down," indicating that a client is having a heart attack, stroke, or some other potentially fatal event. This emphasizes the need for an explicit medical emergency policy in which all staff must be well versed. Such a policy states that staff are certified in first aid and CPR with AED, and are well rehearsed for a timely response in carrying out the multiple duties expected of them, such as who coordinates the scene, who are first and assistant responders, who takes charge of crowd control, who meets and directs paramedics to the scene, and who is responsible for securing the member's file along with notifying the nearest relative. If these policies and procedures are lax, or staff rehearsal is not frequent, the potential for litigation increases exponentially. Therefore, anticipative management is considered not only imperative but also "good insurance" (3).

SUMMARY

The key to the health and safety of facility members is the availability of knowledgeable, skilled, and conscientious fitness instructors capable of establishing a safe exercise environment. This requires that staff members at all levels must not only be appropriately qualified to carry out their respective duties, but also sufficiently motivated to do the job to the best of their abilities.

Today, however, the public is beginning to hold health facilities and fitness instructors more accountable than in the past. As a result, there has been an upsurge in the number of personal injury lawsuits against facilities and instructors along with a concurrent rise in the costs of relevant liability insurance. Even with the obvious deterrent of prospectively executed waivers and releases, the public appears more willing to take their grievances to court.

The current escalation of litigation is a reflection of a serious industry problem regarding client expectations and service delivery. Too frequently individuals are injured as a result of certified instructors not being truly qualified professionals, and too often, individuals die while pursuing a healthier lifestyle because of insufficient screening, ineffective instruction, improper supervision, and/or an inadequate emergency response.

To lessen the possibility of litigation, facility personnel must be capable of thoroughly screening potential members, providing suitable fitness tests, evaluating health assessments and fitness profiles, designing appropriate exercise programs, and attentively supervising member activities. In addition, staff should constantly be aware of potentially dangerous situations and be empowered with the responsibility as well as the accountability to immediately correct hazardous conditions and respond effectively to emergency situations. This can only occur if management is knowledgeable about the field of exercise science and if instructors are properly qualified.

HFSs are typically placed in positions of not only conducting fitness programming but also managing facility operations. Therefore, their knowledge of exercise science must be complemented with a well-rounded knowledge of the many different areas within which management and personnel can become legally embroiled. Too often the many administrative and legal concerns of a health/fitness facility have gone unrecognized or have been misunderstood. The truly knowledgeable HFS recognizes the numerous responsibilities in managing and operating a facility that is totally committed to the health and fitness of its membership as well as the professionalism of the health and fitness industry.

STUDY QUESTIONS

1. What are those incidents in which an HFS would most likely become legally embroiled?
2. Identify major risk management strategies to lessen the chances of litigation.
3. What is the last line of defense in risk management?
4. List some of the municipal, state, and federal administrative requirements in the hiring of personnel and the operation of a fitness facility.
5. List various roles of responsibility in handling a medical emergency such as a sudden cardiac arrest.

REFERENCES

1. ABC News Primetime. *Is Your Health Club Unhealthy?* January 13, 2005.
2. Bates M, editor. *Health Fitness Management.* 2nd ed. Champaign (IL): Human Kinetics; 2008.
3. Eickhoff-Shemek J, Herbert D, Connaughton D. *Risk Management for Health/Fitness Professionals.* Philadelphia (PA): Lippincott Williams & Wilkins; 2009.
4. Earle R, Baechle T, editors. *NSCA's Essentials of Personal Training.* Champaign (IL): Human Kinetics; 2004.
5. Franklin B, editor. *ACSM's Guidelines for Exercise Testing and Prescription.* 6th ed. Philadelphia (PA): Lippincott Williams & Wilkins; 2000.
6. Earle R, Baechle T, editors. *NSCA's Essentials of Personal Training.* Champaign (IL): Human Kinetics; 2004.
7. Cotten D, Cotten M. *Legal Aspects of Waivers in Sport, Recreation and Fitness Activities.* Canton (OH): PRC Publishing Inc.; 1997.
8. Paul E. *Sexual Harassment as Sex Discrimination: A Defective Paradigm.* Vol 8(2). New Haven (CT): Yale Law Review; 1990.
9. Bates M, editor. *Health Fitness Management.* 2nd ed. Champaign (IL): Human Kinetics; 2008.
10. Tharrett S, Peterson J. *ACSM's Health/Fitness Facility Standards and Guidelines.* 4th ed. Champaign (IL): Human Kinetics; 2012.
11. United States Department of Health and Human Services Web site [Internet]. Available from: http://www.hhs.gov.
12. International Health, Racquet & Sportsclub Association. *IHRSA's Standards Facilitation Guide.* 2nd ed. Boston (MA): IHRSA; 1998.
13. United States Equal Employment Opportunity Commission Web site [Internet]. Available from: http://www.eeoc.gov
14. United States Department of Labor Web site [Internet]. Available from: http://www.dol.gov.
15. United States Department of Labor Web site [Internet]. Available from: http://www.dol.gov.
16. United States Federal Trade Commission Web site [Internet]. Available from: http://www.ftc.gov
17. United States Department of Labor Web site [Internet]. Available from: http://www.dol.gov
18. United States Equal Employment Opportunity Commission Web site [Internet]. Available from: http://www.eeoc.gov
19. United States Equal Employment Opportunity Commission Web site [Internet]. Available from: http://www.eeoc.gov
20. United States Equal Employment Opportunity Commission Web site [Internet]. Available from: http://www.eeoc.gov
21. United States Department of Labor [Internet]. Available from: http://www.dol.gov/compliance/topics/hiring-issues.htm

CHAPTER

14 Leadership and Management

Matthew Kutz

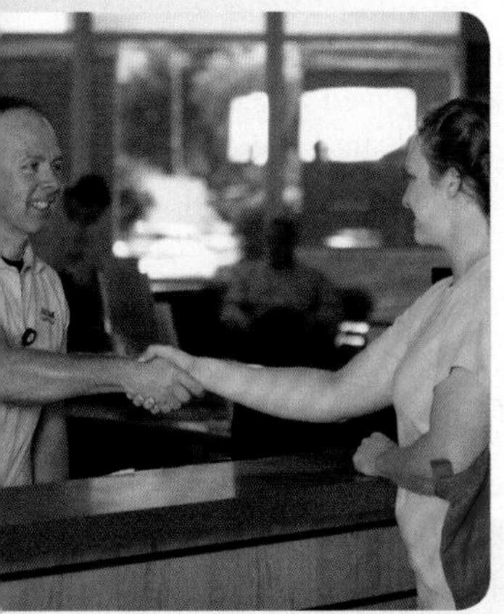

CHAPTER OBJECTIVES

- To address similarities and differences of leadership and management.
- To discuss the past, present, and future of leadership and management research.
- To describe several established leadership behaviors, theories, and styles.
- To identify application of practical management techniques for the HFS.
- To discuss organizational development and strategic planning.

The context of the health and fitness industry is often complex and volatile and, like most other industries, is constantly changing. There is a steady stream of changing regulations, evolving accreditation standards, emerging or reorganized regulatory agencies, new research, and an onslaught of fitness fads. In addition to satisfying many stakeholders (*e.g.*, clients and fitness club owners and peers), there is now the need to have and develop sufficient leadership and managements skills for sustained success.

Leadership has become a fundamental behavior expected of all Health Fitness Specialists (HFSs) regardless of their work context. In 1998, the Pew Commission recommended that all health professionals in the 21st century, whether they seek management positions or not, should practice leadership (31). In other words, leadership behaviors have not only become an industry standard, but also become a professional standard that transcends the work place. Leadership, apart from management, should be practiced consistently and intentionally. The aim of this chapter is to instill a sense of responsibility in the HFS to introduce and cultivate a working leadership philosophy into their professional practice.

DEFINING LEADERSHIP AND MANAGEMENT

The construct of leadership has hundreds of nuances, anecdotes, gradations, and theories. So much literature exists on leadership and its development, making it difficult to sort through and implement. In the past, many of the concepts and ideas concerning organizational effectiveness and motivation focused solely on management techniques. Recently, however, there has been a clear swing toward leadership competencies as a means of achieving organizational effectiveness and employee motivation. Management and leadership, whether independent of each other or in combination, are necessary within the health fitness industry (20). There are clear differences between leadership and management (29) that can be summarized as: in leadership, *people* are led; in management, *resources* are managed. Often, the HFS might fall into the trap of wanting to manage people, and this is an important and central skill set for the HFS; however, management should not be a substitute for leadership. The temptation to manage people is because it is perceived as easier than leading. For example, managing might lead to "punishing" by enforcing established policies and procedures, whereas leading may involve discussion, negotiation, and established new ways of operating.

Operational Definitions

Operationally, leadership is the ability to facilitate and influence others (*i.e.*, superiors, peers, and subordinates) to make recognizable strides toward shared and unshared objectives (20). Management is the ability to use organizational resources to accomplish predetermined objectives (20). Leadership transcends the workplace, whereas management is often confined to the workplace. For example, in a health and fitness setting, leadership is demonstrated when the HFS motivates and inspires clients or patients to make needed lifestyle changes. However, management in this situation may require the HFS to add additional or longer training days, make a referral to other health professionals, or schedule additional consultations. This would require having a well-organized, managed schedule and referral system in place.

Management and leadership are not always different. In fact, it is not unusual for them to have similar outcome objectives and for both to project power and use influence. However, the differences between leadership and management may best be delineated in the examination of intended outcomes and processes (45). The intended outcome of leadership is typically change, vision casting, and innovation; the intended outcome of management is predictability, vision implementation, and maintaining the efficient status quo. These two constructs often require different techniques and operate from fundamentally different frameworks. Dye and Garman (9) describe management as the "science" of mitigating risk, whereas "leadership is the art of taking risks." Therefore, leadership tends to use vision casting, alignment, meaningful communication, self-reflection, and self-assessment to develop willing followers, whereas management uses "planning, organizing, controlling, and coordinating," regardless of its subordinate's willingness (17). Stated another way, management is a function or role within an organization and leadership is a relationship between the follower and the leader, regardless of the organizational context (24).

Another distinguishing factor is that management is required when problems arise of a technical nature, which requires preestablished policies and procedures to be enacted, whereas leadership is required when problems do not have preestablished solutions and instead require adaptability, critical thinking, creativity, and innovation (14).

Although management and leadership are generally accepted as distinct, they are not necessarily exclusive, as both need to exist to efficiently operate at health/fitness facility. Therefore, the HFS should be able to manage a facility (budget, mitigate risk, use policy and procedures, etc.) while also leading people (inspire, communicate, motivate, exhibit empathy and ethical behavior, etc.). Figure 14.1 is an adaptation of a relationship matrix for the integration of leadership and management — the higher the value, the greater the competency.

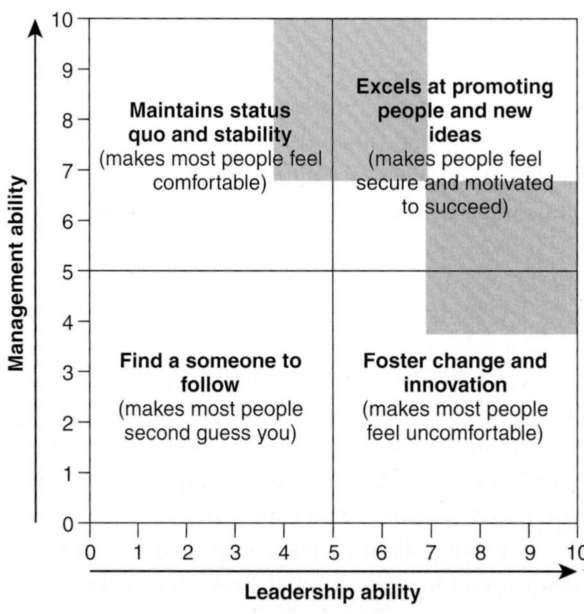

FIGURE 14.1. Integrating leadership and management. (From Kutz MR. *Leadership and Management in Athletic Training: An Integrated Approach.* Baltimore (MD): Lippincott Williams & Wilkins; 2010.)

LEADERSHIP: PAST, PRESENT, AND FUTURE

Although leadership theory is dynamic and continually evolving, four major models of leadership theory are consistently referenced in the literature: classical, transactional, visionary, and organic (1, 2). Collectively, these four leadership models serve as a philosophical foundation from which leadership is practiced.

Through the early 1970s, the classical model dominated leadership theory. Under this model, a leader's power or influence was considered innate and having a vision was not considered necessary to ensure follower support. Often a leader's influence was based on fear or respect. A leader's position or placement was rarely challenged. Of course, as workers became more skilled and knowledgeable, this model became less popular and was less able to motivate subordinates.

Transactional Model

The transactional model also began to gain popularity in the 1970s and signaled the era of the manager. Under this model, vision was neither necessary nor articulated. Instead, influence was based on contractual negotiations of rewards and punishments between the leader and subordinates. Considerable effort was taken by transactional leaders to create "environments" conducive to management intervention. In other words, the focus was on the manager's ability to generate policies and procedures that capitalized on productivity and efficiency. This model rewarded management for generating systems where a manager could intervene. Productivity was considered an outcome of "good" management, and any role employees had in productivity was minimized.

Visionary Model

The visionary model emerged shortly thereafter (mid-1980) and still has many proponents today, although it has lost some popularity. Visionary leadership (also called charismatic or transformational leadership) involves the leader using emotion to inspire and create buy-in of the followers. It is also interesting to note that with the entrance of visionary model, the language changed from "subordinates" to "followers." Within this model, vision became fundamental and followers were encouraged to contribute to the leader's vision.

Organic Model

The most recent model, organic, tends to overlap with visionary. The organic leadership model centers on a collective vision of the group as a team. A vision is important, but it is not "owned" only by the leader, instead the vision is created collectively and the leader helps implement the will of the team. Influence is based on the relationship and mutuality of the team and the endorsement of a leader. Organizational charts from an organic model tend to look like an amoeba instead of the pyramid shape of the other models.

Leadership Theory and Model

As new and more research emerges, leadership models and theories will continue to evolve. As this evolution occurs, there will always be the temptation for leaders to operate out of multiple models, some of which are in conflict with each other. For example, having a personal belief that leadership is something people are born with and is innate (classical model) is very different from the open leadership development programs to anyone interested (organic model) or soliciting feedback on strategic plans from nonleaders (visionary model). Applying different leadership models during the practice of management or leadership is contradictory. However, mixing leadership behaviors or styles is encouraged. It is appropriate to transition between or mix leadership styles when confronted with new or novel problems or situations. For example in a situation or with certain personnel, a leader may have to demonstrate servant leadership and then use a path–goal approach, or situational style in a different situation.

The seminal work of Ralph Stogdill (38)in the 1950s identified 1,800 separate leadership behaviors. Stogdill was eventually able to identify the two key behaviors that were rated by the vast majority of subordinates as critical to leadership: "initiating structure" and "consideration" (8). Initiating structure means organizing and defining relationships in a group (8). Consideration is defined as the degree to which the leader creates an environment of emotional support, warmth, friendliness, and trust (8). These two constructs have served as the foundation for much of how leadership is practiced and understood.

LEADERSHIP BEHAVIORS AND THEORIES

Trait Theory

The "great man" (or woman) theory promoted the idea that being a "superior leader" is an issue of genetics; it is in fact the idea that one is born to lead and has an innate set of leadership qualities and abilities (38). The "great man" ideology still has proponents today; for example, a popular leadership book states, "leadership cannot be manufactured. It cannot be mustered up. It's an innate gifting" (25).

Trait theory postulates two forms — (a) leadership traits are innate or a divine endowment (*i.e.*, great man theory) or (b) an individual can awaken dormant traits over time (44). Regardless if leadership is innate, divine endowment, or learned, those who might have innate leadership ability still must improve their leadership ability through years of practice and experience (9).

Situational Leadership Theory

Situational leadership was originally developed by Blanchard and Hersey in the 1960s. Situational leadership's purpose is to open up communication and to increase the quality and frequency of conversations about performance and development (16). Situational leadership suggests that leadership style is adapted by the leader on the basis of the leader's "diagnosis" of the "development level" of the subordinate (16). The development level or "situation" of a subordinate is based on a relationship between two factors: competence and commitment (16). For example, subordinates with high competence and high commitment (*i.e.*, experts) warrant delegation with little supervision (*i.e.*, a "leader who empowers them to act independently, affirming and confirming their decisions") (30). On the other hand, subordinates who demonstrate low competence but high commitment warrant direction aimed at "developing competence" (16).

Path–Goal Leadership Theory

Path–goal theory was popularized by House in the 1970s and is a modification of contingency or situational leadership. Path–goal involves the leader setting a path to a specific goal for a specific member or team on the basis of that member's personality or team's dynamics (8). Path–goal is about how leaders motivate employees to accomplish their designated goals (30). Path–goal theory draws heavily on motivational theory and emphasizes how the leader's style is influenced by both the work setting and subordinates (30).

Transformational and Transactional Leadership

Burns identified two types of leadership: transformational and transactional (6). Transformational leadership can be summarized as that which inspires and motivates others. Followers are influenced by the leader's creativity, admiration and respect (6). Transformational leaders give respect and admiration to their followers and are likewise typically admired and respected by their followers. Transformational leadership is considered similar to charismatic or visionary leadership (8).

Transformational leaders give "individual attention, inspire others to excel and stimulate people to think in new ways" (19). Stated another way, transformational leadership fosters innovation in coworkers and followers. There are five "practices" associated with transformational leadership: "challenging the process, inspiring a shared vision, enabling others to act, modeling the way, and encouraging the heart" (19).

Transactional leaders view leadership as the process of "exchanging one thing for another" (6). Often transactional leadership comes down to exchanging rewards (salary and benefits) for performance or work (6). Transactional leaders operate under different circumstances and from a different motivation than transforming leaders. Burns pointed out the divergent nature of the two leadership types. Transactional leadership is about the "individual interest" of the leader and is not concerned with the "collective interest of followers"; on the other hand, transformational leadership concerns itself with the follower's interests (6). "The transactional leader's behavior closely resembles that of a manager" (19). It should be noted that transformational leadership is preferred by followers, but is not necessarily the most efficient style.

Lewin's Leadership Styles

In 1939, Kurt Lewin (23) identified three styles of leadership that were commonly used in the decision-making process of managers: autocratic, democratic, and laissez-faire. In the autocratic style, the leader makes decisions on his or her own and typically does not consult with others. Autocratic style often results in the highest level of discontentment among subordinates and followers. An autocratic style typically only works well in an "emergency" situation.

In the democratic style, the leader involves his or her peers and subordinates in the decision-making process. One often-misunderstood aspect of democratic leadership is that consensus or the will of the followers should override the leaders. However, true democratic leadership may still make the unpopular decision; in this style, the leader always reserves the authority to make the ultimate decision. The democratic style is often highly valued by followers. However, a democratic style can be challenging when there are wide ranges of opinions.

The third style is laissez-faire, which virtually eliminates any leadership involvement in decision-making. In other words, followers usually make their own decisions. This is problematic because the "leader" is still ultimately responsible for the group's decisions. This style can work when followers take ownership of the process and are competent and willing to make decisions. However, this style was found to be the least rewarding and often showed low morale of followers.

Servant Leadership

Servant leadership theory was introduced by Greenleaf in the early 1970s, and it shares many traits with transformational leadership (43). The one major difference is that in the decision-making process of servant leadership, the individual's interest is considered. Although transformational leadership implies that the organization is considered first, servant leadership establishes that organizational performance is secondary to the relationship between the leader and the follower (43). The servant leader is said to be a servant first and leader second. Leading and directing are part of their roles and functions, but that role and function is secondary to the desire or need to promote others.

Leader–Member Exchange Theory

Leader–member exchange (LMX) theory centers on the "interactions" between the leader and the follower (30); and was intended to help establish a more mature leadership relationship (12). LMX theory is based on vertical dyad research, which establishes *in-groups* and *out-groups* (30). In-groups are those leader–follower relationships that allow for subordinate's roles to be expanded and negotiated; out-groups are those leader–follower relationships based purely on formal contract

TABLE 14.1 DIFFERENCES BETWEEN LEADERSHIP AND MANAGEMENT

Leadership's Tendencies	Management's Tendencies
• Change oriented	• Predictable
• Vision caster	• Vision implementer
• Innovates	• Maintains status quo
• Motivated to take risk	• Motivated to analyze risk
• Influence/authority transcends the organization	• Influence/authority confined to within the organization
• Solves unexpected and novel problems with creativity	• Solves known and technical problems with established policy and procedure
• Proactive	• Reactive
• Focus on long term	• Focus on short- term
• Identifies opportunities	• Identifies obstacles
• Idea and person centered	• System and plan centered
• Shares information freely	• Shares "need to know" information
• Uses interpersonal skills to handle conflict	• Uses precedent, policy, procedure to handle conflict
• Places emphasis on team accomplishments	• Places emphasis on individual performance
• Works to prevent conflict or problems	• Works to solve existing conflict or problems

HOW TO Identify Emotional Intelligence

Emotional intelligence is a trait that works closely with social, practical, and personal intelligence and allows leaders to accurately perceive others feelings and emotions. To recognize someone with high levels of emotional intelligence, you should note the following four factors:

Internal factors

1. *Self-awareness:* someone who is aware of his or her own emotions and feelings
2. *Self-management:* someone who can regulate his or her own emotions and feelings

External factors

1. *Social awareness:* someone who displays empathy, or is aware of others emotions and feelings
2. *Relationship management:* someone who can successfully regulate emotional aspects of work-related relationships

and predefined roles (30). Followers falling into the in-group category tend to achieve more and receive more of the leader's time and attention (30). Out-group members do what they are told and stick to formal procedures. Typically, out-group members are treated fairly by leaders, but do not get "special attention." Current LMX research is based on how the leader can make relationships with every subordinate so that each one feels he or she is part of the in-group (30).

Emotional Intelligence

Although more of a concept than a theory, emotional intelligence (EI) is recognized as a set of skills (*i.e.*, street smarts) that include awareness of self and others and the ability to handle emotions and relationships (4, 12, 34). EI is the capacity to reason about emotions and use emotions to enhance thinking (26). EI includes the ability to accurately perceive emotions, to access and generate emotions so as to assist thought, to understand emotions and emotional knowledge, and to effectively regulate emotions (26, 34).

Theoretically, EI involves the relationship between cognition and emotion and works closely with other intelligences such as social, practical, and personal (26). Practicing EI involves four critical skills. Those skills are as follows: (a) being able to recognize and perceive emotions of others, (b) using emotions to assist (not hinder) thoughts and thinking, (c) ability to analyze and understand emotions, and (d) managing personal emotions based on personal goals, self-knowledge, and social awareness (26).

Goleman (11) has written extensively on the topic of EI and has popularized its concept. Successful leaders have a high emotional quotient (EQ), which appears to be directly related to EI. In fact, leaders with very high expertise and technical knowledge (*i.e.*, high IQ) fail in certain leadership initiatives because of low EQ (10). The How to Identify EI box shows key elements that must be present to identify a leader with EI.

Contextual Intelligence

Contextual intelligence (CI) is also a concept that has great implications for leadership and management. CI has been described by researchers in psychology, education, and athletic training, as well as by intelligence theorists as the ability to adapt or respond appropriately to any number of different contexts, where the context is determined by environmental factors and stakeholder values (13, 21, 36, 39). CI is a cluster of individual leadership skills that are integrated and demonstrated simultaneously (see Table 14.2). Sternberg is recognized as introducing the term *contextual intelligence*

TABLE 14.2	LEADERSHIP SKILLS ASSOCIATED WITH CI
Future minded	Has a forward-looking mentality and sense of direction and concern for where the organization should be in the future
Influencer	Uses interpersonal skills to ethically and noncoercively affect the actions and decisions of others
Ensures an awareness of mission	Understands and communicates how the individual performance of others influences subordinate's, peer's, and supervisor's perception of how the mission is being accomplished
Socially responsible	Expresses concern about social trends and wissues (encourages legislation and policy when appropriate) and volunteers in social and community activities
Cultural sensitivity	Promotes diversity in multiple contexts, aligns diverse individuals by creating and facilitating diversity, and provides opportunities for diverse members to interact in nondiscriminatory manner
Multicultural leadership	Can influence and affect the behaviors and attitudes of peers and subordinates in an ethnically diverse context
Diagnoses context	Knows how to appropriately interpret and react to changing and volatile surroundings
Change agent	Has the courage to raise difficult and challenging questions that others may perceive as a threat to the status quo
	Proactive rather than reactive in rising to challenges, leading, participating in, or making change (*i.e.*, assessing, initiating, researching, planning, constructing, and advocating)
Effective and constructive use of influence	Uses interpersonal skills, personal power, and influence to constructively and effectively affect the behavior and decisions of others
	Demonstrates the effective use of different types of power in developing a powerful image
Intentional leadership	Assesses and evaluates own leadership performance and is aware of strengths and weaknesses
	Takes intentional action toward continuous improvement of leadership ability
	Has an action guide and delineated goals for achieving personal best
Critical thinker	Cognitive ability to make connections, integrate, and make practical application of different actions, opinions, and information
Consensus builder	Exhibits interpersonal skill and convinces other people to see the common good or a different point of view for the sake of the organizational mission or values by using listening skills, managing conflict, and creating win-win situations

as a subtheme of practical intelligence (36). CI is typically associated with tacit knowledge (41, 42) and is closely associated with wisdom gained from experience; however, recently strategies for teaching and learning CI have also emerged (13, 22). As opposed to academic intelligence, often measured by IQ, CI has been shown to be the best predictor of success in real-life performance situations (18, 37).

CI requires the integration of knowledge gained from a person's total experiences. In other words, problems are solved or solutions are generated on the basis of knowledge built from all experiences (direct and indirect), and this does not exclude experiences that might seem to be unrelated or irrelevant. For the contextually intelligent leader, solutions are based on the use of knowledge acquired in the past and the present, combined with what is currently anticipated about the future. This phenomenon has been described as thinking in three-dimensions or 3D (22). However, there are four obstacles to CI behavior (22), as presented in Table 14.3.

MANAGEMENT TECHNIQUES

Management techniques are viewed as distinct from leadership styles, skills, or behaviors. The term *technique* was chosen because it implies that something can be implemented by anyone in a position to do so, and does not necessarily require any prerequisite skill for the technique to be used. Therefore, management techniques can be applied even if one does not possess leadership skills or demonstrate leadership behaviors. Obviously, the management techniques can be improved, or applied with greater success, if combined with appropriate leadership skills in the management application or implementation.

Management Grid (Blake and Mouton)

The management grid is intended to measure the relationship between one's concern for people and production. The grid allows a manager to identify which of five major styles he or she belongs to better utilize his or her management skills. In addition, the grid takes into account the leader's concern for people, and the concern for production. For the concern of people, the leader considers the needs of team members and their interests when deciding how best to accomplish goals. For the

TABLE 14.3 OBSTACLES AND SOLUTIONS FOR CI

Obstacle to CI	Description	Recommended Solution
The pace of change	Change often happens so quickly that there is no time to respond without some element of guesswork or reflexive reaction	Intentionally "extract" lessons from any and all experiences and be prepared to apply those lessons in seemingly unrelated situations or events
Complexity	The ever-increasing number of external and internal variables that have an impact on people and organizations	Realize that as complexity increases, the amount of information/data required for accurate decision-making decreases
Learned behavior	Past success often creates incredible obstacles to adapting or responding to changing contexts. People are often strongly biased by their existing knowledge and rarely can interpret what they see without that bias	Adopt a new commitment to learn what informs the behaviors and attitudes of self, others, society, and the organization. Do not rely as heavily on precedent or actions that lead to previous success
Inappropriate orientation to time	Most people when faced with a decision will disproportionately pull and apply information from one of three time orientations (past, present, and future), rarely are all three time orientations consulted proportionately	One solution is to think in three-dimensions (3D). Thinking in 3D requires a proportionate awareness of how the past, present, and future are influencing the current context

concern of production, the leader emphasizes efficiency and productivity when deciding how best to accomplish goals. The five major styles identified by Blake and Mouton are as follows:

1. *Improvised management* : A low concern for people and production. The manager's main motivation is to stay out of trouble and maintain the status quo. Effort is at a minimum, and they are satisfied to simply pass orders from superiors.
2. *Country-club management* : High concern for employees, but low concern for production. The goal of the manager is to satisfy needs of employees and provide a friendly atmosphere.
3. *Authoritarian management* : High concern for production and efficiency, but low concern for employees. Managers often perceive personal needs as irrelevant or perhaps even harmful to goals. Often authority is used to coerce subordinates to meet goals.
4. *Middle-of-the-road management* : Moderate concern for production and employee satisfaction.
5. *Team or democratic management* : High concern for both production and morale. Team or democratic managers often try to develop committed work groups and focus.

Scientific Management (Frederick W. Taylor)

Scientific management is the organization and supervision of jobs and duties based on the manager's direct observation of the job. The manager's job was to create rules and procedures on how to do a given job that replaced "rule of thumb," and these were based strictly on the manager's direct and "scientific" observation of that job. Any deviation from the manager's scientifically prescribed procedures is punished. Scientific management's basic tenet was that monetary payment was the only motivation employees needed. In fact, when Taylor published *The Principles of Scientific Management* in 1911, he suggested that sole responsibility of the organization rests with the manager and that only the manager needed to be concerned with working conditions and outcomes. According to Taylor, a manager's responsibility was to provide detailed and specific instructions on how to do the assigned task and that the organization was more important than the individual (27, 33). Scientific management is no longer a popular model; however, remnants of it can be seen in bureaucratic and transactional behaviors. Eventually, the presuppositions that framed scientific management were rejected, but Taylor's contribution to management practice has served as a foundational framework for much of what is practiced today.

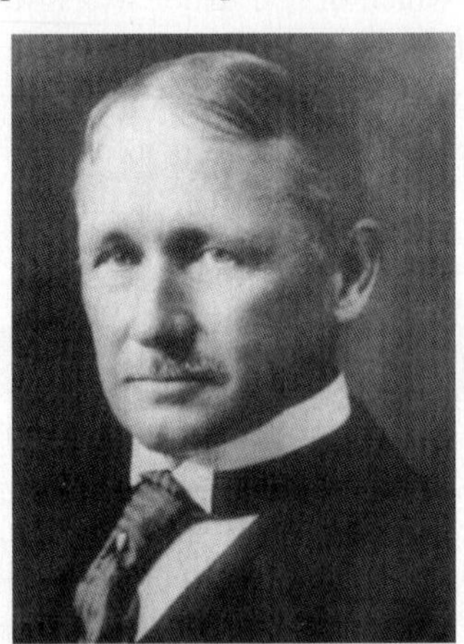

Bureaucratic Model of Management (Max Weber)

Bureaucratic structures are typically formalized and centralized, have a firm hierarchy, and divide labor between specialists (8). Bureaucracy requires standardized rules in the forms of policy and procedure. The benefit of bureaucracy is with an unskilled labor force because it creates a reference point for action and reduces variability. However, critics of bureaucratic management point out that minimized variability is not as effective with today's knowledgeable workers (8). Weber believed bureaucracy to be a set of official functions bounded by rules with a clear division of labor and qualification replaced favoritism as the basis of selection for certain jobs. Bureaucracy, as Weber showed, leveled the playing field for many workers and increased their social equality. Although today elements of bureaucratic management remain, even Weber was able to foresee the risk of bureaucracy and warned of the potential for the organization to dominate policy and individuals.

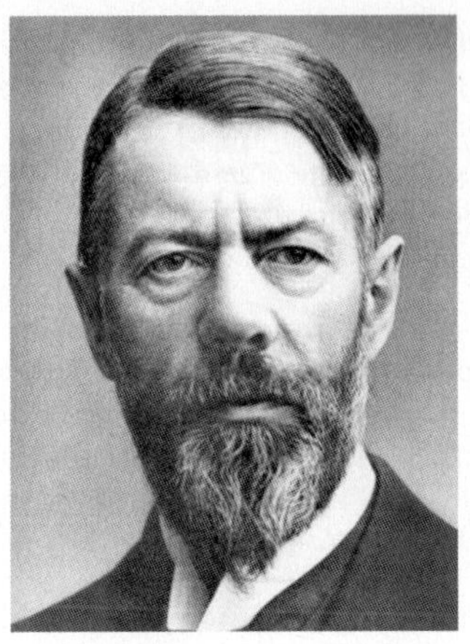

Total Quality Management (W. Edward Deming)

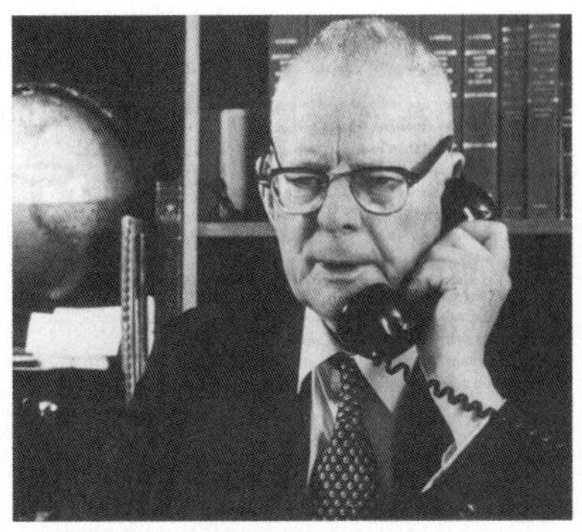

Originally adopted and practiced in Japan, total quality management (TQM) was not favored in the United States until the United States began to fall behind in global competition (44). Deming described TQM as 14 separate aspects of quality management, including such points as "create consistency of purpose for the improvement of product and service," "cease dependence on inspection to achieve quality," and "put everyone in the company to work to accomplish the transformation" (41).

One additional point that is consistently used by HFSs as they work with clients and customers toward reaching their goals is to "remove barriers that rob people of pride and workmanship."

Management by Objective (Peter Drucker)

Management by objective (MBO) was the idea that preestablished objectives should be used in the appraisal of every aspect of an organization and that performance relies on defining and assessing those objectives, and requires collaboration, strategic planning, and goal setting (28). MBO seeks employee buy-in and participative decision making for departmental or organizational objectives. It is not uncommon that MBO managers allow, and even require, employees to develop their own career or job development action plan.

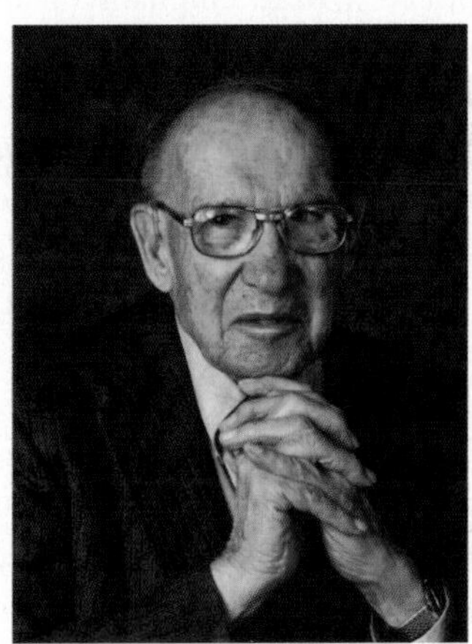

For MBO objectives to work, they must be SMART (specific, measurable, achievement oriented, realistic, and time oriented). Drucker believed that every goal or objective must have each of these five elements of SMART in order to be actionable. Finally, MBO requires appraisal, which is routine clarification and assessment of progress toward previously agreed on goals and objectives. Participating in MBO appraisals is an involved process that includes identifying obstacles that have been hindrances to employees accomplishing their objectives and creating new ones once original objectives have been met.

Motivator-Hygiene Theory (Fredrick Herzberg)

The motivator-hygiene theory was first popularized in business management and states that there are factors that contribute separately to both job satisfaction and dissatisfaction (20). Job satisfaction elements are also known as motivators, which when present add to employee satisfaction. These might include work that is intellectually challenging, recognition of superior performance, and increasingly greater levels of responsibility. Hygiene factors are those that when not present increase worker dissatisfaction. They may include status, job security, salary, and fringe benefits. Hygiene factors do not give satisfaction, but if they are absent, they result in dissatisfaction.

A career as an HFS can serve as a highly satisfying one; there is often a high degree of responsibility and intellectually challenging work. However, there may be hygiene factors, salary and job security, that in spite of the motivators, may lead the HFS to become dissatisfied.

Theory X and Y (Douglas McGregor)

McGregor was a management professor who proposed that human motivation is based on one of two tendencies, which he called X and Y as part of his Theory X and Theory Y of human motivation and management. Theory X is the assumption that most people (followers) are inherently lazy and if given the chance will try to avoid work (20). Belief in Theory

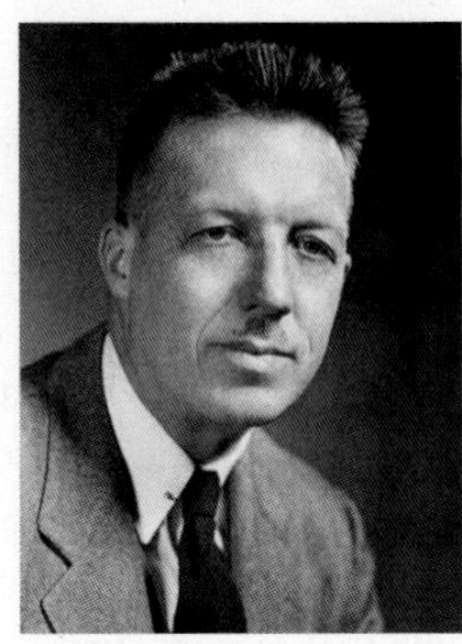

X has a profound effect on how a leader would choose to motivate his or her employees. For example, managers who subscribe to Theory X would need to closely monitor and supervise their employees, likely employing a high degree of micromanagement.

Theory Y is the assumption that employees are self-motivated, desire responsibility, and exercise self-direction (20). Managers who hold to Theory Y tend to believe that if given the chance, employees will be creative and productive. Therefore, managers who subscribe to Theory Y often delegate and share responsibility and can be more transformational leaders.

Behavioral Approach (Mary Parker Follet)

Mary Parker Follett introduced the behavioral model of management and is perhaps the single greatest contributor to how management practice is understood today. Follett was a political scientist and is credited with advancing the democratic style of management. Follett was a "management philosopher" and believed that an organization was a microcosm of society (27, 33). The behavioral model of management placed a large emphasis on the individual's ability to define and shape his or her own roles and lives, and was the precursor to what eventually became known as human resource management (27, 33). Within this model, communication flowed both up and down (vertically), as opposed to the more traditional horizontal communication pathways of the time. Follett was a pioneer who suggested that leadership could be learned, and anyone who did not learn leadership would always remain in a subordinate position. Follet also emphasized how important it was for followers to realize the necessity of the instructions for a job rather than follow instructions blindly or mindlessly. Leaders need to understand the jobs themselves, and need to be able to communicate the short- and long-term aspects of the job from the worker's perspective.

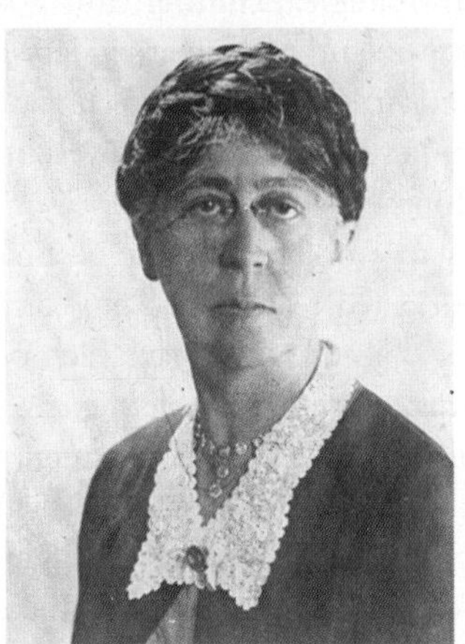

ORGANIZATIONAL BEHAVIOR

Understanding the fundamental management techniques and certain theories of leadership provides a foundation for understanding or effectively navigating organizations. Organizational behavior, similar to human resource management, is the capacity to understand, explain, and improve the attitudes and behaviors of individuals and groups within organizations (7). This brings clarity to why the HFS must be equipped to practice both leadership and management. Many organizational interactions require dealing with human resources, which ultimately require mastery of leadership skills, abilities, and behaviors. Dealing with non–human resources (budgets, facilities, information and knowledge, etc.) requires correct application of different management techniques, with the understanding that there may be overlap or integration of leadership and management.

Colquitt (7) presents an integrated model of organizational behavior that includes five major elements:

1. *Individual outcomes:* These are what happens as a result of the other four elements and include job performance and commitment to the organization. For the HFS, this would represent competency (*i.e.*, proficiency toward HFS Exam Content Outline) and commitment (to his or her customers and employer).
2. *Individual mechanisms:* These consist of five areas that directly impact individual outcomes: (a) job satisfaction — how HFSs feel about their job when not at the job as well as how well they feel in

their day-to-day operations, (b) stress — dealing with the psychological responses to the demands of the job, (c) motivation — the energy HFSs put into their work, (d) trust and ethics — how HFSs believe their employer handles business in terms of honesty and integrity, and (e) learning and decision-making — how HFSs acquire and apply new knowledge and continuing education for their job.

3. *Individual characteristics:* These include HFSs' abilities or skills (*i.e.*, how well they could do their job respective to the expectations and complexity of the job) and personality.
4. *Group mechanisms:* These include how leadership uses power and implements different leadership styles within the HFS's organization.
5. *Organizational mechanisms:* These include the larger concepts of organizational culture and structure.

HFSs should consider all five of these elements when diagnosing how well they fit into an organization, while also realizing that these elements play a critical role in their own individual and organizational success.

Strategic Planning

Strategic planning is another major component of good leadership and management. It is the process of diagnosing the organization's external and internal environments, and includes deciding on a vision and mission, developing overall goals, creating and selecting general strategies to be pursued, and allocating resources to achieve the organization's goals (15). Strategic thinking requires conceptualizing the past, present, and future from the organization's and stakeholder's vantage point. This requires understanding the relevant history of the decision at hand, including the factors that helped or hindered the process up until the present day. Also important is to account for relevant present-day activities that occur locally, professionally, or globally (*i.e.*, perceptions, new research, and changing regulations or reforms). Only after historical information and present day environment have been evaluated can the process of planning for the future begin. Planning for the future must include innovation and a willingness to navigate change.

The overall strategic process is multifaceted process that includes delineating organizational, stakeholder, and individual values; creating vision and mission statements; setting goals and objectives; doing program analysis; and establishing a decision-making process. Therefore, planning is a fundamental aspect of leadership and management, including in the health and fitness context, and should include the following steps:

- *Determining stakeholders:* All enterprises in every industry across the globe have stakeholders. Stakeholders are anyone affected by the actions or plans of an organization, department, or individual. For example, the stakeholders for the HFS in a private health club might include the manager, members, clients, other employees, vendors, sales department, and the neighborhood or community where the club is located. A fundamental component to proper planning is to realize that all decisions and actions are likely to affect most if not all stakeholders.
- *Delineating values:* Values are those practices or attitudes that are predetermined to be celebrated (19). Values are a list of ideals that the organization focuses its time, attention, and resources on; later, it will be these very values that guide the vision and mission statements. Delineating values, therefore, serves a critical role in any organization.
- *Creating a vision:* "Without a vision people perish" (35). A clear and articulate vision is essential for the successful operation of any enterprise and is an ideal image of the future one seeks to create (19, 35). It is the goal or direction an organization, individual, or team strives toward. This concept of vision suggests an orientation toward the future, and a key leadership practice is to visualize an ideal future (5). The HFS can facilitate the advancement of his or her industry and profession by maintaining a clear and articulate vision.

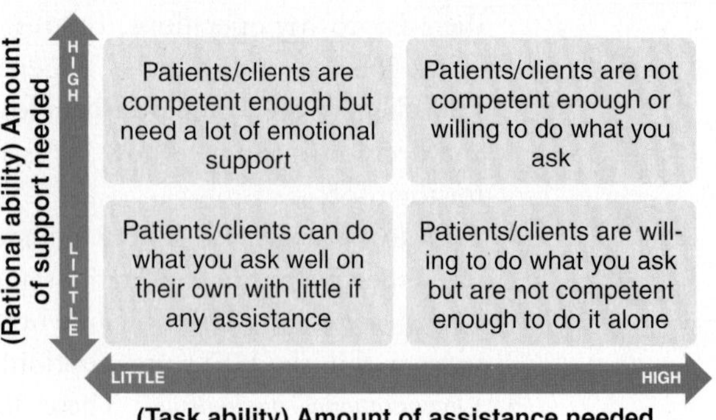

FIGURE 14.2. Situational leadership. (Reproduced with permission from Kutz MR. Toward a conceptual model of contextual intelligence: a transferable leadership construct. *Leadersh Rev.* 2008;8:18–31.)

- *Drafting a mission:* Mission statements expand on the vision by adding "how" the vision will be accomplished. There is a fundamental difference between vision and mission: the vision statement is future oriented and the mission statement is oriented toward current services and conditions — visions challenge, missions anchor (32). The mission statement keeps the HFS focused on who is being serving and how to best serve them. A clearly defined mission can help drive leadership decisions and actions (3, 40).
- *Establishing goals and objectives:* Goals and objectives are critical to tie together all the planning. Objectives are dynamic end points that can stated quantitatively (we want to sell 25% more memberships) or qualitatively (we want to be the best fitness center in the city). The HFS should strive to create SMART goals, each with a realistic objective. Once goals and objectives are identified, actions can be taken toward implementing the strategy. Figure 14.3 is an overall schematic of the strategic planning process.

After strategy is implemented, it is necessary to evaluate the progress. Evaluation is most commonly done with a SWOT analysis (Strengths, Weaknesses, Opportunities, and Threats). Strength and weaknesses are internal factors that identify the good and the bad of what is happening that can be controlled and changed within the organization by leaders and managers. The opportunities and threats are external factors that cannot be controlled. Strengths and opportunities are considered positive, whereas weaknesses and threats are typically negative. All strategic plans must be evaluated regularly, and the HFS should be familiar with the stages of strategic planning and how to perform a SWOT analysis.

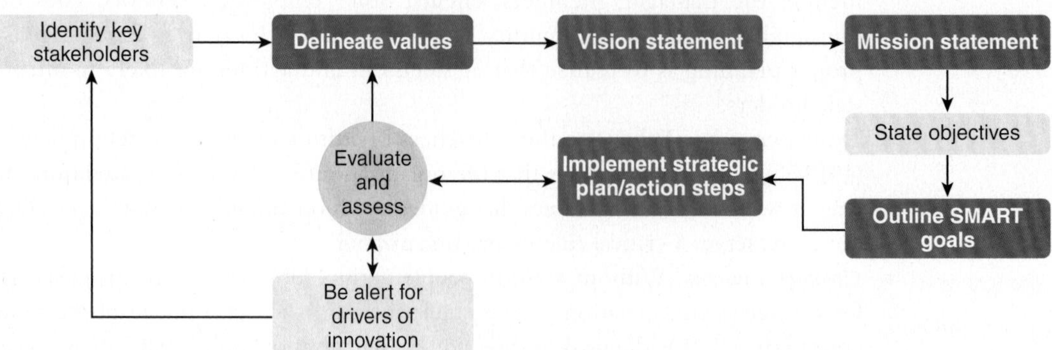

FIGURE 14.3. Strategic planning process. (Reproduced with permission from Kutz MR. Contextual intelligence: Overcoming hindrances to performing well in times of change. *Develop Learn Organ.* 2011;25(3):8–10.)

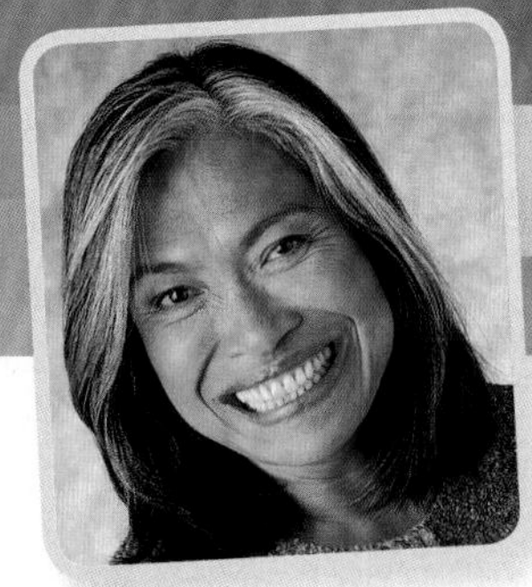

The Case of Jeanie

Submitted by **Carol Jean Dale, ACSM Health Fitness Specialist, North Mississippi Medical Center — Pontotoc Wellness Center, Pontotoc, MS**

Jeanie Dale, an HFS manager and a 25-year veteran of hospital-based wellness operations, has used varying styles of management during the constantly changing outcomes-based expectations for the industry. For Jeanie, management is not just about efficiency but about empowering people to care about their work and the work of others.

Narrative

I work at the Pontotoc Wellness Center, a Medical Fitness Center located in Pontotoc, Mississippi, and at a satellite facility of North Mississippi Medical Center (NMMC), located in Tupelo, Mississippi. NMMC was the 2006 recipient of the Malcolm Baldridge Quality Award, the nation's highest Presidential honor for organizational performance excellence. As a manager, I walk a fine-line to ensure safety and a rigorous standard of care while introducing commercially relevant current trends and meeting the needs of our stakeholders. We want to serve diverse populations while being able to provide the more resource-demanding special populations that are referred by our Exercise Is Medicine (EIM) program.

Initially, we had a medical board of physicians who helped our team set up our EIM program so that we could all be clear about the expectations that the physicians had for us serving their patients. We looked at ease of entry into the program, safety, and reducing physician time. We also considered the educational, nutritional, and exercise components of our services to make it affordable to the clients referred. The referral system has now broadened from physicians to other health care practitioners such as physical therapists, behavioral psychologists, nurse practitioners, and professionals from specialty programs such as our cancer clinics, cardiac, gastric bypass, and pulmonary rehabilitation. The EIM program is a successful venture and continuing to thrive and develop.

I encourage my team to submit ideas for excellence for our department. Although our mission and vision are rooted in the mission of the institution, the organizational plans for wellness services are in continual development. We implemented a dynamic evaluation involving a 90-day action plan process to assess our progress toward achieving our annual goals and outcomes. This organic style of leadership is practiced system-wide and is encouraged by our Director of Wellness Services. The collection of good ideas from everyone helps find the best idea for a particular circumstance and also improves morale of the team at our wellness center.

We also use tools that evaluate our team by having coworkers give feedback to each employee on what we do well and what improvements we need. Because our field is emerging, we need to empower dynamic independent thinkers who can be an important bridge in preventing disease and reducing risk factors. These frontline professionals will directly impact future health care costs and serve to bridge the gap from rehabilitation into improved functional capacity and healthier lifestyles. The transformational leadership style that I try to demonstrate is primarily to encourage individuals to work with autonomy, commitment, and care to improve the quality of life of clients and coworkers. The EIM program provides a framework for us to work as a team to challenge mediocrity and implement evidence-based practices within the context of a medical fitness facility.

Questions

- Provide an example of management and an example of leadership in the implementation of the EIM program.
- How does Jeanie exemplify transformational leadership style?
- Which of the approaches to management and leadership align most closely with the way Jeanie manages the team at Pontotoc Wellness Center?

SUMMARY

Leadership and management are separate constructs that have overlapping outcomes. The two are equally valuable aspects of performance for HFSs, particularly as they seek to advance their career. Leadership is a relationship with people that is based on the ethical use of influence, while management accomplishes goals and objectives by controlling and organizing resources. Leadership research and theory has evolved from a classical approach, which is based on giftedness of the leader, to an organic model, which is a grassroots approach in which everyone can demonstrate leadership. Once HFSs have a grasp on the differences between leadership and management and on the framework for developing their own philosophical underpinnings, they will be well on their way to making a lasting and meaningful difference in their organization and the lives of their customers.

STUDY QUESTIONS

1. Explain why leadership research and theory are important in developing sound leadership practices across different contexts?

2. What are some key applications of a HFS in regard to the different leadership concepts and theories discussed in this chapter?

3. How can CI be used to increase leadership effectiveness in the health and fitness industry?

4. What are the primary differences between leadership and management and how might these differences be seen in the day-to-day operation of a health/fitness facility?

5. Describe which management techniques might be easiest and most difficult to implement in health/fitness facility.

REFERENCES

1. Antonakis J, Cianciolo A, Sternberg R. *The Nature of Leadership.* Thousand Oaks (CA): Sage; 2004.
1. Avery G. *Understanding Leadership.* London (UK): Sage; 2004.
2. Bart C, Hupfer M. Mission statements in Canadian hospitals. *J Health Organ Manag.* 2004;18(2/3):92–110.
3. Bolman LG, Deal TE. *Reframing Organizations.* San Francisco (CA): Jossey-Bass; 2003.
4. Brown MG. Improving your organization's vision. *J Qual Particip.* 1998;21(5):18–21.
5. Burns JM. *Leadership.* New York (NY): Harper and Row; 1978.
6. Colquitt JA, Lepine JA, Wesson MJ. *Organizational Behavior: Improving Performance and Commitment in the Workplace.* New York (NY): McGraw-Hill; 2010.
7. DuBrin AJ. *Leadership: Research Findings, Practice, and Skills.* New York (NY): Houghton Mifflin; 2004.
8. Dye CF, Garman AN. *Exceptional Leadership: 16 Critical Competencies for Healthcare Executives.* Chicago (IL): Health Administration Press; 2006.
9. Fullan M. *Leading in a Culture of Change.* San Francisco (CA): Jossey-Bass; 2001.
10. Goleman D. Leadership that gets results. *Harv Bus Rev.* 2000;78:(2):78–90.
11. Graen GB, Uhl-Bien M. Relationship-based approach to leadership: Development of leader–member exchange (LMX) theory of leadership over 25 years: Applying a multi-level multi-domain perspective. *Leadersh Q.* 1995;6:219–47.
12. Hays KF, Brown CH. *You're on! Consulting for Peak Performance.* Washington (DC): American Psychological Association; 2004.
13. Heifetz R. Anchoring leadership in the work of adaptive progress. In: Hesselbein F, Goldsmith M, editors. *The Leader of the Future 2.* San Francisco (CA): Jossey-Bass; 2006. p. 73–84.
14. Hellriegel D, Jackson SE, Slocum JW. *Management, A Competency-Based Approach.* Cincinnati (OH): South-Western Thomson Learning; 2002.

15. Hersey P, Blanchard KH, Johnson DE. *Management of Organizational Behavior: Leading Human Resources.* Upper Saddle River (NJ): Prentice Hall; 2001.
16. Kent T. Leading and managing: It takes two to tango.*Manag Decis.* 2005;43:(7/8):1010–7.
17. Knight W, Moore M, Coperthwaite C. Institutional research: Knowledge, skills, and perceptions of effectiveness.*Res High Educ.* 1997;38(4):419–33.
18. Kouzes JM, Posner BZ. *The Leadership Challenge.* San Francisco (CA): Jossey-Bass Publishers; 1995.
19. Kutz MR. *Leadership and Management in Athletic Training: An Integrated Approach.* Baltimore (MD): Lippincott Williams & Wilkins; 2010.
20. Kutz MR. Toward a conceptual model of contextual intelligence: A transferable leadership construct. *Leadersh Rev.* 2008;8:18–31.
21. Kutz MR. Contextual intelligence: Overcoming hindrances to performing well in times of change. *Dev Learn Organ.* 2011;25:(3):8–10.
22. Lewin K, Lippitt R, White RK. Patterns of aggressive behavior in experimentally created "social climates." *J Soc Psychol.* 1939;10:271–99.
23. Maccoby M. Understanding the difference between management and leadership. *Res Technol Manag.* 2000; 43:57–9.
24. Maxwell JC. Foreward. In: Kouzes J, Posner B, editors. *Christian Reflections on the Leadership Challenge.* San Francisco (CA): Jossey-Bass; 2004. x p.
25. Mayer J, Salovey P, Caruso D. Emotional intelligence: Theory, findings, and implications. *Psychol Inq.* 2004;15(3):197–215.
26. Miller T, Vaughan B. Messages from the management past: Classic writers and contemporary problems. *SAM Adv Manag J.* 2001;66(1):4–20.
27. Muczyk J, Reimann B. MBO as a complement to effective leadership. *Acad Manag Exec.* 1989;3(2);131–8.
28. Nellis SM. Leadership and management: Techniques and principles for athletic training. *J Athl Train.* 1994;19(4):328–35.
29. Northouse PG. *Leadership: Theory and Practice.* Thousand Oaks (CA): Sage Publications; 2004.
30. O'Neil EH, The Pew Health Professions Commission. *Recreating Health Professional Practice for a New Century.* San Francisco (CA): Pew Health Professions Commission; 1998.
31. Pointer D, Orlikoff J. *The High Performance Board: Principles of Nonprofit Organization Governance.* San Francisco (CA): Jossey-Bass; 2002.
32. Robinson D. Management theorists: Thinkers for the 21st century? *Train J.* 2005:30–1.
33. Salovey P, Mayer JD. Emotional intelligence. *Imagin Cogn Pers.* 1990;9(3):185–211.
34. Senge P. Leadership in living organizations. In: Hesselbein F, Goldsmith M, & Somerville I, editors. *Leading Beyond the Walls.* San Francisco (CA): Jossey-Bass; 1996.
35. Sternberg RJ. *Beyond IQ: A Triarchic Theory of Human Intelligence.* New York (NY): Cambridge University Press; 1985.
36. Sternberg RJ. Intelligence and wisdom. In: Sternberg RJ, editor. *Handbook of Intelligence.* New York (NY): Cambridge University Press; 2000. p. 631–50.
37. Stogdill RM. *Handbook of Leadership.* New York (NY): Free Press; 1974.
38. Teremzini PT. On the nature of institutional research and the knowledge and skills it requires. *Res High Educ.* 1993;34:(1):1–9.
39. Umbdenstock R, Hageman W, Amundson B. The five critical areas for effective governance of not-for-profit hospitals. *Hosp Health Serv Adm.* 1990;35(4):481–92.
40. Wagner RK. Tacit knowledge in everyday intelligent behavior. *J Pers Soc Psychol.* 1987;52:(6):1236–47.
41. Wagner R. Practical intelligence. In: Sternberg RJ, editor. *Handbook of Intelligence.* New York (NY): Cambridge University Press; 2000. p. 380–95.
42. Winston B, Patterson K. An integrated definition of leadership. *Int J Leadersh Stud.* 2005;1(2):6–66.
43. Yoder-Wise P. *Leading and Managing in Nursing.* St. Louis (MO): Mosby; 2003.
44. Yukl GA. *Leadership in Organizations.* Englewood Cliffs (NJ): Prentice-Hall; 2002.

CHAPTER

15 General Health Fitness Management

Diana Ferris • Neal Pire

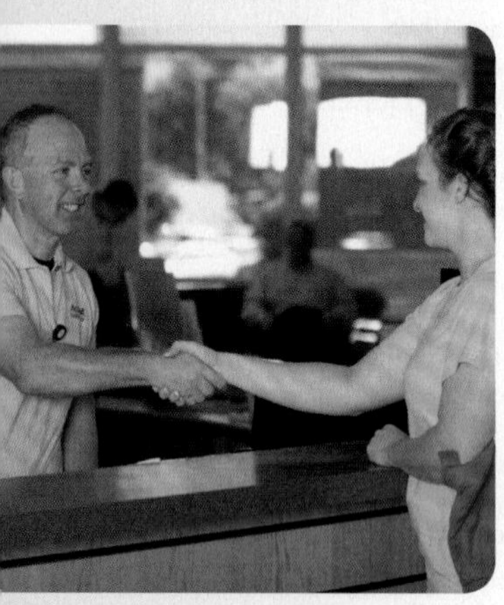

CHAPTER OBJECTIVES

- To know the basics of human resource management, including the procedures necessary to recruit and staff a fitness facility.
- To recognize the relationship between employee training and development and employee performance and retention.
- To identify basic financial statements and their components.
- To recognize revenues, expenses, and different budgets and budget processes.
- To understand the basic elements of the standards and guidelines relating to facility operations and management.

This chapter provides an overview of some general responsibilities involved in managing a fitness-based facility. The role of the manager as a steward of human resources in identifying staffing needs, recruiting, hiring, and empowering employees as valuable assets is covered. Basic financial principles relating to the operation of a fitness center are also presented. In addition, an overview of facility management and operations are presented. Although a manager should have knowledge and experience in the fitness industry, management positions also require expertise in human resources, financial planning and facility operations.

HUMAN RESOURCE MANAGEMENT

One of the most important aspects of any fitness-based business is the team of individuals providing services to the customer. To ensure repeat business, it is critical to build a team of highly qualified individuals who can create strong relationships with customers while providing a friendly and motivating environment.

Staffing and Recruiting

Because every fitness facility is structured differently, the first step to staffing is to determine the service requirements. This will then dictate the types and number of positions needed at different levels throughout the organization. This process should consider the following questions: How many people will it take to complete a job? What staff to member ratio will provide sufficient customer service? What responsibilities will be held by each type of position? How many hours will the facility be in operation each day of the week? What is the membership market? These are just some of the key questions that will help a manger determine the appropriate staffing needs (2).

Types of Positions

Regardless if a facility is corporate, commercial, hospital, or community based, similar positions appear in each type of organization. According to the *2010 Fitness Salary Survey,* conducted by the American Council on Exercise or ACE, the seven most common job titles in the fitness industry are (a) Personal Trainer, (b) Group Fitness Instructor, (c) Fitness Director, (d) Advanced Health and Fitness Specialist, (e) Pilates Instructor, (f) Group Fitness Director, and (g) Club Owner. Table 15.1 provides sample job roles for a few of these positions.

Employee versus Independent Contractor

Many positions in the health fitness industry are filled by hiring employees or independent contractors. According to the Internal Revenue Service Publication 15-A, an individual is an independent contractor if the person for whom the services are performed can only control the result of the work but not the means or methods of accomplishing the result. An employee is an individual who performs services for a client/business that has control over the details of how the services are performed (5). A manager must review the tasks and responsibilities of each job to determine whether it is more appropriate to hire an employee into a position or use an independent contractor, as different situations dictate different practices (see Table 15.2) (11).

TABLE 15.1 COMMON POSITIONS IN THE FITNESS INDUSTRY

Job Position	Job Roles
General manager	Develops core values; creates and implements strategic plan; develops relationship with complimentary business services; oversees annual budget and marketing development and distribution; and manages all on-site directors
Fitness director	Creates and implements member fitness programs; markets fitness services; encourages members to achieve fitness goals through offered programs and services; oversees on-site fitness employees, including personal trainers and group fitness instructors
Group fitness director	Responsible for creation and implementation of group exercise programs; oversees all on-site group fitness instructors
Personal trainer	Markets and sells personal training packages; leads one-on-one or group personal training sessions; performs initial evaluations and reassessments; conducts fitness orientations for all new members; supervises members while circulating fitness floor
Group fitness instructor	Teaches group-based exercises classes and programs for members

TABLE 15.2 FACTORS DEFINING EMPLOYEES AND INDEPENDENT CONTRACTORS

Factors	Employees	Independent Contractors
Behavior control	Subject to the business' instructions about when and where to do work, how to perform the job tasks, what equipment or tools to use, who can assist with the work, where to purchases supplies, what order or sequence to follow, etc.	Typically make their own decisions about how and when to do work, where to purchase supplies/services, maintain their own office or workspace off-site, use personal tools and equipment, etc.
	May be trained to perform services in a particular manner	Use their own methods to complete tasks
Financial control	Most expenses incurred while working for the business are reimbursed	Typically have unreimbursed expenses that occur while work is being completed
	Uses facility and tools owned and maintained by business	Has a significant investment in the facilities/tools used in performing services for someone else
	Work for the business, typically does not market their services/skills to other businesses	Free to seek out business opportunities, advertise, and maintain public business location, and are available to work in the relevant market
	Generally guaranteed a regular wage by hour per week or other period of time	Often paid a flat fee or on a time and materials basis for the job
Type of relationship	Receive employee benefits, such as insurance, pension plan, vacation pay, sick time, etc.	Do not received employee benefits from client
	Indefinite relationship	Relationship lasting for a specific project or period
	Provide services that are a key aspect of regular business activity	Typically provide a one-time service, or service on as-needed basis

Exempt versus Nonexempt

Another consideration for managers when recruiting is whether an employee should be considered exempt or nonexempt. An exempt employee is one who is paid a base salary on a scheduled (weekly, biweekly, monthly, etc.) basis and is typically not eligible for overtime pay. A nonexempt employee is paid on an hourly basis and is usually eligible for overtime pay. The concern of having nonexempt positions may impact financial planning, as overtime pay may pose a significant burden on a facility's budget (8). In addition, it is important not to impose unreasonable working hours on exempt employees, knowing they don't need to be paid overtime, otherwise you may hurt morale and increase employee turnover.

Job Descriptions

Detailed job descriptions are quite important to the staffing and recruiting process for both the interviewer and potential candidates. During the recruiting process, job descriptions define the skills necessary to complete the job and serve as a guide for questions to ask during the interview. Ultimately, this leads to the selection of the best candidate for the position. Once a position has been filled, the job description becomes a guide for employees around which they can base their performance. A detailed job description (see box titled "How to Create a Job Description") should include the job title, main purpose of the job, responsibilities of the job, reporting structure, conditions of employment, and performance measures. Once detailed job descriptions have been written, recruiting efforts can begin (11).

HOW TO Create a Job Description

Creating a job description involved more than just writing down whom you want to hire. There are plenty of variables to consider if you want to attract an outstanding pool of applicants and hire the best possible person for the job. Following is the description of key items to consider when drafting a job description for a General Fitness Manager.

Position Overview

This is the section that will give potential applicants a general sense of the hierarchy within the facility and where they will fit into that scheme. A typical Position Overview could look like this:

> Responsible for supervising the performance of all employees and contractors; Deliver first class fitness experience to all members; Monitor all facility expenses and revenue; Meet monthly, quarterly, and annual goals. This position reports to the Regional Vice President.

Job Responsibilities

Job responsibility is the key to a good job description. It is critical to lay out the specific key aspects of the job so that the applicants know what is expected of them and so that the employer has a solid basis of evaluation. It may not be necessary to list each and every responsibility or potential responsibility, and if not, you should at least state "other responsibilities as they apply" to indicate the list is not comprehensive. The "other responsibilities" should be discussed during any interviews. The Responsibilities should look like this:

> *Supervisory*: Oversee all facility employees including personal trainers, group exercise instructors, front desk staff, spa services staff, and maintenance staff; recruit, hire, and train all staff in facility; conduct performance reviews and create development plans for each employee.
>
> *Facility Operations*: Manage all facility services (group exercise, personal training, day care program); track operating expenses and revenues while monitoring budget guidelines; oversee maintenance and purchase of equipment; coordinate group exercise and personal training programs and schedules; manage employee payroll and benefits; participate and manage daily operations including floor supervision, class instruction, and fitness appointments when appropriate; develop marketing strategies; determine individual and team goals; and review goals on a monthly, quarterly, and annual basis.

Position Credentials

This category can also be called "qualifications," "background," or any number of other words or phrases that makes it clear that this is the background expected of all serious applicants. It is critical to list everything here that you feel necessary to be competitive for this position, as eliminating a candidate based on something not listed can turn into a legal issue regarding inappropriate hiring practices. A typical Credentials section could look like this:

> High School diploma required, Bachelor's degree preferred; 5+ years of relevant work experience; Experience in working in a team environment with the ability to delegate workload and responsibilities; Competence in management skills including quality management, risk management, and achievement of goals; Strong verbal and written communications; Time management and organizational skills; Ability to design, deliver, and evaluate programs and services; Provide exceptional customer service; Knowledge of fitness management

software; Experience in the performance of fitness assessments; Basic computer literacy; Budget tracking and management experience; Current CPR/AED and First Aid certification; Current fitness certification from an accredited organization (*e.g.*, ACSM, ACE, and AFAA)

Employee Status

This section is relatively straightforward and indicates the working hours, including if that is salaried or hourly. The Status section could look like this:

40 hours per week; salaried, exempt

Recruiting

Recruiting refers to the process of finding and attracting new employees. Solid, well-planned recruiting efforts lead to a simplified selection process, allowing a manager to fill positions quickly and with ease.

Recruiting Strategies

The most effective recruiting strategies help fill positions quickly while limiting the cost to the employer. Print and virtual advertising, such as listings posted in the "Help Wanted" sections in local or regional newspapers and advertisements submitted to major Internet job search engines, targets general populations and increases the number of people who see the position, yet decreases the likelihood of reaching qualified candidates. Many companies use professional agencies to save time while recruiting, especially for higher-level management positions, but this method can considerably costlier than others. Internal recruitment, moving or promoting a current employee, can significantly decrease recruitment cost and training time, as the applicant is already familiar with the company and facility. Internal hiring also gives current employees additional work incentive to strive for a higher position. Of course, this method also leaves the company with a new vacancy, although typically at a more entry-level position, which tends to be less costly to recruit and easier to fill. Employee referrals is another low-cost recruiting strategy and gives current employees an opportunity to help the company reach competent applicants, as they often know best the skills required for the position. Colleges and universities have career services centers where current and former students can search local job positions and can be targeted particularly if there is an academic major in health and fitness (8) Many academic institutions offer internship opportunities for students to gain hands-on experience for academic credit. Internship programs allow a company to provide training to a student, and screen a potential future employee. Students who participate in internships tend to have higher grade point averages and are more motivated to find employment after graduation (7).

Attracting the Right Candidates

The key to recruiting is to advertise open positions in areas frequented by the types of individuals needed for that specific job. Positions requiring certifications such as personal trainers or group exercise instructors can be recruited on the career services site at top fitness-related organizations, such as American College of Sports Medicine® (ACSM) and ACE. However, these groups often keep their career services pages limited to individuals already certified, thereby preventing exposure of the job posting to individuals without a baseline qualification. Setting up a booth at the regional conference for a professional organization provides an exposure to local job opportunities for seasoned professionals seeking a change in employment and young professionals ready to enter the field. However, this can come at a great expense.

Selection Process

Once a number of applications have been compiled from recruiting efforts, the selection process can begin. Selection is the process of sorting through the applicants to find qualified individuals who will be taken through the interview process. Depending on the size of a facility, a manager may create a search committee to screen and interview potential candidates. The search committee comprises individuals from key areas within the facility, for example, the Group Exercise Director may have a unique role in the hiring of individuals who may be needed to teach group exercise. Forming a committee also allows for greater collaboration among employees. The first step a manager or committee must take is to create a checklist or matrix of the qualifications and responsibilities needed for the position. Each resume and cover letter should be reviewed within the matrix, looking for past experiences and knowledge that match the crucial items outlined on the matrix. Checking professional references also provides insight into the work habits and skills of the applicant. Applicants whose resumes, cover letters, and references pass the matrix test should be contacted to start the interview process. Sometimes, in larger organizations, the Human Resources department conducts this initial screening and works with the hiring manager to select the most suitable candidates to interview.

Interview Process

A multiple-stage interview process should be applied to each candidate who passes the initial selection process. The first interview may be by telephone. Telephone interviews provide a glimpse of the candidate's interpersonal skills and ability to be prepared. Telephone interviews also allow a search committee to conduct several interviews remotely without incurring additional costs. In situations where a search committee is not warranted, and when the first interview is not by telephone but in person, the immediate supervisor for the position should conduct this interview. The supervisor can gain insight into the candidate's knowledge, skills, experience, and attitude. This interview should be structured with the supervisor using a preplanned checklist of questions to ensure that all necessary information is collected and that all questions asked are legally acceptable. Chapter 13 provides references for employers to check the legality of questions used in the hiring process. A second interview should include team members with whom the applicant will be working. For example, if there is a personal trainer position available, the applicant should be interviewed by the other personal trainers in the facility in an open, team format. The primary focus of the team interview should be on personality and team dynamics to ensure that the applicant is an appropriate fit to the current team in place (11).

Once all candidates have completed the interview process, they should be ranked by both the position's immediate supervisor and the employees in the department in which the open position exists. In the case when there is a search committee, the chair of the committee makes a recommendation to the hiring manager based on the discussion and vote of the committee. In some cases, more than one name can be submitted and the hiring manager makes the final decision. Once the candidates are ranked, an offer should be extended to the applicant with the highest rank first (11).

Compensation

Compensation is not limited to wages. When offering a position to a candidate, it is important to outline the additional benefits that may be included with employment. Organizations vary greatly on what types of supplemental benefits can be offered to augment wages. Some organizations provide professional development funds for employees to support conference attendance or the cost of obtaining additional specialty certifications. Other organizations provide partial or whole health care, dental, eye, or mental health benefits. In addition, child or adult care opportunities, flexible schedules, vacation time, or incentives to earn additional income all provide an attractive package for attractive candidates. For some employees, job security and work-life balance are equally as important as salary (4). Providing opportunities for advancement and professional development aids in recruiting and maintaining a satisfied and qualified workforce.

Employee Orientation, Development, and Training

New employee orientation is important to any facility, as a well-planned orientation will make onboarding easier for the new individual as well as the current staff and members. According to a study published by the Society for Human Resource Management (SHRM) in 2011, more than 80% of organizations have either formal or informal onboarding programs or practices. These programs are used to reduce an employee's uneasiness and anxiety that comes with starting a new position, to prepare the employee to start his or her new position, and to create a strong and positive relationship between the new employee and the organization. If an orientation is effective and successful, it will reduce training time, lower costs related to training, and decrease absenteeism and tardiness (10).

Techniques used to deliver critical orientation information will vary on the basis of position, learning style of the new employee, and teaching style of the immediate supervisor or Human Resources representative. Regardless of the technique used, new employee orientations should include both an overview of company and facility policies as well as teach the new employee job-related skills.

Company orientations, often conducted by a Human Resources or employee personnel department representative, should include the following:

- *The structural and cultural organization of the company, facility, and department:* A discussion should be held regarding the mission statement of the organization, as well as its importance to the new employee and his or her position, and the organizational culture and the expectation it creates. Any employee in a fitness facility must understand the hierarchy and chain of command that exists within the organization, from Chief Executive Officer (CEO) to General Manager, Fitness Director to Personal Trainers, Maintainers, and Desk Staff.
- *Human resource policies and procedures applicable to all employees:* Although information about benefits and compensation is often provided when a position is offered, new employees must be equipped with all company/facility policies and procedures that apply to them and their position. A Human Resources associate or Manager should discuss pay, absenteeism and tardiness, benefits, and the processes the employee needs to follow to access him or her, as well as highlight key areas in the employee handbook, such as job performance and reviews.

Job-specific orientation, typically conducted by an immediate supervisor or department mentor, should the following:

- *Informing the employee of specific job responsibilities and expectations:* A written job description should be given to the new employee, outlining job tasks and responsibilities. At this point, a time frame should be decided on by the new employee and immediate supervisor regarding when the individual will be able to perform the job tasks independently, signifying the completion of the orientation sessions. A probationary period may be used to ensure employee performance in a timely manner.
- *Laying out the workspace to be used by the new employee:* An auqatic exercise class instructor would need an in-depth tour of the pool area and changing rooms, whereas a Health Fitness Specialist (HFS) will need to be shown where equipment is kept, places to find paperwork for members, and a tour of the entire facility before working independently.
- *Including an introduction to immediate coworkers:* Meeting coworkers will allow a new employee to settle in to his or her position quickly and will provide the employee with potential mentors as he or she gains more experience. Group exercise instructors often gain valuable information from other instructors, including member preferences, equipment issues, and class structure — a benefit they will not get from spending time with employees in unrelated positions (7).

Performance Management and Employee Retention

During the onboarding process, new employees should be equipped with the knowledge of what is expected of someone in their position. Expectations must be clearly defined by an organization and the position's immediate supervisor in order for an employee to be successful. For example, if employees on the Membership Sales team do not know that they are expected to sell 50 memberships each month, they will be frustrated when they are disciplined or penalized for selling only 30 memberships. Unknown expectations create a sense of uneasiness amongst employees, and this can lead to poor performance and increased turnover. Instead, make it clear what each employee's specific expectations are, and revise them when needed.

Setting Goals

Expectations should be set with employees on an annual basis, emphasizing the commitment a company has to its employees' development over time. Annual goals give employees insight into where the company plans to be in a year as well as give them guidance as to how they can help the company succeed. It is the responsibility of a manager to meet with each employee, explain the goals of the company, and help the employee determine how his or her position can contribute to the accomplishment of those goals (8).

Goal setting should be a collaboration between the employee and the immediate supervisor. It is important to maintain a distinction between ongoing tasks or responsibilities and goals targeted to improve company standing. Goals should be specific, measurable, achievable, relevant, and time based — five qualities known as the SMART criteria for goal setting (see Table 15.3).

Performance Appraisals

Many companies require formal performance appraisals to be held on an annual basis. Managers, fearing conflict or confrontation, prefer this method to be a more informal process. Instead, regularly scheduled evaluations give the manager an opportunity to gather both positive and negative feedback about employees over the course of the year, and make an informed decision about employee's progress. However, this technique of analyzing and critiquing an employee's performance can often lead to negative experiences for both the employee and the immediate supervisor. For example, a manager observes a front-desk employee ignoring members as he or she enters the facility. If the manager waits months before telling the employee that he or she needs to be acknowledging members while signing in, the employee will continue to perform incorrectly and the manager will become increasingly frustrated. Instead, feedback, both positive and negative, should be delivered to employee on both a regular and as-needed basis (8).

Formal performance appraisals should be held annually, giving the employee and the immediate supervisor a chance to assess the goals set at the beginning of the review year, as well as providing the opportunity for the discussion of future goals. Performance evaluation forms should be completed by the employee first, then by the immediate supervisor. Using this method allows a supervisor to

TABLE 15.3 SMART GOAL-SETTING PRINCIPLE

Specific	A specific goal answers the questions "Who?" "What?" "Where?" "When?" and "Why?" and has a much greater chance of being accomplished since it has definition
Measureable	Goals must be stated with either a quantitative or qualitative assessment. To determine if a goal is measurable, ask "How much? How many? What determines success?"
Attainable/achievable	The goal must be attainable given the employee/employer resources
Relevant	Goals need to relate to an employee and his or her position, and hold some significance or meaning
Time based	A goal needs a time frame in which to be accomplished

understand how the employee thinks he or she has been performing. Performance evaluation forms should include sections for the following:

1. Employee strengths
2. Employee weaknesses
3. Goals from the review period, with explanations of achievement or challenges that were met in the process of achieving success
4. Company-defined skills and competencies

All reviews, whether informal or formal, should be documented by the immediate supervisor, acknowledged by the employee, and kept in the employee's folder (8).

Employee Retention

An effective performance appraisal process can positively affect employee retention. A Gallup Survey completed in 2006 revealed that 32% of employees voluntarily leaving their jobs did so for career advancement/promotional opportunities, whereas another 17% left because of management and general work environment. More frequent performance checks can help maintain strong relations between an immediate supervisor and his or her employees, improving the company's retention rates (9).

Section Summary

The HFS in management positions will typically find themselves involved in staffing or restaffing their facility. It is imperative for the HFS to understand the recruiting, selection, and hiring processes and to collaborate with the appropriate departments (*i.e.*, Human Resources and Talent Acquisition). Good team dynamics and hardworking and dedicated employees are important to running a successful fitness facility.

RISK MANAGEMENT

As the fitness industry continues to grow, the HFS has a great opportunity to work in a variety of settings and make a powerful difference in people's lives. More professional opportunities, however, increase expectations of responsible professional conduct, which means greater potential to liability for failing to act responsibly. Today's HFS must understand these areas of risk exposure and the legal issues and industry standards and guidelines that surround them, and be able to deliver services confidently and proactively.

Risk management is a critical area of concern to any HFS manager and is an initial and ongoing process to identify relevant risks associated with the delivery of a service. This process occurs through the application of various techniques intended to recognize, eliminate, reduce, or transfer risk through the implementation of operational strategies to the program activities designed to benefit both the patients and the program (1).

The role of the HFS manager in creating and maintaining a safe work environment is critical to the success of any fitness facility. It is important to develop a comprehensive and effective risk management plan that minimizes unsafe conditions and practices while maximizing safety by establishing policies and procedures that address safe practices and protect the assets of the company.

Standards and Guidelines for Risk Management and Emergency Procedures

The ACSM has identified eight fundamental standards relating to risk management and emergency procedures (13) (see Table 15.4). Since the HFS may offer services in a variety of locations, including a health and fitness facility, the outdoors, or a client's home, basic precautions should be taken to ensure that every exercise setting is safe.

TABLE 15.4 **ACSM STANDARDS AND GUIDELINES FOR RISK MANAGEMENT AND EMERGENCY PROCEDURES**

1.	Facility operators must have written emergency response policies and procedures, which shall be reviewed regularly and physically rehearsed at least twice annually. These policies shall enable staff to respond to basic first-aid situations and emergency events in an appropriate and timely manner
2.	Facility operators shall ensure that a safety audit is conducted, which routinely inspects all areas of the facility to reduce or eliminate unsafe hazards that may cause injury to employees and health/fitness facility members or health/fitness facility users
3.	Facility operators shall have a written system for sharing information with members and users, employees, and independent contractors regarding the handling of potentially hazardous materials, including the handling of bodily fluids by the facility staff in accordance with the guidelines of the U.S. Occupational Safety and Health Administration (OSHA)
4.	In addition to complying with all applicable federal, state, and local requirements relating to automated external defibrillators (AEDs), all facilities (*i.e.*, staffed or unstaffed) shall have as part of their written emergency response policies and procedures a public access defibrillation (PAD) program in accordance with generally accepted practice, as highlighted in this section
5.	AEDs in a facility shall be located within a 1.5-min walk to anyplace an AED could be potentially needed
6.	A skills review, practice sessions, and a practice drill with the AED shall be conducted a minimum of every 6 mo, covering a variety of potential emergency situations (*e.g.*, water, presence of a pacemaker, medications, and children)
7.	A staffed facility shall assign at least one staff member to be on duty during all facility operating hours who is currently trained and certified in the delivery of cardiopulmonary resuscitation (CPR) and in the administration of an AED
8.	Unstaffed facilities must comply with all applicable federal, state, and local requirements relating to AEDs. Unstaffed facilities shall have as part of their written emergency response policies and procedures a PAD program as a means by which either members and users or an external emergency responder can respond from time of collapse to defibrillation in 4 min or less

Developing an emergency policy includes the organization of a risk management team. A risk management team might consist of a health care professional, a local emergency medical service professional, and key staff members. The emergency response policy should include the procedures for responding to critical incidents such as sudden cardiac arrest or heat illness as well as less life-threatening incidents requiring first aid. Emergency response policies also need to include evacuation procedures in case of fire or natural disaster. The risk management team is charged with the responsibility of training and practicing the emergency response plan so that every employee is prepared in the event of an emergency. Table 15.5 provides additional suggestions for the development and implementation of emergency response plans. The HFSs who are sole proprietors of a fitness business or provide in-home training should also have written emergency policies and procedures.

Risk Management Summary

Risk management is an initial and ongoing process to identify relevant risks associated with the delivery of a service. This occurs through the application of various techniques to identify, eliminate, reduce, or transfer those risks through the implementation of operational strategies to the program activities designed to benefit the clients and program. The HFS is critical in the development of a team of individuals working together to establish and maintain a safe environment for both employees and clients. Although a clearly defined written emergency plan is essential, cultivating meaningful relationships with members and developing a vigilant attitude around safety will create an atmosphere of security and well-being for all. The HFS may also be responsible for facility operations that extend beyond the acute emergency situations.

TABLE 15.5	GUIDELINES FOR RISK MANAGEMENT AND EMERGENCY PROCEDURES
1.	Facilities should use waivers of liability and/or assumption of risk documents with all facility members and users
2.	A facility that delivers or prescribes physical activity programs, primarily or exclusively, to members and users who are considered at an elevated risk for experiencing a health-related event because of their participation in physical activity (*e.g.*, users older than 50 years, individuals with coronary risk factors, diabetes, or clinical obesity) should have a medical director, a medical liaison, or a medical advisory committee provide assistance in reviewing the facility's physical activity screening and programming protocols as well as its emergency response protocols
3.	Facilities should provide the appropriate level of supervision and monitoring for each of the physical activity areas in the facility
4.	All physical activity areas should have a clock, a chart of target heart rates, and a chart depicting ratings of perceived exertion to enable members and users to monitor their level of physical exertion
5.	A facility should extend to each employee and staff the opportunity to receive training and certification in first aid and the use of CPR and an AED
6.	Facilities should have an incident report system that provides written documentation of all incidents that occur within the facility or within the facility's scope of responsibility. Such reports should be completed in a timely fashion and maintained on file, according to the regulatory statute of limitations for the location in which the facility does business

FACILITY MANAGEMENT AND OPERATIONS

Fitness facilities vary greatly in square footage, usage, equipment, layout, and member access. However, there are several key principles of facility management that pertain to every facility regardless of capacity. ACSM's Health/Fitness Facility Standards and Guidelines provide critical information required both to meet industry benchmarks and to comply with NSF International facility accreditation standards. The HFS may be involved in different aspects of facility management. Therefore, a brief description of the role of the HFS from the perspective of operations and equipment usage will be presented.

Operations

In addition to human resource functions relating to scheduling and supervision, facility operations may involve a great variety of tasks relating to supervision of members, access of equipment for members and guests, temperature control, music and sound functions, information technology, and overall facility maintenance. The HFS must always consider the well-being of all members and staff and the overriding principle of creating a safe workplace. Although facility dependent, there are certain operating standards that should be included within all facilities: monitoring entrance/exit and usage of the facility; maintaining proper water temperature and chemical balance for saunas, steam rooms, and/or whirlpools; and employing appropriate supervision for youth programing (13).

The standards are written to ensure that expectations regarding supervision, responsibility and duty are clearly defined. Facilities that are nontraditional in the hours of operation such as 24-hour access sites also have an obligation to provide clear policies and procedures around supervision and access. In addition, creating a safe workplace involves relevant and thoughtfully placed signage that communicates the expectations, responsibility, risks, and actions required to maintain a successful fitness operation. It is also important to consider the policies and procedures around equipment and supplies.

Equipment

Although it is the responsibility of every member and employee to respect equipment, the HFS may be charged with the task of calibrating, inspecting, and maintaining equipment. There are several key questions to ask when considering the care and use of equipment. An equipment checklist is presented below:

1. Is the equipment being used for the purpose it was designed?
2. Is the preventive maintenance schedule adequate given the equipment usage?
3. Is the manufacturer's warranty reasonable given the equipment usage?
4. Is the equipment thoughtfully and safely positioned within the facility?
5. Is the equipment stored properly?
6. Is the equipment being replaced on a reasonable usage cycle?
7. Is the equipment reflective of the mission and character of the facility?
8. Is the equipment user-friendly?

In addition to the responsibility to provide clean and well-functioning equipment to clients, the HFS has a responsibility to provide clear instructions about the use and misuse of equipment. Empowering members with the knowledge of the variety of uses of fitness equipment enables clients to adjust exercise routines and develop additional strategies for adherence and success.

The HFS must understand potential areas of risk exposure and the industry standards and guidelines that surround these facility operations to deliver services confidently and to proactively manage risk. The professionalism that such vigilance requires increases the personal and professional rewards of life as a fitness professional, while also ensuring lasting business success. The most successful HFS will always keep in mind that his or her top priority is to protect the best interests of the participant at all times and in all ways. Protecting the client also means acting with financial integrity.

FISCAL MANAGEMENT

For any fitness facility, accurate financial planning and management are crucial to succeeding in the industry. Fitness managers need a basic understanding of accounting and financial processes to create facility budgets and financial forecasts; the list below defines key accounting terms:

Accounts payable: money the business owes to another individual or business
Accounts receivable: money owed to the business by individuals or businesses
Asset: any property owned by a business that has monetary value
Balance sheet: a financial statement that presents the assets, liability, and equity of a business at a specific point in time
Budget: a plan forecasting expected income and expenses for a given period
Capital: money, goods, land, or equipment that is used to produce other goods and services
Cash flow: movement of money in and out of a business through the collection of revenue and payments of expenses
Depreciation: a decline in the value of any given asset over a period, often because of wear and tear, or age
Equity: the monetary value of a property or an interest in a property in excess of claims or liens against it
Income statement: a financial statement that includes the revenue, expenses, and net income/loss of a business for a specified period
Liability: a debt owed to an individual or business
Net income: gross income less expenses, representing the profit of a business for a specific period
Variance: the difference between an expected and an actual result

Accounting is the process of recording and summarizing business and financial transactions and analyzing, verifying, and reporting the results. These financial records provide information needed to make decisions about the future state of the business.

Basic Accounting Terminology and Principles

A standard method of recording business transactions is necessary to maintain accurate records. The most common methods used in the fitness industry are cash accounting and accrual accounting. In cash accounting, transactions are recorded when money is actually received or paid out. Using this method, membership dues would be recorded on the day the payment was received from the member. In contrast, accrual accounting requires transactions to be recorded when they occur. Therefore, membership dues would be recorded on the day a membership payment is considered due, regardless of if the payment has been received. Accrual accounting tends to be the preferred method in the fitness industry, as it portrays a more accurate depiction of the financial operations of the business (6, 8).

Financial Statements

Financial statements provide a financial summary of a business to owners, accountants, and lending institutions. Balance sheets and profit and loss statements are two of the most important financial statements a manager needs to understand.

Balance Sheet

A balance sheet (Fig. 15.1) indicates the financial status of a business at any given time and is separated into assets, liabilities, and owner's equity. In order for a balance sheet to be accurate, the total assets must always be equal to the total liabilities plus total equity (3).

1. Assets are anything a company owns that has monetary value (*i.e.*, cash, buildings, land, and equipment). Assets are typically divided into two categories: current (short-term) and fixed (long-term).

Balance Sheet for ABC Fitness Center June 30, 20XX		
Assets		
Current assets		
Cash	200,000	
Cash equivalents	90,000	
Inventory	25,000	
Accounts receivable	130,000	
Total current assets	$445,000	
Fixed assets		
Equipment	845,000	
Building	1,500,000	
Land/property	675,000	
Accumulated depreciation		200,000
Total fixed assets	$2,820,000	
Total assets	$3,265,000	
Liabilities		
Current liabilities		
Accounts payable		115,000
Accrued expenses		65,000
Deferred taxes		9,500
Total current liabilities		$189,500
Non–current liabilities		
Notes payable (bank)		1,650,000
Others		120,000
Total non–current liabilities		$1,770,000
Total liabilities		$1,959,500
Owner's equity		
Capital stock		985,000
Retained earnings		215,500
Paid in capital		105,000
Total owner's equity		$1,305,500
Total liabilities and owner's equity		$3,265,000

FIGURE 15.1. Sample balance sheet.

Current assets are those that can and are expected to be turned into cash within the next 12 months. Examples of current assets include the following:

- Cash and cash equivalents
- Inventory
- Accounts receivable
- Prepaid expenses

Fixed assets are those that have been acquired for long-term use by the business. These assets include the following:

- Property (land and buildings)
- Equipment
- Office furniture

2. Liabilities are financial obligations or credits owed by the business. Liabilities are defined as current (short-term) or noncurrent (long-term).
Current liabilities are debts the business is obligated to pay within the next 12 months. Examples include the following:

- Accounts payable
- Income taxes
- Accruals
- Deferred revenue, rent, or taxes

Noncurrent liabilities are debts and expenses that are not due in the next 12 months. Examples include the following:

- Future payments on loans
- Deferred revenue, rent, or taxes

3. Owner's equity is the owner's investment in the business plus any profits or minus any losses. How equity appears on a balance sheet is determined by how the business was established — either as a corporation, limited liability corporation, partnership, or sole proprietorship.

Profit and Loss Statement

A profit and loss statement, also referred to as an income statement (Fig. 15.2), summarizes the financial performance over a specific time (month, quarter, or year). This financial tool includes actual expenses and revenues in the stated time frame as well as a look at how those number compare with a year-to-date plan. Revenues are primarily generated by membership sales, fitness programs, and miscellaneous profit centers, whereas expenses reflect the costs incurred to collect revenue and operate the facility.

Budgeting

Effective financial management relies on a well thought-out budget, created to lay out the allotment of funds spent or brought in by departments and programs. Budgeting, the process of coordinating resources and expenditures required for business function, is essential for any business to survive. Budgets span a minimum of one fiscal year (typically January 1 to December 31 or July 1 to June 30). It is beneficial to a business to be conservative when estimating revenues and liberal when predicting expenses. Underestimating expenses or overestimating sales can put a business in a challenging position, where expenses cannot be paid and profits will not be made.

Types of Budgets

Two of the most common budget processes in the health and fitness industry are zero-based and trend-line. Zero-based budgeting is the process often used when opening a new facility or when

ABC Fitness Center Income Statement for the quarter ending March 31, 20XX

	Actual Year to Date	Forecast YTP	Variance
Revenue			
Membership dues	$397,500	$357,750	$39,750
Enrollment fees	$21,000	$26,250	($5,250)
Personal training	$315,965	$280,860	$35,105
Pilates instruction	$1,527	$2,290	($763)
Pro shop	$2,384	$1,500	$884
Miscellaneous	$11,934	$10,000	$1,934
Total revenue	**$750,310**	**$678,650**	**$71,660**
Expenses			
Payroll and benefits			
Wages	$124,876	$130,000	($5,124)
Commission	$32,000	$30,000	$2,000
Payroll costs	$22,478	$23,400	($922)
Benefits	$18,433	$20,000	($1,567)
Total payroll and benefits expenses	*$197,787*	*$203,400*	*($5,613)*
Fitness			
Locker room supplies	$4,765	$4,500	$265
Equipment maintenance	$5,500	$7,000	($1,500)
Entertainment fees	$1,254	$1,200	$54
Total fitness expenses	*$11,519*	*$12,700*	*($1,181)*
Utilities			
Electricity	$95,988	$100,000	($4,012)
Gas	$17,934	$16,000	$1,934
Water	$16,223	$15,000	$1,223
Total utilities expenses	*$130,145*	*$131,000*	*($855)*
Other			
Advertising	$9,241	$11,500	($2,259)
Office supplies	$1,329	$2,000	($671)
Landscaping	$23,925	$33,320	($9,395)
Total other expenses	*$34,495*	*$46,820*	*($12,325)*
Fixed			
Depreciation	$73,453	$75,680	($2,227)
Insurance	$126,177	$123,725	$2,452
Total fixed expenses	*$199,630*	*$199,405*	$225
Total expenses	*$573,576*	*$593,325*	*($19,749)*
Pretax operating income	**$176,734**	**$85,325**	**$91,409**

FIGURE 15.2. Sample income statement.

making significant changes in operation of an existing facility. This process uses assumptions of business expenses and revenues to develop a budget, rather than relying on previous years' actual numbers. Trend-line budgeting is the most common process used and involves using previous years' financial data to develop the budget for the current and upcoming years. This process makes the assumption that facility expenses and revenues will continue on the trend seen over the past years (8).

Creating a Budget

Once the method of creating the budget has been determined, there are four main steps to follow to develop a complete an accurate budget:

1. *Determine budget expectations:* Any limitations must be determined before starting the development of a budget. Limitations may include restrictions to keep overall expenses close to the previous year's budget or even possibly to cut the expenses to a percentage less than the previous year.
2. *Forecast revenues:* Using previous years' data, a manager can estimate the revenue coming into the facility for the next fiscal year. It is important to include any new sources of revenue that may not have existed in the previous year (*i.e.*, usage fees from a new child care facility opening in the next fiscal year)
3. *Forecast expenses:* Determine operating costs for the upcoming year, making sure to include percentage increases for salaries, increases in maintenance and repairs as equipment ages, etc.
4. *Project profits and losses:* Comparing revenue and expense streams will determine the overall profits or losses for the projected budget. Revisit the first step to ensure that the profits/losses fall within the limitations set for the budget.

It is important to remember that a budget is only a tool; it is a map to follow throughout the fiscal year to ensure the facility can continue to operate and potentially provide a profit. A manager must revisit the budget on a monthly or quarterly basis, reviewing the year-to-date revenue and expenses. On the basis of the direction the finances are headed, adjustments may need to be made for the rest of the fiscal year to stay on track financially (8).

Income Management

All revenue, which is reported on the income statement, must be diligently tracked throughout the year. Areas of revenue include the following:

- *Membership dues:* Membership and entrance fees are generally a facility's main sources of revenue, accounting for 75% to 80% of total revenue (6).
- *Fitness center:* This category would include fees for fitness programs, personal training, specialty group exercise sessions, and locker/towel rentals.
- *Food and beverage:* Often a small profit center, facilities have begun to include a snack/smoothie bar as an incentive to members.
- *Other services:* Depending on the type and size of the facility, a spa department offering services such as massage, youth center, on-site child care, or a pro shop selling clothing or fitness equipment can provide another source of revenue.

Controlling and tracking accounts receivable is critical to the survival of a fitness facility. Decisions must be made on how to collect and manage revenue streams (11). Managing accounts receivables can be a time-intensive task, and most fitness organizations use software programs or third party systems to facilitate the collection of revenue.

The collection of revenue will be fairly straightforward in most instances; however, all businesses must have procedures in place for delinquent accounts. Aged trial balance reports, listing all outstanding balances by category (1–30 d, 31–60 d, 61–90 d, and 90+ d), should be run on a scheduled basis to facilitate the collection of funds (8).

Expense Management

Expenses are nearly as important to a company's financial stability as revenue. If spending is out of control, revenue streams may not be enough to keep a business functioning while still producing a profit. Expenses can be broken down into variable or fixed categories. Variable costs are those that fluctuate on the basis of usage of resources or participation in a program. Possible variable expenses include payroll, benefits, employee education and training, supplies, marketing, equipment maintenance and repairs, and inventory. Fixed expenses are those that are relatively consistent year after year and include insurance, rent, property tax, management fees, and principal and interest owed on any debts or loans (12).

It should be the goal of any manager to eliminate excess spending in any areas within his or her control. Fixed expenses often cannot be negotiated, but most variable expenses can be effectively reduced by following a few guidelines:

1. Obtain at least three quotes from different vendors to find the right price for the best product. Be sure to repeat this process on a regular basis for any items that may be purchased repeatedly to ensure the cost reflects industry norms. Negotiate with vendors to get the best deal on goods and services.
2. Eliminate unnecessary expenses. Examine every cost center and determine its expendability. Fill empty spaces or cost center with profit centers (*i.e.*, make an office or storage closet into a massage room)
3. Contract out services (*i.e.*, landscaping) to limit staff usage, equipment and training expenses, and liability concerns.
4. Use internal resources when possible. A business may prefer to hire a few part-time employees to create and publish all marketing efforts instead of signing a contract with a marketing firm.

Regardless of the methods used, managers must constantly review the budget to keep expenses in control and within the parameters set at the beginning of the fiscal year (8).

Section Summary

Using budgeting and financial planning skills, an HFS can successfully manage a facility's profits and losses. Exposure to different types of facilities will allow managers to develop a variety of financial skills, enhance their ability to accurately forecast a facility's budget, and provide their investors with an annual profit.

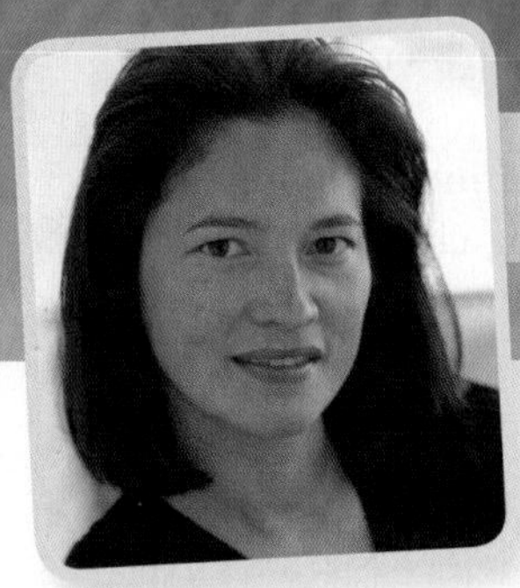

A Day in the Life of an HFS Manager

Submitted by **Nancy Hudson, ACSM-HFS, Baystate Health Employee Fitness Center, Springfield, MA, and Teresa Fitts, DPE, ACSM-HFS, FACSM, Westfield State University, Westfield, MA**

This case focuses on the myriad roles of HFSs who manage facilities. An interview with a Health Fitness Manager is presented.

Background

Based in Springfield, Massachusetts, Baystate Health is a multi-institutional, integrated health care delivery organization serving a population of nearly one million in western New England. With more than 10,000 employees, Baystate Health is the largest private employer in western Massachusetts. Baystate Health's charitable mission is to improve the health of the people in our communities every day, with quality and compassion. The Baystate Health Employee Fitness Center serves the employee population and acts in collaboration with the Department of Health, Wellness & Worklife Solutions. Nancy Hudson, HFS, was interviewed to learn more about her role as a manager.

Interviewer: Tell me a little about your role as a manager?

Nancy: In my position as the supervisor of the Baystate Health Employee Fitness Center, I play a key role to support program design and delivery of wellness and fitness programs for our health system's employees to help build a culture of health and fulfill the organization's charitable mission. The primary role of my position is to effectively and efficiently manage the employee fitness center operation. As the supervisor of a hospital-based facility, I am required to wear many hats and possess a wide range of management skills, including human resource management, financial management, and facility management.

Interviewer: Can you tell me more about what you do in terms of human resources?

Nancy: My role as a human resource manager includes hiring new staff, training, mentoring, staff development and engagement, performance management, policy development, and compensation management. I also develop the schedule of staffing coverage for the fitness center and for group exercise classes.

Interviewer: While no two days are alike, what might you do on a typical day?

Nancy: You are right, there is no such thing as a typical day! One thing I love about my job is that no 2 days are the same. However, let me give you a snapshot of my day last week:

5:15 AM – Open the fitness center. Turn on equipment and check to make sure that the area is clean and orderly.

5:30 – Greet members.

5:40 – Read and respond to e-mails from the previous day.

6:15 – Review the schedule of staff coverage for the week and make adjustments if necessary; e-mail or speak to staff regarding changes in the schedule.

6:30 – Update the fitness center's Web site with current program information.

6:45 – Sign off on payroll.

7:00 – Do a walk-through of the fitness center, ensuring the facility and locker rooms are clean and well stocked with supplies and towels.

7:45 – Prepare for a business meeting with the Manager of Compensation to review the job descriptions for the staff position we will be hiring.

8:00 – Call my recruiter to determine necessary paperwork to fill a staffing shortage. Fill out a temporary staffing position request and submit for approval.

8:30 – Meet with the Manager of Compensation.

9:00 – Call the equipment repair vendor to provide a cost estimate on the replacement of two treadmill belts; review operating budget and expenses to determine timing of repair.

9:05 – Begin developing a group exercise class schedule for the 4th Quarter of the fiscal year; gather staff interest and feedback on my initial thoughts and ideas; e-mail Independent Contractors to discuss their availability for teaching specialty classes and create a basic framework for the group exercise schedule.

9:30 – Travel to management meeting to develop enterprise-wide strategic fitness and wellness initiatives.

11:30 – Provide a tour of the facility and enroll a new member; schedule a fitness assessment and exercise orientation with staff member

12:00 PM – Spend time on the fitness floor talking to members and encouraging them to sign up to participate in an enterprise-wide, team-based physical activity challenge

12:45 – Lead staff in a discussion to develop retention and recruitment strategies; delegate responsibilities

1:45 – Check and respond to e-mails/voicemail

2:00 – Leave for the day.

continues

***A Day in the Life* cont.**

Interviewer: Sounds like a busy day! If you had to name the favorite part of your day, what would it be?

Nancy: I really like the challenge of using our resources to meet the member's needs. The Exercise is Medicine (EIM) initiative is really exciting. We are continually looking for new ways to collaborate and grow. EIM has opened up many opportunities for us.

Interviewer: How would you describe your greatest challenge?

Nancy: My background is in fitness. I needed to learn and get experience in management and financial accounting. Baystate is a great organization, so I was able to get the training and support I've needed to succeed.

Questions

- How does Nancy's role as manager change throughout the day?
- How did Nancy distinguish between different types of staff?

SUMMARY

Managing a fitness-based facility requires experience across many specialties. As discussed in this chapter, managers need expertise not only in the fitness industry, but also in human resources and financial planning in order to be able to maintain an attractive and lucrative facility.

Customer service is such an important draw for potential customers in the fitness industry, such that a manager must make it a top priority to hire and develop a team of individuals with strong communication skills and a positive attitude toward their clients. Building the team and their skills is an ongoing managerial responsibility, as training and development must continually be available to keep staff up-to-date with industry standards and to provide customers with the best experience possible.

Finances touch all aspects of managerial decision making. As such, it is critical to plan and implement budgets when developing a team, creating programs, deciding on marketing tactics, and more. Managers need to take an active role in budget creation to ensure that the facility is run according to the expectations set for by the company. Finally, the development and knowledge of skills in areas other than fitness are crucial for any manager's success in this industry, which can be found throughout other chapters in this text.

STUDY QUESTIONS

1. Provide an example of how employee recruitment strategies utilized by a corporate fitness center may differ from a local commercial fitness center.
2. How can the professional development of employees impact budget decisions? What are some strategies to empower employees to gain additional experience without putting a strain on financial resources?
3. Describe the difference between a trend-line budget and a zero-based budget? When is one budget process more appropriate to utilize?

REFERENCES

1. American College of Sports Medicine. *ACSM's Resource Manual for Guidelines for Exercise Testing and Prescription*. 7th ed. Baltimore (MD): Lippincott Williams & Wilkins; 2013.
2. Bates M, editor. *Health Fitness Management*. 2nd ed. Champaign (IL): Human Kinetics; 2008.
3. Bauer TN. *Onboarding New Employees: Maximizing Success* [Internet]. 2010. Available from: http://www.shrm.org/about/foundation/products/Pages/OnboardingEPG.aspx, November 2011.
4. Bokorney J. Security trumps salary for today's engineers. *Eval Eng.* 2009;48(4):14–7.
5. Collins J, Porras J. *Built to Last: Successful Habits of Visionary Companies.* New York (NY): Harper Business, Division of Harper Collins Publishers; 1994.
6. Department of the Treasury, Internal Revenue Service. Publication 15-A: Employer's Supplemental Tax Guide. 2011.
7. Knouse S, Tanner J, Harris E. The relation of college internships, college performance, and subsequent job opportunity. *J Empl Couns.* 1999;36(1):35.
8. Herbert DL, Herbert WG, Herbert TG. *Legal Aspects of Preventive, Rehabilitative and Recreational Exercise Programs.* 4th ed. Canton (OH): PRC Publishing, Inc.; 2002.
9. Paychex, Inc. *Exempt vs. Non-Exempt: Identifying Employee Classification* [Internet]. Rochester (NY): Paychex, Inc.; 2008. Available from: http://www.paychex.com, October 2011.
10. Perkins T. Basic accounting principles for fitness professionals. *IDEA Fitness J.* 2008;5(7):75.
11. Rockhurst University Continuing Education Center, Inc. *How to Avoid Making a Terrible Hiring Mistake — Participant Notebook.* 2007. Available from: www.nationalseminarstraining.com
12. Spurga, RC. *Balance Sheet Basics.* New York (NY): Penguin Group; 2004.
13. Tharrett S, McInnis K, Peterson JA. *ACSM's Health/Fitness Facility Standards and Guidelines*. 4th ed. Champaign (IL): Human Kinetics; 2007.

CHAPTER

16 Marketing

Mark Nutting • Matthew W. Parrott

CHAPTER OBJECTIVES

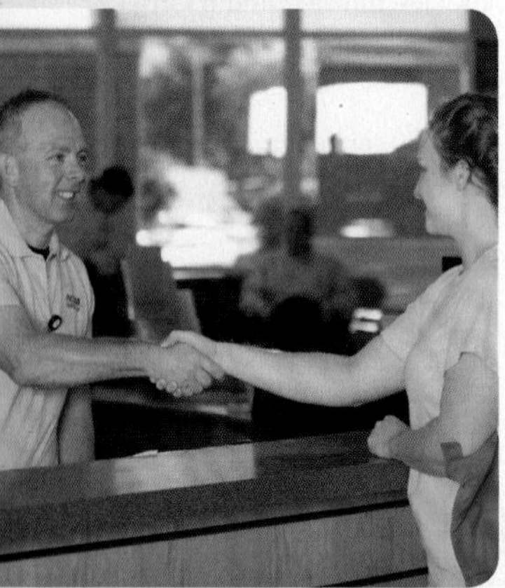

- To identify the different aspects of the marketing mix, including the five P's.
- To recognize the concepts behind the acquisition of new clients and/or participants.
- To apply marketing strategies to business development and growth.

This chapter is designed to provide the Health Fitness Specialist (HFS) with a basic understanding of the marketing mix as it relates to the HFS's specific job profile. An overview of the marketing mix and the application of the strategies that may be used to promote health and fitness services and products will be presented.

MARKETING BASICS

The marketing mix represents a basic building block of marketing for the HFS. At its core, marketing is a function of the aspects that make up product, place, price, and promotion, also known as the four Ps. However, the fitness industry lends itself to one additional "P," representing "people." Knowing and understanding the customers, stakeholders, and target markets enables the HFS to apply a tailored marketing strategy to increase revenues and promote fitness efficiently and effectively. Below is a breakdown of the five Ps:

1. People (not formerly considered part of the marketing mix)
2. Place
3. Product
4. Price
5. Promotion

People

The first function relating to people involves learning more about the individuals and groups who will be served by fitness-related businesses and services. Understanding the demographic, psychographic (attitudes, values, and opinions), and physical activity attributes of potential customers enables the HFS to employ deliberate marketing strategies and build sustainable relationships. For example, once the HFS decides to establish a fitness business, a demographic analysis needs to be performed to better understand the people most likely to frequent the facility. Demographic analyses can provide public information about people residing in any specific geographic area. Researchers have found that individuals who reside within 1 to 5 mile radius of a fitness or recreational facility tend to be more physically active and thus become a target audience (3, 13). Alternatively, a demographic analysis can be performed for an entire trade area or city in an attempt to learn more about a broader client base. Either way, the goal is to evaluate data that can provide information necessary to make good decisions with regard to successful marketing practices. A demographic search can be performed with a variety of online resources, including the U.S. Census Bureau, which is updated every 10 years, providing easily accessed, reliable data, at no cost (http://2010.census.gov/2010census/).

Because of the vast amount of information available, finding a trade area and requesting demographic data can be overwhelming. Therefore, it is important to distinguish which data are relevant to both the industry and the product. In the health and fitness industry, the major factors to examine in a demographic profile are number of people, number of households, household income, and gender breakdown.

The Centers for Disease Control and Prevention (CDC) also provides important information about the exercise and leisure-time habits of individuals. Accessing and synthesizing CDC information enables the HFS to consider both demographic profiles of a particular area and epidemiological data relating to a particular population. For example, almost regardless of the region of the country, approximately 25% of all adults in the United States perform no leisure-time physical activity (CDC 2008) (Fig. 16.1). This segment of the population may be a very difficult target for a new HFS.

However, the remaining 75% of adults are active, and therefore more likely to respond to physical activity marketing. In addition, given that the target population should specifically include those living within 1 to 5 miles of a potential location (20), the HFS can quickly assess the number of potential customers willing to purchase some type of health and fitness services. Having demographic and epidemiological data enables the HFS to make informed decisions about possible services and programs to develop and promote these programs effectively.

Successful program development requires an ability to distinguish between trends and fads. Several organizations provide reliable survey data to help make informed decisions about program development. The annual ACSM Survey of Worldwide Survey of Fitness Trends provides information

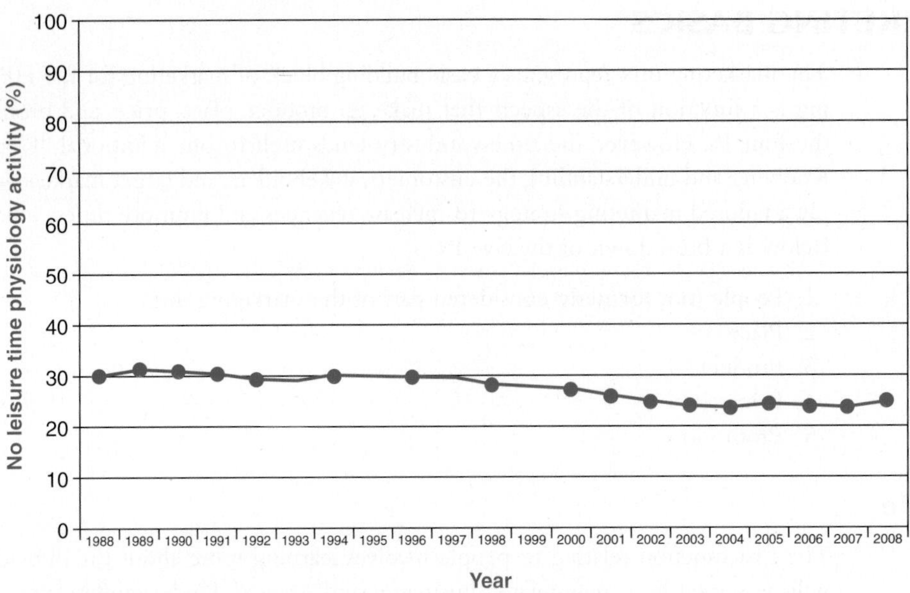

FIGURE 16.1. No leisure-time physical activity 1998 to 2008. (Reproduced from CDC Physical Activity Statistics. Available from: http://www.cdc.gov/nccdphp/dnpa/physical/stats/leisure_time.htm.)

about the top 20 fitness trends within a historical perspective (24). Listed below are the top 10 fitness trends for 2012 (24).

1. Educated, certified, and experienced fitness professionals
2. Strength training
3. Fitness programs for older adults
4. Exercise and weight loss
5. Children and obesity
6. Personal training
7. Core training
8. Group personal training
9. Zumba® and other dance workouts
10. Functional fitness

The International Health and Racquet Club (IHRSA) also provides research reports on industry data and fitness club trends (www.ihrsa.org).

Although these data may seem plentiful, more information is usually needed to determine whether a program can be successful, including issues related to possible competitors and market demand in a particular area. Data about people alone are not enough to develop a comprehensive marketing plan. Therefore, product development and implementation is the next critical component of the marketing mix.

Product

Product can be both tangible (selling a membership) and nontangible (helping someone achieve a fitness goal). Possibly, the most common product of HFSs is personal training services, which can include something to sell (*i.e.*, training sessions) or something to achieve (*i.e.*, increase strength), or both. The HFS might work in a clinical, community, corporate, or private setting, and each of these will determine the type of product available. The product may be an incentive program, educational series, or community-based bootcamp class. Regardless of product type, it is important for HFSs to recognize themselves and their services as an integral part of the product, so they can appropriately market the product in the best possible way. The skills and knowledge required to become a HFS must not be undervalued by the individual who has attained them. As a matter of principle, marketing success begins with believing in the value of the product. Every HFS must first believe in himself or herself.

Practically, one approach might include viewing the product in a different way than originally thought. What is the intention of a client purchasing a fitness-related product and what does the consumer want or expect from the product? The top reasons cited for joining a fitness center are consistently reported as improving health and fitness, and improving appearance (16). The job of the HFS is to market themselves as a professional with the skills and knowledge to help the client achieve these exact results. Although the HFS is continually educating clients about evidence-based practices, it is important not to sell a product purely for the sake of the sale without regard for client interest. Where the product is located can play a pivotal role in the sales and marketing process.

Place

Place refers to where the product can be purchased and/or delivered. For most HFSs, the service will be delivered out of a particular physical location such as a commercial, corporate, private fitness facility, or clinic. However, others may elect to conduct in-home or online personal training services with their clients. In addition, current market practices dictate the need for creating a virtual environment to deliver personal training services over and above the brick and mortar setting. The HFS will need to identify how to properly market his or her services, within a specific environment, whether that be cyberspace, a fitness center, or a client's home.

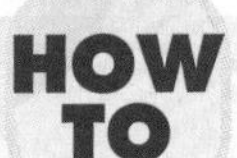

Develop an Incentive Program Incorporating Exercise Is Medicine

As a grassroots effort, Exercise is Medicine (EIM) is a scientifically sound tool that can be used to promote fitness and wellness. As an educational initiative endorsed by many major health, medical, and fitness organizations, EIM initiatives can reach a broad base of consumers across several levels of expertise and engagement. Although the objectives of this program may go beyond a single incentive program, HFSs can focus on one aspect of health, for example, blood pressure, or choose to create a broader connection between fitness and disease prevention. Below are examples of ways to incorporate EIM into programmatic incentives. Creating a team to develop the EIM strategy is the first place to start.

Step 1: Develop Objectives

The vision of EIM to make physical activity and exercise a standard part of a global disease prevention and treatment medical paradigm can be adopted as the vision of any fitness facility.

Objective 1: Increase awareness among members staff, and the local medical community about EIM Initiatives.

Objective 2: Increase member usage of fitness testing programs 25%.

Objective 3: Increase membership of health care professionals 10%.

Step 2: Develop Strategies to Address Objectives

Objective 1: Increase awareness of EIM

Strategy 1: Create an EIM team comprised facility members, human resources representatives, local medical professionals, and local educators.

HOW TO Develop an Incentive Program Incorporating Exercise Is Medicine (continued)

Strategy 2: Provide free blood pressure screening to provide initial information about the connection between exercise and the prevention of hypertension.

Strategy 3: Provide members with a blood pressure form they can bring to their primary care physician.

Objective 2: Increase membership of health care professionals 10%

Strategy 1: Provide trial or discounted memberships to health care professionals.

Strategy 2: Invite health care professionals to "lunch and learn" sessions.

Strategy 3: Develop a strategic partnership with Institute of Lifestyle Medicine (www.instituteoflifestylemedicine.org) to provide educational incentives to health care professionals.

Step 3: Develop an EIM Incentive Program Action Plan

On the basis of the objectives and strategies listed above, develop an action plan to implement the strategies. The resources available for the implementation of an EIM initiative are numerous and are listed at www.exerciseismedicine.org.

Action item: Using the theme of May is EIM month, prepare news releases and other media information relating to exercise and disease prevention to send to local newspapers.

Action item: Develop a reward system for members who access fitness assessment programming.

Action item: Host "lunch and learn" series for local medical professionals to network, and share ideas about exercise as a disease prevention tool.

Action item: Connect with local college or university to enlist kinesiology students as ambassadors of EIM message.

Action item: Use social media to create opportunities to provide information about EIM.

Action item: Organize fitness-related event as culminating EIM month activity.

Step 4: Evaluation

Schedule a meeting of the EIM team as soon as possible after event to discuss ways in which the objectives were met.

Develop simple questionnaire for members about effectiveness of EIM campaign.

Follow up with medical professionals about effectiveness of EIM campaign.

By clearly defining "place," the HFS can better understand his or her market. For instance, if the place is a private fitness center, considerations must be made for the physical environment of the club in terms of how the product is perceived. It is important to consider the impact a place, including physical location or Web site, can have on the perceived value of the product. (7). An easily navigated Web site and/or impeccably clean training studio set forth an image of professionalism, organization, and quality. Consideration should be given to any sensory perception of the place where the product will be delivered. Sensitivity to scents, appropriate music, and comfortable temperatures are just a few of the many factors that relate to a customer's perception of the product as related to the place of delivery. Facility attractiveness and operation has been identified as a key component for customer satisfaction (17). Interconnected with place is the function of price, which involves not only the actual costs of operation but also the perceptions of quality and value.

Price

Determining the appropriate price of the product is multifaceted and critical to the success of any business (3). Basic issues affecting price include cost of developing and/or delivering, profit margin, and market value (real and perceived).

Cost of delivery —The most important factor is the cost of delivering the service. Cost includes marketing, materials (*e.g.*, paper or online), equipment, facility, and the time value of the HFS. Unless subsidized, the price must at least cover the costs of delivery. It is important to be comprehensive in calculating these costs so as not to under- or overprice the product.

Acceptable profit margin —The cost as noted above includes everything except a profit, which is one of the ultimate goals of delivering the product. Therefore, the price above the cost of delivery becomes the actual profit margin. The higher the margin, the more profitable the business. However, set the margin too high, and the product becomes unaffordable to many and overall profit may suffer. An acceptable profit margin varies depending on the type and goals of the business (not for profit vs. for profit) and what the current market will bear. If there are similar products being offered locally, the profit margin should be set with due consideration to competitors pricing. If the price is set too high, many potential customers will be tempted to patronize a lower-priced competitor. If the price is too low, people may be skeptical of the product's quality. Therefore, thoroughly assessing what the local market will bear in terms of overall price becomes critical to the success of the product.

Market value — Another important pricing factor is the balance between perceived value and actual demand for a product. A product with high demand, yet low perceived value ("yes we want it, but we are not willing to pay much for it"), may have to be priced very differently than a product with low demand but great perceived value (a select few want it and are willing to pay handsomely for it). Ideally, develop a product that falls somewhere in the middle such that reasonable demand exists and the product is perceived as valuable. Researchers have found that the consumer behaviors of fitness center members have shifted in the perceptions of the costs associated with fitness club memberships (26), which further emphasize value and perception. In the past, members paid only for programs they would consume. Today, members are more likely than ever to try a new program (25). This may be in part due to the variety of membership options available and the increased popularity of nontraditional programming.

Like many other industries, the pricing of fitness-related services also varies according to region. Facilities located on the West Coast may be able to set pricing at a much higher rate than their Midwest counterparts, which may largely be a function of cost of living differences. Another issue influencing pricing is the demand for access to fitness facilities, and given the West Coast has higher rates of physical activity participation, the demand is also naturally higher. Of course, demand and price are linearly related, which is then reflected in the average income of the HFS (Fig. 16.2).

HFSs who develop marketing plans that incorporate an appreciation of the customer (people) with an understanding of the product and recognition of the perceptions related to price and value are able to apply myriad promotional strategies to achieve and sustain successful business practices.

Promotion

As the fifth "P" in the marketing mix, promotion is an ever-expanding and complex process of educating, presenting, and engaging stakeholders so that consumer loyalty and sustained relationships develop, grow, and are maintained. Following a brief explanation of branding, this section will provide a limited overview of promotional strategies related to the following areas:

1. Advertising
2. Referrals
3. Direct mail/e-mail
4. Internet

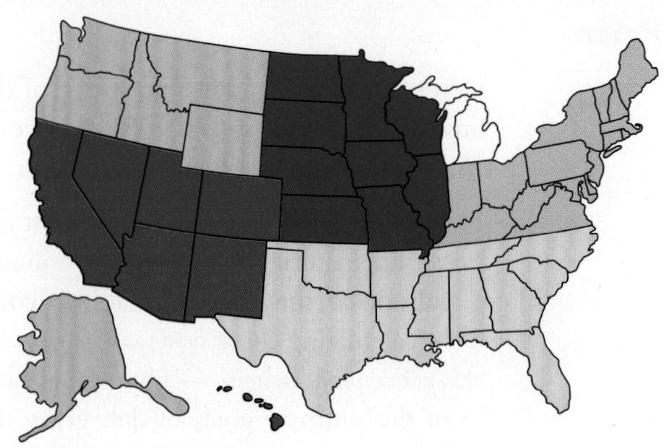

Northwest
PT (FT) - **$41,000 / $35.00**
PT (PT) - **$28,000 / $23.00**
GFI (FT) - **$44,000 / $37.00**
GFI (FT) - **$29,000 / $24.00**

Northcentral
PT (FT) - **$39,000 / $29.00**
PT (PT) - **$26,000 / $25.00**
GFI (FT) - **$36,000 / $22.00**
GFI (FT) - **$25,000 / $23.00**

Northeast
PT (FT) - **$43,000 / $37.00**
PT (PT) - **$21,000 / $30.00**
GFI (FT) - **$47,000 / $37.00**
GFI (FT) - **$21,000 / $26.00**

Southwest
PT (FT) - **$49,000 / $39.00**
PT (PT) - **$25,000 / $33.00**
GFI (FT) - **$41,000 / $33.00**
GFI (FT) - **$21,000 / $28.00**

Southeast
PT (FT) - **$43,000 / $26.00**
PT (PT) - **$26,000 / $31.00**
GFI (FT) - **$36,000 / $28.00**
GFI (FT) - **$25,000 / $24.00**

FIGURE 16.2. Average income of Personal Trainers and General Fitness Trainers by geographic region. (Used with permission from ACE Fitness. Available from: http://www.acefitness.org/salary/default.aspx.)

5. Business to business
6. Sponsorship
7. Personal sales
8. Public relations

Branding

While considering the five Ps, the HFS can also evaluate strategies for reaching the appropriate target market with a suitable message. Deciding how to package the message helps determine the best marketing strategies to implement. Branding is an important consideration for the HFS to convey. What is it not what it is about the product or services that makes them special, unique, or different from other products in the same industry? Why should a potential customer want to purchase fitness services or memberships from you or your facility as opposed to someone else? The HFS working privately has to be able to answer questions about his or her education, experience, and ability in a way that can be successfully branded. If the HFS is employed in a corporate or clinical setting, what is the mission and vision of the organization? What distinctive qualities does the organization have that enables the fitness services to serve a special niche, fulfill a unique need, or carry a particular association? Once these questions are answered, the HFS will have a clearer picture of how to brand the product. As an intangible, brand development is often accomplished by focusing on the health and wellness outcomes associated with fitness. Incorporating vicarious achievement and nostalgia have been found to build brand loyalty (8). In addition, the concept of building a "brand community" has been proposed as an effective mechanism to engage stakeholders both physically and virtually (5). A second consideration in marketing is the image being portrayed. Many fitness professionals create a logo, trade character, or image that relates in some way to health, wellness, and exercise. The logo is another tool to create brand awareness that can be used on business cards and other marketing materials. Increasing brand recognition builds brand loyalty within the target market of potential customers. Creating a professional and unique brand enables the HFS to employ marketing strategies across multiple mediums with a comprehensive design that is easily recognized and identified by stakeholders and potential customers.

Advertising

Advertising can be both a general and a targeted approach to spreading the word about a product. Commonly used advertising mediums in the health and fitness industry include print media such as newspapers, trade magazines, television, radio, and billboard. Social media and directed use of the Internet is fast becoming an effective advertising medium (9). The HFS may consider using one or more of these resources to advertise, although cost needs to be considered. Each advertising medium has unique pros and cons that will vary depending on the goals of the promotion, available resources, and breadth of the marketing plan (23). In addition, word of mouth recommendations have long been considered a highly successful means of promoting products and services, especially in the fitness industry.

Referral

The business of fitness has traditionally been a face-to-face process, although online options are becoming increasingly popular. A rapport built with faithful clientele is deep and long-lasting. Consequently, one of the most effective ways to market services to new clients is to ask for referrals from existing clients. Existing clients are the best sales team because they have experienced the impact of incorporating fitness into their lifestyle and the role a particular HFS can play in bringing about positive change over a period. When clients do refer a new prospect who then becomes a client, it is important to recognize the referring member with some type of reward. A free personal training session or group exercise goes a long way toward future referrals.

Direct Mail/E-mail

Direct mail is an expensive but effective method of reaching a target market because of the ability to select the specific households to pursue. Traditionally, direct mail efforts produce a return rate between 1% and 3%. E-mail marketing has been found to be effective in reaching specific customers with similar interests (21). The key for creating effective e-mail blasts is to compile a list of potential customers. The HFS can build an e-mail list through referrals, existing clients, and if permissible, club e-mail listings. A good e-mail blast can be a powerful message and include images, videos, and coupons that are tailored to a specific type of customer. Typical response rates from e-mail blasts run between 5% and 15%. E-mail marketing has also been found to be an effective strategy for health promotion and behavior change (19). Therefore, carefully crafting the e-mail message is critical to the success of any program or promotion (17). Virtual exchanges provide another opportunity for an HFS to connect with a client or potential client. Facebook, Twitter, and other social network sites provide outstanding mediums to promote the HFS's services.

Internet

Integrated marketing strategies that include e-mail communications and a Web site presence have been found to be more effective than print messages alone (14, 18). Web site development, however, can be complex or simple. Trade magazines relating to health fitness management and Internet businesses offer excellent advice on the choices and process of launching a health fitness Web site (2). A simple Web site would include basic information about the product, place, price, and promotions. More dynamic Web sites can provide a virtual tour and engage a client at a personal level. Interactive Web opportunities can also be developed using social media tools.

Social media can be an excellent marketing tool when used correctly. Facebook, twitter, and other Internet sites have proven useful in referral-based businesses such as fitness because potential clients can make contact quickly and ask questions with relative anonymity. Social media sites can provide an opportunity for exchanges about topics that may be uncomfortable to discuss in face-to-face settings (9, 12).

Business to Business

Like client referrals, business to business (B2B) referrals can be a very inexpensive and powerful way to reach a target audience. Taking the extra time to meet business owners in the area can pay huge dividends in terms of reaching new prospects. The key to developing strategic relationships in the community is to seek out businesses and individuals whose client bases overlap. Some ways to connect with other business professionals may be to attend a chamber of commerce event, host an open house, serve on a city or town committee, or volunteer and/or sponsor a local road race or event. Bartering for services is also an excellent way to build relationships with other professionals. B2B associations provide opportunities for collaboration and growth that can increase profitability with minimal use of resources.

Sponsorship

Sponsorship has been found to be an effective means of promoting fitness-related products and growing B2B connections. Many small business owners seek ways to encourage physical activity for employees (22). Sponsorship enables the HFS to allocate resources toward a specific event and particular target market. Sponsorship also provides an opportunity for the HFS to practice good citizenship by being actively involved in a local community. Sponsorship builds brand recognition with vendors, participants, and spectators; provides a means of distributing print and media communications; and actively engages current fitness club members in the prospect of participating in a cause-related activity. Research has found that corporations primarily use sponsorship as a means of seeking exclusivity and raising public awareness and a positive image (4). Effective sponsorships include an evaluation on the return on investment that enables the sponsor to negotiate tailored packages that best meet the needs of those involved (28). Table 16.1 provides an illustration of the cost/benefit breakdown of common marketing tools.

Personal Sales

When evaluating the performance of fitness center employees, sales revenues are often included in the employee evaluation process (27). Most academic programs do not provide extensive sales training for students majoring in exercise science or kinesiology. However, fitness-related majors tend to be more physically active and appreciate the relationship of physical activity to

TABLE 16.1 COST/BENEFIT BREAKDOWN OF COMMON MARKETING TOOLS

Method	Type	Cost	Impact
Advertising	Internet	Low	Moderate/high
	Television	High	High
	Radio	High	Moderate
	Newspaper/magazine	Moderate	Low
Personal contact	Referrals	Free	High
B2B	Chamber of commerce	Low	High
Sponsorship	Event/cause marketing	Moderate	High

greater quality of life (11). Translating that personal experience to the sale of health and fitness is the key to success for the HFS. Having confidence in the value of the fitness product is important to conveying a genuine attitude. Research cites empathy, ego drive, high energy level, integrity, an ability to learn, positive self-image, and an ability to forge relationships as critical characteristics of successful salespeople (15). To be a maven about a product (1) has also been cited as a significant quality to possess. A maven salesperson is described as someone who has an expertise in a given area or subject, is passionate about the subject, and wants to share that knowledge with others. Confidence in the product coupled with an ability to find and follow leads can lead to a successful career for a HFS.

Finding Leads

In sales, a lead is defined as someone who fits the profile of a target market and has shown an interest in the product or service. The marketing and advertising process is designed almost entirely to help identify leads through e-mail, phone calls, or Web site inquiries. Ideally, leads are individuals who have been exposed to one of the marketing mediums described above and have indicated a desire for more information about the product or service for sale. Each lead is a potential client. For this reason, it is imperative to have a system of managing leads, as each phone call, e-mail, or Web site inquiry that comes in is a potential customer. To be successful, the HFS will develop an organizational plan to include the lead on a spreadsheet and contact the person as soon as possible. The spreadsheet should include all relevant information about the lead, including home address, e-mail address, phone number, and any other personal details the lead provided when he or she responded to the marketing campaign. The more information gathered about the lead, the more personalized response can be provided. The lead spreadsheet should also include the date of each attempted contact and the eventual status of the lead.

Qualifying Prospects

Once a solid lead list is in place, the goal is to turn those leads into prospects. A lead becomes a prospect when he or she has expressed a need for the fitness product or service after an initial contact has been made. Qualifying prospects is a process that involves talking to the prospect and learning as much about the potential client as possible. The key to qualifying the prospect is (a) asking open-ended questions that will allow the HFS to learn the maximum amount possible about the individual ("What do you see as the next action steps?" "What is your timeline for implementing/purchasing this type of service/product?" "What concerns do you have?"), (b) listening to the potential client's responses and remembering relevant information, and (c) helping the prospect realize that what you offer can meet the needs they have expressed. Essentially, the goal is to become familiar with the individual and learn why they are interested in the services and products being promoted.

The Art of the Deal

Many HFSs will be able to positively impact their own compensation by attracting and closing new clients. Learning and adhering to specific sales guidelines should improve closing percentages and overall success.

Closing the deal is an extension of the "qualifying prospects" strategies. At this stage, the HFS will have adequate knowledge of the demographic, psychographic, exercise motivations, and activity goals of the potential client. The key to an effective close is to connect the fitness product or service with a need the prospect mentioned during the qualifying process. For example, a prospect may have identified a need to engage a personal trainer because they have little knowledge in the area of strength training. An appropriate closing strategy would be to reiterate this need verbally to the prospect and then highlight how personal training with you will enhance the prospect's strength training knowledge base. Once the prospect confirms that this benefit serves his or her personal need, the sale is likely to occur. Typically, many needs are uncovered during the prospect qualification process. If possible, try to highlight a second benefit that can be met with the fitness services being promoted and ask the prospect to confirm that the benefit exists. Complimenting a potential customer and engaging in active listening have been found to increase sales of add-on features of fitness equipment (6).

After the prospect has acknowledged at least two needs that can be met with the services being promoted, the groundwork is in place to ask for the sale. At this point, it is important to have some options for the prospect to consider. When asking for the sale, highlight two or three options that fit the prospect needs that were previously identified. The final step is to actually ask the question: "Which of these packages would be the best fit for you?" The framing of this question allows for a positive "either/or" response rather than a "yes or no" response. With proper preparation by really trying to understand where the client is coming from (empathy) and engaging in active listening, the sales process is often more an educational opportunity for both the HFS and the client to learn and understand in greater depth about the challenges and opportunities available for individuals choosing active lifestyles.

Public Relations

Unlike costly advertising, public relations strategies provide an opportunity to promote fitness products and services using minimal financial resources. Although advertising is effective in communicating information about a product or service, public relations gives potential customers an opportunity to consider the product or service at a more emotional level (10). Public relations can be used in several ways from writing a news release to announce a new program or service to writing a weekly column or blog in a local paper or Web site about exercise and physical activity. Both examples provide an opportunity to gain exposure, build brand community, and increase consumer confidence. Although public relations has traditionally been part of a print communication process, online media outlets often utilize expert bloggers to support different content areas. The HFS is qualified and capable of serving as a valuable resource for disseminating evidence-based information about fitness and exercise. Writing is therefore a prerequisite proficiency for preparing quality promotional materials. Seven suggestions for writing simple and effective news releases are provided (19):

1. Identify and address the target audience.
2. Keep it simple and short (never longer than a page).
3. The basics of who, what, when, where, why, and how belong in the first short paragraph.
4. Use short paragraphs and emphasize one major point in each paragraph.
5. Avoid acronyms and technical jargon.
6. With permission, quote authority.
7. Careful and deliberate.

Careful and deliberate use of public relations can support other promotional efforts by providing positive exposure that may create opportunities for future ventures and collaborations.

The Case of the Continuum Performance Center

Submitted by: **Chris Worrell, ACSM-HFS, NSCA-CSCS, and Geoff Sullivan, ACSM-HFS, NSCA-CPT, Continuum Performance Center, East Longmeadow, MA**

A team of certified professionals reinvented themselves to develop a unique brand identity and create a fitness business that defines success by individual client achievement.

Narrative

The Continuum Performance Center (CPC) was created by industry professionals who worked within the confines of an outdated commercial system and witnessed countless active individuals become turned off by the membership structure of "gyms." CPC centers all of its programming around the active individual or those who truly desire to become recreationally involved in activity and movement on a deeper level.

CPC opened its doors with one employee-owner, and has grown to support three full-time and one part-time nationally certified employees who are referred to as "coaches." Within one calendar year, CPC has grown its "subscriber" (title for members) base from 9 unique subscribers to over 160 subscribers who actively train at the facility at least one time every 14 days.

CPC's floor plan is unique in its design. Although constant functional movements are promoted to all subscribers in all training areas at all times, CPC has separate training spaces, totaling 50 square feet. The north end of CPC is dedicated for group programming in a more functional training environment with a large tie into TRX Suspension Training. The south end of CPC offers a more traditional strength environment, but CPC coaches still place a large emphasis on movement.

Branding: Don't Talk About It, Be About It

CPC established itself as the alternative to traditional fitness facilities through its tag line: Don't talk about it. Be about it. By using challenge-oriented Facebook posts, dynamic uploaded video on Vimeo and YouTube, and an information stream from Constant Contact to relay tips, advice, and reminders, CPC has grown 200% within its first year of business. On a daily basis, CPC gets more than 50 hits on Facebook and Twitter and has an 88% open rate on their Constant Contact campaigns. CPC relies solely on social media and e-mail communication with its subscribers to deliver inspiration, motivation, and information. Subscribers have come primarily through word of mouth sales and Facebook "shares."

To keep subscribers involved, CPC rotates programming on a consistent basis to keep interest and motivation high. By having subscribers take ownership of the space and the offerings, it allows CPC to grow at a consistent and positive rate.

Collaboration

Through the CPC 1,500 (a muscular endurance challenge involving 1,500 repetitions of five exercises), TRX Training, and partnerships with other like-minded area small business such as Fit to Ride and Heartsong Yoga Center, members are able to connect to others and take on a physical and mental challenge in a safe, supervised, and challenging environment.

CPC is a neighborhood place for regular people trying to incorporate exercise that is fun, challenging, and variable into their busy lives. Subscribers are from every walk of life, but they have one thing in common – they *want* to be healthy and they've made a commitment to be well. CPC's commitment to the community doesn't stop with its subscribers or other businesses. Giving back to the community is essential to the organizations growth and the core to the mission. Partnering with organizations such as The Western Massachusetts Food

continues

The Case of the Continuum cont.

Bank, Toys for Tots and the American Red Cross, CPC sets a standard of community involvement that resonates with CPC subscribers.

Using social media has enabled CPC to not only reach a broader base of subscribers, but also gain critical feedback about what are the "likes" and "dislikes" of any given demographic. As CPC grows, we hope to continue to be about it and not just talk about it!

Questions

- How does CPC develop the tangible and intangible aspects of their product?
- How has CPC branded itself?
- How does CPC sell its brand?

SUMMARY

This chapter focused on the marketing mix and strategies the HFS can use when initiating and developing a marketing plan for health and fitness related products, services, and programs. An overview of the five Ps of People, Place, Product, Price, and Promotion was provided. Examples of how the HFS could apply strategies to different promotional programs were also presented. Several aspects of the promotions function of marketing were discussed in the context of the experience of the HFS. In addition to personal selling, B2B promotions, sponsorship, and social media promotions, a brief overview of the benefits and uses of public relations as a marketing tool was provided. As a health fitness professional, the HFS is uniquely qualified to act both as an advanced personal trainer and as a manager. As the fields relating to health fitness expand, knowledge and skills relating to management, marketing, and business also expand. The HFS is well positioned to serve in a managerial role, seeking additional training when necessary and building on the competencies and skills inherent in the professional nature of the field.

STUDY QUESTIONS

1. How does advertising differ from public relations? What are the similarities and differences?
2. Explain the five P's of marketing.
3. What role does the mission and vision of an organization have on the development and implementation of fitness services and products?

REFERENCES

1. Adidam P. Mavenness: A non-explored trait of quality salespeople. *Paradigm*. 2009;13(1):6–7.
2. Alsac B. Maximizing your social media investments. *IDEA Fitness J*. 2010(July–August):42–7.
3. Bates M. *Health Fitness Management: A Comprehensive Resource for Managing and Operating Programs and Facilities*. 2nd ed. Champaign (IL): Human Kinetics; 2008. 381 p.
4. Copeland R, Frisby W, McCarville R. Understanding the sport sponsorship process from a corporate perspective. *J Sport Manag*. 1996;10(1):32–48.
5. Devasagayam P, Buff C. A multidimensional conceptualization of brand community: An empirical investigation. *Sport Mark Q*. 2008;17(1):20–9.
6. Dunyon J, Gossling V, Willden S, Seiter JS. Compliments and purchasing behavior in telephone sales interactions. *Psychol Rep*. 2010;106(1):27–30.
7. Ferrand A, Robinson L, Valette-Florence P. The intention-to-repurchase paradox: A case of the health and fitness industry. *J Sport Manag*. 2010;24(1):83–105.
8. Filo K, Funk D, Alexandris K. Exploring the role of brand trust in the relationship between brand associations and brand loyalty in sport and fitness. *Int J Sport Manag Mark*. 2008;3(1/2):39–57.
9. Frimming RE, Polsgrove MJ, Bower GG. Evaluation of a health and fitness social media experience. *Am J Health Educ*. 2011;42(4):2–7.
10. Hoyle LH. *Event Marketing: How to Successfully Promote Events, Festivals, Conventions and Expositions*. New York (NY): John Wiley and Sons; 2002. 4 p.
11. Huddleston S, Mertesdorf J, Araki K. Physical activity behavior and attitudes toward involvement among physical education, health and leisure services pre-professionals. *Coll Stud J*. 2002;36(4):555–73.
12. Gold J, Lim M, Hocking J, Keogh L, Spelman T, Hellard M. Determining the impact of text messaging for sexual health promotion to young people. *Sex Transm Dis*. 2011;38(4):247–52.
13. Kaczynski A, Henderson K. Environmental correlates of physical activity: A review of evidence about parks and recreation. *Leisure Sci*. 2007;29(4):315–54.
14. Marshall A, Owen N, Bauman A. Mediated approaches for influencing physical activity: Update of the evidence on mass media, print, telephone and website delivery of interventions. *J Sci Med Sport*. 2004;7(1 suppl):74–80.
15. Mayer D, Greenberg H. What makes a good salesman? *Harv Bus Rev*. 2006;84(7/8):164–71.
16. Mullen S, Whaley D. Age, gender and fitness club membership: Factors related to initial involvement and sustained participation. *Int J Sport Exerc Psychol*. 2010;8(1):24–35.
17. Papadimitriou D, Karteroliotis K. The service quality expectations in private sport and fitness centers: A reexamination of the factor structure. *Sport Mark Q*. 2000;9(3):157–64.
18. Parrott M, Tennant L, Olejnik S, Poudevigne M. Theory of planned behavior: Implications for an email-based physical activity intervention. *Psychol Sport Exerc*. 2008;9(4):511–26.
19. Perry DJ. Writing for the media. *Tech Commun*. 1992;39(4):638–42.
20. Roux A, Moore L, Evenson KR, et al. Availability of recreational resources and physical activity in adults. *Am J Public Health*. 2007;97(3):493–9.
21. Reed J. Examining the impact of an email campaign to promote physical activity and walking in adult women six-weeks and one-year post-intervention. *ICHPER—SD J Res Health Phys Educ Rec Sport Dance*. 2009;4(1):64–9.
22. Suminski R, Poston W, Hyder M. Small business policies toward employee and community promotion of physical activity. *J Phys Act Health*. 2006;3(4):405–14.
23. Tharrett SJ, Peterson JA. *Fitness Management*. 2nd ed. Monterey (CA): Healthy Learning; 2008. 579 p.
24. Thompson W. Worldwide survey of fitness trends for 2012. *ACSM Health Fitness J*. 2011;15(6):9–18.
25. Wang H, Lin H. An investigation into exercisers at fitness clubs in Dalian. *J Phys Educ Issue*. 2000;14(4):22–4.
26. Wang B, Wu C, Quan W. Changes in consumers behavior at fitness clubs among Chinese urban residents—Dalian as an example. *Asian Soc Sci*. 2008;4(10):106–10.
27. Wen-Yu C, Yuan-Duen L, Tsai-Yuan L. Performance evaluation criteria for personal trainers: An analytical hierarchy process approach. *Soc Behav Pers Int J*. 2010;38(7):895–905.
28. Zinger J, O'Reilly N. An examination of sports sponsorship from a small business perspective. *Int J Sport Mark Sponsorsh*. 2010;11(4):283–301.

CHAPTER

17 Professional Behaviors and Ethics

Teresa Fitts • Randi Lite

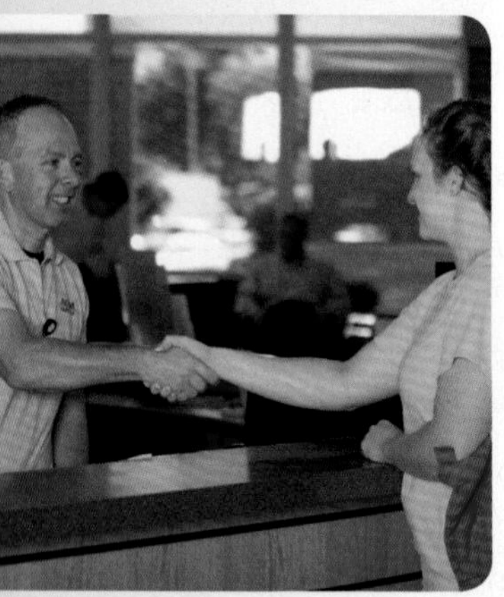

CHAPTER OBJECTIVES

- To briefly trace the historical development and identify the breadth of Certified ACSM Professionals.
- To identify the settings and skills defined in the scope of practice of the Health Fitness Specialist.
- To distinguish boundaries of professional practice among other allied health professions.
- To utilize referral tools for clients outside the scope of practice.
- To demonstrate behaviors that meet professional standards.

Ethics, as a branch of philosophy, can be viewed as an abstract concept focusing on morals and values that inform decisions and behaviors. Ethics is also defined in terms of systematic rules or principles governing right conduct. Each practitioner, upon entering a profession, is invested with the responsibility to adhere to the standards of ethical practice and conduct set by the profession (21). Professional ethics, as it is presented in this chapter, is immensely practical. An initial examination of the historical context with which American College of Sports Medicine® (ACSM) first offered certifications provides an opportunity to consider the development of the profession and the demand for standards of practice. As certified professionals, it is critical to understand the expectations articulated in our code of ethics. To apply the code of ethics to specific challenges facing the Health Fitness Specialist (HFS), the concept of scope of practice is operationalized through several research-based examples. In addition, a useful tool to assist the HFS in ethical decision making relating to scope of practice is provided. Professional ethics encompasses professional practices relating to honesty with others by identifying conflicts of interest as well as disseminating evidence-based information. Professional ethics also includes personal practices relating to responsibility and accountability by staying current and maintaining a certification as well as demonstrating personal behaviors that exemplify the professional nature of the HFS. The need for qualified, competent, and engaged fitness professionals is well documented (24). Professional ethics is the foundation for continuing the tradition of excellence initiated and sustained by the founders and fellows of ACSM.

Therefore, this chapter provides a basic overview of professional ethics as applied to the practice of the HFS. A brief overview of the role ACSM has played in the development of fitness-related certifications is presented, along with a close examination of the ACSM Code of Ethics, with particular focus on the scope of practice for the HFS. Additional areas related to conflict of interest, developing evidence-based practices, maintaining certification, and defining professional behaviors are examined.

HISTORY

Eleven physicians, physiologists, and physical educators founded the American College of Sports Medicine® (ACSM) in 1954 to provide a professional society for individuals sharing a common interest in health and fitness. As part of ACSM's efforts to gain new interest, growth, and visibility, the College hosted an "Invitational Conference on Implementation of ACSM's Exercise Testing and Exercise Prescription Guidelines" in Aspen, Colorado, in December 1974. Here, a small group of ACSM members finalized plans for a proposed certification process for Exercise Program Directors and Exercise Leaders. In May, 1975, ACSM's Guidelines for Graded Exercise Testing and Exercise Prescription were first published. The following month at Pennsylvania State University, ACSM held its first Exercise Program Director's Certification Conference, with 35 professionals earning the first-ever ACSM certification. Later, in September of 1975, 20 individuals were certified by ACSM as Exercise Specialists. The Exercise Test Technician certification began the following year, 1976, with 92 individuals earning certification. ACSM's Health/Fitness Instructor certification started in 1982, followed by the Health/Fitness Director and Exercise Leader certifications in 1986(9). In the 20 years since, ACSM certifications have evolved, and as part of this evolution, some certifications are no longer offered, some are new, and some have been dramatically redefined. All of these changes, however, are a tribute to ACSM's commitment to reflect the current state of the fitness and wellness industry. Figure 17.1 provides a basic timeline as it relates to the development of ACSM certifications, particularly the HFS.

Accreditation

In 2004, ACSM collaborated with six other leading fitness organizations to establish the Committee on the Accreditation for the Exercise Sciences, or CoAES. CoAES is responsible for establishing standards and guidelines for academic programs that prepare students seeking employment in the health, fitness, and exercise industry. In addition, CoAES establishes and implements a process of self-study, review, and recommendation for all exercise science related academic programs seeking accreditation through the Commission on Accreditation of Allied Health Education Programs (CAAHEP). Today, there are three program accreditations through CAAHEP; Bachelor of Science in Exercise Science, Master of Science in Applied Physiology, and Master of Science in Clinical Exercise Physiology. Accreditation, like certification, is a critical component for ensuring a consistent and standardized set of knowledge and skills, which is essential for industry professionals and is conveyed to students through their academic experience.

The need for certified professionals who are competent and proficient in a subject area and who are evaluated through the successful completion of a psychometrically sound, objective examination has grown exponentially. ACSM currently offers five primary certifications and three specialty certifications, with more than 40,000 ACSM certified professionals practicing worldwide. The clinical certifications (Table 17.1) include the Registered Clinical Exercise Physiologist® (RCEP) and the Certified Exercise Specialist® (CES). The fitness certifications (Table 17.1) include the Health Fitness Specialist℠ (HFS), the Certified Personal Trainer℠ (CPT), and the Group Exercise Instructor℠ (GEI). In addition, ACSM offers three specialty certifications that focus on serving individuals with unique needs: ACSM/ACS Certified Cancer Exercise Trainer (CET), ACSM/NCPAD Certified Inclusive Fitness Trainer (CIFT), and ACSM/NSPAPPH Physical Activity in Public Health Specialist (PAPHS).

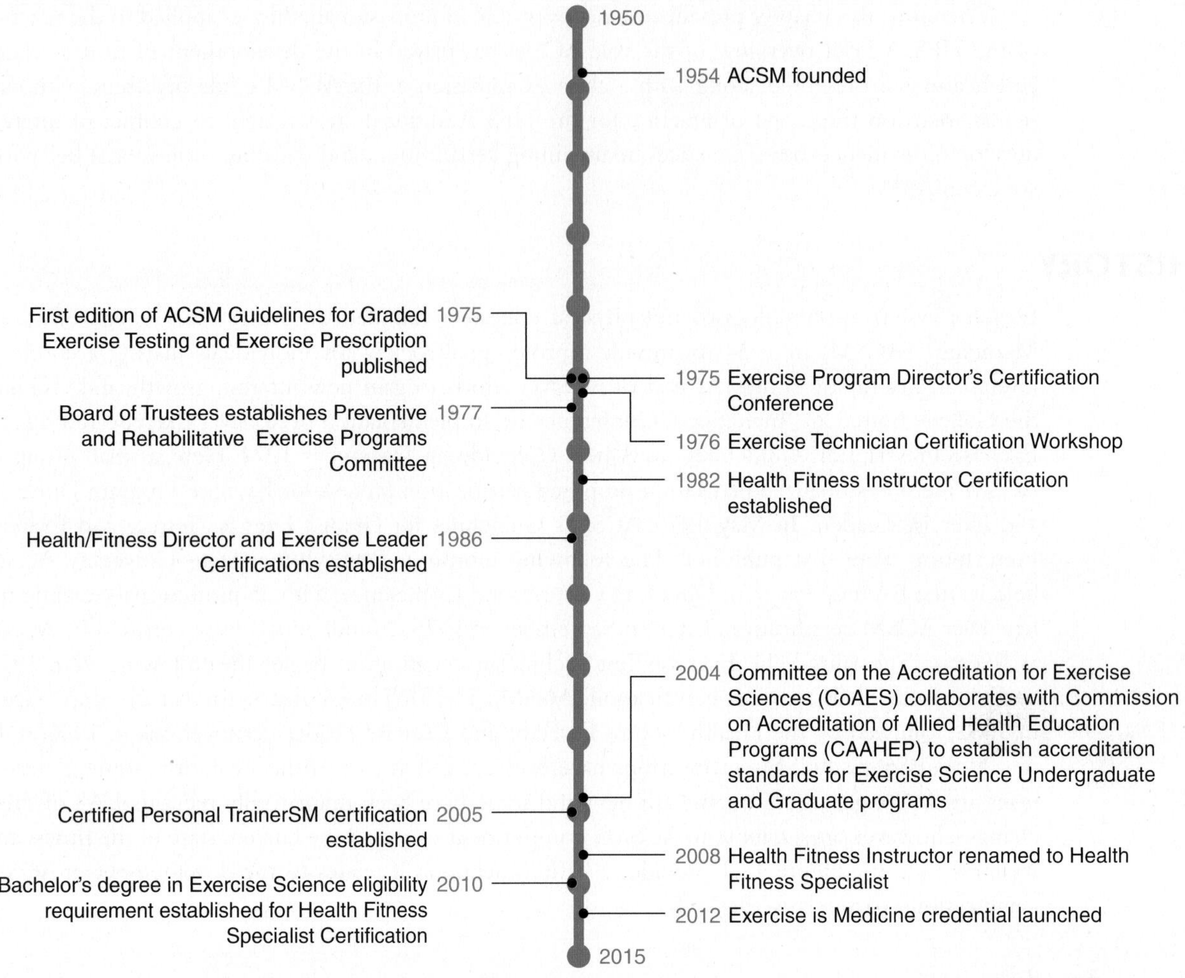

FIGURE 17.1. ACSM historical timeline for certifications and accreditation. (Reproduced with permission from Berryman JW. *Out of Many, One: A History of the American College of Sports Medicine.* Champaign (IL): Human Kinetics; 1995. 283 p.)

What was for many years known as the Health/Fitness Instructor certification was renamed the Health Fitness Specialist, or HFS, in 2008. This change in name better represents the functions of this profession and how it has changed over the years. In addition, the eligibility requirements of the HFS were also changed, in 2010, and now include a Bachelor of Science degree in Kinesiology or Exercise Science. In this way, the ACSM-HFS certification implies specialized training and competencies for degreed individuals to pursue careers in university, corporate, commercial, hospital, and community settings, serving healthy individuals and individuals with controlled conditions released for independent physical activity. The Exercise is Medicine (EIM) credential provides further support for the unique characteristics of the ACSM-HFS.

The EIM credential was developed and launched in 2012 to support the EIM initiative and provide health care providers with an identifiable exercise professional qualified to work with different clients (14). A description of the three-tiered EIM credential is presented in Exercise is Medicine Connection.

Committee on the Certification and Registry Board

The Committee on the Certification and Registry Board (CCRB), a volunteer committee comprised ACSM members, oversees the process of regularly reviewing and revising the job definition, eligibility requirements, and scope of practice for each certification. In addition, each

TABLE 17.1 CURRENT LEVELS OF ACSM CERTIFICATIONS

Registered Clinical Exercise Physiologist (RCEP)	An allied health professional who works in the application of exercise and physical activity for those clinical and pathological situations where it has been shown to provide therapeutic or functional benefit
Clinical Exercise Specialist (CES)	Health care professionals with a Bachelor's degree who typically work in cardiovascular/pulmonary rehabilitation programs, physicians' offices, or medical fitness centers
Health/Fitness Specialist (HFS)	Health and fitness professional qualified to pursue a career in university, corporate, commercial, hospital, and community settings
Certified Personal Trainer (CPT)	Fitness professional who develops and implements an individualized approach to exercise leadership in healthy populations and/or those individuals with medical clearance to exercise
Group Exercise Instructor (GEI)	Fitness professional who works in a group exercise setting with apparently healthy individuals and those with health challenges, who have been cleared by their physicians for independent exercise to enhance quality of life, improve physical fitness, manage health risk, and promote lasting health behavior change

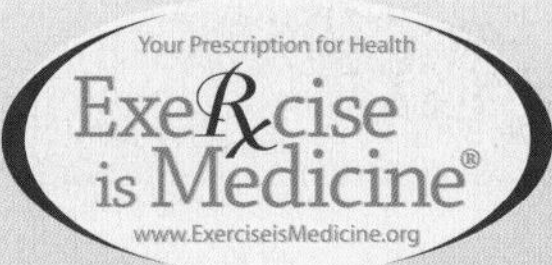

EXERCISE IS MEDICINE CONNECTION

The EIM credential contains three levels based on the health status of the patient referrals. All three levels require exercise professionals to be certified by a National Commission for Certifying Agencies (NCCA) accrediting organization and have obtained a formal education in exercise science (BS or MS degree in Exercise Science).

Level 1: Individuals at low or moderate risk

NCCA accredited fitness professional certification

Successful completion of the EIM credential course and EIM credential examination

Qualifying Certifications

All NCCA accredited fitness professional certifications (EIM course and examination also required)

Level 2: Individuals at low, moderate, or high risk who have been cleared for independent exercise

Exercise science based Bachelor's degree

NCCA accredited fitness professional certification

Successful completion of the EIM credential course and EIM credential examination

Qualifying Certifications

All NCCA accredited fitness professional certifications (EIM course and examination also required)

EIM course and examination exempt for certifications with an emphasis on special populations (ACSM-HFS)

Level 3: Individuals at low, moderate, or high risk, requiring clinical monitoring

Exercise science based Master's degree *or* exercise science based Bachelor's degree plus 4,000 hours of experience in a clinical exercise setting

NCCA accredited clinical exercise certification

Qualifying Certifications

NCCA accredited clinical exercise certifications (ACSM-CES; ACSM-RCEP)

Exempt from EIM credential course and EIM credential examination

Organizations with NCCA Accredited Health Fitness and/or Clinical Exercise Certifications

- Academy of Applied Personal Training Education
- American College of Sports Medicine®
- American Council on Exercise
- The Cooper Institute
- International Fitness Professionals Association
- National Academy of Sports Medicine
- National Council for Certified Personal Trainers
- National Council on Strength and Fitness
- National Exercise and Sports Trainers Association
- National Exercise Trainers Association
- National Federation of Professional Trainers
- National Strength and Conditioning Association
- Training and Wellness Certification Commission

certification undergoes a rigorous external review through the NCCA. The NCCA is a nonprofit, external certifying agency whose mission is to safeguard public safety and well-being through the assessment and evaluation of professional competencies and standards. The NCCA provides accreditation to a broad range of professions, including nursing, respiratory therapy, and counseling. The guiding principle of advancing health through science, education, and medicine that inspired the early community of ACSM members is kept alive today by the ACSM certified professionals who adhere to the ACSM's Code of Ethics through the personal and professional responsibility they practice.

ACSM CODE OF ETHICS

The ACSM Code of Ethics states, "The principal purpose of the College is the generation and dissemination of knowledge concerning all aspects of persons engaged in exercise with full respect for the dignity of people" (2). The Code is further defined by four standards:

Section 1: Members should strive continuously to improve knowledge and skill and should make available to their colleagues and the public the benefits of their professional expertise.

Section 2: Members should maintain high professional and scientific standards and should not voluntarily collaborate professionally with anyone who violates this principle.

Section 3: The College, and its members, should safeguard the public and itself against members who are deficient in ethical conduct.

Section 4: The ideals of the College imply that the responsibilities of each fellow or member extend not only to the individual, but also to the society with the purpose of improving both the health and the well-being of the individual and the community (2).

Although each standard implies many personal and public practices that define the professional nature of an HFS, the following five areas are of great importance:

1. Practicing within one's scope of practice
2. Acknowledging conflicts of interest
3. Providing evidence-based information
4. Maintaining certification
5. Personal characteristics of professional behavior

SCOPE OF PRACTICE

Scope of Practice is the range of responsibility that determines the boundaries within which a profession operates (23). Each phrase in a scope of practice is critical in defining what tasks a professional can do, with whom the professional can work, what settings are appropriate, and what type of oversight is necessary. This textbook is devoted to the knowledge and skills that are needed to practice as an HFS. As such, the text operationalizes the HFS scope of practice. In other words, if a given practitioner in the field adheres to the job tasks and skills described in this text, then he or she is operating within the boundaries of the defined field of the HFS, a requirement for practicing ethically sound behavior. The fundamentals of the scope of practice of the HFS are outlined below in the description developed by the CCRB.

The ACSM Certified HFS is a degreed health and fitness professional qualified to pursue a career in university, corporate, commercial, hospital, and community settings (1). The HFS is skilled in the following:

- Conducting risk classification
- Conducting physical fitness assessments and interpreting results
- Constructing appropriate exercise prescriptions for healthy adults and individuals with controlled conditions released for independent physical activity
- Motivating apparently healthy individuals with medically controlled diseases to adopt and maintain healthy lifestyle behaviors
- Motivating individuals to begin and continue with their healthy behaviors

The HFS Scope of Practice is a living document that is regularly reviewed by ACSM's HFS subcommittee. Each of the ACSM certifications has a subcommittee that operates as part of the CCRB. The components of the Scope of Practice are verified in a systematic manner through a job task analysis (JTA) of practicing HFSs. The JTA is a survey sent to HFS practitioners to gather information about what tasks they are doing in their daily work. On the basis of the survey data, HFS subcommittee members review the Scope of Practice, the knowledge statements (KSs), and the

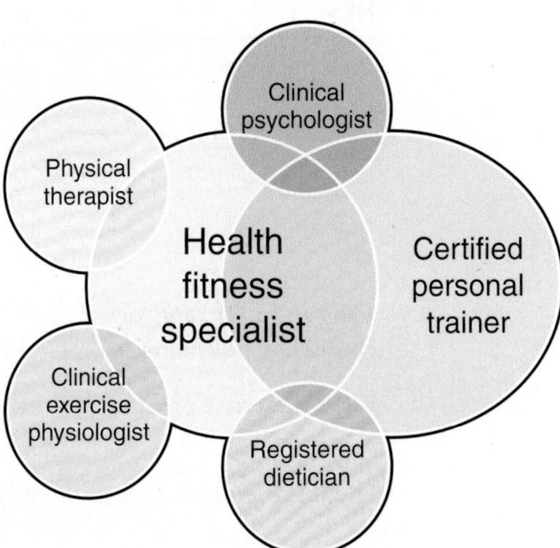

FIGURE 17.2. A visual representation of the overlapping scopes of varying health care, allied health, and health fitness professionals.

content of publications related to HFS work (such as this textbook) to make sure all are in line with the evolution of the profession.

Defining the scope of what an HFS does (*e.g.*, risk classification, fitness assessment, exercise prescription, and lifestyle behavior change), the Scope of Practice also serves as a guide as to what may lie *outside* the boundary of the HFS' scope. Figure 17.2 and Table 17.2 show that although there may be overlap between Scopes of Practice of various professionals working with similar clientele as the HFS, there are distinct areas within which each profession functions. The trick is figuring out where the HFS practice ends and the practice of another professional begins. The purpose of this section is to provide some examples and guidelines so that HFS practitioners can make sound decisions to operate within their defined scope of practice. First, a decision tree will be introduced. Practitioners can use the decision tree to check that the tasks they are performing are firmly within the HFS scope of practice. Then three scenarios will be presented to delineate the boundaries between some of the professions depicted in Figure 17.2 and Table 17.2.

Consider the following scenarios to better understand the complex and delicate issues that arise when faced with Scope of Practice decisions.

Scenario 1

A client asks about recommending a piece of aerobic exercise equipment for his home. The client is a healthy 40-year-old man with hypertension controlled by diet and exercise.

If a practitioner is unsure whether the request in scenario 1 is permitted in his or her scope of practice, then the first place to look might be the most recent HFS JTA. In the 2011 JTA, under Domain II Exercise Prescription and Implementation, Job Task C states "Implement cardiorespiratory exercise prescriptions using the FITT framework (frequency, intensity, time and type) for apparently healthy participants based on current health status, fitness goals, and availability of time" (1).

Figure 17.3 shows a decision tree designed to help the HFS assess whether he or she is practicing within the boundaries of the HFS Scope of Practice (25). Since the client has asked for recommendations on a *type* of exercise equipment, this task is clearly permitted. If the client asked about a specific type of equipment that the practitioner was unfamiliar with, then the HFS must progress further down the decision tree. The HFS knows the task is permitted, but must ask himself or herself question 4 on the decision tree: "Do I personally have the education needed?" If the practitioner is not knowledgeable about that piece of equipment, then he or she needs to gather enough

TABLE 17.2 AREAS OF OVERLAPPING SCOPE OF PRACTICE BETWEEN THE HFS AND OTHER PROFESSIONS

HFS	
Personal trainer	Health screening, exercise assessment, and exercise prescription for apparently healthy individuals and for those with health challenges who are capable of independent exercise
Dietician	Promotion of healthy eating, hydration, and energy consumption to optimize; physical performance, recovery from and adaptation to exercise training and competition, and weight management
Clinical, health, and/or counseling psychologist	Promotion of healthy living through behavior change and cognitive restructuring strategies
Clinical exercise physiologist	Adjusting and adapting exercise training for special populations, including those living with chronic diseases and conditions
Physical therapist	Adjusting and adapting exercise training for special populations, including those living with chronic musculoskeletal and neuromuscular conditions

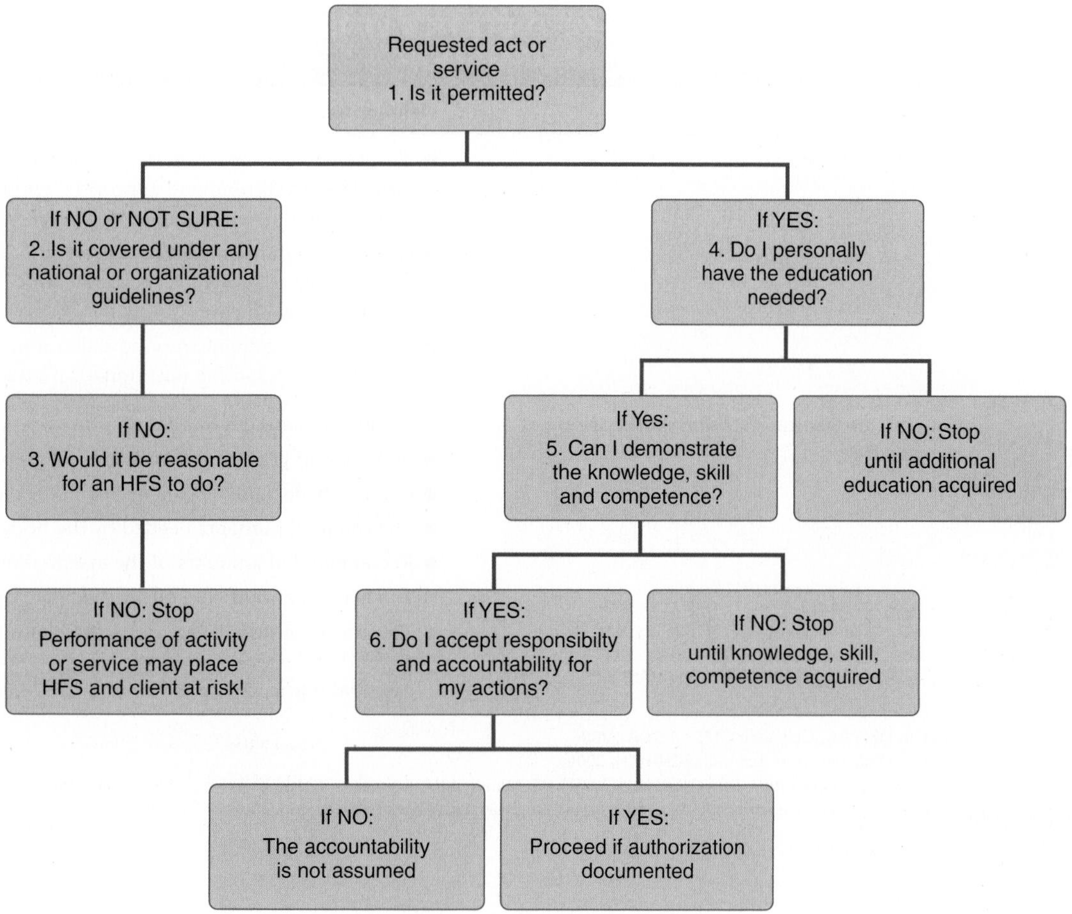

FIGURE 17.3. Scope of practice decision tree. (Reproduced with permission from O'Sullivan-Maillet J, Skates J, Pritchett E. American Dietetic Association: Scope of dietetics practice framework. *J Am Diet Assoc.* 2005;105(4):634–40.)

information to advise the client *or* refer the client to someone else with specific knowledge about that particular piece of equipment.

Nutritional counseling is an area with potential overlap for the HFS, as it is not unusual for clients to request dietary advice. The HFS does have training in basic nutrition, so it seems reasonable that an HFS should be able to work with clients' diets to some extent. In fact, there are 30 knowledge and skill statements in the most recent JTA related to nutrition and weight management. Most of them are KSs under the job task IIF, "Implement a weight management program as indicated by personal goals that are supported by pre-activity screening, health history, and body composition/anthropometrics" (1). The HFS should have knowledge of basic nutritional principles related to weight management, should be able to make referrals to scientifically based resources, and should be familiar with ergogenic aids and supplements and their risks and benefits. However, there is no KS indicating that an HFS should be involved in individual nutritional counseling or therapeutic nutritional advice. Table 17.3 provides clear guidance on what nutritional information is acceptable for an HFS to share with clients.

Scenario 2

The lawsuit *Capati v. Crunch Fitness* provides an instructive example of crossing this line. In 1997, a personal trainer at Crunch Fitness in New York City recommended dietary supplements to Anne Marie Capati. Capati had high blood pressure, and one of the supplements contained Ephedra, contraindicated for those with hypertension. Capati suffered a massive stroke that took her life, hours

TABLE 17.3 THE PRACTICE OF DIETETICS VERSUS GENERAL NONMEDICAL NUTRITIONAL INFORMATION

Activity	Definitions
Practice of dietetics; limited to licensees[a]	• Nutritional assessment to determine nutritional needs and to recommend appropriate nutritional intake, including enteral and parenteral nutrition • Nutritional counseling or education as components of preventive, curative, and restorative health care • Development, administration, evaluation, and consultation regarding nutritional care standards
General nonmedical nutrition information not restricted[b]	Providing information on the following: • Principles of good nutrition and food preparation • Food to be included in the normal daily diet • The essential nutrients needed by the body • Recommended amounts of the essential nutrients • The actions of nutrients on the body • The effects of deficiencies or excesses of nutrients, or food and supplements that are good sources of essential nutrients

[a]Dietetics. Ohio Rev, Code Ann x 4759-2-01(A), 2006.
[b]Dietetics. Ohio Rev, Code Ann x 4759-2-01(M), 2006.
Adapted with permission from Sass C, Eickhoff-Shemek JM, Manore MM, Kruskall LJ. Crossing the line: Understanding the scope of practice between registered dieticians and health fitness professionals. *ACSM's Health Fitness J.* 2007;11(3):12–9.

after a workout at the gym (26, 29). This is an extreme example of what can occur when stepping outside the boundary of scope of practice. Even if the consequences are not life-threatening, exceeding one's scope of practice reflects poorly on one's professional practice and calls to question his or her ethics.

If the personal trainer working with Anne Marie Capati had applied the decision tree to his actions, would this tragedy have been avoided? That is difficult to know, however, following the decision tree provides timely and prudent guidance whenever the task at hand is in question. Question 1 asks: Is it permitted, in this example, to recommend a particular supplement for a client who is trying to lose weight? An HFS would refer to the most current HFS JTA, whereas the personal trainer working with Capati would refer to the current CPT JTA. In either case, the practitioner would have to answer NO to question 2; the service of recommending specific supplements is not covered under the guidelines for CPT's or HFS's. If the practitioner was still unsure, then he could consult the code of ethics for ACSM certified professionals and the licensure laws related to the practice of dietetics in his state. If the answer was still no, then question 3 asks whether it would be reasonable for the practitioner to perform this service. In this case, he might look to position stands, place a call or e-mail to the appropriate certification subcommittee chair, and ask whether the service is routinely performed by other practitioners. In the Capati case, the personal trainer would have found no supporting documentation or practice to support a recommendation of a nutritional supplement to a client.

Looking at this case from a different angle, how might this personal trainer have better handled the query about weight loss supplements? He could have shared evidence-based information about the supplement, including papers that had been published. He could have referred Capati to a registered dietician, especially since one of the job tasks for the HFS is to maintain relationships with other health professionals and to have skill in referral to those professionals.

Scenario 3

Another area that has the potential to be unclear is the differences in scopes of practice between the HFS and the RCEP or clinical exercise specialist.

A 58-year-old woman who is newly diagnosed with heart disease signs up to work with an HFS at a local fitness facility. She had two stents inserted 6 weeks ago, and her doctor told her to exercise. She has Type 2 diabetes and is taking an oral hypoglycemic drug. The client is obese (BMI = 35 kg/m^{-2}) with stage 1 Parkinson disease (PD) and is also taking medication for PD. The HFS working with her is conscientious, so she has already asked the client to get a referral from an MD, which she has supplied. The referral states "OK to exercise." The HFS is unsure as to whether she should be supervised during exercise and whether she should be scrutinized more closely by a clinical exercise professional. This puts the HFS at question 2 in the decision tree: Is it covered under any national or organizational guidelines? The HFS Scope of Practice defines the population that HFSs can work with as "apparently healthy and with controlled conditions released for independent exercise." This client is not apparently healthy as she has a metabolic disease, a cardiovascular disease, and a neuromuscular disease. Are all her diseases in a controlled condition? If the HFS was unsure, then he or she must conservatively answer NO to question 2, and ask herself question 3: Would it be reasonable for an HFS to work with a post-surgical heart disease patient, with two comorbidities? Even with the MD referral, it would probably be wiser for this client to begin in a cardiac rehab program or other clinically supervised program, and then eventually graduate to the services of the HFS. In a best practice scenario, the HFS would contact the referring MD and suggest this alternative.

In most day-to-day situations, the tasks of the HFS will fall squarely within the defined framework for an HFS. Practicing HFSs will not go astray if they are conscientious about using all available professional resources to guide them in scope of practice issues.

CONFLICT OF INTEREST

Acknowledgment and awareness of potential conflicts of interest are coupled with acting within one's scope of practice as hallmarks of professional ethics. The ACSM Ethics and Professional Conduct Committee has defined conflict of interest as "a significant financial interest in a business or other direct or indirect personal gain or consideration provided by a business that may compromise, or have the appearance of compromising, an ACSM member's professional judgment" (3). Conflict of interest has also been defined in terms of a situation in which financial or other personal considerations have the potential to compromise or bias professional judgment and objectivity (28). An example may be an HFS who purchases equipment or services from a friend who in return provides a kickback or "refund." The HFS has not provided fair access for other equipment vendors to bid or offer quotes. In the same way, conflict of interest is apparent in the fitness specialist who will only sell a particular type of nutritional product or clothing without acknowledging the commission base of the sale.

Collaborative models of rehabilitation treatment and fitness training have become more common modes of delivering services to clients. If a company has two divisions in which one provides a referral to the other division for services, this is generally not considered a conflict of interest unless personal gain (commissions) are provided to individual service providers without full disclosure to the customers they serve. In general, the concept of conflict of interest underscores the need to maintain social trust by clearly acknowledging any relationship that may provide personal gain to the professionals involved (10). Disclosure of significant relationships builds client trust and ensures that the professional standards developed to maintain the integrity of the profession are upheld. How information is obtained, discerned, and disseminated is another important aspect of professional ethics.

PROVIDING EVIDENCE-BASED INFORMATION

The National Academy of Sciences identified evidence-based practice as a critical competency of all heath care practitioners (13, 17). Evidence-based practice has been defined in terms of a provision of health care that incorporates the most current and valid research results (16, 20).

Providing evidence-based information is a critical characteristic for the HFS to cultivate and develop. Evidence-based information empowers both the client and the HFS to ask important questions and seek fundamental answers. As a health/fitness professional working with individuals and groups with medically controlled disease, the responsibility to be fully immersed in evidence-based practices is of paramount importance. There are multiple sources of information regarding the explanation and applications of evidence-based practice among allied health and health care providers. Two models of incorporating evidence-based practices among students and young practitioners will be presented.

Amonette, English, and Ottenbacher (5) presented a practical and systematic approach to incorporating evidence-based investigations into the regular practice of the HFS. The four-step process can be used to disseminate scientifically sound information to clients without reliance on anecdotal myths and falsehoods that are so prevalent in fitness and nutrition.

Step 1: Develop a Question

The HFS or the client can inspire questions. Client-driven questions provide important information to the HFS about the level of understanding the client has about his or her physical, emotional, and psychological well-being. Client questions also require that the HFS engage in active listening.

Step 2: Search for Evidence

Evidence can be found in three ways: personal experience, academic preparation, and research knowledge.

Personal Experience

Although personal experience can provide powerful evidence, it is often anecdotal. An HFS may have experience with one client that may not be applicable to another client.

Academic Preparation

Supporting personal and professional experience with academic preparation and research knowledge is helpful in the search for evidence. Every HFS is required to hold a Bachelor's degree in Exercise Science or Kinesiology. The discipline and knowledge gained through the process of obtaining that degree provide the HFS with the tools to seek evidence from appropriate academic sources. However, academic preparation may not always provide the most recent information.

Research Knowledge

Research knowledge is the form of evidence that holds the least amount of bias. With the accessibility of the Internet, peer-reviewed journals can provide ample sources of evidence-based practices that can address a client question. When searching for information, the professional needs to be able to distinguish between quantitative and qualitative research in addition to other types of research studies, for example, a clinical case study or a meta-analysis. In addition, research disseminated at regional and national conferences is cutting-edge and relevant.

Step 3: Evaluate the Evidence

The magnitude of information available makes it difficult to discern appropriate information from inappropriate information. The HFS needs to be able to discriminate the evidence gathered and make thoughtful decisions about the best way to disseminate information to the client.

Step 4: Incorporate Evidence into Practice

The HFS can build on his or her knowledge of the scientific foundations of exercise to use the evidence that best answers the original question. Tailoring the information to the client's needs has

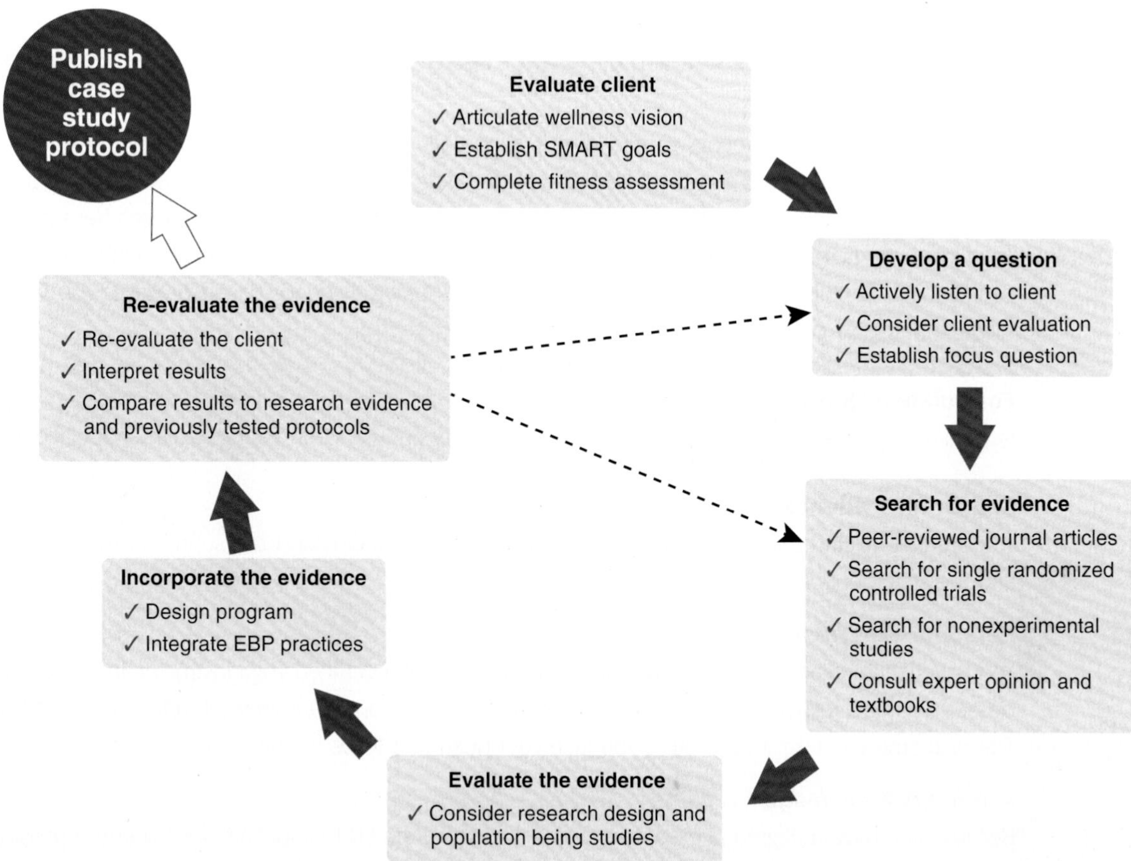

FIGURE 17.4. An example of the application of the evidence-based practice model applied to an individualized exercise prescription. Dashed lines represent alternative or additional steps that may arise. (Used with permission from Amonette W, English K, Ottenbacher K. Nullius in verba: A call for the incorporation of evidence-based practice into the discipline of exercise science. *Sport Med.* 2010;40(6):449–57.)

also been found to be an effective strategy for long-term behavior change (15). A graphic representation of how the four-step process is applied to an exercise prescription is presented in Figure 17.4.

A real life example of the application of the four-step process of evidence-based learning may be found in the How to Incorporate Evidence-Based Practice box. Scott, Altenburger, and Keen (30) also provided an example of an effective application of evidence-based clinical decision-making (EBCD) that has been utilized with physical and occupational therapy students and practitioners. The ability to not only know and understand but also actually apply evidence-based learning principles in a relevant context is supported by researchers in a broad range of disciplines from nursing (11) to education (6). Knowing and understanding the process is not enough. Practicing the skill of integrating EBCD in the context of real clients is necessary. The process, which was divided into three phases, is another application of the process outlined above by Amonette, English, and Ottenbacher with a similar development and progression.

In Phase 1, the students were introduced to the different types of evidence available and given instruction on how to search for evidence and redesign questions using the PICO format (11): P = Population; I = Intervention; C = Comparison; O = Outcome. The therapists generated questions that pertained to real-life problems or practices in their clinics. The student teams selected one question to explore further and seek evidence-based solutions. In phase 2, the students collected evidence and then met with the therapists at the clinic to evaluate the evidence in the context of the question. In phase 3, the students learned about communicating the evidence to the different stakeholders as well as again meeting with the therapists to discuss their findings and get feedback on communication strategies (30).

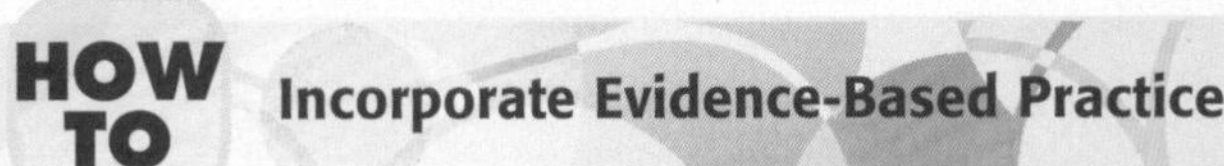

Incorporate Evidence-Based Practice

You have a new client, a young woman who is apparently healthy and whose primary form of exercise is hot yoga four times a week. She tells you that she heard an interview on the evening news debating whether yoga is an adequate means of gaining aerobic health. She is perplexed because her yoga instructor has assured her that her yoga classes are all she needs for complete fitness (aerobic conditioning, flexibility, and whole body strengthening). Using evidence-based practice, you would follow the following steps.

Formulate a Question

Is yoga an effective means of improving cardiorespiratory endurance in young healthy populations?

Search for Evidence

You are able to find a video of the interview online, so you understand the source of the interview and the statements made.

Personal Experience

You have lots of experience with yoga, although you are not a certified yoga instructor. In some yoga classes, you have experienced physical exertion that seems strong enough to elevate your heart rate. The next time you take a yoga class, you take your heart rate twice during the class.

Academic Knowledge

Because you have a degree in exercise science, you know the FITT Guidelines for minimum physical activity levels required for cardiorespiratory adaptation. You know the physiology of the heart, vessels, and respiratory system and understand the dynamics of how exercise at a defined heart rate maximum can produce cellular changes that manifest to improve aerobic capacity.

Research Knowledge

A search for research related to yoga and cardiorespiratory endurance will reveal the current status of the literature. You carefully assess the quality of the studies you find to formulate your conclusions. Are the studies published in peer-reviewed journals? Are there randomized controlled trials generating consistent data across populations?

Evaluate the Evidence

Even if you are able to get your heart rate in range during your yoga classes, this is not strong enough evidence with which to advise your client. Only by looking further into the current research can you reach a conclusion that has clear evidence behind it. The evidence you find may clearly support the claim in the book or it may refute it. Whatever the outcome, your competence as a health fitness professional and your high ethical standards depend on your ability to educate yourself on the basis of the best evidence available at the time.

Incorporate Evidence into Practice

With an understanding of the strengths and the limitations of the current research related to your question, you can answer your client's question with integrity, and create an exercise program for her that is backed by science.

While the Scott, Altenburg, and Keen article cited a collaborative arrangement from physical and occupational therapy settings, the application to the HFS could be made as well (30). The HFS who is working as part of a team of trainers can develop and pose questions to each other on the basis of the issues raised by current or past clients. Many fitness facilities also serve as internship sites for students seeking additional practical experience. The EBCD process can be incorporated into the internship experience through case studies, mentoring, and small group discussions. An example of a real-life application of evidence-based learning in a fitness center setting can be found in the Case Study at the end of this chapter.

Providing evidence-based information enables the HFS to continue to stay abreast of relevant and important information that impacts the health and well-being of clients. Maintaining the HFS certification is another mechanism to stay current and involved with the growing fields of fitness and exercise.

MAINTAINING CERTIFICATION

A profession is often described as a calling or vocation requiring specialized knowledge, methods, and skills, as well as preparation, in an institution of higher learning, in the scholarly, scientific, and historical principles underlying such methods and skills (19). A profession continuously enlarges its body of knowledge, functions autonomously in formulation of policy, and maintains by force of organization or concerted opinion high standards of achievement and conduct. Members of a profession are committed to continuing study, place service above personal gain, and are committed to providing practical services vital to human and social welfare (22). The purpose of ACSM recertification is to ensure that ACSM certified professionals enhance skills and knowledge above and beyond minimum competence. Periodic recertification occurs through the documentation of required continuing educational activities within the 3-year period following successful passing of an ACSM certification exam.

On the basis of the results from the JTA, along with a comprehensive review of recertification policies and procedures of similar credentials from other organizations, the CCRB determined that a 3-year duration was an appropriate window for a certified professional's recertification (4). HFS recertification requirements include the following:

1. Accumulate 60 continuing education credits (CECs).
2. Maintain current CPR certification.
3. Pay the required recertification fee.
4. Have the option to repeat the certification exam (current exam prices apply).

Ways to Earn Continuing Education Credits

There are many ways to earn continuing education credits. Continuing education enables the HFS to build on his or her field experiences and engage in additional networking and scientifically based opportunities that focus and build a professional practice. Table 17.4 provides an overview of ways to earn continuing education credits.

The professional responsibilities of practicing within an appropriate scope of practice, utilizing evidence-based practices, maintaining certification, and adhering to a standard relating to conflict of interest all represent professional ethical behaviors that are informed and nurtured by personal characteristics reflective of a true professional.

PERSONAL CHARACTERISTICS

Cultivating and developing professional practices that reflect the nature of the HFS Certification are critical to growing respect for and continued growth of the health fitness field. Employers in fields aligned with exercise science have articulated specific personal characteristics desirable in potential employees.

TABLE 17.4 WAYS TO EARN CONTINUING EDUCATION CREDITS (CECs)

Obtain a specialty certification	ACSM/ACS Certified Cancer Exercise Trainer (CET) ACSM/NCPAD Certified Inclusive Fitness Trainer (CIFT) ACSM/NSPAPPH Physical Activity in Public Health Specialist (PAPHS)	10 CECs 10 CECs 10 CECs
Attend an ACSM Certification workshop	ACSM Certified Personal Trainer℠ 3-Day Workshop ACSM Certified Personal Trainer℠ 1-Day Workshop ACSM Certified Health Fitness Specialist Workshop ACSM Certified Clinical Exercise Specialist Workshop ACSM Registered Clinical Exercise Physiologist® Workshop	20.75 CECs 7.5 CECs 16.0 CECs 13.25 CECs 15.0 CECs
Participate in an ACSM or approved provider workshop[a]	Weight Management for the Fitness Professional (1 d course) Behavior Change Strategies for Optimal Client Outcomes (1 d course) Business Management for the Fitness Professional (1 d course)	7 CECs 7 CECs 7 CECs
Complete webinars, distance education, other Internet-based continuing education programs on specific clinical or health and fitness related topics		Varies
Attend professional education meetings from ACSM or other nationally recognized organizations		Varies
Take continuing education self-tests that offer CECs, CMEs or CEUs from ACSM or other nationally recognized organizations	*ACSM's Certified News*, ACSM's quarterly newsletter *ACSM's Health and Fitness Journal*	4 CECs per issue 24 CECs per year
Take and receive a passing grade in a health/fitness or exercise science related course from an accredited college or university		10 CECs per credit hour[b]
Author or coauthor books, peer-reviewed journal articles, or accepted abstracts		10 CECs
Teach academic courses; conduct classroom instruction; or present health, fitness, or clinical lectures at an organized professional conference		Varies

[a]A list of approved providers is available at www.acsm.org.
[b]For example, a three-credit-hour course is worth 30 CECs. Course must be health/fitness or clinically related and completed with a grade of "C" or better.
Adapted from American College of Sports Medicine [Internet]. Indianapolis (IN): American College of Sports Medicine; 2007. Renewing your certification. Available from: https://www.acsm.org/Content/NavigationMenu/Certification/ForCertifiedProfessionals/ACSM_Certification_htm

Melton, Dail, Katula, and Mustian (24) interviewed fitness managers from both profit and nonprofit fitness facilities. The managers identified several positive characteristics of personal trainers seeking employment. Trainers who were comfortable interacting and communicated effectively with a variety of individuals, who had a teachable attitude and aptitude, who were fit or provide evidence of engaging in fit behaviors, and who had the discipline and competence to obtain a relevant degree were seen as valuable employees. Likewise, the fitness managers described personal trainers who were arrogant and overconfident or who acted outside their scope of practice specifically around nutritional advice as a liability for the facility. The managers cited the consequences of such negative behaviors in terms of legal liability as well as loss of members, reputation, and revenue (24).

In comparison, the professional characteristics of athletic trainers have also been examined (18). Some of the defining features of quality athletic trainers include being personable, self-confident, mature, assertive, and enthusiastic (18). Likewise, among recreational staff personnel, characteristics such as patience, fun, creative, passionate, and people-oriented define successful professional behaviors (12). Honest, intelligent, and responsible were the top-rated attributes among nurses (27), as were a positive attitude and overall job satisfaction (31). Healthcare professionals are further described in terms of respectful, reflective, and socially responsible (8, 13). In a white paper focusing on the professional characteristics of pharmacy students, behaviors relating to being accountable, being open to new ideas, and being willing to learn were cited as important to individual success (7). Perhaps one of the most cited characteristics of the helping professions is patience, especially in the role of educator and teacher (32). The HFS as a helping health care professional can gain insight into the favorable characteristics cited by professionals from related fields.

The acronym WISE (Wisdom, Integrity, Stewardship, and Enthusiasm) provides a helpful summary of personal characteristics and behaviors important to the success of an HFS.

Wisdom represents the individual seeking answers to sound questions with scientifically based evidence. Integrity signifies the individual respectful of appropriate boundaries while assisting clients in the achievement of holistic and meaningful change. Stewardship represents the individual who values the historical progression of the Exercise Science professions and acts thoughtfully and professionally as a steward of the future. Enthusiasm denotes the individual whose contagious positive attitude inspires others.

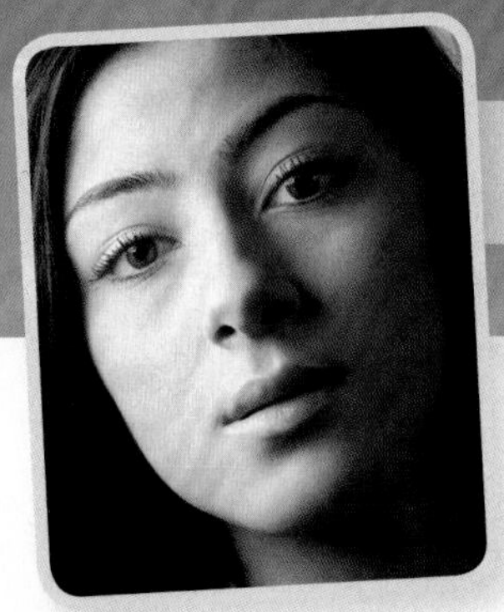

The Case of Marissa, an Undergraduate Intern

Submitted by: **Len Haggerty, Strides Human Performance Institute, Northampton, MA, Melissa Roti, Westfield State University, Westfield, MA**

Students are often overwhelmed when challenged to complete internships and apply scientific knowledge to real-life situations (1). This case provides an example of how utilizing the EBCD method enables a young student to be guided and instructed in a supportive and safe environment.

Narrative

Len Haggerty, owner of Strides Human Performance Institute, believes that education is a key component of both the undergraduate and the professional experience. Strides Human Performance Institute is a fitness and performance facility that offers adult one-on-one sessions and a wide variety of youth classes. The certified trainers focus on functional, sport-specific movements and high energy workouts for energy system development. Len offers a highly competitive internship program for qualified young professionals. Part of the internship process is developing and applying evidence-based decision making within the context of the facility.

Marissa Bonito, a Westfield State University senior, is a student-athlete majoring in Exercise Science and completing her 280-hour internship at Strides. Marissa is an avid runner and is able to focus her evidence-based assignment on an area that is interesting to her. Len provides the structure through an assignment that includes the development of an educational event or program aimed at increasing the understanding of clients on a topic of the intern's choice. Evidence-based decision making provides a framework from which to make appropriate choices for future programming (2, 3).

continues

The Case of Marissa cont.

Phase 1: Generating the Questions

Initially, both Len and Marissa generate relevant questions related to running. From that list, Marissa is able to refine the list and apply the PICO format to redesigning the question to seek appropriate evidence. In phase 1, Len is also able to discern and provide feedback on questions that will apply in the context of Strides. Here is an example of a question that follows the PICO format: Does barefoot running reduce injuries compared with traditional running shoe use, in marathon runners? In this case, the *population* is defined as marathon runners; the *intervention* is barefoot running which is *compared* with classic running shoe use. The *outcome* of interest is injury rate.

Phase 2: Gathering the Evidence

Marissa seeks evidence through peer-reviewed journals and works with Len to further evaluate the evidence and the appropriateness of application for the Strides population. Further questions are often generated in this Phase.

Phase 3: Communicating the Evidence

After review from Len, Marissa disseminates the information through a blog and presentation that is directed toward both Strides members and individuals in broader running community. During the assessment process, Len and Marissa reflect on the value of the evidence and the benefit of generating and seeking appropriate solutions.

Follow-up

Through written and verbal reflections about the internship experience, Marissa is able to consider ways in which evidence-based learning influenced her ability to make choices about programming that benefit Stride's clients. Marissa is also able to identify ways in which the PICO format would enable her to define questions and seek answers in the future.

Questions

- What value does the evidence-based decision-making method have outside a clinical setting?
- Would the answers have been different had a different population been under investigation, for example 5-km runners?
- How can the evidence-based decision-making method empower clients?

References

Casey K, Fink R, Jaynes C, Campbell L, Cook P, Wilson V. Readiness for practice: The senior practicum experience. *J Nurs Educ.* 2011;50(11):646–52. doi:10.3928/01484834-20110817-03. Epub 2011 Aug 17.

Sabas C. The effects of modeling evidence-based practice during the clinical internship. *J Phys Ther Educ.* 2008;22(3):74–84.

Scott PJ, Altenburger PA, Kean J. A collaborative teaching strategy for enhancing learning of evidence-based clinical decision-making. *J Allied Health.* 2011;40(3):120–7.

SUMMARY

The HFS has a personal and professional responsibility to engage in behaviors that "do no harm" (8). After providing a brief history of ACSM Certifications, this chapter has reviewed the ACSM Code of Ethics and provided a more in-depth examination of the professional responsibilities and personal characteristics of the HFS. The professional responsibilities relating to Scope of Practice, Conflict of Interest, Evidence-Based Practice, and Maintaining Certification have been reviewed. Personal characteristics represented by WISE have also been examined in the context of desirable personal characteristics of professionals in the helping professions.

STUDY QUESTIONS

1. The ACSM Certified HFS is qualified to pursue a career in all EXCEPT ________.
   a. local YMCA
   b. hospital cardiac care unit
   c. university fitness and wellness center
   d. clinical research project related to childhood obesity
2. The ACSM Certified HFS Scope of Practice includes
   a. exercise testing of a healthy 76-year-old man with mild osteoarthritis
   b. aerobic training of a 21-year-old acutely anorexic woman
   c. therapeutic exercise to target a cancer survivor's chronic lymphedema of the left arm
   d. interpreting a 12-lead ECG of a CABG patient in a phase 2 cardiac rehab program
3. Henry's business card indicates that he is a certified HFS working as a manager of an employee wellness center. In addition to his management responsibilities, he functions in the role as a personal trainer at the center for employees who want to pay an extra fee to the center for individualized services. Henry has a side business of selling essential oils and nutritional aids for health and longevity. Discuss whether each example is permissible for Henry to engage in.
   a. Henry has a side business of selling essential oils and nutritional aids for health and longevity.
   b. Henry pins his essential oils business card on a bulletin board in the wellness center where other business cards advertise massage services, nutritional counseling, physical therapy, and acupuncture.
   c. Henry gives his essential oils business card and a free sample to every client he works with at the wellness center.
   d. Henry makes essential oils recommendations within the context of a training session for a client at the wellness center.
   e. Henry makes essential oils recommendations within the context of a training session for a private client.
4. List some ways of maintaining one's HFS certification.
5. Discuss personal characteristics that you deem important for professional conduct as an HFS.
6. How do the personal behaviors of an HFS impact the professional integrity of the field?

REFERENCES

1. American College of Sports Medicine. *ACSM's Guidelines for Exercise Testing and Prescription*. 9th ed. Baltimore (MD): Lippincott Williams & Wilkins; 2013.
2. American College of Sports Medicine [Internet]. Indianapolis (IN): American College of Sports Medicine Code of Ethics; 2007 [cited June 12, 2012]. Available from: http://www.acsm.org/join-acsm/membership-resources/code-of-ethics
3. American College of Sports Medicine. *Leadership Manual 2011–2012*. Indianapolis (IN): American College of Sports Medicine. 9 p.
4. American College of Sports Medicine [Internet]. Indianapolis (IN): American College of Sports Medicine. Renewing your certification. Available from: http://certification.acsm.org/renew-your-certification (Accessed: 10/19/2012).
5. Amonette W, English K, Ottenbacher K. Nullius in verba: A call for the incorporation of evidence-based practice into the discipline of exercise science. *Sport Med.* 2010;40(6):449–57.
6. Anderson L, Krathwohl D, editors. *A Taxonomy for Learning, Teaching and Assessing: A Revision of Bloom's Taxonomy of Educational Objectives.* New York (NY): Longman; 2001.
7. APhA-ASP/AACP-COD Task Force on Professionalism. White paper on pharmacy student professionalism. *J Am Pharm Assoc.* 2000;40:96–102.
8. Beach M, Duggan P, Cassel C, Geller G. What does "respect" mean? Exploring the moral obligation of health professionals to respect patients. *J Gen Intern Med.* 2007;22(5):692–5.
9. Berryman JW. *Out of Many, One: A History of the American College of Sports Medicine.* Champaign (IL): Human Kinetics; 1995. 283 p.

10. Brody H. Clarifying conflict of interest. *Am J Bioeth.* 2011;11(1):23–8.
11. Center for Evidence Based Medicine [Internet]. *Asking Focused Questions.* Oxford (UK): CEBM; 2009 [cited 2012 Mar 22]. Available from: http://www.cebm.net/index.aspx?o=1036.
12. Chase D, Masberg B. Partnering for skill development: Park and recreation agencies and university programs. *Manag Leisure.* 2008;13(2):74–91.
13. de Cordova PB, Collins S, Peppard L, et al. Implementing evidence-based nursing with student nurses and clinicians: Uniting the strengths. *Appl Nurs Res.* 2008;21(4):242–5.
14. Exercise is Medicine [Internet]. Indianapolis (IN): The Exercise is Medicine Credential; 2012 [cited 2012 Jun 12]. Available from: http://exerciseismedicine.org/documents/12HFSEEIMcredentialinfo_HR.pdf
15. Eyles HC, Mhurchu CN. Does tailoring make a difference? A systematic review of the long-term effectiveness of tailored nutrition education for adults. *Nutr Rev.* 2009;67(8):464–80.
16. HiltonS, Slotnick H. Proto-professionalism: How professionalisation occurs across the continuum of medical education. *Med Educ.* 2005;39(1):58–65.
17. Institute of Medicine Board on Health Care Services, Consensus Report. Crossing the Quality Chasm: A New Health System for the 21st Century, March 1, 2001.
18. Kahanov L, Andrews L. A survey of athletic training employers' hiring criteria. *J Athl Train.* 2001;36(4):408.
19. Kutz MR. *Leadership and Management in Athletic Training: An Integrated Approach.* Baltimore (MD): Lippincott Williams & Wilkins; 2010. 331 p.
20. Medical Dictionary [Internet]. *Evidence Based Practice.* (n.d.) [cited 2011 Aug 15]. Available from: http://medical-dictionary.thefreedictionary.com/evidence-based+practice
21. Medical Dictionary [Internet]. *Ethics.* (n.d.) [cited 2011 Aug 15]. Available from: http://medical-dictionary.thefreedictionary.com/ethics
22. Medical Dictionary [Internet]. *Profession.* (n.d.) [cited 2011 Aug 15]. Available from: http://medical-dictionary.thefreedictionary.com/profession
23. Medical Dictionary [Internet]. *Scope of Practice.* (n.d.) [cited 2011 Jul 14]. Available from: http://medical-dictionary.thefreedictionary.com/scope+of+practice
24. Melton DI, Dail TK, Katula JA, & Mustian KM. The current state of personal training: Managers' perspectives. *J Strength Cond Res.* 2010;24(11):3173–9.
25. O'Sullivan-Maillet J, Skates J, Pritchett E. American Dietetic Association: Scope of dietetics practice framework. *J Am Diet Assoc.* 2005;105(4):634–40.
26. Perko M, Dennison D. "Does this stuff work?" When health educators discuss dietary supplements. *Int Electr J Health Educ.* 2000;3(1):64–8.
27. Rassin M. Nurses professional and personal values. *Nurs Ethics.* 2008;15(5):614–30.
28. Responsible Conducts of Research Courses Portal [Internet]. *Conflicts of Interest.* New York (NY): Columbia University; [cited 2011 Aug 15]. Available from: http://ccnmtl.columbia.edu/projects/rcr/rcr_conflicts/foundation/index.html#1_1
29. Sass C, Eickhoff-Shemek JM, Manore MM, Kruskall LJ. Crossing the line: Understanding the scope of practice between registered dieticians and health fitness professionals. *ACSM's Health Fitness J.* 2007;11(3):12–9.
30. Scott PJ, Altenburger PA, Kean J. A collaborative teaching strategy for enhancing learning of evidence-based clinical decision-making. *J Allied Health.* 2011;40(3):120–7.
31. Shields MA, Ward M. Improving nurse retention in the National Health Service in England: The impact of job satisfaction on intentions to quit. *J Health Econ.* 2001;20:677–701.
32. Tichenor MS, Tichenor JL Understanding teachers' perspectives on professionalism. *Profession Educ.* 2004;27(1,2):89–95.

APPENDIX A

American College of Sports Medicine Certifications

Note: This appendix is reprinted with permission from *ACSM's Guidelines for Exercise Testing and Prescription*. 9th ed. Baltimore (MD): Lippincott Williams and Wilkins; 2014.

Exercise practitioners are becoming increasingly aware of the advantages of maintaining professional credentials. In efforts to ensure quality, reduce liability, and remain competitive, more and more employers are requiring professional certification of their exercise staff. Additionally, in efforts to improve public safety, mandates for certification by state and/or regulatory agencies (*e.g.*, licensure) as well as third party payers now exist. The American College of Sports Medicine (ACSM) offers five primary and three specialty certifications for exercise professionals. These include the following:

Primary Certifications:

- ACSM Certified Group Exercise Instructor℠ (GEI)
- ACSM Certified Personal Trainer® (CPT)
- ACSM Certified Health Fitness Specialist℠ (HFS)
- ACSM Certified Clinical Exercise Specialist℠ (CES)
- ACSM Registered Clinical Exercise Physiologist® (RCEP)*

Specialty Certifications:

- ACSM/NCPAD Certified Inclusive Fitness Trainer℠
  - NCPAD = National Center on Physical Activity and Disability
- ACSM/ACS Certified Cancer Exercise Trainer℠
  - ACS = American Cancer Society
- ACSM/NPAS Physical Activity in Public Health Specialist℠
  - NPAS = National Physical Activity Society

Advances in the exercise profession have been substantial over the past decade. Specific conditions that are considered essential for a formalized profession to exist are now in place (1). These include:

- A standardized system to develop skills.
- A standardized system to validate skills.
- An organized community to advocate for the profession.

The Committee on Accreditation for the Exercise Sciences (CoAES) under the auspices of the Commission on Accreditation of Allied Health Education Programs (CAAHEP) now validates and accredits university curriculum in the exercise sciences (*i.e.*, standardized skills development). The National Commission for Certifying Agencies (NCCA) provides a standardized, independent, and objective third party evaluation of examination design, development, and performance to ensure certification integrity (*i.e.*, skills validation). ACSM and other organizations such as Clinical Exercise Physiology Association (CEPA), a member of the ACSM affiliate societies, have created professional communities that advocate specifically for the interests of exercise and fitness practitioners.

ACSM CERTIFICATION DEVELOPMENT

The process of developing a certification examination begins with a job task analysis (JTA) (2). The purpose of the JTA is to define the major areas of professional practice (*i.e.*, domains), delineate the tasks performed "on-the-job," and identify the knowledge and skills required for safe and competent practice. The domains are subsequently weighted according to the importance and frequency of performance of their respective tasks. The number of examination test items is then determined based on the domain weight. Each examination reflects the content and weights defined by the JTA. By linking the content of the examination to the JTA (*e.g.*, what professionals do), it is possible to ensure that the examination is practice related.

Examination development continues with question writing. Content experts representing academia and practice are selected and trained on examination item writing. This examination writing team is charged with the task of creating test items that are representative of and consistent with the JTA. Each test item is evaluated psychometrically, undergoing extensive testing, editing, and retesting before being included as a scored item on the examination. Finally, passing scores are determined using a criterion-referenced methodology. Passing scores for each examination are associated with a minimum level of mastery necessary for safe and competent practice. Setting passing scores in this manner ensures that qualified candidates will become certified regardless of how other candidates perform on the examination.

The job definition, domains, and tasks from the JTA for ACSM's five primary certifications are listed in the following sections, and the primary population served, the eligibility criteria, and the competencies for these certifications are found in Table A.1. The complete JTA including knowledge and skill statements for all eight ACSM certifications can be found online at http://certification.acsm.org/exam-content-outlines. Because every question on each of the certification examinations must refer to a specific knowledge or skill statement within the associated JTA, these documents provide a resource to guide exam preparation.

TABLE A.1 AMERICAN COLLEGE OF SPORTS MEDICINE'S CERTIFICATIONS AT A GLANCE

Certification	Primary Population Served	Eligibility Criteria	Competencies
ACSM Certified Group Exercise Instructor[SM]	Apparently healthy individuals and those with health challenges who are able to exercise independently	• ≥18 yr • High school diploma or equivalent • Current CPR and AED certifications (must contain a live skills component) — AED not required for those practicing outside of the United States and Canada	• Develops and implements a variety of exercises in group settings and modifies exercise according to need • Leads safe and effective exercise using a variety of leadership techniques to enhance the motor skills related to the domains of physical fitness
ACSM Certified Personal Trainer®	Apparently healthy individuals and those with health challenges who are able to exercise independently	• ≥18 yr • High school diploma or equivalent • Current CPR and AED certifications (must contain a live skills component such as the	• Identifies health risk factors, performs fitness appraisals and preparticipation health screenings, and develops exercise programs that promote lasting behavior change

TABLE A.1 AMERICAN COLLEGE OF SPORTS MEDICINE'S CERTIFICATIONS AT A GLANCE *(continued)*

Certification	Primary Population Served	Eligibility Criteria	Competencies
		American Heart Association [AHA] or the American Red Cross) — AED not required for those practicing outside of the United States and Canada	• Incorporates suitable and innovative activities to improve functional capacity and manages health risk to promote lasting behavior change
ACSM Certified Health Fitness Specialist℠	Apparently healthy individuals and those with medically controlled diseases	• Bachelor's degree in an exercise science, exercise physiology, kinesiology, or exercise science based degree (one is eligible to sit for the examination if the candidate is in the last term of their degree program) • Current CPR and AED certifications (must contain a live skills component such as the AHA or the American Red Cross) — AED not required for those practicing outside of the United States and Canada	• Applies knowledge of exercise science including kinesiology, functional anatomy, exercise physiology, nutrition, program administration, psychology, and injury prevention in the health fitness setting • Performs preparticipation health screenings and fitness assessments • Interprets assessment results and develops exercise prescriptions • Performs duties related to fitness management, administration, and program supervision • Incorporates suitable physical activities to improve functional capacity • Applies appropriate behavioral change techniques to effectively educate and counsel on lifestyle modification

ACSM Certified Clinical Exercise Specialist℠	Apparently healthy individuals and those with cardiovascular, pulmonary, and metabolic disease	• Bachelor's degree in an exercise science, exercise physiology, kinesiology, or exercise science based degree (one is eligible to sit for the exam if the candidate is in the last term of their degree program)
		• Minimum of 400 h of clinical experience for graduates from a CAAHEP accredited program or 500 h of clinical experience for graduates from a non-CAAHEP accredited program
			• Applies extensive knowledge of functional anatomy, exercise physiology, pathophysiology, electrocardiography, human behavior/psychology, gerontology, and graded exercise testing in the clinical setting
			  • Provides exercise supervision/leadership and counsels patients on lifestyle modification
			  • Conducts emergency procedures in exercise testing and training settings

Continues

TABLE A.1 **AMERICAN COLLEGE OF SPORTS MEDICINE'S CERTIFICATIONS AT A GLANCE** *(continued)*

Certification	Primary Population Served	Eligibility Criteria	Competencies
		• Current certification for the AHA BLS for Healthcare Provider or American Red Cross CPR/AED for the Professional Rescuer or equivalent (must contain live skills component) – AED not required for those practicing outside of the United States and Canada	

ACSM Registered Clinical Exercise Physiologist®	Apparently healthy individuals and those with cardiovascular, pulmonary, metabolic, orthopedic/musculoskeletal, neuromuscular, neoplastic, immunologic, and hematologic disorders	• Graduate degree in clinical exercise physiology with coursework in clinical assessment, exercise testing, exercise prescription, and exercise training (one is eligible to sit for the exam if the candidate is in the last term of their degree program)
		• Minimum of 600 h of clinical experience (external to classroom/laboratory) working with individuals with chronic disease
		• Current certification for the AHA BLS for Healthcare Provider or American Red Cross CPR/AED for the Professional Rescuer or equivalent (must contain live skills component) – AED not required for those practicing outside of the United States and Canada
			• Performs exercise screening and exercise and fitness testing
			  • Develops exercise prescriptions and supervises exercise programs
			• Conducts exercise and physical activity education counseling
			  • Conducts measurement and evaluation of exercise and physical activity-related outcomes

CPR, cardiopulmonary resuscitation; AED, automated external defibrillators; BLS, basic life support.

ACSM'S FIVE PRIMARY CERTIFICATIONS

ACSM Certified Group Exercise Instructor℠ Job Task Analysis

The JTA is intended to serve as a blueprint of the job of a GEI. As one prepares for the examination, it is important to remember that all questions are based on the following outline.

JOB DEFINITION

The GEI (a) possesses a minimum of a high school diploma and (b) works in a group exercise setting with apparently healthy individuals and those with health challenges who are able to exercise independently to enhance quality of life, improve health-related physical fitness, manage health risk, and promote lasting health behavior change. The GEI leads safe and effective exercise programs using a variety of leadership techniques to foster group camaraderie, support, and motivation to enhance muscular strength and endurance, flexibility, cardiorespiratory fitness, body composition, and any of the motor skills related to the domains of health-related physical fitness.

PERFORMANCE DOMAINS AND ASSOCIATED JOB TASKS

The JTA for the GEI certification describes what the professional does on a day-to-day basis. The JTA is divided into domains and associated tasks performed on the job. The percentages listed in this section indicate the number of questions representing each domain on the 100 question GEI examination.

The performance domains are the following:

- Domain I: Participant and Program Assessment — 10%.
- Domain II: Class Design — 25%.
- Domain III: Leadership and Instruction — 55%.
- Domain IV: Legal and Professional Responsibilities — 10%.

Domain I: Participant and Program Assessment

Associated Job Tasks

A. Evaluate and establish participant screening procedures to optimize safety and minimize risk by reviewing assessment protocols based on ACSM standards and guidelines.
B. Administer and review as necessary participants' health risk to determine if preparticipation assessment is needed prior to exercise using Physical Activity Readiness Questionnaire (PAR-Q), ACSM preparticipation health screening, or other appropriate tools.
C. Screen participants as needed for known acute or chronic health conditions to provide recommendations and/or modifications.

Domain II: Class Design

Associated Job Tasks

A. Establish the purpose and determine the objectives of the class based on the needs of participants and facility.
B. Determine class content (*i.e.*, warm-up, stimulus, cool-down) in order to create an effective workout based on the objectives of the class.
C. Select and sequence appropriate exercises in order to provide a safe workout based on the objectives of the class.
D. Rehearse class content, exercise selection, and sequencing and revise as needed in order to provide a safe and effective workout based on the purpose and objectives of the class.

Domain III: Leadership and Instruction

Associated Job Tasks

A. Prepare to teach by implementing preclass procedures including screening new participants and organizing equipment, music, and room setup.
B. Create a positive exercise environment in order to optimize participant adherence by incorporating effective motivational skills, communication techniques, and behavioral strategies.
C. Demonstrate all exercises using proper form and technique to ensure safe execution in accordance with ACSM standards and guidelines.
D. Incorporate verbal and nonverbal instructional cues in order to optimize communication, safety, and motivation based on industry guidelines.

E. Monitor participants' performance to ensure safe and effective exercise execution using observation and participant feedback techniques in accordance with ACSM standards and guidelines.
F. Modify exercises based on individual and group needs to ensure safety and effectiveness in accordance with ACSM standards and guidelines.
G. Monitor sound levels of vocal and/or audio equipment following industry guidelines.
H. Respond to participants' concerns in order to maintain a professional, equitable, and safe environment by using appropriate conflict management or customer service strategies set forth by facility policy and procedures and industry guidelines.
I. Educate participants in order to enhance knowledge, enjoyment, and adherence by providing health/fitness-related information and resources.

Domain IV: Legal and Professional Responsibilities

Associated Job Tasks

A. Evaluate the class environment (*e.g.*, outdoor, indoor, capacity, flooring, temperature, ventilation, lighting, equipment, and acoustics) to minimize risk and optimize safety by following preclass inspection procedures based on established facility and industry standards and guidelines.
B. Promote participants' awareness and accountability by informing them of classroom safety procedures and exercise and intensity options in order to minimize risk.
C. Follow industry accepted professional, ethical, and business standards in order to optimize safety and reduce liability.
D. Respond to emergencies in order to minimize untoward events by following procedures consistent with established standards of care and facility policies.
E. Respect copyrights to protect original and creative work, media, etc., by legally securing copyright material and other intellectual property based on national and international copyright laws.
F. Engage in healthy lifestyle practices in order to be a positive role model for class participants.
G. Select and participate in continuing education programs that enhance knowledge and skills on a continuing basis, maximize effectiveness, and increase professionalism in the field.

ACSM Certified Personal Trainer™ (CPT) Job Task Analysis

The JTA is intended to serve as a blueprint of the job of a CPT. As you prepare for the examination, it is important to remember that all examination questions are based on the following outline.

JOB DEFINITION

The CPT (a) possesses a minimum of a high school diploma and (b) works with apparently healthy individuals and those with health challenges who are able to exercise independently to enhance quality of life, improve health-related physical fitness, performance, manage health risk, and promote lasting health behavior change. The CPT conducts basic preparticipation health screening assessments, submaximal aerobic exercise tests, and muscular strength/endurance, flexibility, and body composition tests. The CPT facilitates motivation and adherence as well as develops and administers programs designed to enhance muscular strength/endurance, flexibility, cardiorespiratory fitness, body composition, and/or any of the motor skill-related components of physical fitness (*i.e.*, balance, coordination, power, agility, speed, reaction time).

PERFORMANCE DOMAINS AND ASSOCIATED JOB TASKS

The JTA for the CPT certification describes what the professional does on a day-to-day basis. The JTA is divided into domains and associated tasks performed on the job. The percentages listed in this section indicate the number of questions representing each domain on the 150 question CPT examination.

The performance domains are the following:

- Domain I: Initial Client Consultation and Assessment — 26%.
- Domain II: Exercise Programming and Implementation — 27%.
- Domain III: Exercise Leadership and Client Education — 27%.
- Domain IV: Legal, Professional, Business, and Marketing — 20%.

Domain I: Initial Client Consultation and Assessment

Associated Job Tasks

A. Provide instructions and initial documents to the client in order to proceed to the interview.
B. Interview client in order to gather and provide pertinent information to proceed to the fitness testing and program design.
C. Review and analyze client data (*i.e.*, classify risk) to formulate a plan of action and/or conduct physical assessments.
D. Evaluate behavioral readiness to optimize exercise adherence.
E. Assess physical fitness including cardiorespiratory fitness, muscular strength, muscular endurance, flexibility, and anthropometric measures in order to set goals and establish a baseline for program development.
F. Develop a comprehensive (*i.e.*, physical fitness, goals, behavior) reassessment plan/timeline.

Domain II: Exercise Programming and Implementation

Associated Job Tasks

A. Review assessment results, medical history, and goals to determine appropriate training program.
B. Select exercise modalities to achieve desired adaptations based on goals, medical history, and assessment results.
C. Determine initial frequency, intensity, time (duration), and type (*i.e.*, the FITT principle of exercise prescription [Ex R_x]) of exercise based on goals, medical history, and assessment results.
D. Review proposed program with client; demonstrate and instruct the client to perform exercises safely and effectively.
E. Monitor client technique and response to exercise modifying as necessary.
F. Modify FITT to improve or maintain the client's physical fitness level.
G. Seek client feedback to ensure satisfaction and enjoyment of the program.

Domain III: Leadership and Education Implementation

Associated Job Tasks

A. Create a positive exercise experience in order to optimize participant adherence by applying effective communication techniques, motivation techniques, and behavioral strategies.
B. Educate clients using scientifically sound health/fitness information and resources to enhance client's knowledge base, program enjoyment, adherence, and overall awareness of health/fitness related information.

Domain IV: Legal, Professional, Business, and Marketing

Associated Job Tasks

A. Obtain medical clearance for clients based on ACSM guidelines prior to starting an exercise program (see Figures 2.3 and 2.4).
B. Collaborate with various health care professionals and organizations in order to provide clients with a network of providers that minimizes liability and maximizes program effectiveness.
C. Develop a comprehensive risk management program (including emergency action plan and injury prevention program) to enhance the standard of care and reflect a client-focused mission.
D. Participate in approved continuing education programs on a regular basis to maximize effectiveness, increase professionalism, and enhance knowledge and skills in the field of health/fitness.
E. Adhere to ACSM's Code of Ethics by practicing in a professional manner within the Scope of Practice of a CPT (see ACSM's Code of Ethics for Certified and Registered Professionals at http://certification.acsm.org/faq28-codeofethics).
F. Develop a business plan to establish mission, business, budgetary, and sales objectives.
G. Develop marketing materials and engage in networking/business exchanges to build client base, promote services, and increase resources.
H. Obtain appropriate personal training and liability insurance and follow industry accepted professional, ethical, and business standards in order to optimize safety and to reduce liability.
I. Engage in healthy lifestyle practices in order to be a positive role model for all clients.
J. Respect copyrights to protect original and creative work, media, etc., by legally securing copyright material and other intellectual property based on national and international copyright laws.
K. Safeguard client confidentiality and privacy rights unless formally waived or in emergency situations.

ACSM Certified Health Fitness Specialist℠ Job Task Analysis

The JTA is intended to serve as a blueprint of the job of an HFS. As one prepares for the examination, it is important to remember that all examination questions are based on the following outline.

JOB DEFINITION

The HFS is a health and fitness professional with a minimum of a bachelor's degree in exercise science. The HFS performs preparticipation health screenings, conducts physical fitness assessments, interprets results, develops exercise prescriptions, and applies behavioral and motivational strategies to apparently healthy individuals and individuals with medically controlled diseases and health conditions to support clients in adopting and maintaining healthy lifestyle behaviors. The academic preparation of the HFS also includes fitness management, administration, and supervision. The HFS is typically employed or self-employed in commercial, community, studio, corporate, university, and hospital settings.

PERFORMANCE DOMAINS AND ASSOCIATED JOB TASKS

The JTA for the HFS describes what the professional does on a day-to-day basis. The JTA is divided into domains and associated tasks performed on the job. The following percentages listed in this section representing each domain on the 150 question HFS examination.

The performance domains are the following:

- Domain I: Health and Fitness Assessment — 30%.
- Domain II: Exercise Prescription and Implementation (and Ongoing Support) — 30%.
- Domain III: Exercise Counseling and Behavioral Strategies — 15%.
- Domain IV: Legal/Professional — 10%.
- Domain V: Management — 15%.

Domain I: Health and Fitness Assessment

Associated Job Tasks

A. Implement assessment protocols and preparticipation health screening procedures to maximize participant safety and minimize risk.
B. Determine participant's readiness to take part in a health-related physical fitness assessment and exercise program.
C. Select and prepare physical fitness assessments for healthy participants and those with controlled disease.
D. Conduct and interpret cardiorespiratory fitness assessments.
E. Conduct assessments of muscular strength, muscular endurance, and flexibility.
F. Conduct anthropometric and body composition assessments.

Domain II: Exercise Prescription and Implementation

Associated Job Tasks

A. Review preparticipation health screening including self-guided health questionnaires and appraisals, exercise history, and physical fitness assessments.
B. Determine safe and effective exercise programs to achieve desired outcomes and goals.
C. Implement cardiorespiratory Ex R_x using the FITT principle (*i.e.*, frequency, intensity, time, and type) for apparently healthy participants based on current health status, fitness goals, and availability of time.
D. Implement Ex R_x using the FITT principle for flexibility, muscular strength, and muscular endurance for apparently healthy participants based on current health status, fitness goals, and availability of time.
E. Establish exercise progression guidelines for resistance, aerobic, and flexibility activity to achieve the goals of apparently healthy participants.
F. Implement a weight management program as indicated by personal goals that are supported by preparticipation health screening, health history, and body composition/anthropometrics.
G. Prescribe and implement exercise programs for participants with controlled cardiovascular, pulmonary, and metabolic diseases and other clinical populations per ACSM protocols.
H. Prescribe and implement exercise programs for healthy and special populations (*i.e.*, older adults, youth, pregnant women).
I. Modify Ex R_x based on environmental conditions.

Domain III: Exercise Counseling and Behavioral Strategies

Associated Job Tasks

A. Optimize adoption and adherence to exercise programs and other healthy behaviors by applying effective communication techniques.
B. Optimize adoption of and adherence to exercise programs and other healthy behaviors by applying effective behavioral and motivational strategies.

C. Provide educational resources to support clients in the adoption and maintenance of healthy lifestyle behaviors.
D. Provide support within the scope of practice of an HFS and refer to other health professionals as indicated.

Domain IV: Legal/Professional

Associated Job Tasks

A. Create and disseminate risk management guidelines for a health/fitness facility, department, or organization to reduce member, employee, and business risk.
B. Create an effective injury prevention program and ensure that emergency policies and procedures are in place.

Domain V: Management

Associated Job Tasks

A. Manage human resources in accordance with leadership, organization, and management techniques.
B. Manage fiscal resources in accordance with leadership, organization, and management techniques.
C. Establish policies and procedures for the management of health/fitness facilities based on accepted safety and legal guidelines, standards, and regulations.
D. Develop and execute a marketing plan to promote programs, services, and facilities.
E. Use effective communication techniques to develop professional relationships with other allied health professionals (*e.g.*, nutritionists, physical therapists, physicians, and nurses).

ACSM Certified Clinical Exercise Specialist℠ (CES) Job Task Analysis

The JTA is intended to serve as a blueprint of the job of the CES. As one prepares for the examination, it is important to remember that all examination questions are based on the following outline.

JOB DEFINITION

The CES is an allied health professional with a minimum of a bachelor's degree in exercise science. The CES works with patients and clients challenged with cardiovascular, pulmonary, and metabolic diseases and disorders, as well as with apparently healthy populations in cooperation with other health care professionals to enhance quality of life, manage health risk, and promote lasting health behavior change. The CES conducts preparticipation health screening, maximal and submaximal graded exercise tests and performs strength, flexibility, and body composition tests. The CES develops and administers programs designed to enhance cardiorespiratory fitness, muscular strength and endurance, balance, and range of motion. The CES educates their clients about testing, exercise program components, and clinical and lifestyle self-care for control of chronic disease and health conditions.

PERFORMANCE DOMAINS AND ASSOCIATED JOB TASKS

The JTA for the CES describes what the professional does on a day-to-day basis. The JTA is divided into domains and associated tasks performed on the job. The percentages listed in this section indicate the number of questions representing each domain on the 100 question CES examination.

The performance domains are the following:

- Domain I: Patient/Client Assessment — 30%.
- Domain II: Exercise Prescription — 30%.
- Domain III: Program Implementation and Ongoing Support — 20%.

- Domain IV: Leadership and Counseling — 15%.
- Domain V: Legal and Professional Considerations — 5%.

Domain I: Patient/Client Assessment

Associated Job Tasks

A. Determine and obtain the necessary physician referral and medical records to assess the potential participant.
B. Perform a preparticipation health screening including review of the participant's medical history and knowledge, their needs and goals, the program's potential benefits, and additional required testing and data.
C. Evaluate the participant's risk to ensure safe participation and determine level of monitoring/supervision in a preventive or rehabilitative exercise program.

Domain II: Exercise Prescription

Associated Job Tasks

A. Develop a clinically appropriate Ex R_x using all available information (*e.g.*, clinical and physiological status, goals, and behavioral assessment).
B. Review the Ex R_x and exercise program with the participant including home exercise, compliance, and participant's expectations and goals.
C. Instruct the participant in the safe and effective use of exercise modalities, exercise plan, reporting symptoms, and class organization.

Domain III: Program Implementation and Ongoing Support

Associated Job Tasks

A. Implement the program (*e.g.*, Ex R_x, education, counseling, and goals).
B. Continually assess participant feedback, clinical signs and symptoms, and exercise tolerance and provide feedback to the participant about their exercise, general program participation, and clinical progress.
C. Reassess and update the program (*e.g.*, exercise, education, and client goals) based on the participant's progress and feedback.
D. Maintain participant records to document progress and clinical status.

Domain IV: Leadership & Counseling

Associated Job Tasks

A. Educate the participant about performance and progression of aerobic, strength, and flexibility exercise programs.
B. Provide disease management and risk factor reduction education based on the participant's medical history, needs, and goals.
C. Create a positive environment for participant adherence and outcomes by incorporating effective motivational skills, communication techniques, and behavioral strategies.
D. Collaborate and consult with health care professionals to address clinical issues and provide referrals to optimize participant outcomes.

Domain V: Legal and Professional Considerations

Associated Job Tasks

A. Evaluate the exercise environment to minimize risk and optimize safety by following routine inspection procedures based on established facility and industry standards and guidelines.

B. Perform regular inspections of emergency equipment and practice emergency procedures (*e.g.*, crash cart, advanced cardiac life support procedures, and activation of emergency medical system).
C. Promote awareness and accountability and minimize risk by informing participants of safety procedures and self-monitoring of exercise and related symptoms.
D. Comply with Health Insurance Portability and Accountability Act (HIPAA) laws and industry accepted professional, ethical, and business standards in order to maintain confidentiality, optimize safety, and reduce liability.
E. Promote a positive image of the program by engaging in healthy lifestyle practices.
F. Select and participate in continuing education programs that enhance knowledge and skills on a continuing basis, maximize effectiveness, and increase professionalism in the field.

ACSM Registered Clinical Exercise Physiologist® (RCEP) Job Task Analysis

The JTA is intended to serve as a blueprint of the job of a RCEP. As one prepares for the examination, it is important to remember that all examination questions are based on the following outline.

JOB DEFINITION

The RCEP (a) is an allied health professional with a minimum of a master's degree in exercise science and (b) works in the application of physical activity and behavioral interventions for those clinical diseases and health conditions that have been shown to provide therapeutic and/or functional benefit. Persons that RCEP services are appropriate for may include, but are not limited to, individuals with cardiovascular, pulmonary, metabolic, orthopedic, musculoskeletal, neuromuscular, neoplastic, immunologic, and hematologic disease. The RCEP provides primary and secondary prevention and rehabilitative strategies designed to improve physical fitness and health in populations ranging across the lifespan.

The RCEP provides exercise screening, exercise and physical fitness testing, exercise prescriptions, exercise and physical activity counseling, exercise supervision, exercise and health education/promotion, and measurement and evaluation of exercise and physical activity-related outcome measures. The RCEP works individually or as part of an interdisciplinary team in a clinical, community, or public health setting. The practice and supervision of the RCEP is guided by published professional guidelines, standards, and applicable state and federal laws and regulations.

PERFORMANCE DOMAINS AND ASSOCIATED JOB TASKS

The JTA for the RCEP describes what the professional does on a day-to-day basis. The JTA is divided into domains and associated tasks performed on the job. The percentages listed in this section representing each domain on the 125 question RCEP examination.

The performance domains are the following:

- Domain I: Clinical Assessment — 20%.
- Domain II: Exercise Testing — 20%.
- Domain III: Exercise Prescription — 20%.
- Domain IV: Exercise Training — 20%.
- Domain V: Education and Behavior Change — 10%.
- Domain VI: Program Administration — 5%.
- Domain VII: Legal and Professional Considerations — 5%.

Domain I: Clinical Assessment

Associated Job Tasks

In this domain, chronic disease(s) includes cardiovascular, pulmonary, metabolic, orthopedic/musculoskeletal, neuromuscular, neoplastic, immunologic, and hematologic disorders.

A. Review patient's medical record for information pertinent to the reason for their visit.
B. Interview patient for medical history pertinent to the reason for their visit and reconcile medications.
C. Assess resting vital signs and symptoms.
D. Collect and evaluate clinical and health measurements including, but not limited to ECG, spirometry, or blood glucose.

Domain II: Exercise Testing

Associated Job Tasks

In this domain, chronic disease(s) includes cardiovascular, pulmonary, metabolic, orthopedic/musculoskeletal, neuromuscular, neoplastic, immunologic, and hematologic disorders.

A. Assess appropriateness of and contraindications to symptom-limited, maximal exercise testing and/or other health assessments.
B. Select, administer, and interpret tests to assess muscular strength and/or endurance.
C. Select, administer, and interpret tests to assess flexibility and/or body composition.
D. Select, administer, and interpret submaximal aerobic exercise tests.
E. Select, administer, and interpret functional and balance tests (*e.g.*, Get Up and Go, Berg Balance).
F. Prepare patient for a symptom-limited, maximal exercise test by providing an informed consent and prepping the patient for electrocardiogram (ECG) monitoring.
G. Administer a symptom-limited, maximal exercise test using appropriate protocol and monitoring.
H. Evaluate results from a symptom-limited, maximal exercise test and report in the medical record and to health care providers.
I. Calibrate, troubleshoot, operate, and maintain testing equipment.

Domain III: Exercise Prescription

Associated Job Tasks

In this domain, chronic disease(s) includes cardiovascular, pulmonary, metabolic, orthopedic/musculoskeletal, neuromuscular, neoplastic, immunologic, and hematologic disorders.

A. Evaluate and document exercise goals and motivations of the patient to design an individualized Ex R_x.
B. Determine and document the Ex R_x for exercise training based on the patient's history, available data, and goals and discuss with the patient.
C. Determine the appropriate level of supervision and monitoring needed to provide a safe exercise environment based on risk classification guidelines.
D. Explain exercise intensity and measures to guide exercise intensity (*e.g.*, target heart rate, ratings of perceived exertion, signs/symptoms, and ability to carry on a conversation) to the patient.
E. Design a home component for an exercise program to help transition a patient to more independent exercise using appropriate behavioral strategies.
F. Discuss the importance of, barriers to, and strategies to optimize adherence.
G. Regularly evaluate the appropriateness of and modify, as needed, the Ex R_x based on the patient's compliance, signs/symptoms, and physiologic response to the exercise program.

Domain IV: Exercise Training

Associated Job Tasks

In this domain, chronic disease(s) includes cardiovascular, pulmonary, metabolic, orthopedic/musculoskeletal, neuromuscular, neoplastic, immunologic, and hematologic disorders.

A. Meet with patient to discuss exercise training plan, expectations, and goals.
B. Identify, adapt, and instruct patient in appropriate exercise modes in order to reduce risk and maximize the development of cardiorespiratory fitness, strength, and flexibility.
C. Monitor and/or supervise patient during exercise based on their level of risk (*e.g.*, cardiopulmonary risk and fall risk) in order to provide a safe exercise environment.
D. Evaluate patient's contraindications to exercise training to make a risk/reward assessment.
E. Evaluate, document, and report patient's clinical status and response to exercise training in the medical record and to their health care provider.
F. Discuss clinical status and response to exercise training with patients and adapt and/or modify the exercise program as needed in order to prevent injury, maximize adherence, and progress toward desired outcomes.
G. Report new or worsening symptoms and adverse events in the patient's medical record and consult with the health care provider.

Domain V: Education and Behavior Strategies

Associated Job Tasks

In this domain, chronic disease(s) includes cardiovascular, pulmonary, metabolic, orthopedic/musculoskeletal, neuromuscular, neoplastic, immunologic, and hematologic disorders.

A. Evaluate patients to identify those who may benefit from mental health services using industry accepted screening tools.
B. Observe and interact with patients on an ongoing basis to identify recent changes that may benefit from counseling or other mental health services.
C. Assess patient for level of understanding of their disease and/or disability, readiness to adopt behavior change, and learning needs.
D. Conduct group and individual education sessions to teach patients about their disease/disability, secondary prevention, and how to manage their condition.
E. Assess knowledge of and compliance with health behaviors and apply behavior change techniques to encourage the adoption of healthy behaviors.
F. Teach relapse prevention techniques for maintenance of healthy behaviors.

Domain VI: Program Administration

Associated Job Tasks

In this domain, chronic disease(s) includes cardiovascular, pulmonary, metabolic, orthopedic/musculoskeletal, neuromuscular, neoplastic, immunologic, and hematologic disorders.

A. Maintain patient records as an ongoing documentation device to provide continuity of care and to meet legal standards.
B. Develop and/or maintain program evaluation tools and report program outcomes.
C. Develop strategies to improve program outcomes.
D. Develop and maintain relationships with referring physicians and other health care providers to enhance patient care.
E. Recruit, hire, train, motivate, and evaluate staff, students, and volunteers in order to provide effective services within a positive work environment.
F. Manage fiscal resources to provide efficient and effective services.
G. Develop, update, and/or maintain policies and procedures for daily operations, routine care, and adverse events.
H. Develop and maintain a safe environment that promotes positive outcomes and follows current industry recommendations and facility policies.
I. Develop and maintain an atmosphere of caring and support in order to promote patient adherence.

J. Promote the program and enhance its reputation through excellent communication and customer service.
K. Regularly conduct departmental needs assessment and develop/modify programs to accommodate changing environment.

Domain VII: Legal and Professional Considerations

Associated Job Tasks

In this domain, chronic disease(s) includes cardiovascular, pulmonary, metabolic, orthopedic/musculoskeletal, neuromuscular, neoplastic, immunologic, and hematologic disorders.

A. Follow industry accepted professional, ethical, and business standards in order to optimize safety, reduce liability, and protect patient confidentiality.
B. Participate in continuing education and/or professional networks to maintain certification, enhance knowledge, and remain current in the profession.
C. Maintain an environment that promotes ongoing written and verbal communication (*e.g.*, insurance providers and patients) and provides documentation of treatment that meets legal standards.
D. Take action in emergencies consistent with current certification, institutional procedures, and industry guidelines.
E. Inform patients of personal and facility safety procedures in order to minimize risk.

THE BOTTOM LINE

Obtaining professional credentials enhances the career development of health/fitness, clinical exercise, and health care professionals conducting exercise programs and exercise testing and improves the delivery of care to the consumer, client, and patient. ACSM offers high quality professional certifications for a variety of health/fitness, exercise, and health care professionals in corporate, health/fitness, and clinical settings.

ONLINE RESOURCES

American College of Sports Medicine Certifications: http://certification.acsm.org/get-certified
American College of Sports Medicine Certifications Job Task Analysis: http://certification.acsm.org/exam-content-outlines
American College of Sports Medicine Code of Ethics for Certified and Registered Professionals: http://certification.acsm.org/faq28-codeofethics
Clinical Exercise Physiology Association: http://www.acsm-cepa.org
Commission on Accreditation of Allied Health Education Programs: http://www.caahep.org
Committee on Accreditation for the Exercise Sciences: http://www.coaes.org
The National Commission for Certifying Agencies under the National Organization for Competency Assurance: http://www.noca.org

REFERENCES

1. Costanzo DG. ACSM Certification: The Evolution of the Exercise Professional. *ACSM Health Fitness J.* 2006;10(4):38–9.
2. Paternostro-Bayles M. The role of a job task analysis in the development of professional certifications. *ACSM Health Fitness J.* 2010;14(4):41–2.

APPENDIX B

ACSM Certified Health Fitness Specialist^{SM} Job Task Analysis

The job task analysis (JTA) is intended to serve as a blueprint for the job of an ACSM Certified Health Fitness Specialist^{SM} (HFS). As you prepare for the exam, it is important to remember that all examination questions are based on this outline.

JOB DEFINITION

The ACSM Certified HFS is a health and fitness professional with a minimum of a bachelor's degree in exercise science. The HFS performs preparticipation health screenings, conducts physical fitness assessments, interprets results, develops exercise prescriptions, and applies behavioral and motivational strategies to apparently healthy individuals and individuals with medically controlled diseases and health conditions to support clients in adopting and maintaining healthy lifestyle behaviors. The academic preparation of the HFS also includes fitness management, administration, and supervision. The HFS is typically employed or self-employed in commercial, community, studio, corporate, university, and hospital settings.

PERFORMANCE DOMAINS AND ASSOCIATED JOB TASKS

The JTA for the ACSM Certified HFS describes what the professional does on a day-to-day basis. The JTA is divided into domains and associated tasks performed on the job. The percentages listed below representing each domain on the 150-question HFS examination.

The performance domains are as follows:

- Domain I: Health and Fitness Assessment — 30%.
- Domain II: Exercise Prescription, Implementation (and Ongoing Support) — 30%.
- Domain III: Exercise Counseling and Behavioral Strategies — 15%.
- Domain IV: Legal/Professional — 10%.
- Domain V: Management — 15%.

DOMAIN I: HEALTH AND FITNESS ASSESSMENT

Associated Job Tasks

A. Implement assessment protocols and preexercise screening procedures to maximize participant safety and minimize risk.

1) Knowledge of:

a. preactivity screening procedures and tools that provide accurate information about the individual's health/medical history, current medical conditions, risk factors, signs/symptoms of disease, current physical activity habits, and medications.

b. the key components included in informed consent and health/medical history.

c. the limitations of informed consent and health/medical history.

B. Determine participant's readiness to take part in a health-related physical fitness assessment and exercise program.

1) Knowledge of:

a. risk factor thresholds for ACSM risk stratification, including genetic and lifestyle factors related to the development of cardiovascular disease (CVD).

b. the major signs or symptoms suggestive of cardiovascular, pulmonary, and metabolic diseases.

c. cardiovascular risk factors or conditions that may require consultation with medical personnel prior to exercise testing or training (*e.g.*, inappropriate changes in resting heart rate and/or blood pressure; new onset discomfort in chest, neck, shoulder, or arm; changes in the pattern of discomfort during rest or exercise; fainting; dizzy spells; and claudication).

d. the pulmonary risk factors or conditions that may require consultation with medical personnel prior to exercise testing or training (*e.g.*, asthma, exercise-induced asthma/bronchospasm, extreme breathlessness at rest or during exercise, chronic bronchitis, and emphysema).

e. the metabolic risk factors or conditions that may require consultation with medical personnel prior to exercise testing or training (*e.g.*, obesity, metabolic syndrome, diabetes or glucose intolerance, and hypoglycemia).

f. the musculoskeletal risk factors or conditions that may require consultation with medical personnel prior to exercise testing or training (*e.g.*, acute or chronic pain, osteoarthritis, rheumatoid arthritis, osteoporosis, inflammation/pain, and low back pain).

g. ACSM risk stratification categories and their implications for medical clearance before administration of an exercise test or participation in an exercise program.

h. risk factors that may be favorably modified by physical activity habits.

i. medical terminology including, but not limited to, total cholesterol, high-density lipoprotein cholesterol, low-density lipoprotein cholesterol, triglycerides, impaired fasting glucose, impaired glucose tolerance, hypertension, atherosclerosis, myocardial infarction, dyspnea, tachycardia, claudication, syncope, and ischemia.

j. recommended plasma cholesterol levels for adults based on National Cholesterol Education Program/ATP Guidelines.

k. recommended blood pressure levels for adults based on National High Blood Pressure Education Program Guidelines.

l. medical supervision recommendations for cardiorespiratory fitness testing.

m. the components of a health-history questionnaire (*e.g.*, past and current medical history, family history of cardiac disease, orthopedic limitations, prescribed medications, activity patterns, nutritional habits, stress and anxiety levels, and smoking and alcohol use).

2) Skill in:

a. the risk stratification of participants using CVD risk factor thresholds; major signs or symptoms suggestive of cardiovascular, pulmonary, or metabolic disease; and/or the presence of known cardiovascular, pulmonary, and metabolic disease status.

b. reviewing preactivity screening documents to determine the need for medical clearance prior to exercise and to select appropriate physical fitness assessment protocols.

C. Select and prepare fitness assessments for healthy participants and those with controlled disease.

1) Knowledge of:

a. the physiological basis of the major components of physical fitness: cardiorespiratory fitness, body composition, flexibility, muscular strength, and muscular endurance.

b. selecting the most appropriate testing protocols for each participant on the basis of preliminary screening data.

c. calibration techniques and proper use of fitness-testing equipment.

d. the purpose and procedures of fitness-testing protocols for the components of health-related fitness.

e. test termination criteria and proper procedures to be followed after discontinuing health fitness tests.

f. fitness assessment sequencing.
g. the effects of common medications and substances on exercise testing (*e.g.*, antianginals, antihypertensives, antiarrhythmics, bronchodilators, hypoglycemics, psychotropics, alcohol, diet pills, cold tablets, caffeine, and nicotine).
h. the physiologic and metabolic responses to exercise testing associated with chronic diseases and conditions (*e.g.*, heart disease, hypertension, diabetes mellitus, obesity, and pulmonary disease).

2) Skill in:

a. analyzing and interpreting information obtained from assessment of the components of health-related fitness.
b. modifying protocols and procedures for testing children, adolescents, older adults, and individuals with special considerations.

D. Conduct and interpret cardiorespiratory fitness assessments.

1) Knowledge of:

a. common submaximal and maximal cardiorespiratory assessment protocols.
b. blood pressure measurement techniques.
c. Korotkoff sounds for determining systolic and diastolic blood pressure.
d. the blood pressure response to exercise.
e. techniques of measuring heart rate and heart rate response to exercise.
f. the rating of perceived exertion (RPE).
g. heart rate, blood pressure, and RPE monitoring techniques before, during, and after cardiorespiratory fitness testing.
h. the anatomy and physiology of the cardiovascular and pulmonary systems.
i. cardiorespiratory terminology, including angina pectoris, tachycardia, bradycardia, arrhythmia, and hyperventilation.
j. the pathophysiology of myocardial ischemia, myocardial infarction, stroke, hypertension, and hyperlipidemia.
k. the effects of myocardial ischemia, myocardial infarction, hypertension, claudication, and dyspnea on cardiorespiratory responses during exercise.
l. oxygen consumption dynamics during exercise (*e.g.*, heart rate, stroke volume, cardiac output, ventilation, and ventilatory threshold).
m. methods of calculating $\dot{V}O_{2max}$.
n. cardiorespiratory responses to acute graded exercise of conditioned and unconditioned participants.

2) Skill in:

a. interpreting cardiorespiratory fitness test results.
b. locating anatomic landmarks for palpation of peripheral pulses and blood pressure.
c. measuring heart rate, blood pressure, and RPE at rest and during exercise.
d. conducting submaximal exercise tests (*e.g.*, cycle ergometer, treadmill, field testing, and step test).
e. determining cardiorespiratory fitness on the basis of submaximal exercise test results.

E. Conduct assessments of muscular strength, muscular endurance, and flexibility.

1) Knowledge of:

a. common muscular strength, muscular endurance, and flexibility assessment protocols.
b. interpreting muscular strength, muscular endurance, and flexibility assessments.
c. relative strength, absolute strength, and repetition maximum (1-RM) estimation.
d. the anatomy of bone, skeletal muscle, and connective tissues.
e. muscle action terms, including anterior, posterior, inferior, superior, medial, lateral, supination, pronation, flexion, extension, adduction, abduction, hyperextension, rotation, circumduction, agonist, antagonist, and stabilizer.
f. the planes and axes in which each movement action occurs.

g. the interrelationships among center of gravity, base of support, balance, stability, posture, and proper spinal alignment.
h. the normal curvatures of the spine and common assessments of postural alignment.
i. the location and function of the major muscles (*e.g.*, pectoralis major, trapezius, latissimus dorsi, biceps, triceps, rectus abdominis, internal and external obliques, erector spinae, gluteus maximus, quadriceps, hamstrings, adductors, abductors, and gastrocnemius).
j. the major joints and their associated movements.

2) Skill in:

a. identifying the major bones, muscles, and joints.
b. conducting assessments of muscular strength, muscular endurance, and flexibility (*e.g.*, 1-RM, hand grip dynamometer, push-ups, curl-ups, and sit-and-reach).
c. estimating 1-RM using lower resistance (2- to 10-RM).
d. interpreting results of muscular strength, muscular endurance, and flexibility assessments.

F. Conduct anthropometric and body composition assessments.

1) Knowledge of:

a. the advantages, disadvantages, and limitations of body composition techniques (*e.g.*, air displacement plethysmography [BOD POD®], duel-energy X-ray absorptiometry [DEXA], hydrostatic weighing, skinfolds, and bioelectrical impedance).
b. the standardized descriptions of circumference and skinfold sites.
c. procedures for determining body mass index (BMI) and taking skinfold and circumference measurements.
d. the health implications of variation in body fat distribution patterns and the significance of BMI, waist circumference, and waist-to-hip ratio.

2) Skill in:

a. locating anatomic landmarks for skinfold and circumference measurements.
b. interpreting the results of anthropometric and body composition assessments.

DOMAIN II: EXERCISE PRESCRIPTION AND IMPLEMENTATION

Associated Job Tasks

A. Review preactivity screening, health appraisal, exercise history, and fitness assessments.

1) Skill in:

a. synthesizing prescreening results and reviewing them with participants.

B. Determine safe and effective exercise programs to achieve desired outcomes and goals.

1) Knowledge of:

a. strength, cardiovascular, and flexibility-based exercises.
b. the benefits and precautions associated with exercise training in apparently healthy participants and those with controlled disease.
c. program development for specific client needs (*e.g.*, sport-specific training, performance, health, lifestyle, functional ability, balance, agility, aerobic, and anaerobic).
d. the six motor skill-related physical fitness components — agility, balance, coordination, reaction time, speed, and power.
e. the physiologic changes associated with an acute bout of exercise.
f. the physiologic adaptations after chronic exercise training.
g. ACSM exercise prescription guidelines for strength, cardiovascular, and flexibility-based exercises for apparently healthy clients, clients with increased risk, and clients with controlled disease.
h. the components and sequencing incorporated into an exercise session (*e.g.*, warm-up, stretching, conditioning or sports-related exercise, and cool-down).

i. the physiological principles related to warm-up and cool-down.
j. the principles of reversibility, progressive overload, individual differences, and specificity of training, and how they relate to exercise prescription.
k. the role of aerobic and anaerobic energy systems in the performance of various physical activities.
l. the basic biomechanical principles of human movement.
m. the psychological and physiological signs and symptoms of overtraining.
n. the signs and symptoms of common musculoskeletal injuries associated with exercise (*e.g.*, sprain, strain, bursitis, and tendonitis).
o. the advantages and disadvantages of exercise equipment (*e.g.*, free weights, selectorized machines, and cardiovascular equipment).

2) Skill in:

a. teaching and demonstrating exercises.
b. designing safe and effective training programs.
c. implementing exercise prescription guidelines for apparently healthy clients, clients with increased risk, and clients with controlled disease.

C. Implement cardiorespiratory exercise prescriptions using the FITT framework (frequency, intensity, time, and type) for apparently healthy participants on the basis of current health status, fitness goals, and availability of time.

1) Knowledge of:

a. the recommended FITT framework for the development of cardiorespiratory fitness.
b. the benefits, risks, and contraindications of a wide variety of cardiovascular training exercises based on client experience, skill level, current fitness level, and goals.
c. the minimal threshold of physical activity required for health benefits and/or fitness development.
d. determining exercise intensity using HRR, $\dot{V}O_2R$, peak HR method, peak $\dot{V}O_2$ method, peak METs method, and the RPE scale.
e. the accuracy of HRR, $\dot{V}O_2R$, peak HR method, peak $\dot{V}O_2$ method, peak METs method, and the RPE scale.
f. abnormal responses to exercise (*e.g.*, hemodynamic, cardiac, and ventilatory).
g. metabolic calculations (*e.g.*, unit conversions, deriving energy cost of exercise, and caloric expenditure).
h. calculating the caloric expenditure of an exercise session ($kcal \cdot session^{-1}$).
i. methods for establishing and monitoring levels of exercise intensity, including heart rate, RPE, and METs.
j. the applications of anaerobic training principles.
k. the anatomy and physiology of the cardiovascular and pulmonary systems, including the basic properties of cardiac muscle.
l. the basic principles of gas exchange.

2) Skill in:

a. determining appropriate exercise FITT for clients with various fitness levels.
b. determining the energy cost, absolute and relative oxygen costs ($\dot{V}O_2$), and MET levels of various activities and applying the information to an exercise prescription.
c. identifying improper technique in the use of cardiovascular equipment.
d. teaching and demonstrating the use of a variety of cardiovascular exercise equipment.

D. Implement exercise prescriptions using the FITT framework for flexibility, muscular strength, and muscular endurance for apparently healthy participants on the basis of current health status, fitness goals, and availability of time.

1) Knowledge of:

a. the recommended FITT framework for the development of muscular strength, muscular endurance, and flexibility.

b. the minimal threshold of physical activity required for health benefits and/or fitness development.
c. safe and effective exercises designed to enhance muscular strength and/or endurance of major muscle groups.
d. safe and effective stretches that enhance flexibility.
e. indications for water-based exercise (*e.g.*, arthritis and obesity).
f. the types of resistance training programs (*e.g.*, total body and split routine) and modalities (*e.g.*, free weights, variable resistance equipment, pneumatic machines, and bands).
g. acute (*e.g.*, load, volume, sets, repetitions, rest periods, and order of exercises) and chronic training variables (*e.g.*, periodization).
h. the types of muscle contractions (*e.g.*, eccentric, concentric, and isometric).
i. joint movements (*e.g.*, flexion, extension, adduction, and abduction) and the muscles responsible for them.
j. acute and delayed onset muscle soreness
k. the anatomy and physiology of skeletal muscle fiber, the characteristics of fast- and slow-twitch muscle fibers, and the sliding-filament theory of muscle contraction.
l. the stretch reflex, proprioceptors, Golgi tendon organ, muscle spindles, and how they relate to flexibility.
m. muscle-related terminology, including atrophy, hyperplasia, and hypertrophy.
n. the Valsalva maneuver and its implications during exercise.
o. the physiology underlying plyometric training and common plyometric exercises (*e.g.*, box jumps, leaps, and bounds).
p. the contraindications and potential risks associated with muscular conditioning activities (*e.g.*, straight-leg sit-ups, double leg raises, squats, hurdler's stretch, yoga plough, forceful back hyperextension, standing bent-over toe touch, and behind neck press/lat pull-down).
q. prescribing exercise using the calculated %1-RM.
r. spotting positions and techniques for injury prevention and exercise assistance.
s. periodization (*e.g.*, macro-, micro-, and mesocycles) and associated theories.
t. safe and effective Olympic weightlifting exercises.
u. safe and effective core stability exercises (*e.g.*, planks, crunches, bridges, and cable twists).

2) Skill in:

a. identifying improper technique in the use of resistive equipment (*e.g.*, stability balls, weights, bands, resistance bars, and water exercise equipment).
b. teaching and demonstrating appropriate exercises for enhancing musculoskeletal flexibility.
c. teaching and demonstrating safe and effective muscular strength and endurance exercises (*e.g.*, free weights, weight machines, resistive bands, Swiss balls, body weight, and all other major fitness equipment).

E. Establish exercise progression guidelines for resistance, aerobic, and flexibility-based activities to achieve the goals of apparently healthy participants.

1) Knowledge of:

a. the basic principles of exercise progression.
b. adjusting the FITT framework in response to individual changes in conditioning.
c. the importance of performing periodic reevaluations to assess changes in fitness status.
d. the training principles that promote improvements in muscular strength, muscular endurance, cardiorespiratory fitness, and flexibility.

2) Skill in:

a. recognizing the need for progression and communicating updates to exercise prescriptions.

F. Implement a weight management program as indicated by personal goals that are supported by preactivity screening, health history, and body composition/anthropometrics.

1) Knowledge of:

a. exercise prescriptions for achieving weight management, including weight loss, weight maintenance, and weight gain goals.

b. energy balance and basic nutritional guidelines (*e.g.*, MyPyramid and USDA Dietary Guidelines for Americans).
c. weight management terminology, including, but not limited to, obesity, overweight, percentage fat, BMI, lean body mass, anorexia nervosa, bulimia, binge eating, metabolic syndrome, body fat distribution, adipocyte, bariatrics, ergogenic aid, fat-free mass, resting metabolic rate, and thermogenesis.
d. the relationship between body composition and health.
e. the unique dietary needs of participant populations (*e.g.*, women, children, older adults, and pregnant women).
f. common nutritional ergogenic aids and their purported mechanisms of action and associated risks and benefits (*e.g.*, protein/amino acids, vitamins, minerals, herbal products, creatine, steroids, and caffeine).
g. methods for modifying body composition, including diet, exercise, and behavior modification.
h. fuel sources for aerobic and anaerobic metabolism, including carbohydrates, fats, and proteins.
i. the effects of overall dietary composition on healthy weight management.
j. the importance of maintaining normal hydration before, during, and after exercise.
k. the consequences of inappropriate weight loss methods (*e.g.*, saunas, dietary supplements, vibrating belts, body wraps, overexercising, very low calorie diets, electric stimulators, sweat suits, and fad diets).
l. the kilocalorie levels of carbohydrate, fat, protein, and alcohol.
m. the relationship between kilocalorie expenditures and weight loss.
n. published position statements on obesity and the risks associated with it (*e.g.*, National Institutes of Health, American Dietetic Association, and ACSM)
o. the relationship between body fat distribution patterns and health.
p. the physiology and pathophysiology of overweight and obese participants.
q. the recommended FITT framework for participants who are overweight or obese.
r. comorbidities and musculoskeletal conditions associated with overweight and obesity that may require medical clearance and/or modifications to exercise testing and prescription.

2) Skill in:

a. applying behavioral strategies (*e.g.*, exercise, diet, and behavioral modification strategies) for weight management.
b. modifying exercises for individuals limited by body size.
c. calculating the volume of exercise in terms of kcal·session^{-1}.

G. Prescribe and implement exercise programs for participants with controlled cardiovascular, pulmonary, and metabolic diseases and other clinical populations with physician clearance for independent exercise.

1) Knowledge of:

a. ACSM risk stratification and exercise prescription guidelines for participants with cardiovascular, pulmonary, and metabolic diseases and other clinical populations.
b. ACSM relative and absolute contraindications for initiating exercise sessions or exercise testing, and indications for terminating exercise sessions and exercise testing.
c. physiology and pathophysiology of cardiac disease, arthritis, diabetes mellitus, dyslipidemia, hypertension, metabolic syndrome, musculoskeletal injuries, overweight and obesity, osteoporosis, peripheral artery disease, and pulmonary disease.
d. the effects of diet and exercise on blood glucose levels in diabetics.
e. the recommended FITT principle for the development of cardiorespiratory fitness, muscular fitness, and flexibility for participants with cardiac disease, arthritis, diabetes mellitus, dyslipidemia, hypertension, metabolic syndrome, musculoskeletal injuries, overweight and obesity, osteoporosis, peripheral artery disease, and pulmonary disease.

2) Skill in:

a. progressing exercise programs, according to the FITT principle, in a safe and effective manner.

b. modifying the exercise prescription and/or exercise choice for individuals with cardiac disease, arthritis, diabetes mellitus, dyslipidemia, hypertension, metabolic syndrome, musculoskeletal injuries, overweight and obesity, osteoporosis, peripheral artery disease, and pulmonary disease.
c. identifying improper exercise techniques and modifying exercise programs for participants with low back, neck, shoulder, elbow, wrist, hip, knee, and/or ankle pain.

H. Prescribe and implement exercise programs for healthy special populations (*i.e.*, older adults, youth, and pregnant women).

1) Knowledge of:

a. normal maturational changes, from childhood to old age, and their effects on the skeletal muscle, bone, reaction time, coordination, posture, heat and cold tolerance, maximal oxygen consumption, strength, flexibility, body composition, resting and maximal heart rate, and resting and maximal blood pressure.
b. techniques for the modification of cardiovascular, flexibility, and resistance exercises based on age, functional capacity, and physical condition.
c. techniques for the development of exercise prescriptions for children, adolescents, and older adults with regard to strength, functional capacity, and motor skills.
d. the unique adaptations to exercise training in children, adolescents, and older participants with regard to strength, functional capacity, and motor skills.
e. the benefits and precautions associated with exercise training across the lifespan.
f. the recommended FITT framework for the development of cardiorespiratory fitness, muscular fitness, and flexibility in apparently healthy children and adolescents.
g. the effects of the aging process on the musculoskeletal and cardiovascular structures and functions during rest, exercise, and recovery.
h. the recommended FITT framework necessary for the development of cardiorespiratory fitness, muscular fitness, balance, and flexibility in apparently healthy, older adults.
i. common orthopedic and cardiovascular exercise considerations for older adults.
j. the relationship between regular physical activity and the successful performance of activities of daily living (ADLs) for older adults.
k. the recommended frequency, intensity, type, and duration of physical activity necessary for the development of cardiorespiratory fitness, muscular fitness, and flexibility in apparently healthy pregnant women.

2) Skill in:

a. teaching and demonstrating appropriate exercises for healthy populations with special considerations.
b. modifying exercises on the basis of age, physical condition, and current health status.

I. Modify exercise prescriptions on the basis of environmental conditions.

1) Knowledge of:

a. the effects of a hot, cold, or high-altitude environment on the physiologic response to exercise.
b. special precautions and program modifications for exercise in a hot, cold, or high-altitude environment.
c. the role of acclimatization when exercising in a hot or high-altitude environment.
d. appropriate fluid intake during exercise in a hot and humid as well as cold environments and high altitude.

DOMAIN III: EXERCISE COUNSELING AND BEHAVIORAL STRATEGIES

Associated Job Tasks

A. Optimize adoption and adherence to exercise programs and other healthy behaviors by applying effective communication techniques.

1) Knowledge of:

a. the effective and timely uses of communication modes (*e.g.*, e-mail, telephone, Web site, and newsletters).
b. verbal and nonverbal behaviors that communicate positive reinforcement and encouragement (*e.g.*, eye contact, targeted praise, and empathy).
c. group leadership techniques for working with participants of all ages.
d. active listening techniques.
e. learning modes (auditory, visual, kinesthetic).
f. types of feedback (*e.g.*, evaluative, supportive, and descriptive).

2) Skill in:

a. using active listening techniques.
b. applying teaching and training techniques to optimize participant training sessions.
c. using feedback to optimize participant training sessions.
d. applying verbal and nonverbal communications with diverse participant populations.

B. Optimize adoption of and adherence to exercise programs and other healthy behaviors by applying effective behavioral and motivational strategies.

1) Knowledge of:

a. behavior change models and theories (*e.g.*, health belief model, theory of planned behavior, socioecological model, transtheoretical model, social cognitive theory, and cognitive evaluation theory).
b. the basic principles involved in motivational interviewing.
c. intervention strategies and stress management techniques.
d. the stages of motivational readiness (*e.g.*, transtheoretical model).
e. behavioral strategies for enhancing exercise and health behavior change (*e.g.*, reinforcement, SMART goal setting, and social support).
f. behavior modification terminology, including, but not limited to, self-esteem, self-efficacy, antecedents, cues to action, behavioral beliefs, behavioral intentions, and reinforcing factors.
g. behavioral strategies (*e.g.*, exercise, diet, and behavioral modification strategies) for weight management.
h. the role that affects mood and emotion play in exercise adherence.
i. common barriers to exercise initiation and compliance (*e.g.*, time management, injury, fear, lack of knowledge, and weather).
j. techniques that facilitate motivation (*e.g.*, goal setting, incentive programs, achievement recognition, and social support).
k. the role extrinsic and intrinsic motivation plays in the adoption and maintenance of behavior change.
l. relapse prevention strategies and plans of action.
m. applying health coaching principles and lifestyle management techniques related to behavior change.
n. strategies that increase nonstructured physical activity levels (*e.g.*, stair walking, parking farther away, and bike to work).

2) Skill in:

a. explaining the purpose and value of understanding perceived exertion.
b. using imagery as a motivational tool.
c. evaluating behavioral readiness to optimize exercise adherence.
d. applying the theories related to behavior change to diverse populations.
e. developing intervention strategies to increase self-efficacy and self-confidence.
f. developing reward systems that support and maintain program adherence.
g. setting effective behavioral goals.

C. Provide educational resources to support clients in the adoption and maintenance of healthy lifestyle behaviors.

1) Knowledge of:

a. the relationship between physical inactivity and common chronic diseases (*e.g.*, atherosclerosis, Type II diabetes, obesity, dyslipidemia, arthritis, low back pain, and hypertension).
b. the dynamic interrelationship between fitness level, body composition, stress, and overall health.
c. modifications necessary to promote healthy lifestyle behaviors for diverse populations.
d. stress management techniques and relaxation techniques (*e.g.*, progressive relaxation, guided imagery, and massage therapy).
e. the ADLs and how they relate to overall health.
f. accessing and disseminating scientifically based, relevant health, exercise, nutrition, and wellness-related resources and information.
g. specific, age-appropriate leadership techniques and educational methods to increase client engagement.
h. community-based exercise programs that provide social support and structured activities (*e.g.*, walking clubs, intramural sports, golf leagues, and cycling clubs).

2) Skill in:

a. accessing and delivering health, exercise, and wellness-related information.
b. educating clients about benefits and risks of exercise and the risks of sedentary behavior.

D. Provide support within the scope of practice of an HFS and refer to other health professionals as indicated.

1) Knowledge of:

a. the side effects of common over-the-counter and prescription drugs that may impact a client's ability to exercise.
b. signs and symptoms of mental health states (*e.g.*, anxiety, depression, and eating disorders) that may necessitate referral to a medical or mental health professional.
c. symptoms and causal factors of test anxiety (*i.e.*, performance and appraisal threat during exercise testing) and how they may affect physiological responses to testing.
d. client needs and learning styles that my impact exercise sessions and exercise testing procedures.
e. conflict resolution techniques that facilitate communication among exercise cohorts.

2) Skill in:

a. communicating the need for medical, nutritional, or mental health intervention.

DOMAIN IV: LEGAL/PROFESSIONAL

Associated Job Tasks

A. Create and disseminate risk management guidelines for a health/fitness facility, department, or organization to reduce member, employee, and business risk.

1) Knowledge of:

a. employee's criminal background checks, child abuse clearances, and drug and alcohol screenings.
b. employment verification requirements mandated by state and federal laws.
c. safe handling and disposal of body fluids, and employee's safety (OSHA guidelines).
d. insurance coverage common to the health/fitness industry, including general liability, professional liability, workers' compensation, property, and business interruption.
e. sexual harassment policies and procedures.
f. interviewing techniques.
g. basic precautions taken in an exercise setting to ensure participant safety.

h. preactivity screening, medical release, and waiver of liability for normal and at-risk participants.
i. emergency response systems and procedures (EAP).
j. the use of signage.
k. preventive maintenance schedules and audits.
l. techniques and methods of evaluating the condition of exercise equipment to reduce the potential risk of injury.
m. the legal implications of documented safety procedures, the use of incident documents, and ongoing safety training documentation for the purpose of safety and risk management.
n. documentation procedures for cardiopulmonary resuscitation (CPR) and automated external defibrillator (AED) certification for employees.
o. AED guidelines for implementation.
p. the components of the ACSM Code of Ethics and the ACSM Certified HFS scope of practice.

2) Skill in:

a. developing and disseminating a policy and procedures manual.
b. developing and implementing confidentiality policies.
c. maintaining a safe exercise environment (*e.g.*, equipment operation, proper sanitation, safety and maintenance of exercise areas, and overall facility maintenance).
d. the organization, communication, and human resource management required to implement risk management policies and procedures.
e. training employees to identify high-risk situations.

B. Create an effective injury prevention program and ensure that emergency policies and procedures are in place.

1) Knowledge of:

a. emergency procedures (*i.e.*, telephone procedures, written emergency procedures, and personnel responsibilities) in a health and fitness setting.
b. basic first-aid procedures for exercise-related injuries, such as bleeding, strains/sprains, fractures, and exercise intolerance (dizziness, syncope, heat and cold injuries).
c. the HFS's responsibilities and limitations, and the legal implications for carrying out emergency procedures.
d. safety plans, emergency procedures, and first-aid techniques needed during fitness evaluations, exercise testing, and exercise training.
e. potential musculoskeletal injuries (*e.g.*, contusions, sprains, strains, and fractures), cardiovascular/pulmonary complications (*e.g.*, tachycardia, bradycardia, hypotension/hypertension, and dyspnea), and metabolic abnormalities (*e.g.*, fainting/syncope, hypoglycemia/hyperglycemia, and hypothermia/hyperthermia).
f. the initial management and first-aid techniques associated with open wounds, musculoskeletal injuries, cardiovascular/pulmonary complications, and metabolic disorders.
g. emergency documentation and appropriate document utilization.

2) Skill in:

a. applying basic first-aid procedures for exercise-related injuries, such as bleeding, strains/sprains, fractures, and exercise intolerance (dizziness, syncope, heat and cold injuries).
b. applying basic life support, first-aid, CPR, and AED techniques.
c. designing an evacuation plan.
d. demonstrating emergency procedures during exercise testing and/or training.

DOMAIN V: MANAGEMENT

Associated Job Tasks

A. Manage human resources in accordance with leadership, organization, and management techniques.

1) Knowledge of:

a. industry benchmark compensation and employee benefit guidelines.

b. federal, state, and local laws pertaining to staff qualifications and credentialing requirements.

c. techniques for tracking and evaluating member retention.

2) Skill in:

a. applying policies, practices, and guidelines to efficiently hire, train, supervise, schedule, and evaluate employees.

b. applying conflict resolution techniques.

B. Manage fiscal resources in accordance with leadership, organization, and management techniques.

1) Knowledge of:

a. fiduciary roles and responsibilities inherent in managing an exercise and health promotion program.

b. principles of financial planning and goal setting, institutional budgeting processes, forecasting, and allocation of resources.

c. basic software systems that facilitate accounting (*e.g.*, Excel).

d. industry benchmarks for budgeting and finance.

e. basic sales techniques that promote health, fitness, and wellness services.

2) Skill in:

a. efficiently managing financial resources and performing related tasks (*e.g.*, planning, budgeting, resource allocation, and revenue generation).

b. administering fitness- and wellness-related programs within established budgetary guidelines.

C. Establish policies and procedures for the management of health/fitness facilities on the basis of accepted safety and legal guidelines, standards, and regulations.

1) Knowledge of:

a. accepted guidelines, standards, and regulations used to establish policies and procedures for the management of health/fitness facilities.

b. facility design and operation principles.

c. facility and equipment maintenance guidelines.

d. documentation techniques for health/fitness facility management.

e. federal, state, and local laws, as they relate to health/fitness facility management.

D. Develop and execute a marketing plan to promote programs, services, and facilities.

1) Knowledge of:

a. lead generation techniques.

b. the four Ps of marketing: product, price, placement, and promotion.

c. public relations, community awareness, and sponsorship and their relationship to branding initiatives.

d. advertising techniques.

e. target market (internal) assessment techniques.

f. target market (external) assessment techniques.

2) Skill in:

a. applying marketing techniques that promote client retention.

b. applying marketing techniques that attract new clients.

c. designing and writing promotional materials.

d. collaborating with community and governmental agencies and organizations.

e. providing customer service.

E. Use effective communication techniques to develop professional relationships with other allied health professionals (*e.g.*, nutritionists, physical therapists, physicians, and nurses).

1) Knowledge of:

a. communication styles and techniques.

b. networking techniques.

2) Skill in:

a. planning meetings.

Index

Note: Page numbers followed by *f* indicate figures; those followed by *t* indicate tables.

L

M

N

O

Q

R

S

T